Respiratory Pharmacology and Therapeutics

IRWIN ZIMENT, M.B., B.Chir., M.R.C.P. (Lond.)

Associate Professor of Medicine,
University of California School of Medicine,
Los Angeles, California;
Chief of Medicine and Director of Respiratory Therapy,
Olive View Medical Center;
Associate Chief, Department of Medicine,
UCLA San Fernando Valley Medical Program,
Van Nuys, California

1978

W. B. SAUNDERS COMPANY   Philadelphia   London   Toronto

W. B. Saunders Company: West Washington Square
Philadelphia, PA 19105

1 St. Anne's Road
Eastbourne, East Sussex BN21 3UN, England

1 Goldthorne Avenue
Toronto, Ontario M8Z 5T9, Canada

Library of Congress Cataloging in Publication Data

Ziment, Irwin.

Respiratory pharmacology and therapeutics.

1. Respiratory organs — Drug effects.   2. Respiratory
agents.   I. Title.

RM388.Z55   615'.72   77–86023

ISBN 0–7216–9700–3

Respiratory Pharmacology and Therapeutics   ISBN   0-7216-9700-3

Last digit is the print number: 9   8   7   6   5   4   3   2   1

TO MY MOTHER
AND
MY WIFE YDA (THILDA)

PREFACE

Five years ago, respiratory pharmacology was a relatively neglected subject, and there was clearly a need for a pharmacology textbook directed at the growing numbers of respiratory therapists and technicians. However, as my efforts to bridge this gap progressed it seemed appropriate to revise my earlier intentions and to expand the scope of the book to provide a more comprehensive text suitable for a wider, international audience, consisting of physicians as well as respiratory therapists, pharmacists, respiratory nurses and perhaps even patients. Numerous tables and summaries have been incorporated to assure the book's usefulness to students, and because the book is an individual statement, controversy has been introduced in the hope that it will stimulate critical thinking about drug usage.

The basic emphasis has been on those drugs which may be of value in the treatment of bronchospasm and abnormal respiratory secretions, with major attention being directed at agents administered by inhalation. A comprehensive description of even seemingly trivial traditional drugs is included, since many of these remain popular although their value may never have been clearly established. In addition, agents used in pulmonary diagnostic studies and drugs which affect respiratory control are included because of their special importance to the patient with respiratory disease.

General anesthetics, although administered by inhalation, have not been considered since they are not primarily used to treat disorders of the lungs. A further limitation has been observed, in that important agents such as anticoagulants, diuretics, cancer chemotherapy drugs and cardiac drugs have not been discussed, since these agents are not given by inhalation and they cannot be regarded as primary respiratory drugs.

Although every effort was made to keep the book accurate and up to date, it is necessary to recognize that pharmaceutical manufacturers change the composition of their products from time to time, and new preparations of old drugs as well as entirely new drugs appear with alarming frequency. Details of drug products should therefore be checked whenever absolute accuracy is an essential requirement. Although my appreciative references to drugs of historical interest should not be taken as an unqualified endorsement of their use, it is hoped that the discriminating reader will agree that all that is new is not necessarily best.

This book was inspired by the many patients who have repeatedly taught me the limitations of pharmacology and the need for good clinical sense and humanistic, understanding compassion. It is hoped that this message has permeated the text, and that readers will recognize that personal interest as well as experience and judgment must always be used synergistically to enhance the therapeutic benefits of the potentially dangerous chemicals that we call drugs.

IRWIN ZIMENT, M.D.

ACKNOWLEDGMENTS

The decision to write this book was based on the encouragement of colleagues, students and friends. Important inspiration was provided during my training by my teachers, Sydney M. Finegold, M.D., who introduced me to pharmacology, and Karlman Wasserman, M.D., Ph.D., who introduced me to respiratory therapy. My research colleague, Stephen N. Steen, M.D., Sc.D., stimulated my interest in bronchodilators, and Jack Lieberman, M.D., encouraged me to think about sputum.

Every reasonable effort has been made to ensure that the information in the book is accurate, and the critical help and advice of a major authority in respiratory pharmacology, Leslie Hendeles, Pharm.D., of the University of Iowa, is gratefully acknowledged, particular help was provided for the chapter on the phosphodiesterase inhibitors. The excellent proofreading by Benji Kremenak was also of immense help.

Many secretaries participated in the arduous tasks of typing the manuscript, but special thanks are due to Dorothy Emley. Original art work was provided by Keith Jasberg and by the Medical Illustration and Graphics Department, UCLA Center for the Health Sciences.

CONTENTS

1

GENERAL PHARMACOLOGY OF RESPIRATORY DRUGS

HISTORY OF RESPIRATORY PHARMACOLOGY

Although inhalation therapy is regarded as a modern subspecialty of American hospital practice, traditional forms of inhalational treatment date back to the earliest surviving records of ancient Hebrew, Chinese, Indian, Greek, Arabic and Roman cultures.[1] The primitive remedies usually consisted of strong smelling aromatic fumes and incenses derived from natural plant essences, or from the burning of organic materials.[2, 3]

Fragrant incenses were used in Biblical times for the treatment of respiratory and other diseases, and they also played a role in the religious and social customs of the Mediterranean tribes of those times. Similar agents with penetrating odors, both pleasant and otherwise, were used by most ancient civilizations, and pungent derivatives, such as vinegar, camphor and eucalyptus, eventually assumed increasing importance in the older medical texts. Many of the early medications derived from natural sources have a long history of popularity in folk medicine, and a large number of them continue in therapeutic usage today.[4]

Inhalational drugs have also been employed throughout history in the treatment or prevention of conditions that were probably not primarily pulmonary abnormalities, although the present-day historian often finds it difficult to determine what specific illnesses some of the ancient writers were attempting to describe. Strong smelling fumes were thought to protect against the evil influences that caused diseases of various kinds, and in the Middle Ages the inhalation of sulfurous and other penetrating chemical fumes was believed to provide relative immunity from the black plague. Medieval European physicians took to wearing protective clothing, complete with a beak like protuberance, which contained cloth permeated with sulfur or other organic substances; the inhalation of their fumes was believed to counteract the noxious ill-defined causes that resulted in the plague.[1] Obviously, these physicians sought to make up in appearance what they lacked in knowledge, and although they had no concept of bacteria, it is possible that their curious bird like garb did actually serve a prophylactic purpose. The birdlike beak may have decreased the direct inhalation of the plague bacillus, and the fumes may have exerted some antibacterial effect. The respiratory therapist of today may find that the illustration of an early birdman of medicine (Fig. 1–1) provides an evocative historical comment on the propensity of ignorance to accouter itself with imposing devices of unproven efficacy.

It is not possible to state at what time in history any specific form of respiratory treatment became established, but it is evident that a number of our modern drugs have been used for hundreds or thousands of years.[5, 6] Steam inhalations were recognized by followers of both Hippocrates (460–370 B.C.) and Galen (A.D. 131–201) to be of value in the treatment of laryngeal and pulmonary disorders. The addition of various aromatic oils, such as the oil of eucalyptus, must date back to similar times,

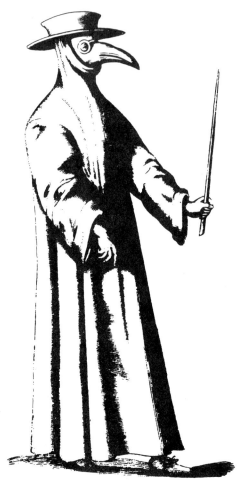

Figure 1–1. Protective costume for an Italian physician during the "pestilence" of 1656—from a book published in 1661. From Marks, G. and Beatty, W. K.: Epidemics. New York, Charles Scribner's Sons, 1976.

hospitals as a steaming vapor for the treatment of respiratory disorders. Oil of camphor, eucalyptus, resinous balms and menthol have centuries of satisfied patients to vouch for the therapeutic respiratory properties of their pungent fumes.

Traditional treatments for pulmonary disorders also include a large number of oral agents, the values of which are often more difficult to discern. One of the longest-established oral respiratory drugs that has withstood the test of time is ephedrine; this drug has been used in China as a bronchodilator and mucosal constrictor for over 5000 years before it entered Western medicine about 50 years ago.[2] Another bronchodilator, khellin, was used by ancient Egyptian physicians, and in recent years the scientific study of this agent brought about the subsequent discovery of the important antiasthma agent cromolyn. Similarly, an ancient Indian drug from the plant *Adhatoda vasica* (Bakas),[2] which has been used as a traditional antiasthma agent, was recently investigated, and this resulted in the development of the modern mucokinetic agent bromhexine. Examples such as these demonstrate that an awareness of the history of respiratory drugs is of relevance today.

MILESTONES IN RESPIRATORY PHARMACOLOGY

Many of the ancient remedies used in the treatment of diseases of the respiratory tract have fallen by the wayside during the course of their centuries of service. However, it is remarkable to find how many of the drugs of early medicine are still in use today, in the United States as well as in other countries throughout the world. In China and India, the contemporary national drug compendia and pharmacopeias still include most of the agents that were introduced thousands of

and gradually, over the course of centuries, some of the traditional nostrums evolved into popular contemporary home remedies, such as Vick's VapoRub. In many countries, tincture of benzoin (friars' balsam) is a long-established favorite aromatic additive that is still inhaled in many homes and

TABLE 1–1. SOME RESPIRATORY DRUGS DERIVED FROM PLANT SOURCES

Chemical Classification	Chemical Description	Examples
ALKALOIDS	Crystalline or oily compound, nitrogenous in nature, usually basic	Atropine, cocaine, ipecac, lobelia, nicotine, opium, strophanthin, xanthines
BALSAMS	Plant exudates that are complex amorphous compounds (resins) mixed with aromatic substances	Benzoin, storax, tolu balsam
GLYCOSIDES	Organic, hydroxycompounds that release sugars on hydrolysis	Digitalis, glycyrrhiza, mustard, squill
OLEORESINS	Resins mixed with volatile oils	Capsicum (cayenne pepper), turpentine, white pine
VOLATILE OILS	Essential oils (responsible for plant odors)	Anise, creosote, eucalyptus, pine

years ago. Many of the respiratory drugs of plant derivation fit into the major chemical classifications of natural drugs that are listed in Table 1-1.

Biblical Drugs

The Old Testament refers to a number of plant derivatives that appear to have been used for the treatment of respiratory disorders. Many of these were strongly scented products that contained aromatic compounds derived from plants. James, in his scholarly book,[6] discusses a number of these products. Oilbanum (Lebonah or Luban, probably frankincense) and myrrh were perhaps the best known. Others included balm of Gilead (also called balm of Mecca), bdellium, storax ammoniacum, and the unpleasant, fetid smelling gum resins, assafoetida and galbanum. Sulfur was also used, both as an oral medication and in the form of sulfurous vapors. Cassia (cinnamon), nitre (potassium nitrate, saltpeter), laudanum (opium), tragacanth, honey, oil, wine and spices were also frequently employed in Biblical times.

Egyptian Drugs

The ancient Egyptian civilization, as well as the other civilizations of Mesopotamia that flourished from 3000 to 1600 B.C., left many detailed records of medical relevance.[1-4] The physicians of these cultures made considerable use of curious and often disgusting remedies of both animal and plant derivation. In addition to using the Biblical drugs, these writers also used the following agents of relevance to respiratory therapy: acacia, anise, benzoin, licorice, mustard, opium, pine oil, squill and turpentine. However, most remedies were utilized in the form of bizarre concoctions, with the liberal addition of synergistic mysticism.

Greek Drugs

The great physician Hippocrates lived in Greece from 460 B.C. until about 370 B.C. He is credited with introducing a more rational and cautious system of medical care into the ancient world, thereby eliminating much of the religious cant that was the usual companion of Near Eastern therapeutics. Respiratory drugs in use in Greek medicine were numerous and varied; they included obscure agents such as opoponax, elemi, copaiba, hellebore, mastic, inula Helenium, oxymel and ptisan, as well as the familiar garlic, pepper, pine fruit and cinnamon.[1-4, 7]

Roman Drugs

The most important physician in the Roman Empire was Galen, who lived from about A.D. 130 to 201. He and other Roman physicians improved on the Greek pharmacopeia by adding drugs such as aconite, anise, belladonna, camphor, ginger and lobelia. Undoubtedly these agents had been used earlier, but the authority of Galen ensured that drugs of this type gained long-lasting respect. Few further additions to the therapeutic armamentarium were considered necessary for several hundred years, and the more important drugs of vegetable derivation came to be known as galenicals. It is of interest that the Greeks and Romans did not appear to employ styrax (benzoin),[8] which was both previously and subsequently used as a major respiratory drug.

Islamic Drugs

The Arabic and Moorish cultures, which flowered from about A.D. 630 to 1030, gave rise to sophisticated alchemists and physicians who made great progress in the arts of pharmacy and therapeutics. In addition to reexamining the older drugs and retaining the best of them, these physicians also favored a number of inorganic minerals and salts, such as ammonium salts, antimony, calcium salts and so on. Although many of these had been used before, the alchemists revitalized interest in them. The Arabs introduced caffeine and candy, not only into medicine, but into everyday life. Similarly, theophylline was in use at this time as one of the constituents of tea and chocolate. It is worth noting that "caffeine" is derived from the Arabic word for "wine," and "theophylline" from the Greek word meaning "divine leaf," in tribute to the tea leaf, which contains a small amount of theophylline. It is also of historical interest that the great twelfth century Jewish physician Maimonides, who practiced in the Islamic court, recommended chicken soup for the "stirring up and ejection of pulmonary phlegm."[9]

Of further interest is a practice in present-day Tanzania. "The Moslem *imganga* (medicine man) may write out a paragraph of the Koran, appropriate to his patient's condition. He writes in a flowing hand with a quill and soluble ink. Then he washes off the ink by pouring water on the paper and bids his patient drink the solution. . . . Or he may decide on inhalation therapy, in which case he will burn the paper on which he painstakingly has written the section of the Koran and the patient will breathe in the resulting fumes."[92]

Eastern Drugs

The Chinese and Indians have always had an extraordinary familiarity with huge numbers of drugs derived from plant and animal sources, such as jinkui shenqui wan (which is composed of Radix aconiti, Carmichaeli praepatate, Cortex cinnamoni, Radix dioscoreae, Cortex moutan radicis, Poria and Rhizoma alismatis), a traditional asthma remedy.[10] The major contribution from China has been ephedrine, which took about 5000 years to find its way into Western medicine.[3] Few other original drugs were contributed to the respiratory pharmacopeia by Far Eastern cultures, and little new progress appears to have been made.[10] Chinese medicine at present consists of a curious mixture of folk medications, acupuncture and political rhetoric, with perhaps all too little of the first two and too much of the latter.

The contemporary Indian Materia Medica[11] lists thousands of drugs that have been used for hundreds of years. Although most of them lack any scientific validation, a number are very familiar, since they are the same as some of the traditional agents that are used in Western medicine. The Indian index lists at least 80 expectorants derived from plants, varying from Abies webbiana (which is related to "Canada balsam") to Zizyphus vulgaris; the list includes more familiar drugs, such as benzoin, camphor, cinnamon, eucalyptus, garlic, glycyrrhiza (which is in licorice), grindelia, lobelia, pepper, prune and scylla. The Indian list of antiasthma drugs is even longer; it contains over 100 drugs, ranging from Abhra bhasma to Zingiber (ginger).

Russian Drugs

It is interesting to consider what the development of respiratory drugs has been in Russia, since this country lies, both geographically and historically, between East and West. Somewhat disappointingly, the current Russian Drug Index[12] lists a mediocre collection of drugs, many of which are used in arbitrary compound mixtures. Some

of the respiratory remedies are obscure, for example Althaea root (marshmallow), primula root extract, tincture of viola, gledischia, Urticaria leaves, equisetum and so on. Other drugs, such as those used in the treatment of asthma, are more familiar: anise, camphor, menthol, eucalyptus, lobelia, sodium nitrate, sodium bicarbonate, sodium iodide and creosote, as well as aminophylline, ephedrine, epinephrine and scopolamine. A number of powerful drugs of dubious benefit are also employed, such as Pituitrin and thymus extract. It should be noted that the British Pharmacoepeia also includes pituitary extracts as bronchodilators, but thymus is possibly a uniquely Russian drug. In general, it would appear that Russia has made no important contribution to respiratory pharmacology over the centuries, although it is probable that a Russian Maimonides has long advocated the use of borsht.

New World Drugs

The European discovery of the American continent in the late fifteenth century led to the subsequent discovery and export of indigenous drugs back into Europe. The most important drugs of respiratory concern were tobacco, ipecacuanha, cocaine and Peruvian balsam. Tobacco over the succeeding several hundred years played an extraordinary role in medicine; initially the smoke was credited with numerous therapeutic powers, and it was advocated by many authorities for the treatment of asthma and similar pulmonary disorders. Currently, there are few physicians who would claim any therapeutic benefits from tobacco, and all respiratory practitioners recognize the evil of this unique drug.

Ipecac was originally used by American Indians as an emetic, and it also was used ritually in some religious practices.[1, 3, 4] It was used extensively in Europe after the seventeenth century, and was credited with numerous therapeutic properties.[2] Early in its use it gained a reputation as an effective expectorant, and this recognition persists. Peruvian balsam also became popular as an expectorant, while cocaine was credited with antiasthma properties before its value as a local anesthetic had been established.

In the eighteenth and nineteenth centuries guaiacol and creosote were popular drugs in the treatment of tuberculosis and other respiratory diseases. These toxic agents fell into disrepute and were replaced by other tar derivatives and glyceryl guaiacolate, which continue to find use.

Recent Pharmaceutical History

Following the Islamic contribution to European medicine, few useful developments occurred in pharmacology until the nineteenth century.

In 1802, the distinguished English physician Herberden advised that asthma should be treated with agents such as Peruvian bark, mustard seed, quicksilver, cinnabar, garlic, squill, opium and tobacco.[12] It is evident that the therapy for asthma had undergone a decline during the preceding 800 years and that most of the new drugs that were introduced were probably of more harm than benefit. When the tobacco smoking habit entered Europe in the seventeenth century, physicians developed a greater interest in the value of inhalational therapy. Some of the inhalational drugs that became popularized for the treatment of respiratory diseases during the seventeenth and eighteenth centuries are listed in Table 1-2. One undoubtedly beneficial outcome of the interest in smoke therapy was the introduction of cigarettes made with herbs containing powerful bronchodilator drugs such as stramonium;[1] when ignited, these plant products release belladonna alkaloids, which can be of marked benefit when inhaled by asthmatic patients. For patients who did not wish to use cigarettes, the ground-up herb was made

into powders that could be burned in a suitable receptacle, which enabled the patient to inhale the liberated fumes.

Ipecacuanha, discovered in South America in the sixteenth century, came to assume an important position in European therapeutics. Numerous physicians reported that the drug was of value in treating asthma and other diseases of the lungs, and there is no doubt that the drug does have expectorant properties. By the time Prosser James wrote his classic book in 1884, *The Therapeutics of the Respiratory Passages*,[6] ipecac had assumed an established place in therapy, and the pharmacologic interest in expectorants was probably at its zenith.

James discussed expectorant and bronchodilator agents under the generic term *pneumatics*. He also provided a meticulous discussion of other drugs that act on the respiratory tract. Agents that acted on the nose, when given topically or by inhalation to produce an increase in nasal discharge, were described as *errhines*. Topical drugs that caused sneezing were labeled *sternutatories* or *ptarmics*. Soothing cough medications that relieved irritation of the throat or larynx were called *bechics*. Those agents that were of primary value in asthma were termed *antispasmodics*, which is the only one of these terms that persists in modern pharmacology.

James and others[14, 15] subclassified expectorant drugs into rather imprecise classes; the terms used included depressants, stimulants and attenuants; and relaxants, emollients, narcotics, tonics, stimulants and astringents. James provided a detailed discussion of historical and traditional agents and described the following Victorian expectorants: potassium iodide, potash, other potassium salts, ammonium carbonate and ammonium chloride; ammonia, sulfur, iodine and other irritant gases; antimony, emetine, apomorphine, pilocarpine, lobelia and tobacco; hot beverages, alcohol, ether, essential oils, terebinthinates, turpentine and oleoresins; scilla, squill and senega; essential oils such as camphor, turpenes, peppermint, cloves, juniper, lavender, cinnamon, caraway, mustard and horseradish; balsams, including benzoin and storax; and alkalis (with some doubt as to the value of sodium bicarbonate). Of the agents discussed by James, two were recommended more than the others: ipecac and iodides. Iodine has had a long history of use in respiratory therapy, and it has probably been inhaled over the course of hundreds of years by

TABLE 1-2. INHALATIONAL DRUGS USED FOR RESPIRATORY DISEASES IN THE SEVENTEENTH AND EIGHTEENTH CENTURIES

Ammonia	Hydrocyanic acid
Ammonium chloride	Iodine
Amyl nitrite	Lobelia, lobeline
Aniline	Marijuana
Apormorphine	Menthol
Arsenic	Mercury
Belladonna (atropine)	Myrtol
Benzene	Opium
Bromine	Phenol
Camphor	Pine oils
Cocaine	Potassium salts
Conium (hemlock)	Pyridine
Creosote	Resorcin
Ether	Silver nitrate
Ethyl iodide	Stramonium
Eucalyptus	Tar derivatives
Guaiacol	Terebinthate
Hashish	Tobacco
Helium	Turpentine

means of burning sponge or seaweed. Although iodine fumes have been credited with expectorant activity, toward the end of the nineteenth century iodine was generally replaced by oral potassium iodide or sodium iodide.

Inhalation therapy had begun to assume a new dimension in the seventeenth century with the discovery of oxygen and other chemical gases. Many physicians concentrated on giving patients inhalations with various gases, most of which failed to retain any creditability in the succeeding years. Toward the end of the eighteenth century a number of other inhalational drugs were also falling into disrepute. Thus, James did not apparently favor a number of the agents that had been advocated just a few years earlier, such as those described by Scudder in his book *On the Use of Medicated Inhalations,* which was published in 1867.[14] Among these remedies were drugs that had been familiar over the centuries, including inhalational drugs derived from hops (tincture of lupuli), chamomile, potassium cyanide, hydrocyanic acid, Conium (hemlock), rose water, aquae caldiae, aquae bullientis, verbascum, chlorine gas and so on. By the end of the nineteenth century, inhalation therapy was

TABLE 1–3. DRUGS USED IN THE TREATMENT OF ASTHMA AT THE BEGINNING OF THE TWENTIETH CENTURY*

Aconite	Ether
Adrenalin	Ethyl iodide
Ammonium salts	Eucalyptus
ammonium chloride	Euphorbia
ammonium carbonate	Grindelia
Amyl nitrite	Heroin
Antimony	Ipecacuanha
Antipyrine	Lobelia
Apomorphine	Morphine, opium
Arsenic and salts	Mustard
Asafoetida	Oxycamphor
Belladonna alkaloids	Oxygen
atropine	Paraldehyde
duboisine	Pilocarpine
hyoscine	Potassium salts
stramonium	potassium chloride
Bromides	potassium iodide
Cannabis (marijuana)	potassium nitrate
Carbonic acid (carbon dioxide)	Pyridine
Carburetted hydrogen	Quinine
Chamomile	Sanguinaria
Chloral	Silver nitrate
Chloroform	Strychnine
Cocaine	Sulfurous acid
Coffee	Tetranitrin
Colchicum	Tobacco

*From Potter, S. O. L.: *Materia Medica, Pharmacy and Therapeutics.* Philadelphia, P. Blakiston's Son & Co., 10th Ed., 1908.

becoming more circumspect, and an attempt to rationalize therapy had been made, although many of the older remedies persisted (Table 1–3).

In 1903, Tissier wrote a tract entitled *Pneumotherapy, Including Aërotherapy and Inhalation Methods and Therapy;* this was published as Volume 10 of Solis Cohen's *A System of Physiologic Therapeutics.*[15] In the section on medicaments suitable for use as vapors the author discussed the following drugs: ammonium chloride, amyl nitrite, aniline, arsenic, benzene, benzoin, bromine, camphor, creosote, eucalyptus, ether, ethyl iodide, guaiacol, hashish, hemlock, iodine, menthol, mercury bichloride, myrtol, opium, phenol, potassium nitrate, pyridine, resorcin, silver nitrate, stramonium, tars, tobacco, turpentine, and a number of similar agents. Some of these agents were used to treat tuberculosis and other infections; at that time phenol (carbolic acid) and similar agents were probably the best antibacterial compounds available. What is of particular interest to the modern reader is the huge number of inhalational drugs that were used, and the careful delineation of the particular disease (be it hay fever, croup, tuberculous laryngitis, diphtheria, bronchitis, asthma or pneumonia) for which each specific agent was believed to be indicated.

Many of these drugs persisted in Western medicine for a number of years. In 1913, Dr. Robin from Paris published *Treatment of Tuberculosis,*[15] in which the following drugs were recommended for inhalation: tannin, alum, turpentine, carbolic acid, benzoic acid, benzoates, creosote, thymol, gomenol, eucalyptol, menthol, sulfurous acid, hydrogen sulfide, chlorine, sulfide of carbon, iodine, iodides, arsenicals, mercury bichloride, aniline, allyl iodide and hydrofluosilicic acid. Of interest is the fact that Robin also advocated the breathing of "air surcharged with nitrogen"; it is unclear what is meant by the author, although one must assume that the mixture was simply air lacking in oxygen! Robin had a somewhat eclectic approach—although he was not averse to giving creosote by inhalation, he particularly advised that it be given by the rectal route.

By 1927, a greater effort was being made to identify the physiologic function of the respiratory drug, and Culbreth[17] provided a useful classification (Table 1–4). Soon after this, the age of scientific pharmacology began to overwhelm the free-ranging imaginations of the respiratory clinicians, and the heyday of inhalation therapy was gradually

TABLE 1–4.   AGENTS LISTED AS ACTING ON RESPIRATORY SYSTEM 50 YEARS AGO*

RESPIRATORY STIMULANTS	apomorphine, atropine, digitalis, emetine, opium, strychnine
RESPIRATORY SEDATIVES	aconite, hydrocyanic acid, opium, etc.
COUGH SUPPRESSANTS	belladonna, codeine, hydrocyanic acid, morphine, opium
NASAL STIMULANTS	ammonia, cubeb, ipecac, quillaga, pepper, etc.
CILIARY EXCITANTS	acacia, ammonium chloride, potassium chlorate, sodium chloride
EXPECTORANTS	ammonia, ammonium salts, apomorphine, balsam of Peru, benzoin, garlic, glycyrrhiza, ipecac, lobelia, onion, pilocarpine, pine tar, saccharine, senega, squill, tartar emetic, tolu, turpentine

*From Culbreth.[17]

succeeded by the conservatism of modern drug therapy. Most of the drugs used in inhalation therapy at present have been introduced during the twentieth century, and the majority of these have been discovered since 1940 (Table 1–5). The practicing respiratory therapist may experience a nostalgic sense of loss when recalling how the glories of a well-endowed inhalational pharmacology of the past have given way to the relatively narrow, albeit scientifically proven, unromantic collection of agents that is acceptable today.

MODERN RESPIRATORY PHARMACOLOGY

Although a large number of the drugs in current use have been used for many years, respiratory therapeutics is being shaped by some of the most innovative and successful of all the drug development efforts of the Western pharmaceutical industry. Many important new drugs have been introduced during the past 15 years that have had a profound effect upon the treatment of respiratory diseases (Table 1–5).[18, 19]

The introduction of any new drug has become a lengthy and expensive undertaking in the United States as a result of legislation that has been introduced with the intent of protecting the public from hazardous or ineffective drugs.[20] In 1938, the Food and Drug Administration (FDA) set up rigorous standards that any new drug had to pass before it was authorized for marketing. Since that time, manufacturers of new agents have had to submit an application containing detailed information about the drug for the FDA to review. Over the years, the FDA has become increasingly more demanding, and in 1962 legislation was enacted that requires manufacturers to carry out extensive, controlled trials to demonstrate the safety and effectiveness of new drugs.[21, 22] Less rigorous standards and far less bureaucratic hindrance in the United Kingdom have enabled the British drug industry, in particular, to harness the creativity of its

TABLE 1–5.   INTRODUCTION OF MAJOR RESPIRATORY DRUGS

Decades and Demidecades	Sympathomimetic Agents	Methylxanthines	Antiasthma Agents	Mucokinetic Agents
1900–1909	Epinephrine	Theophylline		
1910–1919		Aminophylline		
1920–1929	Ephedrine			
1930–1939	Ethylnorepinephrine	Aminophylline (I.V.)		
1940–1949	Isoproterenol Methoxyphenamine		Cortisone Hydrocortisone	
1950–1954	Isoetharine Protokylol	Dyphylline		Alevaire*
1955–1959		Oxtriphylline	Glucocorticoid derivatives	Tergemist*
1960–1964	Metaproterenol Soterenol*		Glucocorticoid derivatives	Acetylcysteine
1965–1969	Fenoterol* Salbutamol* Terbutaline		Cromolyn	Mesna*
1970–1974	Rimiterol*		Beclomethasone* Betamethasone*	Bromhexine* Carbocysteine*
1975–	Carbuterol*			

*Not available in the United States.

experimental pharmacologists and thereby foster a remarkably effective and continuing record of innovations in respiratory therapeutics. In recent years the United Kingdom has made contributions to most areas of respiratory pharmacology and has introduced important drugs such as cromolyn, salbutamol and beclomethasone. In contrast, the pharmaceutical manufacturers of the United States have lagged far behind in ability to produce new agents,[21, 22] and the zealous demands of the FDA have held back established foreign drugs from entry into the American market for astoundingly long periods. Thus, the British bronchodilator salbutamol was available in the United Kingdom in 1968 and yet was not authorized to appear on the United States market even in 1978!

The development of a new drug requires a long and complex interfaceted cooperative effort that involves basic chemists, animal experiments and clinical investigators who are supported in their efforts by the manufacturing pharmaceutical firm that is interested in marketing the eventual product. A new agent is often developed as a result of a chance finding, such as that which characterized the serendipitous discovery by a keenly observant, scientific investigator, that the drug cromolyn has prophylactic value in asthma. Many of the newer drugs have emerged as a result of research that involves a more deliberate and exhaustive examination of the structure and properties of established drugs, which are then subjected to an extraordinary number of scientifically determined chemical manipulations. These procedures are designed to produce a molecule that enhances the therapeutic properties of the original drug while eliminating the undesired side effects. Many of the new sympathomimetic bronchodilators have been synthesized in this deliberate fashion. Other new drugs emerge as a result of alterations in the basic formulation of a marketed product, to improve drug absorption and activity. Some of the newer theophylline products are examples of the same basic drug being formulated in different ways. The drug industry utilizes serendipity, innovative approaches to old drugs, empirical pharmacologic screening of potent chemicals, chemical modification of known active molecules, logical improvements in the formulation of the preparation to be marketed, and a variety of other approaches that characterize the processes of industrial design, development and marketing.[23] A knowledge of the history of pharmacology is relevant to the modern drug industry, and a commitment to the scientific examination of long-established folk medicines of plant origin often leads to the discovery of a potent of new drug.

EVALUATION OF A NEW DRUG

Once a manufacturer has determined, as a result of chemical investigations and animal experiments, that a newly developed chemical has a therapeutic potential, a Notice of Claimed Investigational Exemption for a New Drug (IND) is filed with the FDA.[24] The laboriously assembled information provided in this IND enables the FDA review team to decide whether the drug is suitable for clinical investigation, by qualified researchers using human volunteers; the drug

TABLE 1–6. STAGES IN THE INVESTIGATION OF A NEW DRUG

Stage	Time Taken (YEARS)	Study Process
1. CHEMICAL EVALUATION	Varies	Chemical and physical characterization
2. ANIMAL STUDIES	1–2	Examination of effects and side effects
3. HUMAN STUDIES		
Phase I	2–2½	Initial studies of drug effectiveness and metabolism (in healthy volunteers)
Phase II	1–2	
early		Clinical trial to establish safety in volunteer patients
late		Evaluation of efficacy and safety in large number of volunteer patients
Phase III	1–2	Determination of value of drug in clinical practice, and establishment of criteria for packaging and marketing
4. FDA EVALUATION		If the drug is reviewed favorably by the FDA, it is released on the market.
5. CONTINUING STUDIES		
Phase IV		The drug is subject to continuing evaluation by the manufacturer and the FDA.

trial that follows is known as a Phase I investigation (Table 1–6).

If the Phase I studies establish that the drug appears to be effective, well-tolerated and safe when given to volunteers, the drug is ready to enter Phase II. A number of investigations are then carried out in several medical centers involving volunteer patients who have the specific disease for which the drug is expected to be useful. During the early part of Phase II, information is derived as to the appropriate dosage range and the safety and efficacy of the drug; in the later part of Phase II the results obtained by treating numerous volunteer patients are analyzed statistically to determine the dosage and method of administration that should be used. During both Phase I and Phase II, intensive metabolic studies are carried out to determine how the drug is handled by human organs.

A drug that performs well in Phase II then enters the next part of the clinical investigation. In Phase III a number of carefully monitored trials of the drug in clinical practice are carried out and the information is prepared for the exhaustive review of an FDA team of experts. The detailed results of the preceding years of development and investigation of the drug are assembled in the form of a New Drug Application (NDA) that must be submitted to the FDA.[24] The subsequent review process is lengthy, and if any doubts exist with regard to any aspect of the drug's use, the FDA will request more information. Eventually, if the FDA review is favorable, Phase III is concluded by the release of the drug onto the market. During the course of development and marketing, the drug acquires a number of different names, as is shown for metaproterenol in Table 1–7.

The continuing clinical evaluation of the marketed product constitutes Phase IV; during this period the drug may establish an important niche in the competitive market, or it may fail for reasons of safety or because of its inability to compete. In the future, the FDA is liable to demand a more vigorous evaluation of drugs that are in Phase IV of their development. The exhaustive and costly processes involved in getting a drug established on the market provide a partial explanation for the high cost of even simple drugs.

PRESCRIBING OF DRUGS

A vast number of drugs are available in almost every pharmaceutic category, and most basic agents are formulated, compounded and packaged in a variety of ways. The majority of potent drugs are available to the patient-consumer only by means of a prescription order of a physician. Protection of the public is achieved by having a knowledgeable pharmacist check the prescription and then provide the patient with the medication, appropriately labeled with instructions for usage; information regarding side effects and precautions is provided to the extent that this is judged to be in the patient's interest. A surprising number of potent drugs are available without a physician's prescription, and it is difficult to understand in what way some of these over-the-counter (OTC) medications are safer than prescription drugs. Thus, aerosol preparations of epinephrine are available as OTC drugs, whereas other aerosol bronchodilators are dispensed only on the basis of a physician's prescription, in spite of the fact that there is little to suggest that aerosol

TABLE 1–7. NAMING OF DRUGS

Name	Explanation	Example
Chemical name	Name based on chemical structure	1-(3,5-dihydroxyphenyl)-2-isopropylaminoethanol*
Laboratory designation	Code name adopted by producer	Th-152
Generic names	Common name, usually related to chemical name	metaproterenol, orciprenaline
Official names	May be same as generic name. Names are established by the United States Adopted Names (USAN) Committee, which is a joint nomenclature committee.	metaproterenol (in U.S.) orciprenaline (in Europe)
Trademark names	Proprietary names of marketed products (registered)	Alupent, Metaprel

*An alternative chemical name is also recognized, i.e., $(\pm)$–3,5-dihydroxy-α–[(isopropylamino)methyl]benzyl alcohol.

preparations of epinephine are safer than other aerosol drugs such as isoproterenol. Numerous traditional cough and cold medications are available as proprietary OTC preparations, although the constituents are a mixture of potent drugs and of mild, traditional components whose efficacy is often unproved.[20] While there is no evidence of any important degree of direct public harm resulting from the availability of OTC preparations, it is reasonable to expect that the FDA will eventually attempt to introduce more order into the present illogical marketing system, and in the future it is likely that fewer potent drugs will be readily available to the general public.

In some states, questions have been raised as to who is entitled to mix and administer respiratory drugs, particularly drugs that are given by nebulization. It is clear that licensed physicians and registered nurses are authorized to administer drugs, and they are expected to exercise a measure of individual judgment in so doing. Equally, it is clear that a patient or a family member is entitled to the same privileges when using either an OTC or a prescription drug as an outpatient. On logical grounds there can be no doubt that a duly educated respiratory technician is one of the most highly qualified persons to mix, administer, evaluate and determine correct dosages of aerosolized medications. Furthermore, the respiratory technician who has studied respiratory pharmacology, either during formal schooling or within the framework of continuing education, should be knowledgeable in the use of all major respiratory drugs given by the noninhalational routes. Thus, there should be no quibbling with the concept of the right of the qualified respiratory technician to administer aerosol drugs in a responsible fashion. In all circumstances, the physician who prescribes respiratory drugs and the nurses and technicians who administer them should have a detailed knowledge and understanding of the pharmacology of these agents. Obviously, the dispensing pharmacist should have an equally detailed understanding, and even the patient on chronic drug therapy should have a reasonable level of knowledge concerning the major pharmacologic properties of the drug. Although the physician is the only professional entitled to prescribe drugs, the other members of the health team who are involved with administering the prescription should strive to have as great an understanding of practical pharmacology as that which is expected of the physician.

DRUG FORMULATION

The details of the formulation of individual, marketed drugs are one aspect of drug therapy that is largely unknown to all members of the health team. Although one thinks of a drug as a single, pure entity, all medications are packaged with other chemicals to provide an effective formulation.[25] Many of these additional constituents are disregarded, in the belief that they are inert and have no significant pharmacologic action. A number of additives have been used for so long that even the manufacturers may no longer be able to recall why these chemicals were incorporated in the product; nor can it always be stated what their effects on human tissue might be.[25] Table 1–8 lists some of the common antioxidants and preservatives that are often added to pharmacologic preparations; several of them are used in most drug formulations. It is worth noting that ethylenediamine, the solvent and stabilizer used in aminophylline, can cause asthma! Although this has not resulted in recognized clinical problems, the propensity of ethylenediamine to cause asthma should be borne in mind if an asthmatic patient appears to deteriorate after receiving aminophylline. On the other hand, many antiasthma drugs contain methyl and propyl parabens as preservatives, and although there is contrary evidence,[26] recent work suggests that the parabens have a bronchodilator action.[27]

Additional components contained in formulations of marketed preparations are listed in Table 1–9. It should be recognized that there is lack of uniformity in the classifying terms used to describe the various inert additives, and it is becoming clear that not all classes of additives are as innocuous as had been thought. Of particular current concern are the coloring dyes that are so commonly incorporated both in foods and in medications. In recent years it has been demonstrated that the yellow dye tartrazine (FD and C Yellow No. 5), which is related to acetylsalicylic acid, can cause asthma in patients who are hypersensitive to this chemical. Tartrazine has been used in a considerable number of drug formulations, including many marketed for the treatment of asthma. If an asthmatic patient is believed to be allergic to tartrazine, medications that contain this dye must be avoided. Until recently this could be difficult, as demonstrated by the fact that of 149 bronchodilator products, 29 contained tartrazine, and a

TABLE 1–8. ACTIONS OF SOME SPECIFIC ADDITIVES USED IN RESPIRATORY DRUG FORMULATIONS

	Antioxidant	Antiseptic	Preservative	Solvent	Stabilizer	Other Actions
Alcohol		+	+	+		Tissue irritant
Ascorbic acid	+					Has mucokinetic properties
Ascorbyl palmitate	+				+	
Benzoic acid and benzoates			+			
Cetylpyridinium		+				
Chlorbutanol		+	+			
Ethylenediamine				+	+	Can cause asthma
Ethylenediaminetetraacetate (EDTA)	+					Chelating agent; has mucokinetic properties
Glycerin			+	+		Has humectant properties
Parabens (methyl, propyl)		+	+			May have bronco-dilator properties
Saccharine						Sweetening agent
Sodium bisulfite	+				+	Tissue irritant
Sodium metabisulfite	+					
Sodium chloride				+		Provides tonicity
Sodium citrate						Buffer to adjust pH
Sorbitan trioleate					+	

further 59 contained other azo dyes.[28] An extensive listing of drugs known to contain tartrazine was published in 1976,[29] but since that time almost all manufacturers have discontinued using this dye as a coloring agent in medical products.

INFORMATION ABOUT DRUGS

It can be seen that the patient receives much more than the active drug prescribed by the physician. Furthermore, there is often a question of the comparative bioavailability of the same drug produced by different manufacturers.[30] Occasionally, some brand name drugs resulting in substandard blood levels and inadequate therapeutic responses have been reported. The FDA and other agencies are maintaining a vigilant surveillance to detect and eliminate those preparations that do not meet the standards; there is reasonable certainty that the majority of the

TABLE 1–9. ADDITIVES FREQUENTLY INCORPORATED IN DRUG FORMULATIONS

Additive	Function	Examples
Binders (granulators)	granules that are necessary to bind drugs into tablets	lactose, starch
Buffers	salts and weak acids/alkalis, used to adjust pH	acetates, citrates
Coatings	external layer of oral preparations	gelatin, plastics
Colorants	dyes and pigments, for coloration	azo dyes, tartrazine
Diluents	inert additives, solutions or powders	water, lactose
Disintegrators	additives that help tablet break down in gut	agar, starch
Excipients	various agents used to alter the density or flow characteristics	calcium chloride, lactose
Flavors	agents used to disguise or improve the taste of the drug	many of the traditional expectorants
Humectants (desiccants)	agents that absorb moisture from the environment	propylene glycol, sodium sulfate
Lubricants (surfactants)	agents added to improve manipulation of drug during manufacture	lanolin, oil, talcum
Suspending agents	agents used to suspend drugs that are insoluble in water	acacia, gelatin, tragacanth

prescription drugs in the United States are acceptable.

There has been a tendency for powerful pharmaceutical companies to try to persuade both physicians and the public that the well-known brand name drugs are in some way superior to many of the much less expensive competing brands; the vast majority of these self-serving advertising claims are not justified by the facts.

There are many published guides to help the physician, nurse and therapist obtain information on drug products (Table 1–10). The official compendia provide basic guides to most of the available medications, and the unofficial compendia provide more practical information, including explanations of how drugs should be used and comparisons of various drugs that have similar properties. At least one of the official or nonofficial compendia should be readily available to every professional involved in pharmacologic health care delivery. Each volume has specific features that may make it the book of choice for a particular circumstance, but in general all the books listed in Table 1–10 are of similar quality and each serves well in practice.

In addition to these compendia, standard textbooks can be consulted for theoretic information, and most of the well-known books are treasure houses of information. One additional useful guide to practical therapeutics is the newsletter *The Medical*

TABLE 1–10. MAJOR SOURCES OF DRUG INFORMATION

OFFICIAL COMPENDIA

The Pharmacopoeia of the United States of America (The United States Pharmacopeia, U.S.P., New York)	Listing of proven therapeutic drugs with low toxicity. Provides standards for drugs. Does not provide therapeutic or pharmacologic guidance for drug use. Revised editions published every five years.
The National Formulary (N.F., American Pharmaceutical Association, Washington D.C.)	Lists therapeutic drugs. Also lists drug mixtures, and various substances derived from plants; in these respects the N.F. differs from the U.S.P.
Martindale: The Extra Pharmacopoeia (The Pharmaceutical Press, London)	An extraordinarily comprehensive encyclopedia of drugs, arranged by pharmaceutical class. Provides details of marketed products from many countries, and gives extracts from the literature on many drug actions and side effects.

UNOFFICIAL COMPENDIA

AMA Drug Evaluations (Publishing Sciences Group, Inc., Littleton, Mass.)	A descriptive and detailed catalogue of all categories of drugs, based on therapeutic classification.
American Drug Index (Billups, N. F., Lippincott, Philadelphia)	Dictionary of drug products and dosage forms, cross-indexed. Does not provide commentaries or pharmacologic advice.
American Hospital Formulary Service (American Society of Hospital Pharmacists, Washington D.C.)	Provides monographs on each drug, with advice about use, particularly in hospitals.
Facts and Comparisons (Kastrup, E. K., Facts and Comparisons Inc., St. Louis)	Lists all drugs available, with monographs and discussions of values of individual agents. Provides comparisons of costs of drugs of similar type.
Handbook of Nonprescription Drugs (American Pharmaceutical Association, Washington, D.C.)	Monographs and listing of over-the-counter drugs in various categories, with tabulations of the contents and amounts of constituent agents in mixtures.
Modern Drug Encyclopedia and Therapeutic Index (Lewis, A. J. (Ed.), Yorke Medical Books, New York)	Provides facts about specific medications or classes of therapeutic and diagnostic agents. Provides monographs on many drugs.
Physicians' Desk Reference to Pharmaceutical Specialties and Biologicals (PDR) (Medical Economics, Oradell, N.J.)	Provides information on all drugs, similar to that provided by manufacturers in the leaflets that accompany marketed drugs. Lacks objectivity, and does not compare drugs.
Remington's Pharmaceutical Sciences (Mack, Easton, Pa.)	A comprehensive encyclopedia for pharmacists, which provides a wide range of information, including details and commentaries on most drugs and factors involved in marketing them.
The Merck Index: An Encyclopedia of Chemicals and Drugs (Merck, Rahway, N.J.)	Contains structural formulae, synonyms, and chemical and physical properties of numerous agents, many of which are of therapeutic value. Useful source for information on obscure agents.
The United States Dispensatory (Osol, A. and Pratt, R. (Eds.), Lippincott, Philadelphia)	Provides information on most drugs used in therapeutics, and contains general reviews of pharmacologic classes of drugs. Valuable source of practical therapeutic information.

Letter On Drugs And Therapeutics. This publication is so conservative, however, that the reader may gain the impression that there are few drugs of true value, and that only a minority of the newer drugs offer substantial improvements over the existing products. In actuality, such a view is not unreasonable, but it is important to remember that new drugs provide the physician with an opportunity to utilize a variety of agents in succession when attempting to find the optimal preparation for an individual patient. Experience shows that each patient is likely to find that there is one particular drug of a pharmacologic class, be it old or new, that is most successful in that individual's specific case.

Although the manufacturers are obliged to write their promotional material in accordance with what the FDA determines after evaluation, the dosage recommendations provided in the labeling do not constitute an absolutely rigid requirement for the prescribing physician to follow. The physician is entitled to use any approved drug in any way he chooses as long as he can knowingly justify the prescription. Thus, a drug formulated for intravenous use could be given by aerosol if a physician, who fully understands the pharmacology and the use of the drug, decides that it would be appropriate to prescribe it for administration in this fashion. However, the physician is required to explain the basis for deviating from the prescribing advice provided in the manufacturer's labeling, and a detailed rationale should be entered into the patient's record. Under such circumstances, if the nurse or therapist is satisfied that the drug can safely be given in the dosage or fashion prescribed by the physician, even though this deviates from the standard method of drug delivery, then the drug can be administered with impunity. In all cases, it is incumbent on the nurse or therapist to ensure that the explanation for the deviant method of usage of the drug is written into the patient's record, and careful notation should be kept of the outcome of the therapy.

The drug manufacturer and the FDA regulate the dosage and method of delivery of drugs in order to protect the patient who is being treated by a physician who has an average understanding of a drug. But neither the manufacturer nor the FDA wishes to inhibit the expert physician from using a drug in another fashion when the safety of the method can be guaranteed by the specialist's particular understanding of the pharmacologic consequence of the therapy. Obviously, the specialist physician, who carries out research or attends scientific meetings, and reads the current literature, will have more precise and up to date information about drug therapy than was available when the manufacturer's labeling was prepared.[31]

PHARMACOLOGIC CONSIDERATIONS IN DRUG THERAPY

The rational choice and employment of specific drugs for the treatment of the individual patient necessitate an understanding of some basic pharmacologic principles. General therapeutic principles are reviewed in Table 1–11; the physician should ensure that a chosen drug is optimal for the patient in terms of effectiveness, ease of administration and relative expense. Since alternative preparations abound, some discrimination is always required when selecting a specific preparation. It is also important to realize that patients often appear to derive from a medication a benefit that may be totally inexplicable on the basis of pharmacology; such a response is generally attributable to the *placebo* effect of therapy.[31] The experienced physician uses placebo treatment in an active fashion, knowing that a patient will, for instance, generally appreciate receiving a "cough medicine," even though none of the constituents have any significant pharmacologic effect on the pathophysiology of the cough. Some medications are, however, relatively powerful placebos, and a degree of careful thought must be brought to bear. For example, aerosol therapy, particularly with

TABLE 1–11. SOME GENERAL PRINCIPLES IN THERAPEUTICS

1. Use specific drugs whose main actions and side effects are well known.
2. Choose generic drugs when these are equivalent to more expensive brand name preparations.
3. Use a dosage schedule appropriate to the individual patient's requirements.
4. Avoid combination preparations in general, but recognize the suitability of such preparations for certain patients.
5. Avoid adverse combinations of drugs.
6. Monitor patient clinically for therapeutic response and for adverse effects.
7. Use laboratory tests sparingly, but as required.
8. In chronic drug therapy, be prepared to make changes periodically.
9. Provide the patient with a basic understanding of outpatient drug therapy.
10. When placebo therapy appears to be indicated, use it knowledgeably.

IPPB, often engenders a placebo effect related to the psychologic confidence that a patient invests in this mechanical form of drug administration.[32] Although such treatment is generally safe, it can be dangerous,[33] and must be used with discrimination. Self-medication in the hands of children carries a marked risk of psychologic dependency when the placebo value of therapy is more potent than the primary pharmacologic benefit of the drug. In such circumstances overuse of the drug can occur, and fatalities may result as a consequence of severe side effects.[34]

TIMING OF DRUG ADMINISTRATION

By convention, it is usual to give medications three or four times a day, in proximity to the partaking of meals. In respiratory therapy, the timing of aerosol therapy is often geared to the consideration of convenience; in hospitals, this must be related to staffing patterns and work loads, with wide variations occuring as a result. On pathophysiologic grounds, treatments should be related to the diurnal variations in the abnormal process that is being treated. In many patients with chronic respiratory disorders, symptoms are often worse in the morning because of the lack of therapy during the night; moreover, mucostasis builds up as a result of the inactivity of the coughing mechanism during sleep. Therefore, respiratory treatment should generally be emphasized in the early morning: aerosol therapy sessions should be longer lasting and they should be repeated at closer intervals during the early part of the day (Table 1–12). For an acutely ill patient, drug treatment may be needed continuously, by means of an intravenous drip, or therapy may have to be repeated at frequent intervals. When a patient's condition is stable and there are only minimal symptoms, drugs may be given prophylactically perhaps once or twice a day, or even less frequently. Those patients who develop respiratory problems at predictable times, such as exercise-induced bronchospasm, may need prophylactic drug administration on an infrequent, as-needed basis. Thus, the timing of treatments depends as much upon the patient and the disease process as it does upon the pharmacologic properties of the drug. The best treatment regimen is achieved when the patient understands the objectives of the drug therapy, and participates in making

TABLE 1–12. TIMING OF DAILY TREATMENTS FOR BRONCHIAL DISEASE

A. INITIAL TREATMENT
   Give as early as possible, i.e. soon after awakening.
   Proportionally larger dose may be advisable.
   Maintenance glucocorticoid therapy should be given once a day, before breakfast.

B. SUBSEQUENT TREATMENT
   May be required relatively soon, e.g. within 30–120 minutes.
   Proportionally small dose may suffice.

C. ADDITIONAL TREATMENTS
   Frequency will depend on severity of disease, e.g. in severe bronchospasm, bronchodilator may be needed hourly.
   In milder disease, no additional doses may be needed.
   Dosage intervals should be based on therapeutic half-life of drug. (Usually, retreatments are needed three or four times a day.)

D. NOCTURNAL TREATMENT
   Avoid administration of central stimulators if possible within three hours of hour of sleep.
   Slow-release preparation or a suppository of a theophylline may be useful.
   Some patients will have to interrupt sleep to obtain treatments every 4–6 hours around the clock.

E. TREATMENT SCHEDULES
   Most drugs are needed three or four times a day; the dosages and times should be related to patient's individual needs.
   Dosages should be regulated by the patient, under supervision, on a daily basis.
   Avoid overdosage, particularly with aerosols.
   In some cases (particularly in mild disease) combination preparations are of value.

educated decisions about modifications in dosage.

The pharmacologic basis for intervals between doses should be considered.[23] Although a sophisticated knowledge of the science of drug handling by the body (pharmacokinetics) is not required, a general concept of systemic drug metabolism should be appreciated. Most drugs are given by the oral (*enteral*) route, and the onset of action of an agent depends mainly upon the rate of absorption. Considerable variations in absorptive rates may occur: influential factors include gastric acidity, gastric motility, the integrity of the stomach, the presence of food and water in the stomach and the formulation of the drug preparation. These considerations have been of major concern in theophylline therapy, and numerous new formulations have been introduced in recent years, attempting to improve the rate and completeness of absorption of the drug. However, in patients receiving chronic therapy, with

TABLE 1–13. ROUTES OF ADMINISTRATION OF RESPIRATORY DRUGS

Route	Appearance of Maximal Effect			Formulation	Examples	Main Advantage	Main Disadvantage
	Rapid	Inter-mediate	Slow				
ORAL	+			Elixir	Theophylline	Ease of administration	May irritate stomach
		+		Tablet	Metaproterenol	Ease of administration	Absorption may be erratic
			+	Time release	Aminophylline	Useful at night	Difficult to optimize dose
SUBLINGUAL	+			Aerosol or tablet	Isoproterenol	Dose can be titrated	Results are variable
NASAL	+			Drops or spray	Phenylephrine	Ease of administration	Symptoms may rebound
INHALATION	+			Aerosol	Isoproterenol	Optimal route	Overuse is common
	+			Vapor	VapoRub	Optimal route	May irritate respiratory mucosa
			+	Powder	Cromolyn	Only route	May irritate respiratory mucosa
TRACHEAL INSTILLATION	+			Solution	Acetylcysteine	Optimal route	Irritates respiratory mucosa
		+		Solution	Local anesthetic	Useful with bronchoscopy	May induce some bronchospasm
SUBCUTANEOUS	+			Solution	Terbutaline	For severe bronchospasm	Unsuitable for chronic use
	+	+		Suspension	Epinephrine	Prolonged effect	May result in prolonged side effects
INTRAMUSCULAR		+		Solution	Dyphylline	Very accessible route	Unsuitable for repeated use
		+	+	Solution-in-oil	Epinephrine	Prolonged effect	May result in prolonged side effects
INTRAVENOUS	+			Solution	Aminophylline	Results in maximal effect	Danger of overdose
RECTAL		+		Enema or solution	Theophylline	Useful in emergencies	Irritating to mucosa
			+	Suppository	Aminophylline	Results in potent effect	Irregular absorption

TABLE 1–14. AVAILABLE FORMS OF MEDICATIONS

Products	Description
ORAL	
Liquid	
Aqueous	Drug dissolved in water
Elixir	Sweet, flavored, alcoholic solution of drug
Syrup	Concentrated sugar solution containing drug
Suspension	Undissolved particulate drug in liquid carrier
Solid	
Capsule	Drug enclosed in gelatin shell
Pill	Small, round, compressed mass of drug
Tablet	Compressed mass of drug, often with coating
Sustained-release forms	Capsules and tablets that release medication over course of several hours
INHALATION	
Solution	Aqueous or alcoholic solution of drug
Powder	Drug in micronized powder form
Metered form	Solution or powdered form of drug, with propellant
Vapor	Drug vaporized in steam
INJECTION	
Solution	Aqueous or other solvent (such as ethylenediamine) used to dissolve drug
Suspension	Undissolved particulate drug in liquid carrier
RECTAL	
Enema	Solution forms for rectal administration
Suppository	Drug is incorporated in solid base and is released in rectum

several dosings a day, these concerns are of minor importance since the main object of therapy is to achieve a reasonable blood level throughout most of the day rather than to seek a periodic rapid increase in level following each dosing.

In emergencies, a rapidly absorbed oral preparation would be advantageous, but more rapid absorption can be obtained by giving the drug by the rectal route, or by avoiding the bowel altogether and giving drug therapy *parenterally,* for example, by intramuscular or intravenous administration or by inhalation. Obviously, the intravenous route enables the drug to reach a very high serum level immediately; intramuscular therapy allows a slower entry into the blood stream, but the peak level may be achieved more rapidly than when the drug is given orally. The route of administration and the formulation used have advantages and disadvantages; these factors enter into the physician's decision-making when prescribing a drug (Table 1–13). Most medications are prepared in a number of standard forms to facilitate their administration by the appropriate route (Table 1–14).

METABOLISM AND EXCRETION OF DRUGS

Following its administration, a drug is absorbed and then distributed throughout the body. The medication achieves its effect by acting on specific receptors in the tissues, then most drugs are metabolized by the tissues or by the liver; the degradation products are excreted in the bile or in the urine. Aerosolized drugs have a rapid onset of action, but their effect is usually shorter lived than when the drug is given into the body itself (i.e., by *systemic* administration, as contrasted to *topical* administration). The aerosolized agent is partially degraded in the lung, while part is absorbed into the blood

TABLE 1–15. METABOLIC BREAKDOWN OF DRUGS

Major Degradation Mechanisms	Examples of Drug Substrates
Hydrolysis	barbiturates
Oxidations	
dealkylation	epinephrine, morphine
deamination	amphetamine
dehydrogenation	alcohol
demethylation	barbiturates, diazepam, morphine
hydroxylation	barbiturates, phenytoin
monoamine oxidation	catecholamines, histamine
other oxidation reactions	methylxanthines
Reduction	chloramphenicol, prednisolone
Conjugations	
acetylation	isoniazid, sulfonamides
ethereal sulfatization	epinephrine, isoproterenol
glucuronidation	alcohols, catecholamines
glycine synthesis	salicylic acid
methylation	catecholamines
sulfatization	corticosteroids

stream, and the rest is cleared from the respiratory tract by the mucociliary escalator. Drugs that are given intravenously have a rapid effect, but are relatively rapidly inactivated by metabolic breakdown or excretion. Drugs that are given by other parenteral routes (subcutaneously or intramuscularly) or directly into the gastrointestinal tract are absorbed slowly, and are inactivated gradually. The mechanisms by which metabolic degradation and excretion occur have been intensely studied; the main metabolic degradation processes are listed in Table 1–15.

There is still a deficit in our understanding of the complex mechanisms by which the body handles various drugs in all their marketed formulations, and much of the information available applies to a standard preparation of a drug acting on a normal adult. The metabolic and excretory handling of a drug is governed by numerous complex individual factors, such as the patient's age and genetic constitution, the state of the liver and kidney, prior exposure to the drug, and the effects of other drugs (Table 1–16). Some adverse drug interactions of particular relevance to the respiratory patient are presented in Table 1–17; further details are provided in standard textbooks[23, 24, 31] and compendia (see Table 1–10).

In normal, healthy subjects, it is possible to establish the rate of decline in activity of a drug in the blood by determining serial drug levels in the serum. The time taken for the level to fall to 50 per cent of the peak level is known as the half-life ($T^{1/2}$). When a bronchodilator is given, it is convenient to measure the improvement of a specific airflow function (e.g., FEV_1) as a basis for establishing the physiologic half-life of the drug. Although there is no standard definition for this parameter, the half-life of a bronchodilator is generally considered to be the time that it takes for the increase in a flow measurement such as FEV_1 to decrease by 50 per cent. The importance of half-life measurements arises from the fact that an adequate therapeutic response can be obtained by administering successive doses of the drug at intervals that approximate twice the half-life.

The determinations of serum half-lives and of physiologic half-lives is far from simple in an individual patient. Serum levels are often governed by complex factors, such as the volume of distribution of the drug, the presence of adipose tissue, alterations in blood flow, and secondary pharmacokinetic

TABLE 1–16. FACTORS IMPAIRING DRUG METABOLISM

Factor	Examples of Effects
Genetic	Rapid acetylators of isoniazid may be more susceptible to hypersensitivity hepatitis; slow acetylation may increase susceptibility to peripheral neuropathy.
Age	Very young and elderly metabolize most drugs more slowly.
Pregnancy	May affect metabolism of many drugs; more data required
Cardiac failure	Metabolism of some drugs impaired, e.g. theophylline.
Renal insufficiency	Excretion of many drugs impaired; accumulation may result in toxicity, e.g., antibiotics.
Hepatic insufficiency	Excretion of many drugs impaired; accumulation may result in toxicity, e.g., theophylline.
Cigarette smoking	Smokers may metabolize theophylline more rapidly.
Drugs barbiturates	Induce liver enzymes that accelerate metabolism of corticosteroids
macrolide antibiotics	Delay metabolic degradation of corticosteroids (unknown mechanism)
phenytoin	Induce enzymes that accelerate steroid metabolism
urine acidifiers	Increase clearance rate of pseudoephedrine

processes. Problems in determining the physiologic half-life of a bronchodilator are also encountered, since the results obtained depend, in part, upon the pulmonary function test that is used. Nevertheless, in spite of all these problems, it is possible to categorize the dosing requirement for particular drugs (Table 1–18); the interval between successive doses depends, in part, upon metabolic and excretory factors and, in part, upon the patient's needs (e.g., with the use of prophylactic cromolyn).

In diseased patients, the metabolism and excretion of a drug may be grossly deranged. With most respiratory drugs, the changes in $T^{1/2}$ that may occur in such circumstances are usually of minor importance. However, there is one important exception: theophylline pharmacokinetics is markedly impaired in patients with liver disease, and in such

TABLE 1-17. SOME ADVERSE DRUG INTERACTIONS IN RESPIRATORY PHARMACOLOGY

Class of Drug	Interacting Agents	Possible Effects
SYMPATHOMIMETIC AGENTS	Other sympathomimetics, or theophylline preparations or thyroid preparations	Tachycardia, arrhythmias, changes in blood pressure, nervousness, tremor
	Digitalis glycosides	Ectopic heart beats
	Halogenated anesthetics	Cardiac arrhythmias
	Certain antihypertensive agents (e.g., guanethidine)	Hypertension, or antagonism of hypotensive effect
	Monoamine oxidase inhibitors	Hypertensive crisis, arrhythmias
	Tricyclic antidepressants	Increased sympathomimetic response
	Antihistamines	May increase pressor effects of sympathomimetic agent
	Antidiabetic agents	Increased dosage requirements
	Isoniazid	Increased central stimulation
ORAL EXPECTORANTS	Methylxanthines, digoxin, and other gastric irritants	Nausea and vomiting
ANTIHISTAMINES	Sedatives, tranquilizers	Central nervous system depression
	Monoamine oxidase inhibitors	Potentiation of antihistaminic effects
	Corticosteroids	May potentiate steroid degradation by enzyme induction (barbiturates have similar effect)
ANTITUSSIVES	Sedatives, tranquilizers and antihistamines	Potentiation of central nervous system depression

cases the interval between doses may have to be considerably increased. If dosage adjustments are not made, accumulation of the drug and its active metabolites can occur, and serious side effects may result. Whenever there is doubt as to the $T\frac{1}{2}$ of theophylline, it is advisable to obtain determinations of the serum level. This laboratory test has become readily available, and although it is by no means required to monitor serum levels of theophylline during routine therapy, this is mandatory when unusually large doses are given or when impaired metabolism and clearance of the drug are major concerns.

Primary respiratory drugs do not usually require dosage adjustments in renal insuffi-

ciency, since impaired renal clearance does not have a marked effect on most of these agents. However, impaired renal excretion does have a marked effect on many other drugs, and appropriate alterations in dosage should be made. This is a particularly important requirement in antibiotic therapy, and precise guidelines enable the physician to make the appropriate adjustment in dosage on the basis of the creatinine clearance.[35]

The distribution, handling and metabolism of most drugs in children differ significantly from these processes in adults; as a result, children tolerate different dosages than do adults. Whenever a drug is given to a child, it is essential for the prescribing physician to

TABLE 1-18. DOSING REQUIREMENTS FOR RESPIRATORY DRUGS

Period Between Successive Doses	Class of Drug	Example
Continuous delivery	Gas	Oxygen
Continuous delivery	Methylxanthine	Intravenous aminophylline
1–2 hours	Bronchodilator	Aerosolized isoproterenol
2–3 hours	Mucokinetic	Intratracheal saline
3–4 hours	Bronchodilator	Aerosolized Bronkosol
4–6 hours	Glucocorticoid	Intravenous hydrocortisone
6–8 hours	Most drugs	Routine oral therapy
12 hours	Methylxanthine	Long-acting oral theophyllines
24 hours	Antitubercular	Isoniazid
48 hours	Glucocorticoid	Alternate-day prednisone
As necessary	Prophylactic	Cromolyn before exercise

TABLE 1–19. ADJUSTMENT OF DRUG DOSAGE IN CHILDREN

Age	Weight		Approximate Proportion of Adult Dose	
	KGS	LBS	PER CENT	FRACTION
1 month	3.2	7	12.5	1/8
12 months	10	22	25	1/4
7 years	23	50	50	1/2
12 years	40	80	75	3/4

Young's Rule: Dose $= \dfrac{\text{age (years)}}{\text{age (years)} + 12} \times \text{adult dose}$.

Clark's Rule: Dose $= \dfrac{\text{weight (lbs)}}{150} \times \text{adult dose}$

make sure that the selected dosage is appropriate; each drug must be considered separately, and the manufacturer's guidelines should be followed. The investigational process of determining pediatric dosages tends to be complex; many drugs enter the market before the appropriate dosages for children have been established. In such cases, the labeling points out that the drug is not recommended for children; however, this does not necessarily mean that the drug is unsuitable for children — it usually means that no dosage recommendations have been established. If a pediatrician decides that a drug is indicated for a child, an appropriate dose can be derived from basic pharmacologic principles and from a thorough knowledge of the usage of similar drugs in children. When the physician decides to give a drug to a child in the absence of the manufacturer's recommendations, the dosage can be calculated from the standard adult dosage using various formulas. Two fairly popular rules for dosage are Young's Rule, which is based on age, and Clark's Rule, which is based on weight. Table 1–19 provides approximate guidelines for normal children of average weight at different ages.

ADVERSE EFFECTS OF DRUGS

No drug exerts a simple, isolated, beneficial action solely on the diseased part of an abnormal organ. Every drug has the potential for multiple effects on different organs; the likelihood of these side effects occurring is usually related to the dosage of the administered agent. The safest and most successful drugs are those that produce side effects only when administered in dosages much larger than those normally given; such agents are said to have a high therapeutic:toxic ratio. Nevertheless, all drugs, even when given in precise therapeutic dosage, carry the possibility of toxicity, and many different undesirable effects can occur (Table 1–20). Examples include normal adverse reactions such as tachyarrhythmia secondary to bronchodilator therapy, and nausea caused by methylxanthines. Other reactions are individual hazards that only susceptible patients experience, such as allergy, hypersensitivity and idiosyncratic reactions. The overall incidence of adverse reactions constitutes a serious problem in therapeutics; in many hospitals, 20 to 30 per cent or more of patients experience troublesome reactions.[24] Some occur without warning, but many can be predicted, such as cumulation of theophylline in a patient with liver disease. Scrupulous attention to prescribing the appropriate dosage will prevent many, but certainly not all, adverse reactions. The physician, nurse or therapist must be aware of the particular complications that may occur with each drug that is used, and he or she must monitor the patient faithfully.

One complication associated with drug therapy is the phenomenon of *tolerance* (Table 1–21). The repeated entry of a drug into the body produces metabolic changes of a complex and subtle nature, and the eventual outcome may be one of two kinds of tolerance. On one hand, the drug loses its principal effect and larger doses are required to produce a therapeutic response; this phenomenon is known as *tachyphylaxis,* and is seen with ephedrine and a number of other drugs, especially those with an α-methyl group in the catecholamine side-chain.[36] In contrast, the desired effect of a drug may become so important to the body's functioning that the patient is unable to live comfortably without the drug. In its mildest form, such dependency can even be developed on placebo therapy, but in its most serious form the result is *addiction.*[23] Addiction occurs mainly with drugs that exert an effect on the psyche; it can be a socially devastating problem in the case of narcotic drugs, a community and individual health problem with tobacco, and a personal problem for patients who become addicted to major tranquilizers or glucocorticoids.

One problem that occurs in asthma is a more severe form of tolerance; this is *resistance,* in which the desired pharmacologic response is no longer achieved, even with very large doses. Under such circumstances, an asthmatic patient is liable to

TABLE 1–20. UNDESIRABLE RESPONSES THAT MAY OCCUR DURING COURSE OF DRUG THERAPY

Reaction	Meaning	Examples
ADVERSE REACTION	Direct toxic effect of drug, commonly seen with usual dosage	Tachyarrhythmia from epinephrine
ALLERGY	Development of antibody-mediated reaction following prior exposure to a drug	Asthma and other adverse reactions occurring with penicillin
ANAPHYLAXIS	Severe hypersensitivity reaction, ending in fever, asthma, shock, collapse or death	Reaction occasionally seen immediately after giving penicillin
CUMULATION	Progressive increase in effective amount of drug owing to impaired metabolism or excretion	Build-up of theophylline to toxic level in patient with hepatic insufficiency
HYPERSENSITIVITY	Unusual allergic reaction to a drug that is usually harmless; implies extreme sensitivity to small dose of drug	Severe asthmatic response to aspirin
IDIOSYNCRASY	Rare abnormal reaction to a drug in a genetically susceptible individual *or* Unusual reaction of a patient to an individual drug	Acute porphyria induced by a barbiturate *or* Bronchoconstriction produced by isoproterenol
INTERACTION	Adverse response caused by one drug in presence of another drug	Tachyarrhythmia due to epinephrine in presence of cyclopropane
OVERDOSE	Adverse, potentially lethal, effect from dose in excess of standard	Vomiting induced by guaifenesin
RESISTANCE	Lack of responsiveness to a drug	Status asthmaticus unresponsive to beta-2 adrenergic stimulators
SIDE EFFECT	Significant effect that frequently occurs, but not desired	Nausea induced by standard dose of a methylxanthine
TACHYPHYLAXIS	Development of rapid tolerance to effect of drug, necessitating increasing dosages for effectiveness	Tolerance to standard dose of ephedrine that appears after a few days
TOLERANCE	Unusual resistance to standard dose of a drug (may be inherent or acquired)	Requirement of greatly increased dosage of a theophylline for effectiveness
TOXICITY	Dose-related adverse effect occurring in all individuals	Cardiac arrhythmia from isoproterenol

TABLE 1–21. FORMS OF TOLERANCE TO DRUGS

Abnormality	Characteristics	Examples
TACHYPHYLAXIS	Diminished response to a drug, necessitating increased dosage for therapeutic effect	Dosage of ephedrine must often be increased in asthmatics if a prolonged course is administered.
RESISTANCE	Almost total loss of primary therapeutic response to a drug	Loss of bronchodilator effect of sympathomimetic agents in status asthmaticus (extrapulmonary side effects may persist)
DEPENDENCY	Inability of patient to cease using a drug without experiencing severe secondary withdrawal symptoms	Steroid-dependency often develops in patients who take moderately large doses of glucocorticoid for more than a few weeks
ADDICTION	Psychic dependency on a drug, liable to result in antisocial behavior	Dependency on drugs with strong psychic effects, such as diazepam or cocaine
PARADOXICAL EFFECT	Production of an effect by a drug that is the converse of the usual effect	Bronchospasm is occasionally caused by isoproterenol and other bronchodilators.
REBOUND PHENOMENON	Development of marked reversal of initial therapeutic effect	Nasal obstruction may worsen after initial relief when mucosal constrictors are used excessively.

develop status asthmaticus, when routine sympathomimetic bronchodilator drugs fail to produce bronchospasmolysis even in dangerously large doses—these doses may produce adverse extrapulmonary effects, such as cardiac arrhythmias. With the onset of this form of resistance (sometimes referred to as "locked lungs"), it is necessary to administer another type of drug, such as a glucocorticoid. Some asthmatic patients develop resistance to a bronchodilator and the drug may actually cause more bronchospasm; such an effect is known as a *paradoxical response*.[37] The incidence of this dangerous complication appears to be small, and the mechanism involved has not been clearly established. However, should this problem develop, it is important to withdraw the offending drug and to avoid related agents. A similar adverse effect occurs in the nose following the use of mucosal constrictor drugs; prolonged use may lead to the development of *rebound* mucosal congestion, also treated by withdrawing the responsible agent.

Modern respiratory therapy has turned increasingly to the scientific administration of topical inhalational drugs in an effort to avoid some of the side effects discussed previously. The main pharmacologic concept of inhalational drug therapy is comparable to that of dermatologic therapy: the application of small amounts of a drug topically, where it is needed, obviates many of the risks of side effects involving other organs, which might result from the introduction of larger amounts of the drug into the body as a whole.

AEROSOL THERAPY

Topical pulmonary therapy is administered mainly by aerosols. An aerosol is defined as a suspension of a liquid or a solid in the form of fine particles dispersed in a gas. The size of a particle that can be thus suspended is believed to range from 0.005 μ to 50 μ in diameter.[38] The unit of measurement that is employed is the micron, which is symbolized by the Greek letter μ (pronounced "mew"); the micron is one-millionth of a meter, or one-thousandth of a millimeter. The diameter of a terminal airway is about 0.5 to 1 mm, and that of an alveolus is about 200 to 300 μ (0.2 to 0.3 mm).[38] Therapeutic aerosols appear to be most efficacious when they have particle diameters of about 0.5 to 5 μ. To put these sizes in perspective, it should be noted that

TABLE 1–22. SOME TECHNIQUES USED IN MEASURING SMALL PARTICLE SIZE

Adsorption
Cascade impacter
Centrifuge
Electrical conductivity
Electroformed sieves
Electron microscope
Electrostatic precipitation
Elutriation
Impaction
Impingers
Inertia
Light scattering
Light microscope
Nuclei counter
Permeability
Scanners
Sedimentation
Spectroscopy
Thermal precipitation
Turbidimetry
Ultracentrifuge
Ultramicroscope
X-ray diffraction

the particles in cigarette smoke, before they enter the respiratory tract, have a diameter range of 0.1 to 0.4 μ. The exhaled particles are larger because they contain water molecules. The difference in size accounts for the difference in color between inhaled and exhaled smoke.

Aerosol behavior is extremely complex,[39] and numerous methods have been used to establish the size of the particles (Table 1–22). When attempts are made to study the movement and fate of particles in the respiratory tract, the problem is much more complicated, and there is enough disagreement in the findings of various workers to produce a confusing literature.[39–42] Nevertheless, a number of general principles and many approximations provide a basic understanding of aerosol particle behavior.

PRODUCTION OF AEROSOLS

Aerosols can be created by both natural and artificial means.[43] Therapeutic aerosols can be produced by *combustion* of solid plant derivatives; the smoke that is produced contains aerosolized droplets and solid particles of various sizes. More specific and therapeutically valuable are the aerosols produced from solutions of drugs. The simplest and crudest forms of inhalation therapy employ coarser particles that result from condensation of vapor around droplet nuclei to form *mists;* examples are those generated by showers and steam kettles, or by simple household humidifiers and nebulizers. The more sophisticated medical devices employ evaporation, dispersion and fragmentation of solutions to generate finer particles, followed by baffling to remove the larger droplets. A number of different principles are used to generate the aerosol: spinning discs, aerodynamic or jet generators, centrifugal generators, hydrodynamic generators, ultrasonic vibrators and pressurized cartridges.[44]

In clinical practice, most hospitals use a variety of jet, positive pressure, hydrosphere and ultrasonic nebulizers; for individual therapy, pressurized cartridge dispensers are commonly used. Additionally, some medications are aerosolized in the form of fine powders; usually a coarser, inert powder is incorporated to improve the flow characteristics of the inhaled drug. In general, there is little important difference between the particle sizes of the aerosols delivered by the well-known devices of each category, although the amount of medication nebulized in unit time and the density of the aerosol may differ. The ultrasonic devices produce a high density, relatively stable mist of appropriately sized particles, but there is little to suggest that these nebulizers have any additional value.[45] In practice, the differences between various types of nebulizing units are of less importance than factors such as gas flow rate, baffling systems, length of tubing, patient's breathing pattern and so on.[26, 38–47]

Effective devices for aerosolization have been available for over 100 years, and although considerable advances have been made in recent years, the actual improvements with respect to therapeutic outcome are relatively unimpressive. There has been little work of true significance in practical aerosol therapy since Dautrebande published his classic book in 1962.[26]

PARTICLE SIZES AND DEPOSITION

The usual therapeutic aerosol that enters the respiratory tract consists of particles in the size range of 0.5 μ to 10 μ; many manufacturers claim that the majority of particles produced by their individual nebulizers have a mass mean diameter of about 5 μ.[48] Various studies suggest that the optimal size for aerosol particles for the deposition of bronchodilator drugs in the human lung lies between 2 μ and 4 μ, when the usual type of clinical nebulization therapy is administered by the oral route to patients with mild to moderate bronchospasm.[40, 41]

Numerous efforts have been made to establish the fate of particles of different sizes, and much of the accepted information has recently been summarized by Gross.[42] However, the information is largely based on theoretical considerations rather than on analysis of what occurs in the clinical setting (Table 1–23). Nevertheless, it can be concluded that maximal distal deposition is obtained by patients who use slow, deep breaths with large tidal volumes. Particles of about 2 μ diameter deposit most successfully under such breathing conditions, whereas very large particles (more than 15 μ) do not reach the distal lung, and particles less than 0.5 μ tend to be exhaled. Suspended particles smaller than 0.2 μ in diameter tend to behave as a gas rather than as an aerosol, and most patients exhale the majority of these particles. However, if a nebulizer produces an aerosol in which the majority of the particles are less than 0.5 μ in size, the sheer

TABLE 1–23. DEPOSITION OF AEROSOL PARTICLES IN VARIOUS PARTS OF HUMAN RESPIRATORY TRACT*

	Particle Sizes				
	20 μ	6 μ	2 μ	0.6 μ	0.2 μ
Mouth	14–18%	0–1%	0%	0%	0%
Trachea	10–19	1–3	0	0	0
Tertiary bronchi	9–21	9–20	2–5	0	0–1
Terminal bronchioles	1–6	9–24	3–8	2–4	4–6
Respiratory bronchioles	0	3–12	2–11	2–6	4–6
Alveoli	0	5–18	0–17	0–9	0–10
Total Deposition	93–100	83–95	41–82	16–38	22–47
Deposition in lower respiratory tract	0	41–44	30–70	11–34	15–40

*Based on information provided by Gross.[42]

TABLE 1–24. DEPOSITION OF AEROSOL PARTICLES IN A PATIENT BREATHING THROUGH THE MOUTH

Particle Size (MICRONS)	Maximum Retention (PER CENT)	Site of Maximal Retention
>10	100	Pharynx, larynx, trachea
6	95	Larynx, bronchi, bronchioles
4	90	Bronchioles, acini
2	80	Bronchioles, acini
1	60	Acini
0.6	35	Alveoli (>60% may be exhaled)
0.1	Variable	Alveoli (>50% may be exhaled)
<0.1	?	(Evaporate or coalesce)

immensity of the numbers of these particles in the aerosol will result in an appreciable drug effect although only a small percentage of the particles will deposit.[41] To illustrate this point, 1 ml of a nebulized solution would produce less than two billion particles of 10 μ diameter, whereas a million times as many particles of 0.1 μ diameter would be produced. Therefore, even if only a small percentage of these latter particles is deposited, the number of drug-laden droplets that can activate receptor sites in the distal lung is immense.

Table 1–24 illustrates the maximum retention and the sites of deposition for particles of different sizes, according to generally accepted information. However, not all experts would accept all these figures.[44] There is general acceptance of the concept that particles in the size range of 0.1 to 1 μ are minimally deposited.

The deposition of aerosols is governed by physical principles that apply to particles of different sizes (Table 1–25).[42] The larger ones settle as the result of inertial impaction, or are filtered out by the nose (if nasal breathing is used), or at the sites of division of the large airways, since the turbulent flow produced by anatomic angulations results in the impaction and deposition of high velocity droplets. The remaining particles settle mainly under gravitational force by sedimentation, and this occurs in the more distal airways where most pulmonary pathology is located. The very small particles behave more like a gas, and they become effective only if they are given a chance to be absorbed by the alveolar mucosa: such a process, which relies on Brownian motion, is time-dependent, and occurs only to an appreciable extent during breath-holding.

When one reads the numerous and often contrasting accounts of particle deposition, one is forced to conclude that the evidence presented by daily clinical practice is vastly more relevant than the arguments of theoreticians. In practice, it is obvious that most patients can obtain adequate therapy with all types of nebulizing units and with any of the various types of polydisperse aerosols.[44, 49] Thus, there is at present no clear clinical evidence that any particular type of nebulizer or any theoretical range of particle size offers a premium form of therapy. Certainly, pharmacologically oriented therapists will find it more relevant to concentrate on using specific drugs in an optimal fashion with the nebulizing units that are available to them rather than to ponder too deeply about the aerosol particle sizes. Nevertheless, certain variables deserve an appropriate degree of concern. These are considered as follows:

TABLE 1–25. PHYSICAL FACTORS IN AEROSOL DEPOSITION

Physical Factor	Types of Particles Most Affected	Site of Deposition in Airways	Other Controlling Factors
Inertial impaction	High density aerosols, 10 μ size and larger.	Nose and larger airways, at angulations	Favored by high velocity flow and obstruction in airways.
Gravitational sedimentation	High density aerosols; particles 1–6 μ in size.	Smaller airways.	Favored by deep, slow breathing.
Diffusion	Particles less than 1 μ in size.	All parts of tracheobronchial tree, including terminal bronchioles and acini.	Favored by breath-holding (i.e. zero airflow).

OPTIMAL AEROSOL THERAPY

The deposition of an aerosol depends on numerous factors in addition to the type of nebulizer and the size of the particles that it delivers. Since aerosols are generally used to treat abnormal airways, much of the theory regarding their behavior in models that simulate the normal lung is not relevant. Thus, a patient whose distal airways are obstructed as a consequence of bronchospasm, mucosal inflammation and bronchial secretions may have difficulty in depositing any of the aerosol where the drug is most needed. Furthermore, the dyspneic patient may be incapable of using the optimal breathing pattern required to produce maximal deposition. Whenever aerosol therapy is used, it is important that the patient be instructed and encouraged to breathe slowly and deeply, and to hold the breath at the end of inspiration.

The quality of the aerosolized drug also has an influence on the fate of the particles. Solutions containing salts or chemical substances that exert an osmotic effect have a marked effect on the stability and behavior of particles once they enter the respiratory tract.[45, 49] If the particles are hypertonic, they will attract water molecules from the humid atmosphere in the airways, and grow in size; this growth will result in particles becoming larger, and they will tend to deposit more proximally. As a result, very hypertonic particles may provide effective therapy for the large airways, but are inefficient for treatment of distal areas of the lung. In contrast, particles of low tonicity tend to evaporate and grow smaller, and therefore are more likely to deposit distally. However,

a further factor intervenes—namely, the tendency of particles to collide and coalesce. Thus, even the smallest particles may grow by coalescence, and therefore deposition may occur more proximally than their initial size would suggest. The balance of evaporative and coalescent changes can markedly alter the destiny of particles, the theoretical fate of which may undergo a complete change during their dynamic passage through a patient's airways.

Some workers feel that by adding a hygroscopic substance to a solution that is to be nebulized the stability of the particles is enhanced.[40, 50] In theory, a hygroscopic particle will be less susceptible to evaporation, and may therefore be more likely to successfully deposit in the larger airways; however, the value of hygroscopic additives in clinical practice is questionable.[51] In any case, scientific planning of aerosol characteristics for optimal deposition in a particular part of the lower airway may be irrelevant, since it is rarely known which part of the bronchial tree is most in need of treatment. Thus, bronchospasm and mucus retention may be maximal almost anywhere in the bronchial or bronchiolar airways, and even the best diagnostician will find it impossible to specify in a given patient which level of the airways has the greatest need for aerosol deposition. It is therefore generally impractical to try to make a careful scientific decision concerning the optimal qualities that an aerosol prescription should provide for an individual patient with airway disease.

Nevertheless, there are a number of reasonable conditions that should be satisfied whenever aerosol therapy is used (Table

TABLE 1–26. FACTORS AFFECTING DEPOSITION OF AEROSOL PARTICLES IN BRONCHI

Variables	Conditions Favoring Deposition
AEROSOL FACTORS	
Particle size	Optimal size lies in the range of 0.6–6 μ.
Droplet constituents	Hygroscopic particles are more stable; they tend to grow in size and deposit more proximally.
Uniformity of droplets	Uniformly sized droplets are more stable; this favors distal deposition.
Density of aerosol cloud	More deposition occurs with dense aerosols.
Temperature of aerosol	Droplets at body temperature are more stable and do not evaporate.
Electrostatic charge	Negatively charged droplets are more stable and may deposit more distally.
Helium as a carrier gas	Low density carrier may enhance distal deposition.
PATIENT FACTORS	
Depth of breathing	Slow, large volume breathing favors deposition.
Inspiratory hold	End-inspiratory breath hold favors deposition.
Mouth breathing	Aerosols penetrate through mouth to distal lung.
Airway patency	Patent airways allow distal penetration.
Nonreactive airways	Control of cough and bronchospasm improves aerosol deposition.

1–26). The breathing pattern of the patient should be coached by the therapist to ensure effective deposition throughout the lower airways. The solution to be aerosolized should be near isosmotic in general, or should be hypertonic if more proximal deposition is required. The addition of glycerol or propylene glycol may confer advantageous hygroscopic properties. Ideally, the aerosol should reach the patient's respiratory tract at body temperature; this important condition is rarely attained, because there are considerable mechanical problems involved in heating the aerosol to above room temperature. Some workers feel that a negative electrostatic charge improves aerosol stability and enhances deposition; however, this is controversial, and the evidence is far from sufficient to justify the expense and inconvenience of ensuring that an aerosol receives a negative charge.[26, 40, 41] Similarly, although some authorities consider that the use of helium as a carrier gas improves aerosol penetration and deposition in the lung,[52, 53] this concept is unacceptable in general practice, since the modality is both controversial and costly.

One of the major considerations in aerosol therapy is whether intermittent positive pressure respirators produce more effective aerosol deposition. For many years there has been a remarkable tendency to assume that IPPB offers the best aerosol therapy, in spite of evidence to the contrary.[54, 55] However, this statement should not be construed as a total condemnation of IPPB nebulization therapy, since, as Muir points out, this modality offers a convenient method for helping patients with airways obstruction to breathe deeply.[45] Thus, IPPB may be advantageous for those individuals who are unable to provide the type of optimal breathing pattern in the absence of the orchestration that the respirator can impose.

PRACTICAL PROBLEMS IN AEROSOL THERAPY

Although aerosolization of respiratory drugs has become enormously popular in North America, the production and utilization of aerosols is much more costly and complex than the delivery of similar medications by simple oral administration. The main advantage of aerosol therapy is that a drug given in this fashion produces a more rapid pulmonary effect with fewer side effects than result from giving the drug by any other route. There are a number of other advantages, but the numerous disadvantages are more impressive (Table 1–27). First, side effects are not entirely obviated by using inhalational administration, since a significant proportion of the nebulized drug is deposited in the mouth and pharynx when most forms of nebulization are employed. Various studies have revealed that aerosolization with positive pressure devices

TABLE 1–27. ADVANTAGES AND DISADVANTAGES OF INHALATIONAL ADMINISTRATION OF DRUGS

Quality	Advantages	Disadvantages
Dosage	Small dosage required	Precise dosage impossible
Onset of action	Rapid therapeutic effect	Rapid relief encourages overuse.
Side effects	Minimal extrapulmonary effects; especially important with bronchodilators	Tachyphylaxis to bronchodilator may occur with relative increase in extrapulmonary effects.
Availability of route	Inhalational route is almost always available	Very young or very dyspneic patient cannot inhale correctly.
Titration of dose	Can be achieved with careful observation	Standard dosage may be difficult to establish.
Delivery system	Can be simple, e.g. hand-actuated nebulizer	May be extraordinarily complex and expensive.
Ease of administration	Can be very simple, if self-administered	Very complex in hospital, requiring respiratory technicians, etc.
Cost-effectiveness	Self-therapy is economical	Administered therapy (by IPPB, etc.) is very expensive.
Psychological factors	Provides oral-inhalational satisfaction	Patient may become over-dependent on nebulizer.
Quality control	Provided by responsible patient or therapist	Poor control is a major problem in respiratory therapy.
Technician role	Can be very supportive to patient	May constitute an excessive expense in many cases

results in as little as 20 per cent of the drug in the nebulizer being deposited in the body; the rest remains in the nebulizer and tubing, or is breathed out into the room air.[32, 45, 56] Of the 20 per cent or so that may remain in the body, less than half is deposited in the lower respiratory tract; the greater portion is absorbed through the oral mucosa, or is swallowed and is liable to be partially absorbed by the stomach. Inefficient or inappropriate use of IPPB will result in a smaller amount being deposited in the lung, and a relatively greater proportion may be absorbed systemically. When a simple jet nebulizer or a metered spray is used, most of the aerosol enters the body; only about 10 per cent is deposited in the airways, but a significant proportion impacts on the oropharyngeal mucosa and may be absorbed there, or after swallowing. A considerable decrease in systemic absorption can be achieved by rinsing out the mouth following nebulization therapy, and in this fashion the incidence of systemic effects can be diminished.

The actual amount of drug deposited in the distal part of the lungs is partly dependent on the nebulizing unit used. However, no comparative studies have been carried out to determine the fate of equal doses of different drugs aerosolized by the various types of metered nebulizers and by positive pressure devices. One study, however, has clearly demonstrated the marked variability of different manufacturers' products of pressurized inhalers containing suspensions of isoproterenol.[57] The dose delivered by six different units varied from 89 to 461 μg of drug per actuation of the valve, and the amounts actually differed by as much as 22 per cent from the dose that the manufacturer claimed the device delivered. The proportion of the dose that was believed to enter the respiratory tract varied from 3 per cent to 36 per cent! Factors that determine the therapeutically effective proportion of the dose

TABLE 1–28. FACTORS AFFECTING PROPORTION OF METERED DOSE OF A DRUG THAT PRODUCES A THERAPEUTIC ACTION IN THE PATIENT

Variables	Factors Influencing Therapeutic Outcome
PATIENT VARIABLES	
Position of nebulizer with respect to airway	Keeping nebulizer 2 cm from open mouth may increase inhaled dose.
Rate of airflow during inspiration	More rapid airflow (i.e., unobstructed airway) increases proportion of dose entering lungs.
Patient coordination	Good coordination increases dose entering lungs.
NEBULIZER VARIABLES	
Formulation of drug with the propellant	Micronized *suspensions* may result in more efficient dosing than do *solutions* of drug.
Adjuvants and excipients	Propylene glycol, lactose, etc. are added to improve aerosol deposition in lungs.
Valve reliability	May be very variable, e.g., optimal dosing requires a clean orifice.
Vapor pressure of propellant	Optimal pressure in nebulizer results in suitable aerosol characteristics.
Homogeneity of contents	Shaking container before use is necessary for standard dosage.
Environmental factors	Temperature can affect aerosol production.
Repeated use of nebulizer	Dosage released by partially empty container may differ from dosage obtained when container is full.
DRUG VARIABLES	
Epinephrine, isoproterenol, Bronkosol	Partially absorbed in mouth and stomach
Fenoterol, metaproterenol, salbutamol, terbutaline	Effective when swallowed into gastrointestinal tract
Cromolyn	Not absorbed by oral/gastrointestinal mucosa
Water-soluble glucocorticoids	Effective when swallowed into gastrointestinal tract
Beclomethasone, betamethasone	Not effective if swallowed
CLEARANCE FACTORS	
Mouth rinsing after nebulization	Decreases oral or gastrointestinal absorption
Coughing	Decreases deposition in lower respiratory tract
Effective mucociliary activity	Decreases persistence of drug effect in lung
Favorable V/Q relationships in lungs	Decreases persistence of drug effect in lung

The variables affect the relative proportions entering the lungs and the gastrointestinal tract. The properties of the particular drug determine whether the portion deposited in the mouth or stomach results in a therapeutic effect.

TABLE 1–29. COMPARISON OF AMOUNTS OF ISUPREL THAT MAY BE DEPOSITED IN THE LUNGS WHEN USING MANUFACTURER'S RECOMMENDED DOSES*

Method of Delivery and Recommended Dose	Dosage Nebulized (Milligrams)	Amount Deposited in Airways (Per Cent)	(Micrograms)
Metered aerosol, 4 puffs (Mistometer II)	0.5	10	50
IPPB with mouthpiece (0.25 ml 1:200 Isuprel)	1.25	10	125
IPPB with endotracheal tube (0.25 ml 1:200 Isuprel)	1.25	20	250

* Based on product information of Winthrop Laboratories.

The estimates of the amounts deposited in the airways are based on the approximate retention that can be expected in the airways using standard nebulization techniques. See References 35, 56 and 62, and Table 1–30.

released from the inhaler are listed in Table 1–28: these include variations in the patient's lung status and in the technique of using the nebulizer,[58-62] product factors such as the valve mechanism and the nature of the product formulation, and other, more subtle considerations. The evidence suggests that micronized particles, either in the dry form (as with cromolyn) or suspended in the propellant (as with most epinephrine and some isoproterenol products manufactured in the United States), constitute more reliable and reproducible aerosol mists than those resulting from alcoholic or water-based solutions of drugs.[57]

Table 1–29 compares the possible outcomes of nebulizing standard doses of a single drug (isoproterenol), using the manufacturer's FDA-approved dosage recommendations, by metered aerosol, IPPB with a mouth-piece or IPPB through an endotracheal tube. If one assumes excellent deposition in the airways by the mouth breathing techniques, then about 10 per cent of the nebulized dose given by the first two methods will be retained in the lungs.[56] If the

TABLE 1–30. PROPORTIONS OF DIFFERENT DRUGS THAT COULD HAVE PHARMACOLOGIC EFFECT WHEN GIVEN BY DIFFERENT METHODS OF NEBULIZATION

Site of Deposition	Maximal Deposition	Bronchodilators Catecholamines e.g., Isoproterenol	Catecholamine Derivatives e.g., Metaproterenol	Glucocorticoids Water-soluble e.g., Dexamethasone	Insoluble e.g., Beclomethasone	Cromolyn
METERED DEVICE						
Percentage lost in room air and apparatus	10–20					
Percentage deposited in lower airways	5–15	5–15	5–15	5–15	5–15	5–15
Percentage deposited in mouth/stomach (30–90% of deposited drug may be absorbed from stomach)	75–90	15–25*	30–70†	30–70†	0‡	0‡
Total percentage of dose that may be effectively deposited.		20–40	35–85	35–85	5–15	5–15
IPPB WITH MOUTHPIECE						
Percentage lost in room air and apparatus	40–65					
Percentage deposited in lower airways	5–15	5–15	5–15	5–15	5–15	5–15
Percentage deposited in mouth/stomach (30–90% of deposited drug may be absorbed from stomach)	5–20	1–5*	2–15†	5–15†	0‡	0‡
Total percentage of dose that may be effectively deposited.		6–20	7–30	10–30	5–15	5–15

These figures are only *estimates*. They illustrate the varying proportions of nebulized doses of different respiratory drugs that might be responsible for a therapeutic effect in a patient.

* Drugs may be partially absorbed through the oral/gastrointestinal mucosa.

† Drugs may be fully absorbed through the oral/gastrointestinal mucosa.

‡ These drugs are not absorbed through the oral/gastrointestinal mucosa. (These products are not given by IPPB in the United States at present.)

aerosol does not have to traverse the mouth, pharynx and larynx (e.g., if the aerosol is administered through a wide tracheostomy tube), then the third method could be expected to result in greater deposition—perhaps at least 20 per cent of the nebulized dose. Such a comparative study does not appear to have been carried out, but it would seem evident that nebulization directly down the trachea would result in a significantly greater delivery into the lungs. It is probable that standard dosages result in 500 per cent greater dose of bronchodilator when the drug is nebulized by the third method as compared to the first (see Table 1–29).

A further consideration is that a significant proportion of a nebulized drug, when given by a metered aerosol or a pressure nebulizer, is deposited in the oropharynx. Unless the mouth is rinsed out, most of this drug is either absorbed through the oral mucosa or swallowed. Isoproterenol can readily be absorbed through the sublingual mucosa, and a significant proportion can be effectively absorbed in the stomach. Thus, a systemic effect is added to the direct topical effect, and this may account for most of the extrapulmonary side effects that accompany isoproterenol nebulization. With drugs such as metaproterenol, all the aerosol that enters the stomach can be absorbed. Since metered metaproterenol releases about 0.65 mg of the drug per actuation, four breaths can introduce 2.6 mg into the mouth and lungs, and usually most of this enters the stomach. Since the effective oral dose is only about 10 mg, the amount obtained by swallowing all the nebulized dose is not inconsequential. If metaproterenol is well-absorbed sublingually (information on this is lacking), it is possible that a significant bronchodilator effect could be obtained by simply nebulizing 16 puffs from the metered aerosol under the tongue, without any inhalation into the lung being required!

In Table 1–30, a speculative accounting is provided of the possible total therapeutic dosages that could be achieved either by using a metered aerosol or IPPB with a mouthpiece: the approximate information is derived from many sources.[32, 56, 57, 63] There is reason to believe that up to 90 per cent of the metered dose enters the stomach, whereas only up to 20 per cent of the dose given by IPPB reaches the gastrointestinal tract. For drugs such as isoproterenol, which can be at least partially absorbed through the oral or gastric mucosa into the blood stream,

perhaps 15 to 25 per cent of the metered dose and maybe 1 to 5 per cent of the IPPB dose can enter the systemic circulation; the total proportion entering the body and therefore being available for bronchodilation by one route or another could amount to 40 per cent of the original dose released by the metered inhaler, and perhaps up to 20 per cent of the IPPB dose. Such variables in effective dosing when giving various drugs by different techniques emphasize the imprecise nature of inhalational dosage recommendations. Physicians and therapists should give due consideration to this evidence, which points accusingly at the extreme lack of certainty and the excess of confusion in the field of aerosol therapeutics.

The additional complexities and practical disadvantages that militate against precision in the use of inhalational administration of drugs are analyzed in detail in Table 1–31. The provision of complex mechanical devices and skilled technicians or nurses who are required to operate and maintain the equipment results in further problems and expenses in inhalational therapy. In contrast, the taking of a tablet or other simple oral medication is almost devoid of complexity (Table 1–32).

Inhalation therapy enjoys its greatest use in countries that can afford to provide a luxurious standard of health care, whereas patients in poorer countries make do with simpler methods—and perhaps attain com-

TABLE 1–31. CAUSES OF INACCURACY IN AEROSOL DELIVERY

DELIVERY SYSTEM PROBLEMS
  Nebulization equipment may be inefficient or unreliable.
  Flow rate of carrier gas may be inappropriate.
  Particle size may be inappropriate.
  Tonicity of particles may be inappropriate.
  Hygroscopic properties of droplets may be inappropriate.

PROBLEMS RELATED TO PATIENT
  Patient may fail to use technique of slow, deep breathing with end-inspiratory breath-hold.
  Patient may be unable to coordinate inhalation with nebulization.
  Aerosol particles may cause bronchospasm/coughing.
  Patient may overuse self-therapy, and may become overdependent on nebulization mystique.

PROBLEMS OF THE HEALTH DELIVERY TEAM
  Lack of reliable information on particle physics makes rational therapy difficult.
  Accurate monitoring of drug dosage is impossible.
  Inadequate information on pharmacology of aerosol drugs results in incorrect prescribing.

TABLE 1-32. DISADVANTAGES OF AEROSOL THERAPY COMPARED TO ORAL THERAPY (WITH A TABLET OR LIQUID MEDICATION)

Aerosolization requires complex and costly apparatus, whereas oral medications require no unusual equipment.

A high degree of patient cooperation is required for effective aerosol therapy—or the patient has to be intubated.

It usually requires skilled personnel to provide aerosol therapy and to service the equipment.

Accurate dosing is almost impossible with nebulizing devices.

The nebulizing device may become contaminated and can transmit infection.

Accurate knowledge of aerosol pharmacology is not readily available.

The common side effects of a drug are not always eliminated by administering it as an aerosol.

Additional side effects may result from nebulization, e.g. gagging, gastric insufflation, over or under oxygenation, pulmonary hyperinflation, bronchospasm.

Patients are more likely to overtreat themselves with aerosol therapy.

Aerosols may fail to reach the diseased part of the lung.

Poorly administered aerosolization constitutes a complex method of introducing the drug into the stomach.

parable results![32] At present, the uncertainties and confusion regarding the use of IPPB[54] and other nebulization methods, as well as the problems related to lack of information regarding the optimal use of metered aerosols,[58-63] are both annoying and challenging, but they must not be allowed to obscure the clear practicality of the successful results achieved in millions of respiratory patients who appear to be satisfied by inhalational administration of drugs. The conclusion for the individual practitioner must be that whereas a standard, narrow range of dosages suffices for orally administered drugs, the dosages of aerosols are subject to extreme variability, and necessitate careful individual experimenting and adjusting in each case.

SOME FALLACIES IN AEROSOL THERAPY

There is a tendency to credit aerosols with theoretically valuable properties that are actually of little practical importance. Thus, it is often implied that a nebulizer that produces particles of less than 2 μ in size is required for effective treatment at the acinar or alveolar level of the lung. There are several fallacies in this reasoning: (1) Although the particles may initially be smaller than 2 μ, if they are hypertonic (as therapeutic aerosols often are) they will absorb water in the tracheobronchial tree, and they will grow and tend to coalesce so as to produce even larger particles, which will tend to deposit more proximally.[45] (2) In a patient with diseased airways, the poor airflow in the mid-lung and the turbulence that is caused will tend to result in more proximal deposition of particles of all sizes. (3) Even if the particles do reach the alveolar level, their ability to effect a therapeutic outcome will be very limited, since most pathologic conditions that are treatable by inhalation therapy (i.e., bronchospasm, mucosal edema, retained secretions and mucociliary impairment) are located more proximally, in the middle-sized and smaller bronchioles. For these reasons, one should be very skeptical when a manufacturing company boasts that its brand of nebulizer produces optimal particles for alveolar deposition.

A related fallacious claim credits ultrasonic nebulizers with properties that exceed those of the simpler forms of nebulizers. It is true that ultrasonic nebulization produces a denser, and perhaps more stable, cloud of droplets, but the size range of the particles does not differ significantly from the range produced by simpler nebulizers. The dense cloud also carries a serious disadvantage: many patients who have reactive airways develop some bronchospasm and experience mucosal irritation when they inhale an ultrasonic aerosol. Furthermore, it has not been shown that most inhalational medications are effectively nebulized by ultrasonic devices. There is a suspicion that the aerosol that is produced may initially contain more solvent, and that a progressively greater proportion of the dissolved salt or drug is aerosolized as the nebulization process continues;[49] eventually, some precipitated solute may remain in the reservoir. It is also possible that some drugs undergo chemical breakdown when exposed to ultrasonic vibration.

The concept that aerosolization allows precise treatment of lungs with minimal treatment of extrapulmonary organs is a clinical fallacy. It is likely to hold true if the aerosol is delivered directly through an endotracheal tube, but it is certainly not the case when the patient takes an average aerosol treatment. Since the "average" treatment varies from casual self-medication with a hand-actuated aerosol unit to a professionally supervised IPPB session using an endotracheal tube or a face mask, the range of doses delivered both to the lower respiratory tract and to the upper airway and gastrointestinal tract is obviously susceptible to considerable variation. At its best, aerosol therapy may result in empirical success; at its worst, it is simply an expensive and cumbersome method of administering a drug into the stomach.

Finally, although aerosol therapy is supposed to allow effective pulmonary therapy with minimal side effects, many patients do obtain significant cardiovascular side effects from bronchodilator aerosols. Indeed, the overuse of such aerosols can produce fatalities.[36] Similarly, the aerosol treatment of asthma with water-soluble glucocorticoids can produce cushingism, while attempts to treat pulmonary infections with antibiotics such as penicillin may result in induced hypersensitivity to the drug. The administration of certain agents by nebulization may cause direct adverse effects; thus some aerosolized mucokinetic agents can cause gagging, nausea, vomiting, airway irritation and bronchospasm. Drugs of the theophylline series, which can be very toxic when given by the oral or parenteral route, should be ideal for aerosol administration. Unfortunately, aerosols of these agents are not only relatively ineffective, but they may induce bronchospasm. Aerosol therapy is indeed a very mixed blessing. The major faults of aerosol therapy are summarized in Table 1–32, in which the aerosol administration of a respiratory drug is contrasted with oral administration of a tablet or solution.

DRUGS THAT ARE GIVEN BY AEROSOL THERAPY

Although bronchodilators and mucokinetic agents are the main groups of drugs that are conventionally administered by inhalation, a number of other drugs have been given by this means. Most of the agents reported to have been effective when given by the inhalational route are included in Table 1–33. These drugs are of two types: those given for treatment of pulmonary conditions, and those given via the lungs for their extrapulmonary effects.[15, 17, 39, 40, 64, 65]

The important drugs given for their pulmonary action are those used in the treatment of bronchospasm, and those given to loosen mucus or to constrict the respiratory mucosa. Some antimicrobial agents are also effective when administered topically into the lungs. Respiratory gases are also used either for therapeutic purposes, or as carriers or propellants for other aerosolized drugs. Finally, various diagnostic tests of lung structure and function involve the inhalation of provocative agents or quantifiable tracers into the airways.[66]

Although few drugs are administered by the pulmonary route for their systemic effect, the lung is an absorptive organ, and thus provides access for drugs into the systemic circulation. The most important group of agents given by this means is the anesthetic gases and vapors; local anesthetics can be given in excessive amounts into the lung, and can thereby achieve a systemic effect. Many hormones can be delivered into the body through the lungs. Epinephrine and glucocorticoids are, of course, given for their effects on the lungs, but a systemic effect can readily be attained. Insulin can be given by this route, but such a mode of administration has not been exploited. Hormones derived from the pituitary are given by inhalation, both for this systemic effect and for their antiasthma effect.

A person can be immunized by delivering a suitable antigen into the lungs. This has been reported to be effective when BCG is given to immunize patients against tuberculosis. Other antigenic agents have also been given by this route.[39]

Respiratory stimulants can be administered by inhalation. Sal volatile (smelling salts) is a mixture of ammonium bicarbonate and ammonium carbonate. In Victorian times, no lady could indulge herself in a drawing room swoon without being subjected to a whiff of this ubiquitous, household restorative agent. Amphetamine, in the form of Benzedrine inhaler, used to be popular as a nasal mucosal constrictor, but it was perhaps all too popular because of its central stimulating effect. Carbon dioxide is still in use as a respiratory stimulant, since its inhalation increases the $PaCO_2$, resulting in stimulation of the respiratory center; the same approach is one of the many suggested treatments for hiccups.

One of the most recently described uses of the pulmonary route is for anticoagulation by means of aerosolized heparin.[67] Agents like calcium chloride, caffeine and digoxin have been given by inhalation, but such a method of administration is not likely to be employed currently. Vasoactive drugs, such as amyl nitrite, are still given by inhalation for the treatment of angina; this drug has also recently gained a reputation for its psychic effect, but since its use is likely to be ac-

TABLE 1–33. AGENTS THAT HAVE BEEN GIVEN BY INHALATION

Class of Agent	Category	Examples
AGENTS THAT ACT ON THE LUNGS		
Bronchodilators	Catecholamines and related agents	Isoproterenol, epinephrine, terbutaline, etc.
	Methylxanthines	Aminophylline, Microphyllin
	Anticholinergics	Atropine, stramonium
	Antihistamines	Methapyrilene, thenyldiamine
Antiasthma agents	Bischromones	Cromolyn
	Glucocorticords	Beclomethasone, betamethasone
	Alpha-blocking drugs	Phentolamine
Mucokinetic agents	Water	Droplets, steam, etc.
	Electrolyte solution	Sodium chloride, ammonium chloride
	Mucolytics	Acetylcysteine, iodides
	Enzymes	Trypsin, hyaluronidase, dornase
	Detergents	Tyloxapol, ethasulfate
	Humectants	Glycerol
	Demulcents	Propylene glycol, VapoRub
	Volatile oils	Cedar leaf oil, eucalyptus
Mucosal constrictors	Alpha-adrenergic agents	Phenylephrine, cyclopentamine
Antimicrobial agents	Antibiotics	Gentamicin, polymyxin, streptomycin, kanamycin, tobramycin, neomycin
	Antifungal agents	Amphotericin, nystatin
	Antituberculous agents	Paraminosalicylic acid, streptomycin
	Antiseptics	Hydrogen peroxide, urea peroxide
	Chemotherapeutic agents	Sulfonamides
Respiratory gases	Therapeutic	Oxygen, carbon dioxide
	Carrier	Helium
Propellants, etc.	Carrier	Fluorocarbons, lactose
Diagnostic agents	Antigens	Dust, spores, pollens
	Cholinergics	Pilocarpine, methacholine
	Histaminergics	Histamine
	Industrial agents	Platinum salts, toluene diisocyanate
	Radioisotopes	Technetium-99 m, albumin-^{131}I
	Contrast agents	Dionosil, barium sulfate, tantalum
	Inert agents	Glass spheres
	Tracer gases	Carbon monoxide, argon, helium
Miscellaneous		Chlorophyll, phenosulfonphthalein
AGENTS WITH SYSTEMIC EFFECTS		
Anesthetics	Local anesthetics	Lidocaine, cocaine
	General anesthetics	Halothane, ether
	Depressants	Barbiturates
Hormones	Pituitary extracts	Antidiuretic hormone, pituitrin
	Pancreatic hormone	Insulin
	Corticosteroids	Dexamethasone, hydrocortisone
Immunizing agents	Vaccines, etc.	BCG, smallpox vaccine, polio antigen
Analeptics	Respiratory stimulants	Ammonia, nikethamide
	General stimulants	Amphetamine, strychnine, Benzedrine
Miscellaneous	Acidifying agents	Calcium chloride
	Anticoagulants	Heparin
	Cardiotonics	Digitalis glycosides
	Diuretics	Caffeine
	Hydration	Water, electrolyte solutions
	Vasoactive drugs	Amyl nitrite, sodium nitrite; epinephrine, ergotamine
	Vitamins	Vitamin B_{12}, ascorbic acid
	Undesirable agents	Tobacco smoke, glue, Freon
	War gases	Phosgene, chlorine
	Germs	Various bacteria, fungi and spores

companied by a severe headache, other psychic stimulants enjoy a greater following. Vitamins, such as B_{12}, have been given by the inhalational route and are probably just as effective a placebo by this means as when administered intramuscularly.

Unfortunately, the lung provides an easy port of entry for all sorts of undesirable agents, varying from the unpleasantness of smog and industrial dusts, to the ridiculous use of agents such as glue, Freon or acetone for psychic thrills, to the horrors of phosgene and similar toxic gases employed in warfare. Bacteria, viruses and other microbiologic agents could also be used in germ warfare, but this form of inhalational assault is so terrifying that, as yet, no warring faction has been malevolent enough to employ it.

Potentially harmful inhalational exposure is given under laboratory control to investigate individual bronchial reactivity. A large number of drugs and agents have been used in such bronchial provocation tests, and some of these bronchoconstrictors are of value today, especially those used in the evaluation of a patient with industrially determined bronchospasm.[68] Many such bronchoconstrictors have been reported over the years (Table 1–34), and a few continue to be used in sophisticated pulmonary function laboratories.

To conclude on an optimistic note, it is possible that the lung will be used as a source of delivery into the body of many agents that cannot readily be given by other routes, for instance when oral or routine parenteral administration is technically unfeasible. However, the pharmacokinetics of absorption and distribution through the lung will require more detailed understanding than exists at present. Certainly, water and electrolytes can readily be administered through the lungs to create a positive fluid or salt balance. It is only a matter of time before a sophisticated pharmacopeia of aerosolized agents for systemic therapy is developed as a new outgrowth of scientific inhalation therapy.

METERED NEBULIZERS AND PROPELLANTS

The technological developments in the aerosol industry have resulted in a huge variety of drugs, cosmetics, household materials and industrial products being packaged as aerosols. The convenience of these products, in spite of the imprecision associated with their use, accounts for the great popularity of metered aerosols in respiratory therapy. In the case of certain drugs, such as glucocorticoids, the advent of an aerosol formulation has been associated with a considerable improvement in the therapeutic management of patients who require these agents. At present, there is good reason to believe that metered aerosols will maintain an important place in respiratory therapy, although the dangers, not only of the drugs themselves but also of the propellants, have caused considerable concern. However, it is difficult at present to envisage a better way of delivering potent agents in small, precisely metered doses other than by the successful dispensers currently in use. In fact, it is possible that the metered containers will find increasing use if they are attached to a positive pressure respirator to facilitate delivery of the required dose to a patient who has difficulty employing the deep, coordinated breathing pattern that is required; the cartridges of many manufacturers can be attached to the delivery tubing of most respirators and can be actuated during the respiratory cycle.

Most drugs in metered dispensers are solutions of the active agent; alcohol is probably the most frequently used solvent. The propellant is generally Freon. The cartridge contains a two-phase system: the liquefied Freon forms one phase; the second is the solution of the drug and dissolved Freon. Other drugs are packaged as suspensions of fine (micronized) powders in the Freon liquid.[69]

TABLE 1–34. SOME DRUGS THAT CAUSE BRONCHOCONSTRICTION WHEN GIVEN BY INHALATION*

Adrenolytics	Histamine (and related agents)
Antihistamines	Irritants (fumes, gases, etc.)
(e.g., Benadryl)	Meperidine
Bradykinin	Nicotine
Caffeine	Parasympathetic agents (e.g.,
Chloroform	acetylcholine, pilocarpine)
Chloropicrin	Percaine
Dibucaine	Phosgene
Dolophine	Potassium chloride
Enzymes	Serotonin
Ether	Sodium metabisulfite
Furmethide	Xanthines
Glycerine	

*See references 39, 40, 64, 68. Additional agents may be given as part of a bronchial challenge evaluation to discover whether a patient is susceptible to a potentially provocative environmental contaminant. Many therapeutic inhalational agents may also cause some bronchospasm, e.g. acetylcysteine, beclomethasone, cromolyn.

When a pressurized cartridge is actuated, the valve allows the escape of a metered dose, consisting of both phases, from the container. The release of pressure results in Freon issuing as a gas, and the solution or powder of the drug exits forcefully as a spray. The subsequent fate of the active drug is far from clear. Some evaporation of an alcoholic solvent will occur, and therefore the particles diminish in size, but once they are inhaled they may grow again by absorbing water molecules. Many of the particles that are forcefully ejected from the cannister impinge on the oropharyngeal mucosa and, in many patients, perhaps less than 10 per cent is deposited in the lungs.

Metered nebulizers usually contain a number of pharmaceutical excipients (additives with suitable properties) as well as Freon (see Table 5-3). Some of these leave a marked taste in the mouth, or cause irritation of the throat; these experiences may result in patients' preferences or dislikes for particular brands, which are quite unrelated to the bronchodilator or other intended pharmacologic properties. The excipient incorporated in the marketed capsules of cromolyn powder is lactose; this is present as larger particles that improve the flow characteristics of the inhaled preparation. The lactose impacts on the pharynx and in the trachea, and causes irritation in many patients; in susceptible subjects the powder may induce reflex bronchospasm. In general, it appears that micronized powders are more irritating than aerosol solutions, and although a few aerosol bronchodilators are marketed in the form of powders with lactose as an excipient (see Table 5-15), they are relatively unpopular. Indeed, it is possible that cromolyn, which is presently used in powder form, will eventually be marketed as a solution; such a formulation has already been made available in the United Kingdom.

Metered aerosols have certainly received a great deal of criticism. Some physicians have condemned them because they engender over-reliance and a tendency to over-medication in many patients. Aerosols of isoproterenol have been particularly controversial because of the reported dangers associated with their misuse. Since isoproterenol is a short-acting bronchodilator with poor specificity, it is now obsolete in many countries.[70] On the other hand, aerosol therapy in the management of asthma continues to occupy a very important place in the opinions of most experts, and the newer aerosol drugs will probably enhance the popularity

TABLE 1-35. FREON PROPELLANTS

Propellant.	Chemical Name	Formula
FC11*	Trichlorofluoromethane	CCl_3F
FC12*	Dichlorodifluoromethane	CCl_2F_2
FC113	Trichlorotrifluoroethane	$C_2Cl_3F_3$
FC114*	Dichlorotetrafluoroethane	$C_2Cl_2F_4$
FC115	Chloropentafluoroethane	$CClF_2CF_3$

*These propellants are commonly used in cartridge preparations and are listed in the National Formulary.

of this form of therapy.[70, 71] The claims that the administration of various aerosol drugs prevents exercise-induced asthma and that oral drugs (when available) are much less effective provide a further powerful argument for favoring aerosol therapy in most asthmatic patients.

Although most asthmatic patients throughout the western world receive bronchodilators or other antiasthma drugs by aerosol, the use of metered inhalers continues to provoke controversy[72] because of the potential hazard imposed by the propellants to the patient and the environment.[73, 74]

Freon (known as Arcton in England) consists of a mixture of haloalkanes (fluoralkanes) that are known as fluorocarbons; they are derivatives of methane and ethane. The main agents in common use are known as FC11, FC12 and FC114 (Table 1-35). Aviado[75] places the Freon propellants into four classes (Table 1-36). The most toxic is FC11, which can cause cardiac toxicity and respiratory depression. FC12 is somewhat less toxic, although it has the same adverse effects, and it can cause bronchoconstriction. Large doses of these propellants, when given by inhalation to experimental animals, can result in a blood level that can produce fatal cardiac stimulation, hypotension or apnea. The third most commonly used fluorocarbon is FC114, which is also less toxic than FC11. In England, FC113 has also been used in bronchodilator preparations,[76] although its high toxicity makes it particularly undesirable. Some other propellants, such as FC115, have low toxicity; these fluorocarbons would be more suitable for aerosol therapy.[77]

In general, manufacturers have chosen to use a mixture of an aerosol that has a low (e.g., $-30°$ C) boiling point with one that has a high (e.g., $+24°$ C) boiling point. Such a mixture allows easier manufacture and does not require exposure of the workers to high pressure or extreme cold.[76] The mixture also

TABLE 1-36.   CLASSIFICATION OF FLUOROCARBON PROPELLANTS*

Class	Pressure	Toxicity	Myocardial Irritability (TACHY-CARDIA)	Cardio-vascular Depression (HYPO-TENSION)	Respiratory Depression	Broncho-constriction	Examples
1	Low	High	+++	+++	±	±	FC11, FC113
2	Low	Intermediate	+	+	−	++	FC114
3	High	Intermediate	+	+	++	++	FC12
4	High	Low	±	±	−	+	FC115

*Based on animal studies.[75]

results in a lower vapor pressure within the container and thus reduces the risk of the unit exploding or the valve assembly being expelled. In practice, the marketed respiratory aerosol cartridges are safe when handled sensibly.

Many studies have been carried out to determine whether the fluorocarbon propellants expose respiratory patients to a significant risk. Although large doses of these agents can have fatal effects on animals, and probably on humans, Dollery's conclusion seems to be appropriate; that is, that there is not likely to be a hazard from the propellants when the inhalers are used in recommended fashion, but there could be a health risk if an excessive dose of aerosol is inhaled.[76] If, for instance, a patient were to take an inhalation of bronchodilator accompanied by propellant gas with every breath for several minutes, a toxic blood level of fluorocarbon could undoubtedly be achieved,[78] and this might sensitize the myocardium to the possibility of exercise-induced or catecholamine-induced arrhythmia. Of course, the excessive dose of the bronchodilator itself could cause cardiovascular toxicity and the adverse action of the Freon may not be separable in such cases. Perhaps some deaths in patients with severe asthma, who in desperation grossly overused their aerosols, can be attributed to the combined effects of toxic levels of propellant and bronchodilator in the blood stream.[79]

The concerns regarding fluorocarbon toxicity have been exacerbated by ecologists who fear that propellants can destroy the ozone layer in the stratosphere. There are valid arguments for finding alternative methods for aerosolizing the host of commercial products currently packaged in cartridges that use fluorocarbon propellants,[80] but experience and rationality lead one to conclude that, at present, the metered aerosol respiratory drugs are a necessity rather than a threat. If used appropriately, these valuable aerosolized drugs are not harmful to the patient,[81, 82] and they cannot be considered a threat to the environment. Other fears, such as the possibility of fluorocarbons damaging lung surfactant, have been considered, but are certainly of no clinical relevance.[83] Nevertheless, there is a good case for the pharmaceutical industry to strive to develop a less controversial method of providing metered doses of respiratory drugs, and to entirely eliminate volatile propellants from less essential household and industrial products.

RESPIRATORY MEDICATIONS

The average respiratory patient who requires chronic therapy is often treated with more than a dozen drugs. Some of the commonly prescribed drugs for chronically ill patients are needed for secondary complications of the respiratory condition; the victim of advanced asthmatic bronchitis is susceptible to heart failure, and may need cardiac drugs, diuretics, antibiotics and psychoactive agents in addition to the prime respiratory drugs. However, if one isolates drugs that are used most commonly for the management of lung diseases, it is possible to categorize these pharmaceutic agents into a number of groups (Tables 1-33 and 1-37). The most important agents are bronchodilators, antiasthma drugs, mucokinetic agents and drugs used in the treatment of coughs and colds. Most of these groups contain several agents that are given primarily by the inhalational route, although many of them can also be given by other routes. Some are not suitable for inhalational use; the usual properties that preclude them from administration by nebulization are their lack of solubility or their direct tissue-irritating qualities.

Some agents, such as local anesthetics and antibiotics, are sometimes given by the inha-

TABLE 1–37.   MAJOR CLASSES OF DRUGS USED IN RESPIRATORY THERAPEUTICS

Classes	Examples INHALATIONAL	NONINHALATIONAL
MAJOR RESPIRATORY DRUGS		
Brochodilators		
Sympathomimetics	Isoproterenol	Ephedrine
Phosphodiesterase inhibitors	Papaverine	Theophylline
Anticholinergics	Atropine	
Antiasthma Drugs		
Glucocorticoids	Beclomethasone	Prednisone
Bischromones	Cromolyn	
Mucokinetic Agents		
Expectorants	Saline	Sodium iodide
Mucolytics	Acetylcysteine	Carbocysteine
Enzymes	Dornase	
Mucosal Constrictors		
Antihistamines	Thonzonium	Antazoline
Sympathomimetics	Phenylephrine	Pseudoephedrine
Antitussives		
Narcotics		Codeine
Non-narcotics		Benzonatate
Respiratory Depressants		
Narcotics		Morphine
Physiologic agents	Oxygen	
Respiratory Stimulants		
Analeptics	Ammonia	Doxapram
Physiologic agents	Carbon dioxide	Progesterone
DRUGS PRIMARILY NONRESPIRATORY		
Anesthetics		
Local anesthetics	Lidocaine	Lidocaine
General anesthetics	Halothane	Rectal ether
Antibiotics	Neomycin	Penicillin
SPECIAL DRUGS		
Bronchoconstrictors	See Table 1–34	Propranolol
Carrier gases	Helium	
Diagnostic agents	Xenon	Labeled albumin

lational route, although this is not their prime means of administration. General anesthetics are the main drugs administered by inhalation for their systemic effects, whereas their action on the lung is mostly detrimental. A further group of inhalational drugs are those given for diagnostic purposes or for the investigation of airway dynamics; a large number of potential bronchoconstrictor agents have been identified (Table 1–34), and some (such as methacholine) are occasionally used in provocation tests to determine whether the airways are hyper-reactive—a test for latent asthma.

Other groups of drugs that may be considered as respiratory agents are those that act primarily on the respiratory center of the brain, either to stimulate respiration or to depress it. Most of these drugs have other central actions, but some of the stimulants have a preferential effect on the respiratory center.

The classes of agents listed in Table 1–37 will be described in detail in subsequent chapters. Those that have a primary effect on the lungs will be given major consideration, with special emphasis on agents administered by aerosols. Aerosolized agents are the pharmaceutic basis of inhalation therapy.

RESPIRATORY DRUG PRESCRIPTIONS

Since many respiratory medications are given by inhalation, the practitioner who prescribes or administers these drugs must possess a particular awareness of the dosing system used in aerosol therapy. Most drugs are made available as solutions in water or another solvent, and the percentage strength is recorded as a concentration, by weight, of solute in a standard volume of the solvent. A 100 per cent solution consists of 1 gram per 1

TABLE 1–38. PERCENTAGE CONCENTRATIONS OF SOLUTIONS
(WEIGHT IN VOLUME)

Percentage	Ratios	g/l	g/100 ml	g/ml	mg/100 ml	mg/ml
100	100:100, or 1:1	1000	100	1	100,000	1000
10	10:100, or 1:10	100	10	0.1	10,000	100
5	5:100, or 1:20	50	5	0.05	5,000	50
1	1:100, or 10:1000	10	1	0.01	1,000	10
0.5	5:1000, or 1:200	5	0.5	0.005	500	5
0.1	1:1000	1	0.1	0.001	100	1

Example
A mixture of 0.25 ml 1:200 isoproterenol in 2.5 ml water contains
  0.25 ml of 0.5% isoproterenol
  = 0.25 ml of a solution containing 5 mg/ml
  = 0.25 × 5 = 1.25 mg isoproterenol.
Thus, the mixture contains 1.25 mg isoproterenol in 2.75 ml solution.

ml, and all derivations can be made from this basic measure (see Table 1–38). Frequently, physicians order that a certain amount of the solution should be diluted by a specific amount of additional solvent, and it is necessary for the therapist or nurse not to lose sight of the absolute amount of active drug in the combination. Thus, a mixture containing 0.25 ml of a 0.5 per cent solution will contain 1.25 mg of drug irrespective of how much diluent is added.

In Table 1–39 the various common measuring systems that are used in pharmacologic prescribing are compared. Both liquid and solid drug measurements are usually made in the metric system, but the imprecise and confusing apothecary system is often used also. Since the apothecary system has different values in some countries, it is preferable to use only the internationally standardized metric system. The avoirdupois system of ounces and pounds is still used in everyday life, but it is scheduled for eventual replacement by the metric system, and therefore it should no longer be employed in pharmaceutics. It is often convenient to prescribe medications for use at home on the basis of everyday, household measures; however, these values are so unstandardized that a patient may easily obtain 100 per cent more or less of the drug than was intended. Presumably, the old-fashioned concept of prescribing drugs by the teaspoon or tablespoon will soon fade into oblivion when the precision of the metric system becomes common in daily life.

One major consideration for the respiratory therapist to bear in mind is that the

TABLE 1–39. PHARMACEUTICAL MEASUREMENTS

Liquid Measure		Household Measure*	WEIGHT		
Metric	Apothecary*		Avoirdupois	Metric	Apothecary*
1000 ml (1 l)	1 quart (2 pints)		2.2 lb	1000 g (1 kg)	
500 ml	1 pint (16 fluid ounces)†	2 tumblerfuls		500 g	7680 gr
360 ml	12 fluid ounces (1 pound)‡	3 teacupfuls	1 lb (16 oz)‡	454 g	5760 gr
30 ml	1 fluid ounce (8 drams)§	2 tablespoonfuls	1 oz (437 gr)§	29 g*	480 gr§
4 ml	1 dram (60 minims)	1 small teaspoonful		4 g	60 gr
1 ml	15 minims	¼ teaspoonful		1 g (1000 mg)	15 gr
0.06 ml	1 minim‖	1 drop (aqueous)	1 gr	60 mg*	1 gr
				1 mg (1000 μg)	1/60 gr

l = liter	℥ = ounce		lb = pound	kg = kilogram	gr = grain
ml = milliliter	ʒ = dram		oz = ounce	g = gram	
cc = cubic centimeter	m = minim		gr = grain	mg = milligram	
(1 cc = 1 ml)				μg = microgram (mcg)	

*Approximate equivalents.
†More accurately, 1 pint should be regarded as equivalent to 473 ml.
‡The apothecary pound contains 12 ounces, whereas the avoirdupois pound contains 16 ounces.
§The apothecary fluid ounce (480 grains) is heavier than the avoirdupois ounce (437 grains); the grain is the same in both systems.
‖A minim does not weigh 1 grain, and is not necessarily equivalent to 1 drop.

TABLE 1–40. SOME USEFUL EQUIVALENTS

WEIGHT		LENGTH	
1 microgram (μg, mcg)	= 0.000,001 gram (g)	1 micron (μ)	= 0.000,001 meter
1 milligram (mg)	= 0.001 gram	1 millimeter (mm)	= 0.001 meter = 1,000 μ
1 kilogram (kg)	= 1,000 gram	1 centimeter (cm)	= 0.01 meter
	= 2.2 pound (lb)	1 meter (m)	= 39.4 inch (in)

VOLUME

1 gallon = 3,785 milliliter (ml)
1 liter = 1,000 ml
1 pint = 473 ml
1 ounce = 30 ml (approx)
1 ml = 16.23 minims

TABLE 1–41. PHARMACOLOGIC ABBREVIATIONS

$\bar{a}$	Ante	Before
a.c.	Ante cibos	Before meals
ad lib.	Ad libitum	At pleasure, unrestricted
aq.	Aqua	Water
b.i.d.	Bis in die	Twice a day
cap.	Capsula	Capsule
$\bar{c}$	Cum	With
et	Et	And
gtt.	Gutta(e)	Drop(s)
h.s.	Hora somne	At bedtime
neb(ul.)	Nebula	A spray
p.o.	Per os	By mouth
p.c.	Post cibos	After eating
p.r.n.	Pro re nata	When necessary
q.(h.)(d.)	Quaque (hora)(die)	Each (hour)(day)
q.i.d.	Quater in die	Four times a day
q.s.	Quantum satis	As much as is sufficient
℞	Recipe	Prescription, prescribe
rept.	Repetatur	Let it be repeated
$\bar{s}$	Sine	Without
sol.	Solutio	Solution
sat. sol.(SS)	Solutio saturata	Saturated solution
sig.	Signa	Write on the label
stat.	Statim	Immediately
supp.	Suppositorium	Suppository
tab.	Tabella	Tablet
t.i.d., or t.d.	Ter in die	Three times a day

"drop," so often used in prescribing inhalational solutions, is a very imprecise measure. Although it is correct that one drop of water is almost equivalent to 1 minim, the latter measurement is precise (being equal to 0.06 ml), whereas the drop is variable. The size of a drop is influenced by many factors, such as the construction of the dropper, whether it is used in the vertical position or not, the temperature and consistency of the solution, and so on. The most important factor controlling the volume of a drop is the viscosity of the solution: a drop of an alcoholic solution of low viscosity may be only half the size of an aqueous drop, whereas an oily or syrupy solution can result in a drop that is about twice the volume of a drop of water.

Table 1–40 provides some useful equivalent measurements of weight, length and volume. In Table 1–41, the most common abbreviations used in drug prescribing are listed.

RECOMMENDED PHARMACOLOGY TEXTBOOKS

Avery, G. S. (Ed.): Drug Treatment: Principles and Practice of Clinical Pharmacology and Therapeutics. Acton, Mass., Publishing Sciences Group, Inc., 1976.

Aviado, D. M.: Kranz and Carr's Pharmacologic Principles of Medical Practice. Baltimore, The Williams and Wilkins Company, 8th ed., 1972.

Bergerson, B. S.: Pharmacology in Nursing. St. Louis, The C. V. Mosby Company, 13th ed., 1976.

Bevan, J. A. (Ed.): Essentials of Pharmacology: Introduction to the Principles of Drug Action. Hagerstown, Md., Harper and Row, 2nd ed., 1976.

DeKornfeld, T. J.: Pharmacology for Respiratory Therapy. Sarasota, Glenn Educational Medical Services, Inc., 1976.

DiPalma, J. R. (Ed.): Drill's Pharmacology in Medicine. New York, McGraw-Hill Book Company, 4th ed., 1971.

Falconer, M. W., Ezell, A. A., Patterson, H. R., and Gustafson, E. A.: The Drug, the Nurse, the Patient. Philadelphia, W. B. Saunders Company, 6th ed., 1978.

Falconer, M. W., Patterson, H. R., and Gustafson, E. A.: Current Drug Handbook, 1976–78. Philadelphia, W. B. Saunders Company, 1976.

Fields, L. J., Williams, T. J., and Gavavaglia, M. M. (Eds.): Pharmacologic Review for Intensive Cardiopulmonary Therapy. Sarasota. Glenn Educational Medical Services, Inc., 1975.

Foye, W. O. (Ed.): Principles of Medicinal Chemistry. Philadelphia, Lea and Febiger, 1974.

Goodman, L. S. and Gilman, A. (Eds.): The Pharmacological Basis of Therapeutics. New York, Macmillan Publishing Company, Inc., 5th ed., 1975.

Mathewson, H. S.: Pharmacology for Respiratory Therapists. St. Louis, The C. V. Mosby Company, 1977.

Modell, W. (Ed.): Drugs of Choice 1978–1979. St. Louis, The C. V. Mosby Company, 1978.

Wilson, C. O., Gisvold, O. and Doerge, R. F. (Eds.): Textbook of Organic Medicinal and Pharmaceutical Chemistry. Philadelphia, J. B. Lippincott Co., 7th ed., 1977.

REFERENCES

1. Tiersten, S.: R T pharmacology: where has it been and where is it going? Respir. Therapy 4:23-26, Jan., 1974.
2. Trease, G. E.: A Textbook of Pharmacognosy. London, Baillière, Tindall and Cox, 8th ed., 1961.
3. Leake, C. D.: An Historical Account of Pharmacology to the 20th Century. Springfield, Ill., Charles C Thomas, 1975.
4. Sperber, P. A.: Drugs, Demons, Doctors and Disease. St. Louis, Warren H. Green, Inc., 1973.
5. Paterson, J. W. and Shenfield, G. M.: Bronchodilators, Part 1. B.T.T.A. Rev. 4:25, June, 1974.
6. James, P.: The Therapeutics of the Respiratory Passages. New York, William Wood and Company, 1884.
7. Major, R. H.: Classic Descriptions of Disease. Springfield, Ill., Charles C Thomas, 3rd ed., 1945, p. 561.
8. Claus, E. P., Tyler, V. E. and Brady, L. R.: Pharmacognosy. Philadelphia, Lea and Febiger, 6th ed., 1970.
9. Kleinerman, J. In New Directions in Asthma, M. Stein (Ed.). Park Ridge, Ill., American College of Chest Physicians, 1975, p. 52.
9a. Anon: In Tanzania, the road to medicine is paved with magic. Hosp. Practice 9:133–157, April, 1974.
10. Departments of Traditional Medicine, Internal Medicine and Biochemistry, Shanghai First Medical College: Treatment of bronchial asthma with traditional Chinese medicine. China's Medicine 3:230–235, 1967.
11. Nadkarni, A. K.: Indian Materia Medica. Bombay, Popular Book Depot, 3rd ed., 1954.
12. Jablonski, S.: Russian Drug Index. Bethesda, Md., U.S. Department of Health, Education and Welfare (Public Health Service), 1967.
13. Rosenblatt, M. B.: History of bronchial asthma. In Bronchial Asthma: Mechanisms and Therapeutics, E. B. Weiss and M. S. Segal (Eds.). Boston, Little, Brown and Company, 1976.
14. Scudder, J. M.: On the Use of Medicated Inhalations in the Treatment of Disease of the Respiratory Organs. Cincinnati, Moore, Wilstach and Baldwin, 2nd ed., 1867.
15. Tissier, P. L.: Pneumotherapy Including Aërotherapy and Inhalation Methods and Therapy, Vol. X. In A System of Physiologic Therapeutics, S. Solis Cohen (Ed.). Philadelphia, P. Blakiston's Son and Co., 1903.
16. Robin, A.: Treatment of Tuberculosis. Ordinary Therapeutics of Medical Men. New York, The Macmillan Company, 1913.
17. Culbreth, D. M. R.: A Manual of Materia Medica and Pharmacology. Philadelphia, Lea and Febiger, 7th ed., 1927.
18. Grover, F. W.: Oxtriphylline glyceryl guaiacolate elixir in pediatric asthma: with a theophylline review. Ann. Allergy 23:127–147, 1965.

19. Aviado, D. M. and Salem, H.: Sympathomimetic bronchodilator preparations available in the United States. Rev. Allergy 24:441–450, 1970.

20. Burack, R. and Fox, F. J.: The New Handbook of Prescription Drugs. New York, Ballantine Books, revised edition, 1975.

21. Wood, M.: Evaluating our drug regulation system. Respir. Therapy 4:41–44, July, 1974.

22. Wardell, W. M.: Introduction of new therapeutic drugs in the United States and Great Britain: an international comparison. Private Practice, Nov. 1973, pp. 61–73.

23. Levene, R. R.: Pharmacology: Drug Actions and Reactions. Boston, Little, Brown and Company, 1973.

24. Martin, E. W. (Ed.): Hazards of Medications. Philadelphia, J. B. Lippincott Company, 1971.

25. Wood, M. and Ziment, I.: Additives and combinations. Respir. Therapy 4:19–24, Sept., 1974.

26. Dautrebande, L.: Microaerosols: Physiology, Pharmacology, Therapeutics. New York, Academic Press, 1962.

27. Geddes, B. A. and Lefcoe, N. M.: Respiratory smooth muscle relaxing effect of commercial steroid preparations. Am. Rev. Respir. Dis. 107:395–399, 1973.

28. Buswell, R. S. and Lefkowitz, M. S.: Oral bronchodilators containing tartrazine. J.A.M.A. 235:1111, 1976.

29. Smith, L. J. and Slavin, R. G.: Drugs containing tartrazine dye. J. Allergy Clin. Immunol. 58:456–470, 1976.

30. Koch-Weser, J.: Bioavailability of drugs. N. Engl. J. Med. 291:233-237, 503–506, 1974.

31. Melmon, K. L. and Morrelli, H. F. (Eds.): Clinical Pharmacology: Basic Principles in Therapeutics. New York, The Macmillan Company, 1972.

32. Ziment, I.: Why are they saying bad things about IPPB? Respir. Care 18:677–689, 1973.

33. Karetzky, M. S.: Asthma mortality: an analysis of one year's experience, review of the literature and assessment of current modes of therapy. Medicine 54:471–484, 1975.

34. Halpern, S. R.: Management of childhood asthma. J.A.M.A. 229:819–820, 1974.

35. Ziment, I. and Koppel, M. H. J.: Antimicrobials when kidneys can't cope. Current Prescribing 2:32–43 Aug., 1976.

36. Goldstein, A., Aronow, L. and Kalman, S. M.: Principles of Drug Action: The Basis of Pharmacology. New York, John Wiley and Sons, 2nd ed., 1974.

37. Jenne, J. W. and Chick, T. W.: "Unresponsiveness" to isoproterenol. Chest 70:691–693, 1976.

38. Stuart, B. O.: Deposition of inhaled aerosols. Arch. Intern. Med. 131:60–73, 1973.

39. Kanig, J. L.: Pharmaceutical aerosols. J. Pharm. Sci. 52:513–535, 1963.

40. Dautrebande, L.: Physiological and pharmacological characteristics of liquid aerosols. Physiol. Rev. 32:214–275, 1952.

41. Morrow, P. E.: Aerosol characterization and deposition. Am. Rev. Respir. Dis. 110 # 6 Pt. 2:88–99, 1974.

42. Gross, P.: The deposition of aerosol particles in the respiratory tract: the factors governing their distribution and their clearance from the lungs. In Bronchial Asthma: Mechanisms and Thera-

peutics. E. B. Weiss and M. S. Segal (Eds.). Boston, Little, Brown and Company, 1976.

43. Cushing, I. E. and Miller, W. F.: Nebulization therapy. In Respiratory Therapy. P. Safar (Ed.). Philadelphia, F. A. Davis Company, 1965.

44. Gorman, W. G. and Hall, G. D.: Inhalational aerosols. In Current Concepts in the Pharmaceutical Sciences: Dosage Form Design and Availability. J. Swarbrick (Ed.). Philadelphia, Lea and Febiger, 1973.

45. Muir, D. C. F. (Ed.): Clinical Aspects of Inhaled Particles. Philadelphia, F. A. Davis Company, 1972. Chs. 1 and 9.

46. Mercer, T. T.: Production and characterization of aerosols. Arch. Intern. Med. 131:39–50, 1973.

47. Sheldon, G. P.: Nebulized bronchodilators in obstructive lung disease. Ann. Allergy 30:24–35, 69–85, 1972.

48. Wood, M.: Production of therapeutic aerosols. Resp. Therapy 5:19–22, Jan., 1975.

49. Ferron, G. A., Kerrebijn, K. F. and Weber, J.: Properties of aerosols produced with three nebulizers. Am. Rev. Respir. Dis. 114:899–908, 1976.

50. Miller, W. F.: Aerosol therapy in acute and chronic respiratory disease. Arch. Intern. Med. 131:148–155, 1973.

51. Muir, D. C. F.: Physiological aspects of ultrasonic aerosols. Respiration Suppl. 27:185–190, 1970.

52. Barach, A. L. and Segal, M. S.: Helium-oxygen therapy in bronchial asthma. In Bronchial Asthma: Mechanisms and Therapeutics. E. B. Weiss and M. S. Segal (Eds.). Boston, Little, Brown and Company, 1976.

53. Loehning, R., Milai, A. S. and Safar, P.: Intermittent positive pressure breathing therapy. In Respiratory Therapy. P. Safar (Ed.). Philadelphia, F. A. Davis Company, 1965.

54. Ziment, I.: Intermittent positive pressure breathing. In Respiratory Care: A Guide to Clinical Practice. G. G. Burton, G. N. Gee and J. E. Hodgkin (Eds.) Philadelphia, J. B. Lippincott Company, 1977.

55. Smelzer, T. H. and Barnett, T. B.: Bronchodilator aerosol: comparison of administration methods. J.A.M.A. 223:884–889, 1973.

56. Davies, D. S.: Pharmacokinetics of inhaled substances. Postgrad. Med. J. 51(Suppl.7):69–75, 1975.

57. Bell, J. H., Brown, K. and Glasby, J.: Variation in delivery of isoprenaline from various pressurized inhalers. J. Pharm. Pharmac. 25:32P–36P, 1973.

58. Modell, J. H.: Uses and abuses of aerosol therapy. Respir. Care 20:356–361, 1975.

59. Connolly, C. K.: Method of using pressurized aerosols. Br. Med. J. 3:21, July, 1975.

60. Coady, T. J., Stewart, C. J. and Davies, H. J.: Use of pressurized aerosols by asthmatic patients. Br. Med. J. 2:833, April, 1976.

61. Pavia, D., Thompson, M. L., Clarke, S. W. and Shannon, H. S.: Effect of lung function and mode of inhalation on penetration of aerosol into the human lung. Thorax 32:194–197, 1977.

62. Orehek, J., Gayrard, P., Grimaud, G. and Charpin, J.: Patient error in use of bronchodilator metered aerosols. Br. Med. J. 1:76, Jan., 1976.

63. Asmundsson, T., Johnson, R. F., Kilburn, K. H. and Goodrich, J. K.: Efficiency of nebulizers for depositing saline in human lung. Am. Rev. Respir. Dis. 108:506–512, 1973.

64. Abramson, H. A.: Present status of aerosol therapy of the lungs and bronchi. *In* Progress in the Science of Allergy. New York, Karger, 1949, pp. 84–124.

65. Dittmer, D. S. and Grebe, R. M. (Eds.): Handbook of Respiration. Philadelphia, W. B. Saunders Company, 1958.

66. Wagner, H. N. Jr.: The use of radioisotope techniques for the evaluation of patients with pulmonary disease. Am. Rev. Respir. Dis. 113:203–218, 1976.

67. Jaques, L. B., Mahadoo, J. and Kavanagh, L. W.: Intrapulmonary heparin: a new procedure for anticoagulant therapy. Lancet 2:1157–1161, 1976.

68. Aas, K.: The Bronchial Provocation Test. Springfield, Ill., Charles C Thomas, 1975.

69. Mintzer, H.: Aerosols. *In* Dispensing of Medications (Formerly Hsua's Pharmaceutical Dispensing). E. W. Martin (Ed.). Easton, Pa., Mack Publishing Company. 7th ed., 1971.

70. Woolcock, A. J.: Inhaled drugs in the prevention of asthma. Am. Rev. Respir. Dis. 117:191–194, 1977.

71. Tashkin, D. P.: Therapeutic advantages of the newer bronchodilator compounds. Chest 71: 125–126, 1977.

72. Editorial: Fluorocarbon aerosol propellants. Lancet 1:1073–1074, 1975.

73. Frank, R.: Are aerosol sprays hazardous? Am. Rev. Respir. Dis. 112:485–489, 1975.

74. Bernstein, I. L.: Medical hazards of aerosols. Postgrad. Med. 52:62–77, 1972.

75. Aviado, D. M.: Toxicity of aerosol propellants in the respiratory and circulatory systems. X. Proposed classification. Toxicology 3:321–332, 1975.

76. Dollery, C. T.: The toxicity of propellant gases. *In* Evaluation of Bronchodilator Drugs. D. M. Burley et al. (Eds.). Published by The Trust for Education and Research in Therapeutics (England), 1974, pp. 183–190.

77. Aviado, D. M. and Drimal, J.: Five fluorocarbons for administration of aerosol bronchodilators. J. Clin. Pharmacol. 15:116–128, 1975.

78. Dollery, C. T., Williams, F. M., Draffan, G. H., Wise, G., Sahyoun, H., Paterson, J. W. and Walker, S. R.: Arterial blood levels of fluorocarbons in asthmatic patients following use of pressurized aerosols. Clin. Pharmacol. Therap. 15:59–66, 1974.

79. Aviado, D. M.: Toxicity of aerosols. J. Clin. Pharmacol. 15:86–104, 1975.

80. Aviado, D. M.: Toxicity of propellants. Prog. Drug Res. 18:365–397, 1974.

81. Brooks, S. M., Mintz, S. and Weiss, E.: Changes occurring after Freon inhalation. Am. Rev. Respir. Dis. 105:640–643, 1972.

82. Silverglade, A.: Asthma deaths and bronchodilator aerosols. Am. Rev. Respir. Dis. 107:1076–1078, 1973.

83. Modell, J. H., Gollan, F., Giammona, S. T. and Parker, D.: Effect of fluorocarbon liquid on surface tension properties of pulmonary surfactant. Chest 57:263–265, 1970.

2

PATHOPHYSIOLOGY AND PHARMACOLOGY OF SPUTUM

Sputum, or phlegm, is an abnormal, viscous, excretory product of the diseased respiratory tract. The healthy respiratory mucosa produces a bathing layer of secretions that continually moves up the airways as a result of ciliary activity. The normal adult may produce over 100 ml of respiratory tract (or bronchial) secretions a day;[1] all of this is gradually propelled cephalad, into the pharynx where it is swallowed without awareness. When a patient is aware of excessive secretions and either swallows or spits out (expectorates) the material, then we realize that sputum is being produced. Usually, the expectorated product is contaminated by oropharyngeal cells, bacteria, food particles and saliva; thus sputum will differ from lower respiratory tract fluid, unless the material is obtained by aspiration through a tube that bypasses the oropharynx. "Normal sputum" is a contradiction in terms, since it is not "normal" to expectorate sputum.[2]

Although the words "sputum" and "mucus" are often used interchangeably, sputum is, by definition, a lower respiratory tract product, whereas mucus is produced by all mucous membranes. Mucoid fluid expectorated from the mouth is not necessarily "sputum," since it could originate from the nose or sinuses. Patients are not always able to differentiate such secretions (sometimes described as "postnasal drip") from true sputum. Clinicians and therapists must take care to determine whether an expectorated specimen is truly sputum.

Unfortunately, sputum is a relatively neglected biologic fluid, and it is surprising to find a gaping deficit in established knowledge about this product of respiratory disease.[3] At present, no entirely acceptable definition of either sputum or mucus exists, and the available descriptions of the biochemical and other components of this fluid are in a state of confusion. Sputum will be defined here as a nonhomogeneous, semisolid, viscous, adhesive fluid containing water, mucus and other components, derived from the lower respiratory tract. Although much remains unknown about the production and composition of sputum, there is a basis of information upon which rational approaches to pharmacologic alterations of sputum can be built.

THE CONSTITUENTS OF SPUTUM
(Table 2–1)

The most important constituent of sputum is mucus, a proteinaceous material consisting mainly of mucopolysaccharides (identified as "mucin" in stained specimens), in the form of long, interconnected, fibrous molecules within a gel (Fig. 2–1).[4] In the respiratory tract, the secretions tend to layer out into a more superficial gel-layer and a deeper, less viscous, sol-layer. The amount of water in the sol-layer and incorporated into the gel-layer is an important determinant of the overall viscosity of the material; the absolute level of viscosity is clearly related to the concentration of acid glycoprotein.[2, 5]

The often characteristic heaviness and coloration of infected sputum are related to the presence of strands of molecules of deoxyribonucleic acid (DNA), which are derived from the breakdown of leucocytes, mucosal cells and bacteria, and to the presence of other constituents in the cellular

TABLE 2–1. MAJOR CONSTITUENTS OF SPUTUM

Class	Main Components	Functions
Water		Constitutes 95% of sputum
Glycoproteins (also called mucopolysaccharides, mucoprotein, mucin, "mucus")	Fucomucin (+ N-acetyl neuraminic acid)	Main contributor to viscosity
	Sialomucins	Contribute to viscosity
	Sulfomucins	Bind virus particles
Nucleic acids	Deoxyribonucleic acid (DNA)	Presence suggests infection
Lipoprotein	Dipalmitoyl lecithin	Main constituent of surfactant
Serum proteins	Immunoglobulins	Contribute to humoral defense
	Albumin	Contributes to viscosity
	Transferrin, lactoferrin	No special role in sputum
Enzymes	Lysozyme	Participates in inflammatory reaction
	Proteases	Intrinsic proteolytic digestion of mucoprotein
Cellular debris	Polymorphs	Contribute to cellular defense
	Macrophages	Contribute to cellular defense
	Eosinophils	Produce Charcot-Leyden crystals
	Epithelium	Ciliated cells are hallmark of tracheobronchial secretion
Electrolytes	Calcium	May contribute to viscosity
	Sodium, potassium, magnesium	Contribute to appropriate osmotic environment for cilia
Saliva	Enzymes, oral mucosal cells, microbes, food particles	Must be carefully distinguished from expectorated tracheobronchial secretions

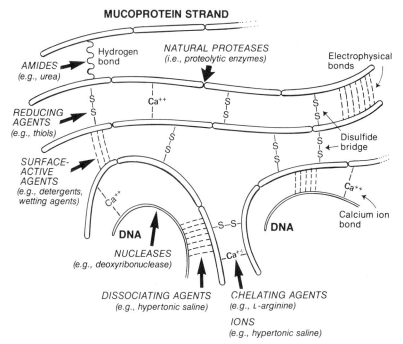

Figure 2–1. Structure of mucus. The mucopolysaccharide chains are interconnected by numerous chemical and physical bonds. These can be broken by appropriate chemicals and drugs, which thereby reduce the viscosity of the mucus. (From "Secretions of the Respiratory Tract: Physiology and Pharmacology" by Irwin Ziment, Projects in Health, Inc., 1976.)

debris. Fresh, purulent sputum is usually yellow, but it is reddish or brownish if red blood cells are present. Secretions that stagnate in the lungs before expectoration gradually become greenish, apparently because of oxidation catalyzed by the enzyme myeloperoxidase (also called verdoperoxidase), which is derived from leucocytes.[6] Not all green or yellow sputum is necessarily "purulent," because pus cells (polymorphs) are not always present in it. In asthma, the sputum may be yellow even in the absence of polymorphs, because the characteristic presence of eosinophils or Dietrich's plugs (granular, fatty debris from cells and bacteria) can also impart this color.

Among the simplest components in sputum are various electrolytes; it is possible that their role may be much more important than has previously been thought. Calcium, in particular, may be a major factor in conferring viscosity to sputum;[7, 7a] it is found in highest concentrations in sputum from patients who have bronchiectasis or cystic fibrosis. The calcium, as well as proteins and DNA, may contribute to the characteristically high viscosity of sputum in these diseases.

The pH of sputum may be an important factor in viscosity, but this has not been studied adequately, and reports on the pH of infected and normal sputum are contradictory.[8, 9, 10] However, there is evidence that an alkaline environment is associated with a decrease in the viscosity of sputum.[11]

The functions of respiratory tract fluid are mainly protective. The fluid traps inhaled particles, and is essential for the self-cleansing protective mechanism of the lung. The secretions provide a defense against invasion by microorganisms: phagocytes, immunoglobulins and other humoral antimicrobic agents move freely in the fluid environment to the site of infection. The mucous layer protects the epithelium from drying out, and it provides a demulcent bath for the ciliated cells.

THE MUCOCILIARY BLANKET

The respiratory tree from the larynx to the terminal bronchioles is lined with a mucosa that bears *cilia*, each about 6 μ in length (Fig. 2–2). The cilia are not under neurologic control, but nevertheless they beat in coordinated fashion, generating a propulsive wave cephalad towards the larynx.[7a, 12] The

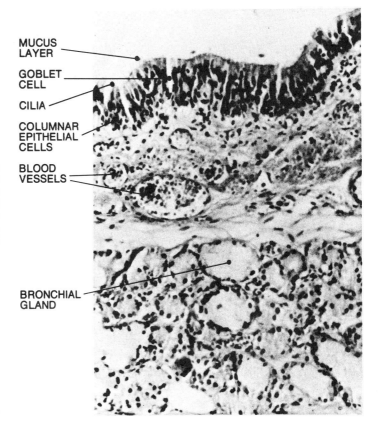

Figure 2–2.   Cross-section through a respiratory airway. The superficial mucous layer overlies the submucosa, which contains blood vessels and bronchial glands. Deep to this layer, and not shown in this photomicrograph, is the unstriped muscle layer. (After Ziment)

MUCUS LAYER

GOBLET CELL

CILIA

COLUMNAR EPITHELIAL CELLS

BLOOD VESSELS

BRONCHIAL GLAND

cilia normally beat at the amazing rate of over 1000 times per minute; although the mechanism controlling the autonomous activity of the cilia is poorly understood, it is known that various agents can slow the rate of the beat.[7a] Such inhibitors are listed in Table 2-2 and include alcohol, irritant dusts, fumes and smoke (including cigarette smoke), inflammatory agents such as noxious gases, viruses and bacterial infections; local anesthetics in high concentrations;[13] intravenous serotonin;[14] cuffed endotracheal tubes;[15] high concentrations of inspired oxygen;[14, 16] high concentrations of histamine, codeine, nicotine and pentobarbital;[17] and methysergide and phentolamine.[17] Except for oxygen and endotracheal cuffs, these potential ciliodepressants are not often encountered in therapeutic management.

TABLE 2-2. FACTORS THAT IMPAIR CILIARY ACTIVITY

MECHANICAL and ENVIRONMENTAL
Endotracheal tubes
Extremes of temperature
High oxygen concentration
High carbon dioxide concentration
Dusts, fumes, smoke (cigarette and other)
Lack of humidity
Over-liquefaction of mucus

INFLAMMATION
Trauma (e.g. suctioning)
Chemical and physical burns
Bacterial and viral infections

DRUGS (in relatively high concentration)
Local and general anesthetics
Codeine
Pentobarbital
Alcohol
Acetylcysteine
Tyloxapol
Nicotine
Cromolyn

EXPERIMENTAL
Histamine (aerosol)
Atropine, other anticholinergic agents (?)
Methysergide
Phentolamine, phenoxybenzamine
Serotonin (intravenous)
Dinitrophenol

HISTOTOXIC
"Pollutants" (oxides of nitrogen and sulfur)
Cyanide
Monoiodoacetic acid
Formaldehyde

PATHOLOGIC
Viruses
Chronic bacterial infection
Serum factor in fibrocystic disease patients
Mucostasis (due to dehydration, impaired clearance mechanics, etc.)

The mucosal epithelium contains *goblet cells* in addition to the ciliated cells; about 20 per cent of the epithelial cell layer in the trachea consists of goblet cells, but the frequency decreases to 1 or 2 per cent in the bronchioles. These cells are packed with secretory granules, and they periodically discharge their contents in the form of gelatinous mucus. The goblet cells do not have any autonomic innervation, and the means by which their activity is regulated have not been elucidated. However, they do respond to topical irritation, and chronic exposure to irritants such as cigarette smoke increases the size, number and activity of goblet cells. In chronic bronchitis there is an enormous increase in goblet cell population in the distal respiratory tree.

The submucosa of the cartilaginous airways, down to about the fifteenth bronchial level, contains tracheobronchial tubulo-acinar glands. These *bronchial glands* are similar to the salivary glands in several respects. They are exocrine-glands and they secrete a relatively watery fluid through ciliated ducts onto the surface of the ciliated epithelium. They are under autonomic control; vagal (or parasympathomimetic) stimulation causes them to discharge their contents. Aerosol drugs and irritant fumes can stimulate the bronchial glands, as can various blood-borne drugs.

The ciliated epithelium of the tracheobronchial tree is bathed by the mucoid fluid secreted by the bronchial glands and the goblet cells. There is an extraordinarily precise structural organization of the mucociliary blanket, and normal mucus clearance depends upon the maintenance of this finely controlled relationship.[12] The fluid is usually 5 to 10 μ thick, and it is made up of two distinct layers. The deeper, more watery layer accounts for about 4 to 8 μ of the total thickness, and it is essentially an electrolytic solution containing relatively little mucopolysaccharide: this is the *sol-layer*. Superficially, and seeming to float on the sol-layer, is the 1 to 2 μ thick, gelatinous *gel-layer*, which serves to trap foreign materials on its sticky surface. The cilia beat freely in the sol-layer, and the metachronal wave is transmitted cephalad by the tips of the cilia to the gel-layer,[12, 18] which is propelled along the underlying sol-layer like a covering of scum moved by ripples on the surface of a lake. Because of this finely balanced dynamic relationship, the gel-layer is kept in constant motion, being propelled up the respiratory tree against the force of gravity.[19]

TABLE 2-3. ANATOMIC FACTORS IN MUCOCILIARY FUNCTION

Factor	Stimulated By	Inhibited By
Cilia	Bronchodilator aerosols	Irritants, infection
Goblet cells	Irritants, infection	
Bronchial glands	Vagus, bronchomucotropics	Anticholinergics
Capillaries	Vasodilators, hydration, inflammation	Dehydration
Alveolar type II cells	Stretching of cells	Shallow breathing
Clara cells	Catecholamines	?
Microvilli	?	?
Airway patency	Sympathomimetic agents	Airway disease

The whisking action of the cilia appears to help bring about the separation of the gel-layer from the sol-layer, a phenomenon known as thixotrophy.[3]

It is, without doubt, too simplistic to consider the sol-layer as originating from the secretions of the bronchial glands, and the gel-layer as derived entirely from the goblet cells, although this simple model enables one to understand the movement of respiratory tract secretions. Actually, the structure of the mucociliary blanket of fluid is controlled by a highly complex mechanism (Table 2–3). It is thought that part of the sol-layer derives also from transudation from the mucosal capillaries and from the additional secretions of the *alveolar type II cells* and the *Clara cells*[20] (nonciliated epithelial cells of uncertain function in the terminal bronchioles), and that the bronchial glands contribute to both layers. The ciliary epithelium is thought to contain fine microvilli projecting from the surface of the ciliated cells and from specialized brush cells; these are believed to play a role in the regulation of the depth of the sol-layer.[12] Obviously, the mucociliary blanket, which is a fundamental factor in most chronic obstructive pulmonary disorders, requires a great deal more investigation. But it is evident that the finely woven tapestry of cilia and mucoid fluid layers does constitute the lung's security blanket.

MUCOKINESIS

The production of sputum involves a complex chain of coordinated events.[4] Expectoration can occur only if the secretory mucosa produces an excessive amount of material of appropriate consistency. If the secretions are too thin, the watery fluid may gravitate toward the alveoli; if too thick they will tend to remain in the small airways and become inspissated. The cilia must function appropriately, and the two-layer relationship

of the secretions must be maintained—otherwise the cilia will not be able to waft the material toward the mouth. The airways must be patent, and adequate humidity must be present, otherwise the secretions will tend to thicken, since reabsorption of fluid occurs during the ascent up the mucociliary escalator.[12] Finally, the complex cough mechanism must be intact, either as a voluntary or as a reflex response. This requires functioning chest muscles and diaphragm, which coordinate with appropriate vocal cord activity; sufficiently rapid airflow must be generated by this integrated mechanism to permit an effective blast of air to propel the secretions out of the trachea. The neural interrelationship between the various involved muscles and the brain must also be intact.

Abnormalities at any stage will interfere with successful expectoration, which is the final act in the process of producing and moving secretions from the lung. The whole sequence of events involves much more than coughing and spitting, which is what constitutes "expectoration." A more appropriate word for the complex process of moving mucus would be "mucokinesis."[21] Similarly, any drug or procedure that results in the removal of sputum from the respiratory tree can be described as "mucokinetic." Using this terminology, drugs such as saline and potassium iodide can be called "mucokinetic agents"; techniques such as postural drainage and suctioning can be called "mucokinetic procedures."

ACTIONS OF MUCOKINETIC DRUGS

In patients who have abnormal or excessive respiratory secretions, expectoration may occur freely or with difficulty. If easy expectoration occurs, and if this does not cause the patient any problem (as is the case in many people with mild chronic bronchitis), then a mucokinetic is not necessarily

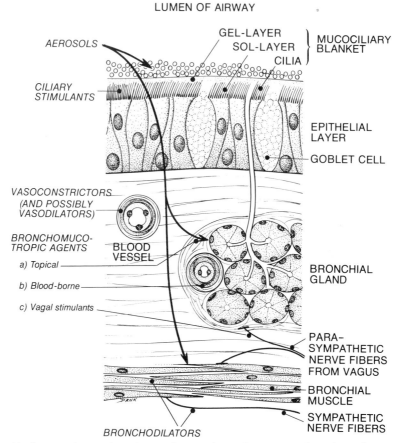

Figure 2–3. This diagram of a cut through a respiratory airway demonstrates how the various mucosal elements contribute to the production of the mucociliary blanket. Drugs can affect the structure of the blanket, either through their effects on specific structures in the mucosa or directly by topical action.

required, although the underlying abnormality may demand another form of therapeutic intervention. On the other hand, if expectoration occurs only with difficulty and is associated with airway obstructive problems for the patient, a mucokinetic may be of considerable help.

In the patient with excessive or altered mucus production, and difficulty with expectoration, therapy may have to be directed at one or more of the several stages involved in mucokinesis. The following factors are involved (see Fig. 2–3).

The Goblet Cells. In many respiratory diseases, the goblet cells increase in number and, perhaps, in activity. As a result, an excessive amount of viscous mucus is secreted. Unfortunately, the goblet cells do not appear to be under nervous or hormonal control, and therefore they are not readily susceptible to pharmacologic therapy. Goblet cell overactivity is a direct consequence of irritation resulting from infection, allergy,

or the breathing of noxious fumes, and treating or removing the cause may allow the goblet cells to return to a less active status. However, there are no drugs that result in a decrease in number or activity of the goblet cells as a direct pharmacologic action.

The Bronchial Glands. The mucosal glands of the tracheobronchial tree are thought to secrete a more watery fluid than do the goblet cells. Although this has not been proved, indirect evidence suggests that increased bronchial submucosal gland activity often results in improved mucokinesis. The watery secretions can serve in two ways to decrease the mucus problem: first, the secretions enter the sol-layer, bathing the cilia, and thereby provide a favorable medium for ciliary activity, thus increasing the effectiveness of the ciliary beat; second, the secretions may enter the gel-layer, thereby directly reducing the viscosity of this thick, gelatinous, mucoid material.

Most oral "expectorants" are believed to

act either directly or reflexly on the bronchial glands to increase the volume of their secretions.[22] These glands are under parasympathetic nervous system control,[23] and thus they are susceptible to the effects of many cholinergic drugs that act on the respiratory branches of the vagus nerves. Other drugs can directly stimulate the glands to secrete; these agents act independently of the nervous supply, either by a direct topical effect or following systemic administration.

The Mucosal Blood Vessels. Serous fluid can transude (under the influence of pressure) or exude (when inflammation is present) out through the blood vessels into the interstitial tissues and, if the process continues, into the airways. Fluid may be derived by these means from the alveolar capillary bed, which arises from branches of the pulmonary artery; if the secretion of fluid is pronounced, pulmonary edema results. The airways proximal to the alveoli are supplied by blood vessels of the bronchial circulation; if the blood flow in these vessels is increased, transudation into the mucosal tissue and possibly into the airways may result. There is little information about the role of these mucosal blood vessels in normal respiratory secretion production, but it is probable that certain drugs can stimulate an increased output from the vessels, thereby resulting in the addition of serous fluid to the mucoid secretions in the airways.

Other Secretory Cells. The Clara cells and the type II cells are believed to contribute to the sol-layer; both these cell-types may also produce surfactant. The type II cells are responsible for producing a thin alveolar layer of fluid, which is distinctly different from the double-layered mucus blanket that extends distally only as far as the respiratory bronchioles. The mechanism controlling the secretion of the Clara cells and type II cells remains to be elucidated.

The Mucus Blanket. The relationship between the two component layers of mucus bathing the cilia can be altered by stimulating the bronchial glands. Alterations in the viscosity of the gel-layer and in the depth of the sol-layer can be achieved by topical therapy with water and other drugs introduced directly into the airways.

Various drugs can also be given by topical administration to produce direct alteration of the mucopolysaccharide molecules of the gel-layer. Drugs can be given topically or systemically to bring about depolymerization of the complex mucoproteins and deoxyribonucleic acid (DNA). Several different agents are used in this fashion to decrease the viscosity of sticky secretions.

The Cilia. Although the mechanisms that control ciliary activity are poorly understood,[18] it is known that many drugs have direct and indirect effects upon the cilia. Improved mucokinesis is achieved by using agents that increase the rate and coordination of ciliary activity, and such drugs may be given systemically or topically.

The Airways. Bronchoconstriction, expiratory airway collapse and anatomic distortion interfere with mucokinesis. The bronchial muscles, which form a spiral continuum along the airways, undergo tonic changes during the respiratory cycle. By constricting during expiration, they narrow the airway diameter, thereby resulting in augmentation of the airflow; this activity probably helps to "milk" the respiratory secretions up the airways toward the mouth. Drugs are of considerable value as a means of reversing the pathophysiologic processes that result in bronchoconstriction, but mechanical methods (such as the temporary use of expiratory retard) may be required to help correct airway collapse and distortion. Various pharmacologic agents are also of value in decreasing the mucosal edema, which is often a contributory factor in obstructive airway disease; such mucosal constrictants improve mucokinesis.

The Cough Reflex. Patients with impaired or diminished cough may respond to various cough stimulants, which thereby improve mucokinesis. If there is muscular inadequacy, severe airway obstruction, or absent neurologic function, all efforts to obtain effective coughing may be without success, and mechanical methods (such as suctioning or postural drainage) will be required to achieve mucokinesis. Similarly, a normal cough center in the brain is a requisite for normal coughing, whereas an abnormal center may result in excessive coughing or absence of the cough. This center is thought to be located in the dorsolateral portion of the medulla, adjacent to the rootlets of the vagus, and it is intimately related to the respiratory center.[24]

Motivation. To a large extent, sputum expectoration results from voluntary coughing. The poorly motivated, exhausted or uncooperative patient may retain sputum simply because of inability or unwillingness to make the exertion required for an effective cough. Stimulation, exhortation, instruction and other techniques directed at the patient's psyche may achieve successful mucokinesis when pharmacologic agents are unsuccessful.[25]

FAILURE OF MUCOKINESIS

If excessive or abnormal respiratory tract secretions are produced in the airways, then abnormalities of ciliary activity, defects in airflow or alterations in cough effectiveness will result in sputum retention. Most of the clinical problems of obstructive pulmonary disease are related to either bronchospasm or failure of the mucokinetic mechanism. In patients with chronic obstructive airway disease, the bronchospastic component can often be treated by bronchodilator drugs, and in such cases it is the numerous other factors responsible for impairment of mucokinesis that result in respiratory failure. Most patients with bronchitis and emphysema who are admitted to intensive care units require special efforts to compensate for the impairment in mucokinesis. Since much of the compensatory treatment involves mechanical techniques, these patients demand a considerable amount of help from nursing and respiratory therapy personnel.

Pharmacologic methods aimed at decreasing sputum viscosity may be unsuccessful if ciliary activity, airflow dynamics and coughing are inadequate for moving secretions against gravity. In such situations, decreasing the viscosity of the secretions may even be detrimental, since the loosened fluid will tend to run more freely along the gravitational incline deeper down the tracheobronchial tree. Indeed, the use of agents that markedly decrease the viscosity of the retained mucoid fluid may result in the patient drowning in these secretions. However, when suctioning or gravity can be used therapeutically, the concomitant addition of pharmacologic thinning of the respiratory secretions will offer a valuable adjuvant contribution.

MUCOKINETIC DRUGS

Most drugs that improve mucokinesis achieve their results by causing thinning of hyperviscous secretions; others act by improving either ciliary activity or airway mechanics. No drug can actually improve the cough mechanism, and most so-called "cough medicines" are used to suppress, rather than enhance, coughing.

Pharmacology has a long history of therapeutic efforts to improve mucokinesis by inhalational methods.[22] The exposure of patients to various aromatic vapors and burning incenses, or simply to steaming water, dates back to the early days of folk medicine, and many of the methods used today have hundreds of years of use behind them. The pharmacologic therapy of retained respiratory secretions is still largely based upon inhalational remedies.

In the past hundred years or so, oral agents have become popular, and although such drugs are well-recognized and are

TABLE 2–4. CLASSIFICATION OF MUCOKINETIC DRUGS*

Class	Action	Examples

Agents that increase the depth of the sol-layer	Topical diluents
	Bronchial gland stimulators:
	    direct
	    blood-borne
	    vagal action
	Hyperosmotic agents
		Water, electrolyte solutions
		Bronchomucotropic agents:
		    inhaled irritants
		    iodides
		    subemetic doses of emetics
		Bronchorrheics, e.g. hypertonic saline

Agents that decrease the viscosity of the gel-layer (usually "mucolytics")	Agents that split disulfide bonds
	Enzymes
	Agents that break mucoprotein-DNA
	    complexes
	Agents that alter mucoprotein production
	Activators of proteases
	Reducing agents
	Agents that break hydrogen bonds
	Agents that chelate with calcium
		Thiols, e.g. acetylcysteine
		Dornase, trypsin
		Hypertonic salts, e.g. saline, sodium
		    bicarbonate
		S-carbocysteine, bromhexine
		Iodide, electrolytes
		Ascorbic acid + copper
		Urea, 1-arginine
		1-arginine, hypertonic saline

Agents that decrease the adhesiveness of the gel-layer	Wetting agents Surface-active agents	Water, sodium ethasulfate Tyloxapol, sodium bicarbonate, propylene glycol

*Mucokinetic drugs that stimulate ciliary activity are listed in Table 2–6.

pharmacologically classified as expectorants, their ability to induce or improve expectoration is often lacking in convincing proof.

The pharmacologic management of respiratory secretions is based upon four broad concepts:

1. Increasing the depth of the sol-layer
2. Altering the consistency of the gel-layer
3. Decreasing the adhesiveness of the gel-layer
4. Improvement of ciliary activity.

It is not always certain that a given drug has an action that can be classified on the basis of these concepts, but in the following discussion the concepts will be explained and simplified to help provide a rational basis for drug therapy (Table 2–4).

DRUGS THAT INCREASE THE DEPTH OF THE SOL-LAYER

Many patients with respiratory distress and sputum retention are relatively dehydrated. This occurs as a result of rapid or deep breathing, which increases the amount of water vapor lost in the expirate, or because of anxiety or fever, which cause sweating, or it follows from decreased fluid intake secondary to dyspnea and exhaustion. As a result, there is a decrease in the serous component of bronchial gland secretions; these glands and the goblet cells exude more viscous secretions. Under such conditions, the sol-layer becomes decreased in depth, and the gel-layer becomes thicker.

The appropriate relationship between the two layers of secretions overlying the cilia can be improved by adding water to the sol-layer. This can be achieved by nebulizing or instilling *water* or an *electrolyte solution* into the bronchial tree; the water rains out and becomes incorporated into the gel-layer, which becomes less viscous, and some of the water enters the sol-layer, increasing its depth. Electrolytes may have a specific depolymerizing effect on the complex proteins in sputum,[7] and their osmotic effect draws water into the sol-layer from the mucosa.

The sol-layer can also be increased in depth by stimulating the bronchial glands to

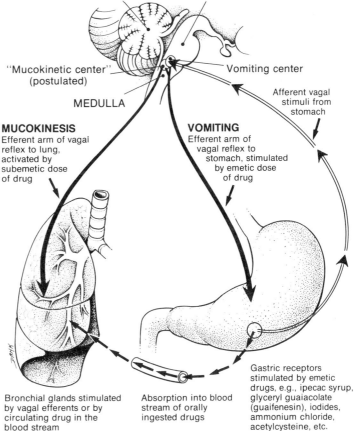

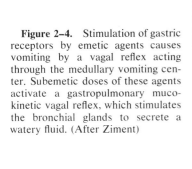

Figure 2–4. Stimulation of gastric receptors by emetic agents causes vomiting by a vagal reflex acting through the medullary vomiting center. Subemetic doses of these agents activate a gastropulmonary mucokinetic vagal reflex, which stimulates the bronchial glands to secrete a watery fluid. (After Ziment)

CEREBELLUM   PONS

"Mucokinetic center" (postulated)

Vomiting center

MEDULLA

Afferent vagal stimuli from stomach

MUCOKINESIS
Efferent arm of vagal reflex to lung, activated by subemetic dose of drug

VOMITING
Efferent arm of vagal reflex to stomach, stimulated by emetic dose of drug

Bronchial glands stimulated by vagal efferents or by circulating drug in the blood stream

Absorption into blood stream of orally ingested drugs

Gastric receptors stimulated by emetic drugs, e.g., ipecac syrup, glyceryl guaiacolate (guaifenesin), iodides, ammonium chloride, acetylcysteine, etc.

secrete more actively. Boyd[22] has referred to agents that act in this fashion as *broncho-mucotropic agents,* but this term has fallen into disuse. Increased bronchial gland secretion can be achieved by improving the patient's general hydration, which will make fluid more readily available to the glands. The administration of oral or intravenous fluids can thus help restore the appropriate depth to the sol-layer.

Most so-called oral expectorants are believed to act by stimulating the bronchial glands to secrete. The majority of oral expectorants act on the gastric mucosa to initiate reflex stimulation of the vagal efferent nerve supply to the bronchial glands.[26] The brain center for vomiting is in the lateral reticular formation of the medulla oblongata,[28] in close association with the center for coughing. An *emetic* drug stimulates vagal afferents through gastric receptors, and thereby activates the vomiting (emetic) center. If the reflex is completed through the efferent vagal nerve to the stomach, vomiting will result. A weaker afferent stimulus seems to result in activation of vagal efferents to the pulmonary plexus,

which supplies the bronchial glands. In this fashion, a subemetic dose of an emetic drug results in reflex stimulation of the bronchial glands, causing them to secrete, thereby improving mucokinesis. This reflex can be termed the *gastropulmonary mucokinetic vagal reflex* (Fig. 2–4), and it may be postulated that there is a mucokinetic center in the medulla oblongata close to the vomiting center.[4] This explains why vomiting is often accompanied by throat-clearing and expectoration. It has long been known that asthmatics (particularly children) with inspissated respiratory secretions improve if they are made to vomit; that is, they "vomit" from their lungs as well as from their stomachs.

Expectorants that act through the mucokinetic reflex will, in larger doses, cause sufficient gastric irritation to result in vomiting; thus, expectorant drugs in excessive dosage act as emetics (Fig. 2–5). It is possible that natural emetics, such as mustard and concentrated salt solution, may improve mucokinesis. It would be expected that mustard, horse-radish, garlic, chiles, curry and peppers, which cause increased

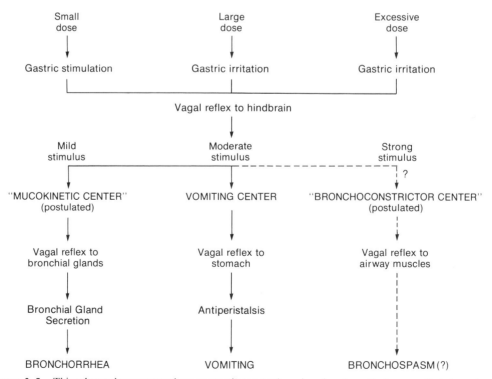

Figure 2–5. This scheme demonstrates how an emetic agent when given in subemetic dose results in bronchorrhea. Theoretically, an excessive emetic dose could stimulate the vagal efferents to the airway muscles, thereby causing bronchoconstriction.

salivation and nasal mucosal irritation (with consequent nasal secretion and sneezing), and which may also act as emetics, would augment bronchial gland secretion.[28] Indeed, there is a suspicion that respiratory patients belonging to ethnic groups that eat "hot" foods and condiments may have less trouble with inspissated secretions complicating bronchitis.[29] Those who eat such diets rarely seem to require intubation or tracheostomy to facilitate management of secretions during the course of their chronic obstructive disease.

Finally, some drugs are believed to act directly on the bronchial gland once a suitable blood level is obtained following oral or intravenous administration. *Iodides,* in particular, appear to stimulate bronchial gland secretion by direct action. Good evidence for this effect is provided by the frequent occurrence of excessive nasal and parotid gland secretions following iodide therapy. In fact, one of the unpleasant toxic manifestations of iodide administration is parotid swelling, resembling mumps, caused by excessive stimulus to the salivary gland, which secretes more fluid than can be drained out by the parotid duct.

The bronchial glands can be stimulated to secrete by a variety of noxious inhalational agents. The most obvious example is tobacco smoke, which many chronic smokers consider to be a morning requirement to help them expectorate the night's accumulation of thick secretions. If a chronic bronchitic stops smoking, expectoration may be quite difficult for the next few days; relief takes two to three weeks, when the inflamed respiratory mucosa will have had an opportunity to recover and goblet cell activity will have diminished. Other noxious fumes and vapors, such as smog, poison gases or industrial fumes, can result in irritative activation of the bronchial glands. Water or saline solutions delivered by aerosol may have a lesser effect, which, however, appears to be entirely therapeutic.[30] The increased irritation associated with ultrasonic aerosol use may not be completely benign;[31] bronchospasm may be induced and adverse mucosal changes may occur, particularly when hypertonic solutions are nebulized. Pathologic stimulation of bronchial gland secretion may result in excessive amounts of secretions of low viscosity; this fluid is termed bronchorrhea. It is often difficult to distinguish bronchorrhea from mucolysis after nebulizing certain solutions of mucolytic drugs, as will be explained later.

DRUGS THAT ALTER THE CONSISTENCY OF THE GEL-LAYER

When the gel-layer becomes thickened by dehydration or biochemical changes or by the addition of the products of inflammation, the viscosity increases and cephalad propulsion of the mucociliary blanket is impeded. When thickened mucus reaches the larynx, further progress depends upon coughing, and it is at this level that the secretions frequently accumulate in the patient with chronic obstructive disease.[19]

The causes of the increase in viscosity are not clear, but it is believed that increased numbers of complex molecular strands with intermolecular bonding accounts for much of the hyperviscosity of abnormal sputum. The admixture of cellular debris and DNA causes increased purulence and may result in increased viscosity.[32, 33] Effective treatment of the underlying process, by the use of antimicrobial agents for instance, will eventually return the gel-layer to its normal consistency.

More immediate thinning of the viscous gel-layer requires the topical application of water, which hydrates and thins out the gelatinous mucus, or of drugs that break down the complex molecular strands. Agents able to alter the molecular composition of mucopolysaccharides, DNA or cell debris are called *mucolytics.*[34] Three classes of mucolytic drugs can be defined:

1. Agents that rupture disulfide bonds
2. Proteolytic enzymes
3. Miscellaneous mucolytics.

Agents That Rupture Disulfide Bonds. The viscosity of sputum is correlated with the presence of disulfide bridges between the long mucopolysaccharide strands, resulting in a network of matted molecules.

Breakage of disulfide bonds results in a marked decrease in the viscosity of mucus, and the most successful mucolytic agents that have been investigated appear to produce their effects by this mechanism. In 1963, Sheffner[35] reported on L-cysteine and its congeners, which have viscosity-reducing properties for both mucoid and purulent sputum. The quality possessed by all agents tested by Sheffner was the presence of a free *sulfhydryl group,* which participates in a sulfhydryl-disulfide interchange reaction, thereby rupturing the disulfide bridges of mucoproteins, resulting in depolymerization (see Fig. 3–1). Such agents are classified as *thiol compounds.* The most suitable of the sulfhydryl compounds tested proved to be the N-acetyl derivative of L-cysteine, *acetylcysteine* (Mucomyst). L-cysteine, although of similar potency to that of acetylcysteine, is not suitable for nebulization, since it is readily oxidized in the lungs to form relatively insoluble cystine, which precipitates from solution.

Although the main effect of thiol compounds on mucus is that of disulfide bond oxidation, these agents are believed to have other important properties. The molecular configuration of the protein substrate and the spatial interaction of the sulfhydryl group with the molecule determine the overall effect. The manufacturers of the thiol compound *S-carboxymethylcysteine* (carbocysteine, Mucodyne), which has a blocked sulfhydryl group, claim that its apparent mucolytic effect is indirect, being related to its ability to stimulate the direct secretion of mucus containing an increased content of the less viscous sialoglycopeptides and sulfoglycopeptides. Many sulfhydryl compounds are also capable of disrupting the polymerization bonds of DNA, thereby reducing the viscosity of purulent sputum.

A number of other compounds possessing a free sulfhydryl group have been tested for mucolytic properties. The most active include *dithiothreitol* (which is more effective but more toxic than acetylcysteine), *2-mercaptoethane sulfonate* (Mesna, Mistabron), *N-acetylcysteamine, 2-mercaptoethanol, β-mercaptoethylamine* as well as L-cysteine.[36] Several of these are capable of reacting with and binding metals such as calcium (an action termed chelation); compounds related to 2-mercaptoethanol (such as dimercaprol, also known as British antilewisite or BAL) are used in the treatment of metal poisoning. Toxic elements such as copper, mercury and arsenic act with and inhibit essential enzymes that possess sulfhydryl bonds; certain thiol compounds with free sulfhydryl groups, such as BAL, are thought to compete for the metal, thereby protecting the enzymes. Mercaptoethanol, unlike the thiol compounds used in respiratory therapy, is very susceptible to oxidation by oxygen.

The binding of calcium by other chelating agents has been shown to decrease sputum viscosity. Thus, Lieberman[7] found that *sodium versenate* (the sodium salt of ethylenediaminetetraacetic acid, EDTA), used clinically in the management of hypercalcemia and lead poisoning, reduces the viscosity of purulent sputum in vitro. *Tetrasodium versenate* is more mucolytic than disodium versenate, perhaps because it has greater affinity for binding calcium. So far, chelating agents have not found practical application as mucolytic agents apart from their experimental use. However, it is of interest that the commercial preparation of acetylcysteine contains EDTA to protect the mucolytic agent from oxidation by oxygen, but the amount present appears to be insufficient to contribute to mucolysis.

In the U.S., the only sulfhydryl mucolytic in clinical use is acetylcysteine, but in Europe 2-mercaptoethane sulfonate and S-carboxymethylcysteine are available. *Dithiothreitol* (1, 4-dithiomesoerithritol, Riker 746, Cleland's Reagent, Sputolysin) is used as a laboratory agent for reducing sputum viscosity; it is used to homogenize sputum since it does not inhibit the microflora nor does it alter cellular morphology in cytologic specimens. Although L-cysteine is an effective mucolytic, other amino acids have not proved to be as successful.

Proteolytic Enzymes. Enzymes are proteins derived from animals, plants or bacteria. They act specifically on substrates to bring about a rapid biochemical change, as occurs in the normal processes of digestion and decay. The enzymatic breakdown of complex protein substrates usually results in the production of smaller, more soluble molecules that are more readily transported within the body.[37] Enzymatic degradation of respiratory tract fluid proteins results in products that are less viscous than the original mucoproteins and DNA.

Sputum undergoes spontaneous change due to natural proteolytic enzymes released by leucocytes, bacteria and other cells in the material, but this normal digestive process is relatively slow and unimpressive. The addition of topical enzymes to sputum in vitro produces a much more dramatic breakdown; several enzymes have been used therapeutically for this purpose. The main inhalational enzymes are derived from animal or bacterial sources, but some plant enzymes have also been reported to be effective. The inhalational enzymes are all highly purified, but they are capable of causing unpleasant toxic reactions, either directly or by traces of impurities. In particular, they may cause febrile reactions when introduced into closed cavities, possibly because pyrogenic molecules are produced during the enzymic degradation of the complex substrates. Thus,

TABLE 2–5.   EFFECT OF DNA ON SPUTUM VISCOSITY

DNA:Mucoprotein Ratio	Intrinsic Proteolytic Enzymes	Effect on Viscosity	Comment
High	Inhibited	Increased	Viscosity can be reduced by hypertonic saline, which dissociates DNA-muco-protein complexes
Low	Active	Reduced	Similar effect achieved by removing DNA by dornase or hypertonic salt solutions

enzymes are relatively unsuitable for the topical treatment of empyemas, and they are hazardous when introduced into abscess cavities in the lung.

Various proteolytic enzymes have been used to decrease the viscosity of both purulent and nonpurulent sputum. Lieberman[7, 38] studied the effects of 12 enzymes on respiratory tract secretions from patients with cystic fibrosis. Only four of these had marked mucolytic effects: trypsin, chymotrypsin, deoxyribonuclease and elastase. The most effective agent was *trypsin,* which has a nonspecific proteolytic effect, and therefore can digest both mucoprotein and DNA. Trypsin, and to a lesser extent *chymotrypsin,* catalyze the cleavage of the peptide bonds of the mucoprotein molecule, resulting in liquefaction of mucoid sputum; these enzymes are less effective at liquefying purulent sputum. *Leucine aminopeptidase,* on the other hand, causes mucolysis of purulent but not mucoid sputum.

Purulent sputum contains proteolytic enzymes (proteases) released from disintegrating leucocytes and bacteria. There is evidence that DNA, a characteristic component of purulent sputum, inhibits natural proteolytic enzymes and protects the mucoprotein from spontaneous digestion.[32, 34] This might explain the observed resistance of purulent sputum to inherent proteolytic liquefaction, and the restoration of proteolytic activity that follows when DNA is inactivated (Table 2–5).

A number of agents have been found to potentiate the natural proteolysis in sputum. The most important of these are *iodides,* which enhance proteolytic breakdown to a greater degree than do other inorganic salts such as hypertonic sodium chloride.[39] It has been suggested that proteolysis results from the ability of iodides to split glycoproteins, thereby making them more susceptible to proteolytic enzyme action. Certain organic compounds containing iodine, which had been reported by Lieberman as being

even more effective inducers of proteolysis (thyroxine and several of its analogues), were subsequently retested and were found to be devoid of mucolytic properties.[7]

The enzyme *deoxyribonuclease* (DNAase, pancreatic dornase, Dornavac) causes depolymerization of DNA, and results in a marked decrease in viscosity of pus-containing secretions. This effect, however, might depend more on the fact that DNAase, by breaking down DNA, permits the intrinsic proteases to induce secondary liquefaction.[5, 17] Purulent sputum is usually, but not always, more viscous than mucoid sputum:[40] in patients with chronic sputopathies (nonspecific sputum production), who are free of active respiratory tract infection, the sputum may, in fact, be expectorated with relative ease. Therefore, enzyme therapy is not indicated for the stable patient with bronchitis whose sputum appears purulent, unless there is concomitant marked hyperviscosity.

Although DNAase is the most effective agent for digesting DNA, the viscosity of sputum that contains DNA can also be reduced by other proteolytic enzymes and by simpler agents. Thus, *hypertonic salt solutions* cause dissociation of nucleoprotein complexes, and alkalinization of sputum decreases the inhibition of both natural and therapeutic proteases by DNA.[32]

Two other enzymes are available for clinical use, and they have been employed as mucolytics. These are *streptodornase* and *streptokinase;* they are natural enzymes obtained from certain streptococci. Streptodornase is similar to pancreatic dornase, and it functions as a deoxyribonuclease. Streptokinase is an activator of the plasma factor plasminogen, and it can activate the fibrinolytic enzymes in human plasma, thereby resulting in the breakdown of fibrin and fibrinogen. Although fibrin and fibrinogen may be present in mucus, streptokinase has not been shown to have mucolytic properties. These enzymes are irritating to tissue and they release pyrogens; therefore they are not considered to be suitable for clinical use.[41]

A number of other enzymes have mucolytic activity.[42] *Lysozyme,* a natural enzyme in mucoid secretions, has been shown to reduce the viscosity of nasal secretions. *Helicidin,* an extract from snail mucus, has been of benefit when nebulized into children with whooping cough. High concentrations of *bromelain* (a mixture of proteolytic enzymes from the pineapple plant), and *papain* and *ficin* (plant enzymes) may be capable of digesting sputum.[7] What is more important is that papain can digest living tissues; in fact, it is given experimentally by nebulization to produce emphysematous changes in the lungs of animals. Certain bacteria produce enzymes such as mucinases and hyaluronidase, and myxoviruses produce neuraminase; these mucolytic enzymes may enable pathogens to breach the respiratory tract mucus barrier. The use of all these various enzymes as mucolytics has no place at present in clinical practice.

The proteolytic enzymes do not alter cellular components in secretions; therefore they are of value in the laboratory for homogenizing sputum specimens submitted for cytologic examination. Although most of them do not attack living tissue, none are used as routine mucolytics in clinical situations, because they are irritating to the respiratory tract. Moreover, since they are proteins, they may also stimulate the production of antibodies, thereby provoking sensitization reactions. There is a theoretical fear that proteolytic enzymes may be damaging to the lungs of patients who have α_1-antitrypsin deficiency,[34] but this adverse effect has not been seen in practice.

Miscellaneous Mucolytics. A number of agents have been reported capable of causing mucolysis by splitting up mucoprotein molecules.

Various *mucolytic amides* have a liquefying effect on proteins,[43] and it is possible that mucolysis is caused by the breakage of mucoprotein molecules into smaller and less asymmetrical components. The in vitro addition of *urea* (carbamide) can induce liquefaction of mucoid and purulent sputum, but the amounts required are too large for clinical application in the respiratory tract. Urea is also said to have mist-stabilizing properties, and bacteriostatic qualities. However, although it might be a useful adjunct in aerosol therapy, it has not gained acceptance.

Ascorbic acid (vitamin C) in the presence of oxygen causes depolymerization of mucopolysaccharides; the action is catalyzed by cupric ions. A freshly made solution of ascorbic acid, sodium percarbonate and copper sulfate (known variously as oxymist, Ascumist, Ascoxal and Gumox) had been claimed to be an effective mucolytic. The compound releases nascent oxygen that reacts with ascorbic acid (Asc-Ox reaction), and this was believed to result in the depolymerization of mucopolysaccharides. It is possible that the relatively high osmolality of the oxymist aerosol stimulates a nonspecific exudation of fluid from the respiratory mucosa, thereby resulting in dilution of the mucus, rather than in depolymerization of the mucoproteins. This consideration also applies to other inhalational mucolytic agents, for which in vitro effectiveness cannot be disputed, but whose in vivo action may depend on their hypertonicity, which produces bronchorrhea rather than mucolysis. Some workers suggest that the mucolytic action of oxymist depends on the low pH of the ascorbic acid; this, however, is controversial.

Hyperosmolar salt solutions have a proteolytic effect, and various hypertonic electrolyte solutions have been shown to aid in producing mucolysis.[7, 32] Hypertonic solutions of saline, ammonium chloride and sodium bicarbonate can decrease mucus viscosity when applied topically by nebulization or by instillation into the respiratory tract.[11, 45] Lieberman[7] has shown that monovalent ions (such as sodium chloride, sodium iodide and sodium thiocyanide), in strengths greater than molar, reduce the viscosity of purulent sputum in vitro; however, mucoid sputum is not affected. Bivalent ions (such as magnesium chloride, calcium chloride and ammonium sulfate) are effective in less concentrated solutions, such as half-molar. Lieberman found that two-molar ammonium sulfate causes almost instantaneous liquefaction. He also noted that certain electrolyte solutions seemed to cause an initial increase in sputum viscosity prior to liquefaction. The mucolytic action of these electrolyte solutions results from the ions causing dissociation of nucleoprotein-mucoprotein complexes, thereby rendering the mucoprotein available for the proteolytic action of the natural proteases in the purulent sputum (see Table 2–5). Mucoid sputum, which lacks DNA and proteases, is not affected by electrolytes in this way. A further possibility is that monovalent ions may exchange with calcium in cross-linkages in the mucoprotein molecular strands, thereby leading to a dissociation of the fibrillar network; thus, mucoid sputum may be lysed to some extent.

DRUGS THAT DECREASE THE ADHESIVENESS OF THE GEL-LAYER

A major problem with thick or sticky respiratory tract secretions is increased adhesiveness, which makes it difficult to detach the mucoid material from the walls of the airways. Secretions may be thick and viscous, yet may have relatively little adhesiveness. On the other hand, some sputum specimens show a remarkable degree of adhesiveness to glass and plastic; this property may also be manifested by unexpectorated sputum in the airways. Pharmacologic agents that exert a surface effect may decrease adhesiveness without causing any change in the macromolecular structure of the sputum. Such agents have been called wetting agents or detergents, and can be classified as surface active agents or *surfactants:* they produce a decrease in surface tension of respiratory tract secretions.[42, 45, 46]

Such agents reduce the tendency of solutions to form cohesive drops, thereby resulting in a spreading out of the fluid as a film of larger surface area. If a glass slide is coated with such a surfactant, sticky mucus on the slide will move more readily under gravity than it would if no surfactant were present. It is thought that surfactants can reduce the cohesive forces in respiratory tract secretions, facilitating the penetration of topical medications into the mucoid material.

Surfactants are classified as anionic, cationic, nonionic or amphoteric.[47] The nonionic surfactants include the inhalational agents *glycerol, propylene glycol* and *tyloxapol*. *Ethasulfate* is an anionic surfactant. Although all these drugs have been marketed in combination preparations for the inhalational treatment of viscous secretions, few controlled trials have been carried out to determine the value of the individual agents. In fact, much of the experience that has been obtained suggests that the surfactants contribute little of therapeutic significance, and they have not gained the popularity that early reports forecasted. Certainly, such agents do not have any mucolytic activity.[7]

DRUGS THAT IMPROVE CILIARY ACTIVITY
(Table 2–6)

Patients who have inflammatory diseases of the respiratory tract may be at double jeopardy with regard to mucus. Not only are the respiratory tract secretions excessive and of increased viscosity, but the damage to the mucosa is liable to impair ciliary function. Improvement of ciliary function results in an important contribution to effective mucokinesis. Although little is known about either normal ciliary activity or the various factors associated with abnormal function, it is probable that the following are important: rate and force of beat, direction of metachronal wave and coordination of cilia.[12, 14, 18] In some ways, the functional behavior of the cilia resembles that of heart muscle cells, and although the cilia do not appear to be under nervous system control, it has been postulated that a "pacemaker" mechanism may control their activity. It is possible that certain drugs that improve mucokinesis act on this hypothesized pacemaker to cause a more effective ciliary beat.

Relatively few experiments have been carried out to evaluate the response of cilia to aerosolized medications, but the findings are of interest. Parasympathomimetic drugs are known to impair mucokinesis, but they seem to achieve this by impairing mucus

TABLE 2–6. DRUGS THAT STIMULATE CILIARY ACTIVITY*

Class	Examples
Sympathomimetics	Isoproterenol, terbutaline, etc.
Phosphodiesterase inhibitors	Theophylline
Ions	Sodium, calcium, potassium
Salts	Potassium iodide, sodium chloride, ammonium chloride
Cholinergic agents	Acetylcholine, pilocarpine
Alkaloids	Veratrum, strophanthin, digitalis
Local anesthetics†	Tetracaine, dibucaine, cocaine
General anesthetics†	Ether, chloroform, cyclopropane
Mediator	Serotonin (aerosol only)
Antimediator	Prednisolone
Smoke and pollutants	Tobacco, sulfur dioxide (in some subjects)
Volatile oils	Terpene

*In general, aerosols are most effective, but many of these agents have a significant effect when administered by other routes
†Low concentrations

production rather than by decreasing ciliary activity. In contrast, *sympathomimetic drugs* seem to primarily affect the cilia, and many of them increase the rate of mucus transportation along the tracheobronchial tree. *Isoproterenol, epinephrine, racemic epinephrine, terbutaline* and *carbuterol* have been found to increase ciliary activity when administered by nebulization or parenterally, to animals or humans with airway disease.[13, 14, 48–50] Other drugs that improve ciliary activity include *prednisolone, potassium iodide, ammonium chloride, acetylcholine, pilocarpine* and *aminophylline*.[17]

Histamine, in moderate or low concentrations, does not affect the cilia, but certain other messengers, including *serotonin* and *ATP,* when given by aerosol, improve ciliary activity.[13, 14] The "anti-messenger" drug cromolyn may slightly decrease mucociliary transport.[48] It is disappointing that some of the popular mucokinetic drugs, such as acetylcysteine, tyloxapol and alcohol, when given by aerosol, markedly slow ciliary transport of mucus; other surface-active agents may have a similar effect[14].

Certain ions improve the ciliary beating action; although normal saline has little direct effect on the cilia, there is evidence that *calcium* and *iodides* do have such an action.[13] It is believed that this effect constitutes a further reason for favoring potassium iodide or sodium iodide as mucokinetic drugs. Unfortunately, there is no information as to the effect on cilia of other popular "expectorants," such as glyceryl guaiacolate and ipecacuanha. It is of interest that *strophanthin (ouabain)* and other *digitalis derivatives,* drugs used for their powerful effect on heart muscle, have a stimulatory effect on cilia;[13, 14] however, no therapeutic effect on mucus transport has been noted clinically as yet, although it is possible that cardiac glycosides improve ciliary transport depressed by hypoxia.[51]

Rather surprisingly, some *local anesthetics,* such as tetracaine and dibucaine, when given in low concentration, result in ciliary stimulation.[13] Other agents, such as lidocaine and procaine, however, result in uncoordination of the ciliary beat; hexylcaine has a particularly long lasting, inhibitory effect. Certain noxious gases and fumes have a similar toxic action, but carbon monoxide, carbon dioxide and nicotine do not seem to directly affect the cilia. An acidic environment is said to inhibit ciliary activity;[52] thus, secretions with a low pH may contribute to mucokinetic impairment.

Fiberbronchoscopy will enable more exact studies of ciliary activity to be carried out. Various drugs claimed to have stimulatory effects on cilia (such as iodides, catecholamines and veratrum) will undoubtedly be subjected to more careful observations, and the range of mucokinetic drugs that stimulate the cilia is likely to be extended.

EVALUATION OF MUCOKINETIC AGENTS

The effectiveness of a diuretic can be readily determined, since it is easy to collect and quantify urine output, and the fluid can be accurately evaluated both chemically and physically. Unfortunately, respiratory tract secretions are difficult to collect, and efforts at quantification by weight or volume are frustrating and inaccurate. Moreover, chemical and physical examinations are unreliable at best, and unavailable in general. Thus, most physicians and therapists subjectively evaluate the effectiveness of a mucokinetic by judging qualitatively whether the expectorated material has increased in amount and decreased in stickiness.

Various techniques have been developed to help quantify the physical characteristics of sputum. Such rheologic tests usually examine the consistency or viscosity of the material, or the response of the fluid to shearing stress. Since sputum is a nonhomogeneous fluid (i.e., it is non-Newtonian) it shows a changing viscosity in response to changes in the rate of shear. "Consistency" might be a more accurate measure of sputum's fluid character than is "viscosity." Instruments that have been used in quantitative evaluations include consistometers, viscosimeters, consisto-viscosimeters and capillary shearing systems.[3, 7, 36, 53–56] There is, no standardized methodology or instrumentation for measuring the "viscoelastic" properties of sputum. Lieberman, who has done some of the best work on sputum, considers the cone-plate viscosimeter to be the most valuable instrument for measuring changes in viscosity.[7, 56] However, numerous other methods have been reported to be of value in the rheologic evaluation of sputum[57] (Table 2–7).

Chodosh[58] recommends studying the flow of sputum in an inclined tube, and points out that the adhesiveness or stickiness of the material is the most important parameter in practice. However, Hirsch and Kory[39] contest the value of such measurements of

TABLE 2–7. TECHNIQUES FOR RHEOLOGIC EVALUATION OF SPUTUM

U-tube viscometer
Falling-sphere viscometer
Concentric-cylinder viscometer
Cone-plate viscometer
Other fluid consisto-viscosimeters
Perforated disc
Chemical balance rheometer
Magnetic rheometer
Rheogoniometer (oscillation)
Rheogoniometer (creep testing)
Inclined tube (flow)

---

consistency and, in common with most other investigators, they prefer the use of the fluid consisto-viscosimeter.

Unfortunately, much of the experimental work on sputum pharmacology has been hampered by the lack of agreement or standardization in the field. Some workers simply evaluate an expectorant by measuring the volume expectorated following delivery of the drug; this approach may be of more practical value than the sophisticated measurements of flow characteristics. However, there is always concern that the expectorated materials are not true lower respiratory tract secretions, but that they consist mainly of oropharyngeal secretions.

Sophisticated instrumentation is rarely available as a guide to pharmacologic therapy in most hospitals and clinics, but physicians and therapists should nevertheless attempt to determine the effectiveness of the therapy that they employ. In general, it is possible to make a collection of a patient's

TABLE 2–8. EXAMINATION OF SPUTUM

QUANTITY – should be evaluated every eight hours.

TIME OF MAXIMUM EXPECTORATION –
  should be correlated with treatments

COLOR – white: suggests no significant cellular
             content
         yellow: suggests polymorphs or eosinophils
         green: suggests infection, with stagnation
         red or brown: suggests blood

ODOR – anaerobes, *Pseudomonas,* and urea-splitting
  organisms are readily detected

ADHESIVENESS – most relevant rheologic test

ALTERATIONS IN ADHESIVENESS – with
  mucokinetic agents can be grossly tested at
  bedside

HOMOGENEITY – best evaluated by allowing
  sample to stand in test tube and layer out

MICROSCOPY – allows detection of macrophages,
  other cells, structural components, microorganisms

---

sputum, which can be quantified daily. The use of an inclined tube also enables the average practitioner to determine, in a gross fashion, whether or not there has been a change in the sputum consistency and adhesiveness.

Rational mucokinetic therapy can only be achieved if drug administration is correlated with the results.[21] Thus, every time a course of treatment is given, the respiratory therapist should regard it as his or her responsibility to make observations on the patient's sputum.[60, 61] The quantity should be recorded, and color, homogeneity and stickiness should be noted (Table 2–8). The therapist is also in a position to judge which of several possible topical agents might be most suitable. Whenever feasible, the expectorated sputum should be divided into a number of specimens of about 0.5 ml (using a syringe, or wooden sticks or forceps), and the samples should be placed in plastic or glass cups, or on slides. To each of the specimens, a few drops of an agent (e.g., saline, sodium bicarbonate, alcohol, acetylcysteine) should be added, and the specimens agitated gently. After one or two minutes it should be possible to determine whether the agent had an appreciable effect on the sputum consistency and viscosity.

Such tests do have limitations, unfortunately. First, sputum is difficult to maneuver into aliquot specimens and, of course, glass or plastic hardly represents the respiratory mucosa. The few drops of drug represents a considerably greater surface contact than would be achieved by nebulizing a few ml of the agent into the patient's lungs, and a more dramatic effect may be expected in the in vitro test situation. Usually, this test shows that acetylcysteine has the most marked effect; this is not unexpected, since all the studies on laboratory specimens have shown that this drug is an outstanding mucolytic. Again, one cannot be sure that success in the laboratory or at the bedside will guarantee successful mucolysis in a particular patient. However, the important observations in these bedside tests are: first, whether acetylcysteine has a definite mucolytic effect on the sputum specimen; and second, whether any other agent has an equivalent or a more marked effect. Quite often, the bedside test shows that an agent such as sodium bicarbonate has a more definite effect on decreasing a particular sputum's adhesiveness than does acetylcysteine. Findings such as this can provide a more rational basis for selecting an agent for nebulization.

REFERENCES

1. Editorial: Bronchial secretions. Brit. Med. J. 2:51, April, 1975.
2. Charman, J., Lopez-Vidriero, M. T., Keal, E. and Reid, L.: The physical and chemical properties of bronchial secretions. Brit. J. Dis. Chest 68: 215–227, 1974.
3. Dulfano, M. J. (Ed.): Sputum. Springfield, Ill., Charles C Thomas, 1973.
4. Ziment, I.: Secretions of the Respiratory Tract. New York, Projects in Health, 1976.
5. Iravani, J. and Melville, G. N.: Mucociliary function in the respiratory tract as influenced by physiochemical factors. Pharmac. Therap. B. 2:471–496, 1976.
6. Robertson, A. J.: Green sputum. Lancet 1:12–15, 1952.
7. Lieberman, J.: Measurement of sputum viscosity in a cone-plate viscometer. An evaluation of mucolytic agents in vitro. Am. Rev. Respir. Dis. 97:662–672, 1968.
7a. diSant'Agnese, P. and Davis, P. B.: Research in cystic fibrosis, Part 3. N. Engl. J. Med. 295:597–602, 1976.
8. Palmer, K. N. V.: The effects of solutions of varying pH on in vitro sputum viscosity. Bull. Physio-path. Respir. 9:433–435, 1973.
9. Palmer, K. N. V.: Sputum liquefiers. Brit. J. Dis. Chest 60:177–181, 1966.
10. Yeager, H.: Tracheobronchial secretions. Am. J. Med. 50:493–509, 1971.
11. Lieberman, J. and Kurnick, N. B.: Influence of deoxyribonucleic acid content on the proteolysis of sputum and pus. Nature 196:988–990, 1962.
12. Kilburn, K. H.: A hypothesis for pulmonary clearance and its implications. Am. Rev. Respir. Dis. 98:449–463, 1968.
13. Okeson, A. C. and Divertie, M. B.: Cilia and bronchial clearance: the effects of pharmacologic agents and disease. Mayo Clin. Proc. 45:361–373, 1970.
14. Laurenzi, G. A., Yin, S., Collins, B. and Guarneri, J. J.: Mucus flow in the mammalian trachea. Proc. Tenth Aspen Emphysema Conf. 1967. PHS Publication 1787, pp. 27–40.
15. Sackner, M. A., Hirsch, J. and Epstein, S.: Effect of cuffed endotracheal tubes on tracheal mucous velocity. Chest 68:774–777, 1975.
16. Sackner, M. A., Hirsch, J., Epstein, S. and Rywlin, A. M.: Effect of oxygen in graded concentrations upon tracheal mucous velocity. Chest 69:164–167, 1976.
17. Iravani, J. and Melville, G. N.: Effects of drugs and environmental factors on ciliary movement. Respiration 32:157–164, 1975.
18. Satir, P.: How cilia move. Sci. Am. 231:44–52, 1974.
19. Boma, B.: Pathophysiology of the cleaning mechanism of the lung. Progr. Respir. Res 6:51–65, 1971.
20. Ebert, R. V. and Terracio, M. J.: Observation of the secretion on the surface of the bronchioles with the scanning electron microscope. Am. Rev. Respir. Dis. 112:491–496, 1975.
21. Ziment, I.: Mucokinesis – the methodology of moving mucus. Respir. Therapy 4:15–20, Mar./Apr., 1974.
22. Boyd, E. M.: Expectorants and respiratory tract fluid. Pharmacol. Rev. 6:521–542, 1954.
23. Chakrin, L. W., Baker, A. P., Christian, P. and

Wardell, J. R.: Effect of cholinergic stimulation on the release of macromolecules by canine trachea in vitro. Am. Rev. Respir. Dis. 108: 69–76, 1973.
24. Chou, D. T. and Wang, S. C.: Studies on the localization of central cough mechanism: site of actin of antitussive drugs. J. Pharmacol. Exp. Therap. 194:499–505, 1975.
25. Lagerson, J.: The cough – its effectiveness depends on you. Respir. Care 18:434–448, 1973.
26. Gunn, J. A.: The action of expectorants. Br. Med. J. 2:972–975, 1927.
27. Borison, H. L. and Wang, S. C.: Physiology and pharmacology of vomiting. Pharmacol. Rev. 5: 193–230, 1953.
28. Ziment, I.: What to expect from expectorants. J.A.M.A. 236:193–194, 1976.
29. Ziment, I.: Why folk remedies for bronchitis persist. Patient Care 9:25, Aug., 1975.
30. Lovejoy, F. W. and Morrow, P. E.: Aerosols, bronchodilators and mucolytic agents. Anesthesiology 23:460–472, 1962.
31. Malik, S. K. and Jenkins, D. E.: Alterations in airway dynamics following inhalation of ultrasonic mist. Chest 62:660–664, 1972.
32. Lieberman, J.: Inhibition of protease activity in purulent sputum by DNA. J. Lab. Clin. Med. 70:595–605, 1967.
33. Lopata, M., Barton, A. D. and Lourenco, R. V.: Biochemical characteristics of bronchial secretions in chronic obstructive pulmonary disease. Am. Rev. Respir. Dis. 110:730–739, 1974.
34. Lieberman, J.: The appropriate use of mucolytic agents. Am. J. Med. 49:1–4, 1970.
35. Sheffner, A. L.: The reduction in vitro in viscosity of mucoprotein solutions by a new mucolytic agent, N-acetyl-L-cysteine. Ann. New York Acad. Sc. 106:298–310, 1963.
36. Hirsch, S. R., Zastrow, J. E. and Kory, R. C.: Sputum liquefying agents: a comparitive in vitro evaluation. J. Lab. Clin. Med. 74:346–353, 1969.
37. Sherry, S. and Fletcher, A. P.: Proteolytic enzymes: a therapeutic evaluation. Clin. Pharmacol. Therap. 1:202–226, 1960.
38. Lieberman, J.: Enzymatic dissolution of pulmonary secretions. Am. J. Dis. Child. 104:342–348, 1962.
39. Lieberman, J. and Kurnick, N. B.: The induction of proteolysis in purulent sputum by iodides. J. Clin. Invest. 43:1892–1904, 1964.
40. Dulfano, M. J. and Adler, K. B.: Physical properties of sputum. Rheologic properties and mucociliary transport. Am. Rev. Respir. Dis. 112:341–347, 1975.
41. Lyons, H. A.: Use of therapeutic aerosols. Amer. J. Cardiol. 12:461–464, 1963.
42. Sheffner, A. L. and Lish, P. M.: Acetylcysteine and other mucolytic agents. In International Encyclopedia of Pharmacology and Therapeutics, H. Salem, and D. M. Aviado, (Eds.). Volume III. New York, Pergamon Press, 1970.
43. Lieberman, J.: In vitro evaluation of the mucolytic action of urea. J.A.M.A. 202:694–696, 1967.
44. Dulfano, M. J. and Glass, P.: An effective mucolytic aerosol in chronic bronchitis. J.A.M.A. 207:1310–1314, 1969.
45. Levine, E. R.: A more direct liquefaction of bronchial secretion by aerosol therapy. Dis. Chest 31:155–168, 1957.
46. Finley, T. N.: Pulmonary surface activity and the

problems of atelectasis, wetting, foaming and detergency in the lung. Anes. Analg. 42:35–42, 1963.

47. Blacow, N. W. (Ed.): Martindale: The Extra Pharmacopoeia. London, The Pharmaceutical Press, 26th Edition, 1972, pp. 385–391.

48. Blair, A. M. J. N. and Woods, A.: The effects of isoprenaline, atropine and disodium cromoglycate on ciliary motility and mucus flow measured *in vivo* in cats. Brit. J. Pharmacol. 35: 379P–380P, 1969.

49. Cruz, R. S., Landa, J., Hirsch, J. and Sackner, M. A.: Tracheal mucous velocity in normal man and patients with obstructive disease; effects of terbutaline. Am. Rev. Respir. Dis. 109:458–463, 1974.

50. Sackner, M. A., Epstein, M. and Wanner, A.: Effect of beta-adrenergic agonists aerosolized by freon propellant on tracheal mucous velocity and cardiac output. Chest 69:593–598, 1976.

51. Newhouse, M. T.: Factors affecting sputum clearance. Thorax 28:262, 1973.

52. Negus, V. E.: Ciliary activity. Thorax 4:57, 1949.

53. Adler, K. B., Wooten, O. and Dulfano, M. J.: Mammalian respiratory mucociliary clearance. Arch. Environ. Health 27:364–369, 1973.

54. Adler, K., Dulfano, M. J. and Wooten, O.: Physical properties of sputum. Am. Rev. Respir. Dis. 109:490–493, 1974.

55. Reid, L.: The bronchial mucous glands and their acid glycoproteins. Progr. Respir. Res. 6:29–42, 1971.

56. Lieberman, J.: Measurement of sputum viscosity in a cone-plate viscometer. Characteristics of sputum viscosity. Am Rev. Respir. Dis. 97: 654–661, 1968.

57. Davis, S. S.: Rheological examination of sputum and saliva and the effect of drugs. *In* Rheology of Biological Systems. H. L. Galebnick and M. Litt (Eds.). Springfield Ill., Charles C Thomas, 1973.

58. Chodosh, S. and Medici, T. C.: Expectorant effect of glyceryl guaiacolate. Chest 64:543–544, 1973.

59. Hirsch, S. R. and Kory, R. C.: Expectorant effect of glyceryl guaiacolate. Chest 64:544–545, 1973.

60. Chodosh, S., Baigelman, W. and Pizzuto, D.: Examining sputum. Am. Fam. Physician 12: 116–121, Sept. 1975.

61. Epstein, R. L.: Constituents of sputum: a simple method. Ann. Intern. Med. 77:259–265, 1972.

CHAPTER
3
MUCOKINETIC AGENTS

It is difficult to classify mucokinetic agents according to their pharmacologic properties, since the exact mechanism by which they work is not always known. However, they can be broadly classified according to their method of administration, and subclassified on a pharmacologic basis as in Table 2–4. In this chapter, the more important agents will be considered according to the following classification:

A. Inhalational agents (may also be effective when given orally)
  1. Water
  2. Saline solutions — hypotonic, isotonic, hypertonic
  3. Hygroscopic agents — propylene glycol
  4. True mucolytics
    a) Thiols — acetylcysteine, 2-mercaptoethane sodium sulfonate
    b) Enzymes — deoxyribonuclease, trypsin, chymotrypsin, streptodornase and streptokinase
  5. Surfactants — Alevaire, sodium bicarbonate, ethanol, ethasulfate
  6. Volatile agents
    a) Balsams
    b) Other volatile oils
B. Oral agents (sometimes given by inhalation)
  1. Vagal stimulants — salt solutions, creosote derivatives, terpenes, ipecacuanha
  2. Direct mucokinetics — iodides, bromhexine, carbocysteine, others
C. Secondary agents — including additives and synergists.

INHALATIONAL MUCOKINETIC AGENTS

The traditional forms of inhalation therapy still have a large following of appreciative patients, but the development of modern respirators, humidifiers and nebulizers has made the simpler techniques less popular. Most traditional, expectorant, inhalational remedies for sputopathies were added to water, which was used as a carrier base in the form of a vapor or as droplets. The favored expectorants used in the past were, in general, easily volatilized solid or liquid drugs, and they usually had a "medicinal" odor. Often, the therapeutic mixture was essentially no more than aromatic water vapor. The modern inhalational agents still employ water as a carrier vehicle, but the drugs are usually present in substantial concentrations and exert a definite pharmacologic effect.

Although many drugs and placebos have been given by inhalation throughout the ages, relatively few have survived during the era of scientific pharmacology. In Europe, specific pharmaceuticals to improve mucokinesis are rarely administered by inhalation, whereas in the United States the tremendous growth of inhalation therapy has favored extensive use of inhalational drugs. However, even in the U.S., the number of acceptable specific agents is surprisingly small. Moreover, most of these agents have gained little acceptance in countries such as Great Britain, where sputum is by no means an unknown entity. Some of the disadvan-

TABLE 3–1. PROBLEMS ASSOCIATED WITH INHALATIONAL MUCOKINETIC THERAPY

ADMINISTRATION	Requires relatively expensive apparatus.
	Requires skilled personnel.
	Requires cooperative patient.
QUESTION OF EFFECT	Laboratory proof of value does not necessarily imply effectiveness in patient.
	Effect in patient is difficult to quantify.
	A "mucolytic" agent may cause increased expectoration only because its irritant effect or hypertonicity results in bronchorrhea.
	Nebulized agents are also swallowed, and the resulting gastric stimulation may be the major cause of any improved mucokinesis (via vagal reflex).
OVER-EFFECTIVENESS	Loosened secretions may impact distally if patient does not cough or drain out the material.
	Some patients become more hypoxic when loosened material is redistributed in airways.
SIDE EFFECTS	Bronchospasm and irritation of mucosa may be produced.
	Unpleasant side effects may result in patient refusing adequate dosage.

tages of inhalational mucokinetics are listed in Table 3–1.

The major problems in the use of inhalational mucokinetics are the special requirements of personnel and equipment; this form of therapy is difficult, time-consuming and expensive, and is only acceptable as routine in a country that can afford it. The second major problem is the difficulty in determining whether specific drugs, that have a desirable effect on sputum in the laboratory are beneficial when introduced into the respiratory tree. In Chapter 2 it was recommended that bedside evaluations be made. However, the demonstration of the effectiveness of a drug in vitro is no guarantee that success can be achieved in the patient; therefore, much of the available theoretic and laboratory data may give misleading impressions about the effectiveness of various drugs.

The more effective mucolytic agents irritate the respiratory mucosa, and appear to cause some degree of bronchospasm and ciliary inhibition; they may even result in low-grade mucosal inflammation. The increased production of respiratory secretions with a lower viscosity, that is a favorable outcome of the therapy, may represent *bronchorrhea,* resulting from the outpouring of serous fluid from the irritated tracheobronchial tree. Thus, post-therapy expectoration does not necessarily indicate that distally impacted secretions have been mobilized. Further problems in ensuring effective mucokinesis were discussed in Chapter 2.

The negative aspects of economic and scientific considerations explain the relative disenchantment with inhalational mucokinetic therapy in many parts of the world, and there recently has been a waning of enthusiasm for this form of therapy in the U.S. The

following section will discuss, in detail, the individual agents commonly employed by American physicians and respiratory therapists, who may still feel that there is adequate clinical experience to justify continued use of many of these controversial inhalational preparations.

WATER

Water is certainly the most valuable agent in inhalation therapy. It may be given as a mist (steam) or as a vapor (aerosols), or it may be directly instilled into the tracheobronchial tree. It can be given alone, or with various, medically active constituents, including electrolytes, volatile oils and more specific drugs. However, there are those who argue that water is best reserved for administration by mouth rather than by inhalation.

When water is given as hot or cold steam, it appears to soothe inflamed mucous membranes: this is its *humectant* or *demulcent* action. There is doubt about how much mist deposits in the lower airways, and there is little evidence that it actually alters the consistency of respiratory secretions.[1, 2] Nevertheless, patients often report benefit from the steam, and there is evidence that humidity can decrease sputum viscosity.[3] Some patients prefer heated mist, others prefer it cold; this sometimes depends on the temperature of both the patient and the environment, but the optimal mist can be determined only by individual trial. Treatment may be given as an individual therapy for the patient, or the room or the bed environment can be humidified on a continuous basis. Steam therapy seems to be particularly appreciated by many patients with upper and middle respiratory tract inflammation or infection, and by children with croup.

Alternatively, water can be given in droplet form by nebulization.[4] Plain water droplets can become incorporated into the gel-phase of mucus, and thereby decrease its viscosity; however, large amounts of water are required to effect any measurable change.[5] On the other hand, excessively large amounts of water simply dilute the mucoid fluid. It is clear that small amounts of water, such as can be provided by the usual aerosol treatment, have less effect on sputum viscosity than do comparable amounts of true mucolytic drugs. Although water has a time-honored role in the treatment of respiratory disease, more information is needed about its effects on tracheobronchial mucus.

Many patients find that nebulized water is irritating (particularly if given as a dense aerosol); coughing and bronchospasm may be induced.[2] During inhalation, the smaller particles of water tend to evaporate, and then recondense on larger particles by the process of isothermal distillation.[5, 6] Thus, particles either disappear or become larger, and the latter droplets tend to precipitate in the more proximal reaches of the airways. Few particles of pure water given by aerosol are deposited in the terminal bronchioles or alveoli. If an ultrasonic aerosol of plain water is administered, the small droplet particles would tend to become even smaller by evaporation, or larger by coalescence; the resulting particles would either be exhaled without deposition, or would impact proximally. Thus, ultrasonic nebulization of water does not produce optimal deposition in the distal airways. If a hygroscopic substance, such as a fatty alcohol, is added to the water, the droplets tend to be more stable, and greater precipitation can be expected in the distal airway.[6]

Plain water can be given by direct instillation, but saline is generally preferred. However, if a patient is on salt restriction, plain water would be advisable, since the instilled solution could be absorbed through the respiratory mucosa into the systemic circulation. Bacteriostatic water is the cheapest available wetting agent, and it is the obvious choice for use with home humidifiers of all degrees of sophistication: the simple steam kettle remains an active veteran of untold domiciliary battles against respiratory disease. In the hospital, it is customary to seize on such simple practices and complicate

them to the point of dubious benefit. Thus, it is more usual to administer a few ml of water in the form of an aerosol by a nebulizer with or without IPPB for 10 to 30 minutes several times a day. Furthermore, plain water is too lacking in glamor to be accepted as an optimal drug, and thus the simple breathing of steam is a comparatively rare form of inhalation therapy.

Untoward Effects. Water is relatively harmless when given in small amounts by mist or nebulization, or even by direct instillation, but inappropriate use can cause adverse effects.[7] Larger amounts of pure water (short of drowning, however!) may be well-tolerated, although mucosal engorgement may be produced by absorption of the hypotonic fluid. Patients with reactive airways may develop bronchospasm following bland nebulization; a prophylactic bronchodilator is usually advisable. Care is needed with patients who are on fluid restriction, since substantial amounts of water may be absorbed, particularly if an ultrasonic mist is administered for long periods at frequent intervals. A respiratory patient's response to humidification is individualistic, and some patients with airway disease find that a humid atmosphere makes breathing more uncomfortable, and leads to an increase in the work of breathing. Some individuals may tolerate cold mist, but not hot steam: there is marked variability, particularly in patients with reactive airways.

Administration. Water can be given in a variety of different ways, utilizing the full range of inhalational equipment. The only special requirement is that the water should be free of microorganisms. *Distilled water* is not necessary; in fact, it may be even more irritating than the relatively impure *sterile (bacteriostatic) water,* which contains small amounts of dissolved constituents. *Tap water* can be used by domiciliary patients, but it should first be boiled. It is regrettable that individual-dose packaging of water has elevated this simple fluid to the status of a relatively costly medication.

Dosage and Recommendations. One to 5 ml of water can be nebulized several times a day for its humectant effect. Larger amounts, particularly if given by an ultrasonic nebulizer for 15 to 30 minutes, can be used to induce a sputum specimen. Plain water can be instilled directly down the trachea; 5 to 10 ml is a reasonable dosage, and it can be given several times a day. Plain water can be used on its own or as a diluent for other drugs given by aerosol, but it is more irritating than saline, which is always preferable except in the rare case when electrolyte administration is contraindicated. Nebulization sessions, with or without IPPB, should probably last a minimum of 20 minutes to produce a definite mucokinetic result. During treatment sessions, coughing and expectorating should be encouraged; if necessary, physical therapy or endotracheal suctioning should be performed at the end of the session.

Various devices can be used for nonindividual therapy, such as an inexpensive room-humidifier, or even a hot shower in a small bathroom; the latter offers a useful source of humidification at home for a child with acute croup. Individual therapy can be administered by various mist tents or aerosol canopies, or by a variety of steamers, humidifiers, nebulizers and aerosolizers, with or without positive pressure. A bowl of steaming water can be used for inhalation therapy by enclosing the head and upper trunk in a simple tent improvised from a large towel. Simple methods of providing humidity may be far more reasonable for the domiciliary patient with chronic respiratory disease than are the complex and frequently overused hospital modalities of IPPB and ultrasonic nebulization. These latter require more care and attention and often result in no greater benefit than the much more available and less expensive, traditional, home methods of taking the vapors. Hospital steam tents, in particular, have been criti-cized in recent years,[2] and at present they must be regarded as providing a generally obsolete form of moisture therapy. Since inhalation therapy with plain water is of disputable value, complex, unproved modes of delivery cannot be defended as valid means of improving mucokinesis.

SALINE SOLUTIONS
(See Table 3–2)

Topical sodium chloride in low concentration decreases the viscosity of sputum by simple dilution. Hypertonic solutions have an additional osmotic effect.

Isotonic Saline

Normal saline (0.9% sodium chloride) is also known as isotonic or physiologic salt solution, since it exerts the same osmotic pressure (tonicity) as serum. One liter of the solution contains 154 milliequivalents (mEq) of sodium (Na) and an equal amount of chloride (Cl); it has an osmotic pressure of 308 milliosmols (mOs). When given by nebulization or instillation into the respiratory tract, this concentration of salt is relatively inert. The particles are stable, and deposition may occur in the more distal airways, thereby resulting in hydration of the respiratory secretions. The aerosol or mist resulting from normal saline is "bland," and it is usually very well-tolerated.

TABLE 3–2.   WATER AND ELECTROLYTE SOLUTIONS USED IN INHALATION THERAPY

	pH	Concentration of Electrolytes (mEq/ml)				
		Na^+	K^+	Cl^-	HCO_3^-	I^-
AEROSOL						
Sterile water	6.0					
Sodium chloride (saline):	4.5–7.0					
0.45% (half normal)		0.077		0.077		
0.9% (isotonic, "normal")		0.154		0.154		
3.0% (hypertonic)		0.513		0.513		
5.0% (hypertonic)		0.855		0.855		
15.0% (hypertonic)		2.565		2.565		
Sodium bicarbonate:	7.0–8.5					
1.4% (1/6 molar, near isotonic)		0.167			0.167	
5.0% (0.6 molar)		0.595			0.595	
7.5% (0.9 molar)		0.893			0.893	
8.4% (molar)		1.0			1.0	
NONAEROSOL						
Sodium iodide (intravenous)						
10% solution		0.67				0.67
Potassium iodide, oral (SSKI)			6.0			6.0
100% solution						

Hypotonic Saline

Hypotonic saline (half-normal, 0.4% saline) is often used in inhalation therapy. This concentration of saline is thought to be particularly suitable for ultrasonic nebulization. Evaporation probably occurs in the airway, with removal of water from the salt nuclei until the droplets become almost isotonic. Thus, these particles tend to become smaller, which suggests that they would tend to impact in the more distal airways or in the alveoli.[5] Although it is said that deeper penetration therapy is provided by ultrasonic nebulization of hypotonic saline, this claim requires substantiation.

Hypertonic Saline

Hypertonic saline (twice-normal saline, 1.8 per cent sodium chloride, or higher concentrations up to 20 per cent) is said to provide an aerosol that is particularly effective for stimulating a productive cough. The particles would tend to absorb moisture from the airways, resulting in dilution of the saline toward isotonicity. During this process, the particles would grow in size, and therefore impaction would tend to occur in the upper airways. Hypertonic particles depositing on the respiratory mucosa are irritating; thus, such an aerosol readily induces coughing. The hypertonic solution osmotically attracts fluid out of the mucosa, thereby adding water to the respiratory secretions. Thus, hypertonic saline has an osmotic bronchomucotropic effect, and it improves mucokinesis.

TABLE 3-3. MUCOKINETIC ACTIONS OF HYPERTONIC SALINE

ORAL—Effect on oral and gastric mucosae.
  Stimulation of salivation and gagging, thereby
    encouraging patient to expectorate
  Reflex vagal stimulation causing bronchial gland
    secretion

TOPICAL—Effect on mucociliary blanket.
  Osmotic effect resulting in increased secretion of
    watery fluid into mucus.
  Adds water to gel phase, directly decreasing
    viscosity.
  Dissociates DNA-mucoprotein complexes,
    making the mucoprotein available to proteolytic
    enzymes.
  Activates proteases, increasing mucoprotein
    digestion.
  May undergo ionic exchange with calcium in
    cross-linkages, decreasing mucoprotein
    intramolecular bonding.
  Reflex stimulation of coughing through effect on
    cough and irritant receptors in pharyngeal and
    tracheobronchial mucosae.

The more concentrated the saline, the greater the osmotic effect; in fact, bronchorrhea might be produced (see Table 3-3). Additional benefits of hypertonic salt solutions on mucoprotein and DNA are discussed in Chapter 2.

USAGE OF SALINE SOLUTIONS

Untoward Effects. Solutions of saline may irritate the face, mouth, throat and airways; moreover, the hypertonic solutions can damage equipment as well. Productive coughing is usual and desirable, but the use of hypotonic and hypertonic (and sometimes even isotonic) saline may cause bronchospasm. The salty taste of hypertonic solutions may cause gagging, choking or nausea, and vomiting might ensue, although most patients tolerate up to 20 per cent saline by nebulization without difficulty.

Administration of large amounts of saline could be hazardous to a patient with congestive cardiac failure since absorption of the fluid can readily occur, and may worsen the underlying cardiovascular problem. The respiratory tract can absorb saline, and thus an appreciable amount of fluid with a significant sodium load can enter the circulation. Care should be taken to not exceed a patient's daily sodium requirement when there is a need for sodium restriction, such as is frequently the case when a patient has hypertension or cardiac, renal or hepatic disease. The use of hypertonic saline in such patients may result in an increased total body fluid load, and peripheral edema may occur; this risk is increased if the patient is on steroid therapy. Large amounts of hypertonic saline can draw fluid into the lung, and may even result in fluid blocking the airways. If bronchospasm is also induced by the aerosol, atelectasis may result.

Hypertonic saline does not damage cytologic specimens, but it is inhibitory to the growth of most bacteria; however, it is not harmful to mycobacteria, and can therefore be used to induce sputum specimens for the diagnosis of tuberculosis.

Administration. Salt solutions are commonly used to dilute bronchodilators, mucolytics and other inhalational drugs. They are also given alone as humectants, or as cough inducers or mucokinetics. Superheated hypertonic saline (5 to 15 per cent), at a temperature of 105 to 185°F (40.6 to 85°C), is useful for inducing sputum production for cytologic examination or for mycobacteriologic and fungal cultures, although superheated steam can be unpleasant for the patient.

Saline may be administered by any nebulization equipment or by direct instillation. Half-normal saline is thought to be the optimal drug for use with ultrasonic nebulizers.

The addition of a hygroscopic agent, such as propylene glycol, may result in a more stable and effective aerosol for penetration into the distal airways. Thus, the combination of twice-normal saline (2N NaCl) with 2.5 per cent propylene glycol may result in a useful aerosol for inducing productive coughing; some authorities recommend higher concentrations, such as 15 per cent sodium chloride with 20 per cent propylene glycol. Any greater concentrations would probably be capable of extracting fluid from a prune, and the sputum specimens would be unsuitable for microbiologic studies. Thus, if the specimen is to be submitted for routine culture, 2N saline with 2.5 per cent propylene glycol is a more suitable combination for the usual patient.

Dosage and Availability. It is usual to give 0.5 to 2 ml by nebulization several times a day. Larger amounts may be given to induce sputum production. For direct instillation 5 to 10 ml is usually used, but as much as 1 liter at a time of normal saline can be poured repeatedly into a lung through a Carlen's catheter during a lavage procedure for pulmonary alveolar proteinosis. Various concentrations of sodium chloride solutions are packaged in vials or bottles varying in content from 3 ml to 1 liter. The smaller sized rubber-stoppered vials are suitable for inhalation therapy. Most commercial preparations of saline are acidic, with a pH of 4.5 to 7.0. For home patients, ten 1 gm tablets of sodium chloride can be dissolved in 2 pints of boiled water to provide approximately normal saline.

Recommendations. Hypotonic saline is indicated for use with ultrasonic nebulization; it may also be advisable as a diluent for use in patients on restricted sodium intake. **Normal saline** is the most suitable salt solution for routine nebulization therapy, either on its own or as a diluent of other medications. It is also the most suitable for routine irrigation by direct instillation into the intubated respiratory tract. **Hypertonic saline** solutions are not recommended for routine aerosol therapy; they are mainly of value for cough stimulation or sputum induction. When hypertonic saline is used, side effects (nausea, vomiting, irritation of skin or

TABLE 3–4. USES OF SALINE IN MUCOKINETIC THERAPY

HYPOTONIC SALINE (0.45% or ½ N.NaCl)
  For droplets that deposit more distally
  For use with ultrasonic nebulization
  As diluent for use in patient on salt-restricted diet

NORMAL SALINE (0.9% or N. NaCl)
  For general use as a wetting agent
  For general use as a diluent or dry solvent
    a. in inhalation therapy
    b. in systemic or oral therapy
  For irrigation of the lungs (instillation or lavage)

HYPERTONIC SALINE (2–20% NaCl)
  For particles that deposit more proximally
  For inducing bronchorrhea (i.e., sputum induction)
  Can be given as a superheated aerosol to obtain
    specimens for cytology or for fungal or
    mycobacterial culture

mucosa, bronchospasm, hypernatremia, edema) must be watched for. Not more than four treatments a day for a few days with this irritating drug should be required by the average patient. Nebulization equipment should be carefully cleaned following aerosolization of hypertonic saline to prevent corrosion of metal parts or accumulation of salt crystals in the capillary tubing of the nebulizer.

For sputum induction, it is generally advisable to use a normal saline aerosol; concentrations of sodium chloride greater than 5 per cent should be avoided in those circumstances, where recovery of some organisms may be hampered by hypertonic saline. However, higher concentrations can be used for inducing expectoration for mycobacterial culture, and for cytologic studies since the cellular morphology is not adversely affected even by 15 per cent saline.

The current lack of definitive information about the effects of water and salts on the properties of mucus makes it difficult to provide meaningful advice on the use of various types of saline solutions for improving mucokinesis. The previous discussion offers a guide to the practical concepts currently utilized in many hospitals, but it is clear that the popularity of these agents in respiratory therapy greatly exceeds both the available theoretic and practical information on which their use is based. Table 3–4 summarizes the uses of saline.

HYGROSCOPIC AGENTS

These agents are able to absorb water, and they resist dehydration. They are, therefore, allegedly capable of producing droplets of increased stability; they have the additional advantage of providing a symptomatic soothing effect in the respiratory tract. Hygroscopic agents can be added to other pharmacologic agents as adjuvants, or they can be administered alone. The only important agent in this class is propylene glycol; glycerin is also used, mostly as an adjuvant in proprietary mixtures.

Propylene Glycol

Glycols are dihydric alcohols that have hygroscopic properties and a low evaporation rate. Propylene glycol (1-2-propanediol) is the least toxic glycol.[8] It is a clear, colorless, odorless, viscous liquid that is similar but preferable to glycerol; it behaves like a combination of glycerol and alcohol. Being hygroscopic it absorbs moisture, and is freely soluble in water. It has a sweet taste, and is well tolerated on the skin as well as by the stomach and respiratory tract. Propylene glycol has long been employed in inhalation therapy,[9] both for stabilization of droplets and as a humectant or demulcent. It has the added possible value of being a disinfectant, since it can kill many bacterial species in a concentration as low as one part in 2 million; it does not kill bacterial spores, and is unlikely to kill mycobacteria or fungi. Furthermore, it is claimed that propylene glycol has the ability to break hydrogen bonds in mucoprotein molecules, thereby acting as a weak mucolytic agent[10] (see Table 3–5). It may also have weak bronchodilator properties.[10a]

A 2 per cent solution in water is isosmotic with serum, and is therefore nonirritating to the airways. Low concentrations of propylene glycol (2 to 5 per cent) are used in various aerosol mixtures to help produce more uniform droplets with greater stability, but it is not certain that these deposit more effectively in the distal airways. A solution of 10 per cent propylene glycol in distilled water has been recommended for nebulization therapy in patients suffering the pulmonary consequences of cystic fibrosis.[11] Higher concentrations of the drug may irritate the airways; the hyperosmolar, hygroscopic effect draws tissue fluid into the lumen. Thus, propylene glycol, in concentrations of 15 to 20 per cent, is often used alone or in combination with hypertonic saline, to induce coughing, with subsequent production of a sputum specimen.[9] Concentrations of up to 80 per cent have been used by

TABLE 3–5.   PROPYLENE GLYCOL

PROPERTIES
   Hygroscopic agent (humectant) with sweet taste and demulcent (soothing) qualities
   Has droplet-stabilizing properties; may improve aerosol deposition
   Antibacterial, antifungal and antiviral effects; not likely to kill mycobacteria or fungi in sputum specimens obtained for culture
   Does not alter cellular morphology
   Can break hydrogen bonds in mucoprotein

USES OF AEROSOL
   Reduces irritant effects of other aerosol drugs
   Suitable for inducing sputum specimens for cultures and cytologic studies
   Potentiates mucolytic actions of other mucokinetic agents
   Can be used to help sterilize ambient air

CONCENTRATIONS AND DOSAGES
   2–5% used alone or in combination for most types of aerosol therapy
   5–15% can be used alone or with hypertonic saline to cause coughing and to induce sputum production
   Concentrations of 15–20% can be used to loosen very viscous secretions
   Aerosol dose varies from 1–10 ml
   Used in concentrations of up to 80% in some proprietary mixtures for inhalational use, e.g., Aerolone.

Dautrebande.[10a] Sputum specimens obtained by nebulizing propylene glycol–hypertonic saline mixtures, especially if superheated to 140 to 185°F (60 to 85°C) are of value in the diagnosis of coin lesions, since the expectorated material is suitable for cytologic studies[9]; however, fungi and mycobacteria could be inhibited by propylene glycol. In practice, it seems that propylene glycol results in the production of sputum that is suitable for culture in spite of theoretic disadvantages.

Untoward Effects. Propylene glycol is very safe when given in conventional, therapeutic dosages, although higher concentrations may cause excessive coughing and may result in irritation of the upper airways and the lungs. However, the drug has no serious toxicity in concentrations of up to 80 per cent, and may serve as a weak bronchodilator for some patients, although this is of no practical significance.

Recommendations. The addition of propylene glycol should be considered whenever inhalation therapy with an aerosol drug seems to produce less than the optimal result. Thus, 1 to 2 ml of 2 per cent propylene glycol can be added to bronchodilator or mucokinetic aerosols with complete safety, and the enhanced stability of the droplets may result in more optimal distal airway deposition. Higher concentrations are used in many proprietary preparations (e.g., 80 per cent in Aerolone), in which the drug serves as an excipient.

Moderate concentrations of propylene glycol (e.g., 10 to 20 per cent) can be nebulized to help raise very viscous secretions or to induce a sputum specimen for cytologic studies. If a 20 minute therapy session is unproductive, subsequent treatments with the addition of 10 per cent sodium chloride could be administered for 20 to 30 minutes two to three times a day for a few days. The mixture can be given at room temperature, but better results are obtained if the solution is heated to 105° F (40.6° C) or even as high as 185° F (85° C). Ultrasonic nebulization of such a solution is poorly tolerated by most patients, and there is little to recommend this practice. Following aerosol treatments, the apparatus must be carefully cleaned, using alcohol as a solvent, to remove any viscous propylene glycol that may have impacted in the tubing.

Glycerin(e) is similar to propylene glycol, but is said to be more irritating to the respiratory tract. It could be used in a similar fashion to propylene glycol; however, it is more viscous and more toxic. Currently, there appears to be no basis for preferring glycerin.[8]

TRUE MUCOLYTICS

Mucolytic agents are capable of breaking mucoprotein molecules into smaller, more soluble and less viscous residues. The important drugs are acetylcysteine and the various inhalational enzymes. Several other agents have been claimed to possess true mucolytic properties (including iodides, salt solutions, propylene glycol and ascorbic acid), but their effectiveness in vitro is less than that of the agents that will be considered here.

Thiols

Acetylcysteine

Acetylcysteine (N-acetyl-L-cysteine, Mucomyst) is the most popular proprietary mucokinetic agent for administration into the respiratory tract to loosen secretions. It was introduced in the early 1960s following the demonstration that L-cysteine has mucolytic properties. L-cysteine is used as the basis of Cytoclair, which is employed as a laboratory mucolytic in the cytologic examination of sputum. Acetylcysteine is the N-acetyl derivative of L-cysteine, and it is the best-tolerated congener for therapeutic use.

Mode of Action. The free sulfhydryl group of acetylcysteine interacts with the disulfide bridges of mucoprotein, thereby breaking the complex protein network into less viscous strands (Fig. 3–1). Acetylcysteine is a reducing agent, and it is broken down by oxidizing reagents. When it reacts with mucoprotein, it is broken down to acetate and cysteine; some hydrogen sulfide is liberated and causes the characteristic malodor of the drug.

Acetylcysteine is extremely effective in the laboratory as a liquefier of mucoprotein. There is no evidence that the drug can break down DNA, and it does not have any action on fibrin or blood clots.[12] There is clinical evidence that acetylcysteine can reduce the viscosity of purulent as well as mucoid sputum, but there is no clear explanation of

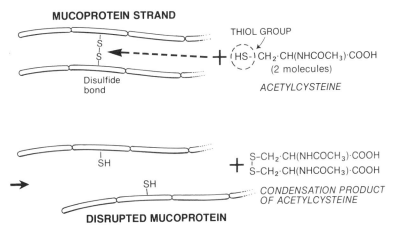

Figure 3–1. (From "Secretions of the Respiratory Tract: Physiology and Pharmacology" by Irwin Ziment, M.D., Projects in Health, Inc., New York, 1976.)

how this occurs. The manufacturer claims that it is the salt effect of sodium acetylcysteine that breaks down DNA; no evidence is offered that acetylcysteine itself depolymerizes DNA. It is probable that any mucolytic effect of the drug on purulent sputum is caused by the acetylcysteine breaking down the mucoprotein component; the use of a salt as the diluent probably serves to help break down the DNA and the mucoprotein. It is, therefore, completely inappropriate to credit acetylcysteine with special ability to break down purulent sputum. The suggestion that the drug has an excellent lytic effect on pus[12] is not quite correct, since the sodium in the salt or in the diluent appears to be responsible for at least a part of the lysis. The evidence suggests that the drug is an effective mucolytic for mucoid secretions but less so for other types of sputum. The various qualities of acetylcysteine that may account for its mucolytic properties are listed in Table 3–6; its antimucokinetic properties are also listed.

The drug is most effective at a pH between 7 and 9, and it can produce marked mucolysis within a few minutes in the laboratory. It is less effective if introduced into an acidic environment in the lung; this should be given consideration when adding a relatively large proportion of a solution with a low pH (such as is the case with most bronchodilators).

When administered into the respiratory tract, acetylcysteine is capable of producing liquefaction of sputum, and a marked increase in expectoration may occur. It is not always clear whether the mucokinesis results from mucolysis or from stimulation of the mucosa by direct irritation by the acetylcysteine or liberated hydrogen sulfide, or by the outpouring of mucosal fluid of low viscosity (bronchorrhea) caused by the hypertonicity of the drug.[12a] Several careful studies have revealed the difficulty of evaluating the effectiveness of acetylcysteine in sick patients.[13, 14] Indeed, the use of acetylcysteine in subjects with chronic obstructive airway disease does not usually lead to improvement in pulmonary function tests; the 20 per cent solution may actually cause some deterioration.[13, 19] Any improvement that does occur may, in fact, be attributable to the bronchodilator that is usually given with the acetylcysteine to prevent bronchospasm.[19]

Absorption of acetylcysteine can occur through the respiratory mucosa, but no harmful effects result, since the drug is metabolized by the liver; it is deacetylated to cysteine, which enters normal metabolic pathways. The drug is relatively free of any serious systemic side effects, and it has not been found to be harmful even in patients with liver disease.

Uses. Topical administration of acetylcysteine may be of value in a variety of disorders characterized by retention of sputum. It can be used to loosen viscous mucoid secretions in chronic bronchopulmonary diseases such as bronchitis, asthma and emphysema, but it is probably less effective in conditions associated with purulent spu-

TABLE 3–6. ACTIONS OF MUCOMYST (SODIUM ACETYLCYSTEINE)*

Property of the Drug	Effect
MUCOKINETIC ACTIONS	
Free sulfhydryl group	Rupture of disulfide bridges
Salt effect, owing to sodium in the drug or in the diluent	Lysis of mucoprotein and of DNA (due to breakdown of complexes and activation of intrinsic proteases)
Alkalinity of the preparation (enhanced by adding sodium bicarbonate)	Decreases adhesiveness of secretions and activates proteases
Hypertonicity of the preparation	Stimulates bronchorrhea
Stimulation of vagal reflex via receptors in pharynx, airways and stomach	Increases secretion of bronchial glands (bronchomucotropic effect)
Stimulation of cough and irritant receptors in the airways	Cough induction
ANTIMUCOKINETIC ACTIONS	
Induces bronchospasm	Traps secretions, and decreases effectiveness of cough
Inhibits ciliary activity	Impairs mucociliary escalator
Stimulates goblet cells	Causes secretion of viscous mucus
Loosening of secretions in weak patient	Secretions gravitate to bases of lungs (unless coughing, postural drainage or suctioning follows drug administration)

*Mucomyst is available as the sodium salt, and it is usually used as a 10% solution by diluting the 20% solution with an equal volume of saline or sodium bicarbonate or even sterile water.

tum such as bronchiectasis and pneumonia. It has also been claimed to dissolve mucoid sputum from certain patients with alveolar proteinosis, although this has not been substantiated. Its value in cystic fibrosis remains controversial, although it seems to be of use in selected cases.[12, 16, 17] Unfortunately, many of the studies involving both short-term and long-term therapy with acetylcysteine in the management of chronic sputopathies fail to demonstrate convincing evidence of substantial or even worthwhile benefit.[13, 14, 18, 19]

Acetylcysteine has been of particular value in the treatment of atelectasis caused by inspissation of secretions or by impaction of a mucoid plug; it has been advocated for use during anesthesia and in the preparation of patients for procedures such as bronchography. A particular value of the drug may be in the treatment of the nonspecific sputopathy that usually occurs in a patient with a tracheotomy or an indwelling endotracheal tube.

Other Uses of Acetylcysteine. The drug may also be given orally (in a cola beverage, to disguise its taste) in a dosage of 5 ml of the 10 per cent solution one to four times a day to help loosen mucus in the bowel of a patient with cystic fibrosis who has abdominal pains caused by inspissated intestinal contents. A similar result with acetylcysteine has been achieved by administering the drug by enema.[17]

It has been reported that oral administration of acetylcysteine in doses of 500 mg/kg a day may be an effective antidote in paracetamol poisoning.[20, 21] Cysteine, a precursor of glutathione, combines with paracetamol to form a conjugate that is excreted by the kidney. Acetylcysteine appears to be a more acceptable alternative to cysteine, and preliminary work suggests it can be effective in accelerating the rate of removal of paracetamol.[21] In the U.S. paracetamol is known as acetaminophen, and it is present in analgesics such as Tylenol. Poisoning with this drug is becoming more common, and acetylcysteine may have an important role in the management of this problem.[21a]

Untoward Effects. Adverse reactions are more frequent with the higher concentration (20 per cent) product than with the more dilute (10 per cent) preparation.[15] The drug may produce a burning sensation in the trachea, and the sulfurous taste and odor may result in nausea and anorexia with gagging or even vomiting. The breath may have an odor for some time after adminis-

tration of the drug; this can be lessened by rinsing the mouth or washing the teeth following each treatment.

Many patients develop coughing when acetylcysteine is nebulized; lower concentrations may be needed for effective treatment. Asthmatic patients and other subjects with hyperreactive airways may develop bronchospasm; this potentially serious effect can be prevented or treated by nebulizing a sympathomimetic bronchodilator prophylactically or therapeutically. Another possible danger to be watched for is the development of marked bronchorrhea, which can present a particular hazard to the patient who is unable to cough effectively. The continued use of acetylcysteine may be less successful once inspissated or impacted viscous secretions have been removed. The fact that acetylcysteine has an adverse effect on ciliary activity has not been correlated with any clinical detriment as yet. However, if mucus is loosened or bronchorrhea is caused, in a patient with a poor cough or with impaired cilia, the secretions may move downward into the more distal airways, resulting in a worsening of gas exchange.

Persistent use of the drug may irritate the oral mucosa, resulting in stomatitis. Similarly, rhinitis, laryngitis and tracheitis may be produced and severe hoarseness, rhinorrhea or hemoptysis may occur. Acetylcysteine is not, however, irritating to the skin or eyes, even when given in a mist tent. True sensitization is not a problem, since acetylcysteine does not liberate potentially antigenic polypeptides from mucoprotein, although chills and febrile reactions have been reported to occur occasionally. In spite of all these problems, many patients are able to tolerate daily nebulization of acetylcysteine for at least many months.[18]

Administration and Dosage. Acetylcysteine may be nebulized with or without positive pressure, using a mouthpiece or a face mask: aerosolization without IPPB is generally less effective. Ultrasonic nebulization can be utilized but is not recommended, since the resulting aerosol is too irritating. The mouth should be rinsed and the patient should gargle or drink water, if possible, after each treatment, to relieve any unpleasant taste or dryness of the mouth. Following treatment with a mask, the face should be washed to remove sticky residue. Acetylcysteine should not be aerosolized from a heated nebulizer chamber, since it is broken down under such circumstances.

Acetylcysteine may be administered to

patients in oxygen tents, head tents, or croup tents: up to 300 ml a day may be required, but the results do not appear to justify this expensive form of therapy. The drug is most effective when directly instilled into the respiratory tract, and results are much more impressive than those obtained by nebulizing the drug.[19] It can be given either through an endotracheal tube, a tracheostomy, a transtracheal catheter or a bronchoscope; the patient should be kept well oxygenated. When administered in this fashion, it may provoke coughing, which tends to disseminate the solution throughout the tracheobronchial tree; the drug should be allowed to act for a couple of minutes before the loosened sputum is suctioned out. If the patient is unable to expectorate, then the loosened secretions may cause a deterioration in the pulmonary condition, unless postural drainage or suction is used.

Favorable pulmonary results have been reported in Europe when acetylcysteine is given in dosages of up to 600 mg a day by the oral or intravenous route. It is alleged that adequate mucokinesis can be produced by giving the drug by either of these routes, and no significant side effects are caused.[13]

The drug is usually given in a dose of 2 to 5 ml of the 10 per cent solution or 1 to 5 ml of the 20 per cent solution by nebulization, but the dosage varies from 1 to 20 ml, and the drug can be given every two to six hours, depending on need. It should be remembered that prolonged nebulization of a large dose of the 20 per cent solution increases the concentration of the acetylcysteine remaining in the nebulizer, which may then become more difficult to aerosolize and more irritating; the manufacturer suggests that diluent be added when three quarters of the initial dose has been aerosolized. See Table 3-7.

Availability and Compatibility. N-acetyl-L-cysteine is marketed as the sodium salt; currently it is available as Mucomyst, but it was formerly also marketed as Respaire and is known as Airbron in some other countries. It is packaged in vials containing 10 to 30 ml, as 10 per cent and 20 per cent solutions, and either strength may be further diluted by administering the drug with saline, sodium bicarbonate or a bronchodilator. The drug is supplied as the sodium salt, and the chelating agent disodium edetate (EDTA, 0.05 per cent) is added to prevent oxidative break down of acetylcysteine. The pH of the solution is adjusted to 7.0 with sodium hydroxide.

Once a bottle has been opened, it should be kept refrigerated. However, if air is allowed into the bottle, the drug undergoes breakdown, and a marked loss of effectiveness occurs after a few days. If the unopened bottle is stored at $20°$ C ($68°$ F), potency is maintained for at least two years, but the opened bottle should be used within four days. Oxidative breakdown occurs if the drug is autoclaved.

Acetylcysteine may be used with most other inhalational agents. However, it is incompatible with tetracyclines, ampicillin, erythromycin, amphotericin, Lipiodol, hydrogen peroxide, trypsin and chymotrypsin. These agents react with acetylcysteine and produce a color change, a precipitate, or an odor. A light purple color may develop spontaneously, but this is not untoward. The drug is a reducing agent, and it is incompatible with oxidizing agents such as hydrogen peroxide. If possible, the drug should not be mixed with an acid solution, since there is a decrease in its effectiveness at a pH of less than 7. Contact with metals such as copper and iron or with rubber should be avoided, since acetylcysteine is partially broken down by such contact, with release of hydrogen sulfide. See Table 3-8.

Recommendations. At present, acetylcysteine can be regarded as the most effective inhalational mucolytic drug available in the U.S. It is indicated when sputum retention persists despite an adequate trial of simpler mucokinetic drugs. Acetylcysteine should be evaluated in vitro using the individual patient's sputum, and a trial of therapy carried out if the tests suggest the drug is superior to water or salt solution. It is

TABLE 3-7.   METHODS OF ADMINISTERING ACETYLCYSTEINE

INHALATION e.g., 2–5 ml 20% solution with 2 ml N. saline.
> As an irritant—main effect may be to produce bronchorrhea and apparent mucolysis

INSTILLATION e.g., 5 ml 20% solution with 5 ml 5% NaHCO$_3$.
> Produces mucolysis–useful in treatment of atelectasis, or to loosen very viscous secretions

ORAL e.g., 5 ml 10% solution (up to 600 mg/day).
> To loosen inspissated bowel contents in patients with cystic fibrosis
> Following absorption, may cause mucolysis in the lungs
> For treatment of acetaminophen poisoning (e.g., 500 mg/kg/day)

INTRAVENOUS
> Investigational form of administration in mucokinetic therapy

TABLE 3–8. GENERAL PRECAUTIONS WITH ACETYLCYSTEINE

Use only when simpler mucokinetics have been shown to be less effective (in vivo or in vitro).
When given by nebulization:
    dilute with equal volume of saline or sodium bicarbonate;
    incompatible with tetracyclines, amphotericin, Lipiodol, hydrogen peroxide, trypsin, etc.;
    when nebulizing, dilute remaining drug in nebulizer when only 25% original volume remains.
When given by instillation:
    dilute with equal volume sodium bicarbonate;
    position patient so that drug gravitates to area of lung requiring mucolysis.
Always use with a bronchodilator to prevent bronchospasm.
Do not give by ultrasonic nebulization.
Store opened bottle in refrigerator, and use within a few days.
Avoid contact of drug with rubber or metals.
Slight discoloration does not disqualify for use.
Patient must be monitored for adverse reactions, e.g., gagging, nausea, bronchospasm, "drowning" in loosened secretions, hypoxemia.
Apparatus (and patient, if necessary) should be cleaned following nebulization.

of particular value in the management of inspissated, adhesive, mucoid sputum, but it may also improve the expectoration of purulent sputum. There is little difference in effectiveness between the 10 per cent and 20 per cent solutions for most patients; the undiluted 20 per cent solution is rarely required. The drug is most effective when instilled directly into the trachea in a dosage of 2 to 5 ml as often as once an hour. Nebulization of the drug appears to be much less effective, but it can be given by an air compressor or, if need be, with IPPB three or four times a day, although the dosage and frequency of administration should be decided on the basis of its effect in individual cases. However, there is little support in the literature for long-term acetylcysteine therapy. Therefore, acetylcysteine should be given by aerosolization only to selected patients.

In general, 1 to 2 ml of the 20 per cent solution should be given, with an equal amount of 2 to 5 per cent sodium bicarbonate, in company with a standard dose of a bronchodilator, such as isoproterenol, to prevent bronchospasm: the alkalinity of the sodium bicarbonate produces an optimal pH for the activity of acetylcysteine. Side effects should be watched for during treatment and any severe reaction should be an indication for discontinuing use of the drug. The therapist should encourage the patient to rinse out the mouth and throat following administration of the aerosol by the oral route. If a face mask is used, the therapist should clean the patient's face following the treatment. Similarly, the nebulizer and tubing should be immediately rinsed out to remove sticky residues.

2-Mercaptoethane Sodium Sulfonate

2-Mercaptoethane sodium sulfonate (MESNA, Mistabron) has been used extensively in Europe[13, 22] but is still in the investigational stage in the U.S. The drug is a thiol derivative with a free sulfhydryl group; its similarity to acetylcysteine is shown in Fig. 3–2.

This mucolytic has been recommended for use as a 20 per cent solution for nebulization. It appears to be more effective than acetylcysteine[14, 23] and it has a less objectionable taste and odor. Investigations in the U.S. suggest that it is well-tolerated by patients with chronic bronchospastic disorders,[24] although it might be expected to induce bronchospasm in some susceptible individuals, as does acetylcysteine. Further evaluation of this drug would be justified, but it is doubtful whether it can offer enough advantages to displace acetylcysteine.

Enzymes

Although enzymatic dissolution of purulent secretions has been advocated for many

$$HS \cdot CH_2 \cdot CH \cdot COOH \quad\quad ACETYLCYSTEINE$$
$$\underset{NH \cdot COCH_3}{|}$$

$$HS \cdot CH_2 \cdot CH_2 \cdot SO_3Na \quad\quad MERCAPTOETHANE\ SODIUM\ SULFONATE$$

$$HOOC \cdot CH_2 \cdot S \cdot CH_2 \cdot CH \cdot COOH \quad\quad CARBOXYMETHYLCYSTEINE$$
$$\underset{NH_2}{|}$$

Figure 3–2. Thiol mucolytics with free sulfydryl groups (acetylcysteine and mercaptoethane sodium sulfonate) and with blocked sulfhydryl group (carboxymethylcysteine).

years, the expense, toxicity and relatively minor benefits of enzyme therapy have led to a marked decline in their popularity.

Deoxyribonuclease (Dornase)

Deoxyribonuclease (desoxyribonuclease, pancreatic dornase, Dornavac) is the most frequently employed of the various inhalational enzymes used to loosen purulent sputum. The drug, introduced in the late 1940s, has been largely superseded by acetylcysteine for potent mucolysis.

Mode of Action. Dornase is a proteolytic enzyme, and it specifically depolymerizes deoxyribonucleic acid (DNA), thereby decreasing the viscosity of these long molecules that are characteristic components of purulent sputum. Dornase has little effect on mucoprotein and none on fibrin.[12] The drug does not have any action on living cells, and it is safe for patients with alpha$_1$-antitrypsin deficiency. It had been feared that these patients might not be able to break down dornase in the lungs, thereby allowing the enzyme freedom to digest the living pulmonary tissue, but there is no evidence that this occurs.

Lieberman[25] has shown that DNA can combine with natural trypsin, and that it inhibits the proteolytic enzymes present in normal respiratory tract secretions. The depolymerization of DNA by dornase permits intrinsic pulmonary proteolytic activity to occur, causing breakdown of mucoprotein. Moreover, dornase liberates mucoprotein that is combined with DNA, making the mucoprotein more accessible to proteolysis.[26] Thus, the administration of dornase may result in considerable liquefaction of sputum, both by direct digestion of DNA, and by indirectly enhancing natural proteolysis of mucoprotein. It is possible that this secondary effect is the major factor in the success of dornase as a mucokinetic agent. This composite action of dornase suggests that the drug is a particularly rational form of therapy for purulent secretions, although, in practice, acetylcysteine (which does not directly break down DNA) appears to be equally effective in most cases.

The sputum of a patient with chronic respiratory disease may actually become less viscous when it becomes purulent than it would be if it remained mucoid, owing to the liberation of bacterial and leucocytic proteolytic enzymes that digest the mucoprotein. However, purulent sputum may be very viscous, possibly as a consequence of excess DNA. Furthermore, DNA may bind basic antibiotics, thereby rendering topical therapy with these drugs less effective. Thus, in certain circumstances, the assorted disadvantages resulting from DNA may be reversed by treatment with dornase, qualifying this drug as a particularly effective mucokinetic agent in selected cases.

Uses. Although dornase may be deemed of value in the treatment of viscid, purulent, inspissated secretions, there are few pulmonary conditions in which the drug has been of proven benefit, and there is less enthusiasm for the drug than there was prior to the introduction of acetylcysteine.[27] The average patient with bronchitis or pneumonia does not appear to require dornase, although the drug may be indicated when mucokinesis cannot be achieved satisfactorily by simpler means. Dornase is considered to be of particular value in certain patients with bronchiectasis, lung abscess, cystic fibrosis or in other situations in which chronic infection persists in the respiratory tract.[28] If treatment with antibiotic nebulization is contemplated, prior treatment with dornase may be advisable. Immediate improvement may not occur, and the dornase therapy may have to be given for two to three days before any benefit appears.

Inhalation therapy with dornase may be of value when given by the nasal route for the treatment of infections of the paranasal sinuses. The drug can also be nebulized into tracheotomized patients to help loosen infected, encrusted secretions that sometimes develop in the trachea (and, in severe cases, may result in tracheitis sicca). Other uses for dornase have been found beyond the inhalational domain. The drug has been successfully employed in the irrigation of purulent wounds and for decreasing the viscosity of infected material draining from the kidney or bladder. Some surgeons introduce dornase into empyemas in the pleural space, but this may cause severe febrile reactions, and the practice is no longer advocated.

Untoward Effects. Dornase is usually given by aerosolization, and it is suitable for ultrasonic nebulization, since it is less irritating than acetylcysteine administered in this fashion. Pharyngeal and sometimes tracheal irritation may be produced, although a burning sensation in the mouth is generally the main complaint. The addition of propylene glycol as a diluent may result in a less irritating aerosol, and helps ensure more distal deposition in the lung. If the aerosol is too concentrated, pharyngeal irritation may cause coughing, and poor distal deposition will result.

Dornase does not digest living tissue, and it does not cause metaplasia, although, on occasion, hemoptysis has been a complication of treatment. Febrile and asthmatic-like reactions, or anaphylactoid reactions, may rarely occur in susceptible patients if therapy is prolonged. Furthermore, it is possible that dornase loses its effectiveness if nebulized for more than a few days in succession; prolonged use may result in the production of antibodies against beef protein. For these reasons, a treatment course with this drug should be limited, and its administration is contraindicated in patients known to be hypersensitive to beef protein.

Administration and Dosage. See Table 3–9. The recommended method of giving dornase for inhalational purposes is by nebulization with a simple nebulizer or IPPB, or with an ultrasonic nebulizer. The drug can be given by direct instillation into the tracheobronchial tree; this is the usual method for administration into the paranasal sinuses, an empyema or the urinary tract. When given for the treatment of paranasal sinus infection, it is recommended that the

TABLE 3–9. DORNASE (DEOXYRIBONUCLEASE, DORNAVAC)

ACTIONS
   Proteolytic breakdown of DNA (present in purulent secretions)
   Permits endogenous proteases to lyse mucoprotein
   Enables antibiotics in secretions to work more effectively

INDICATIONS
   Viscid, purulent secretions (e.g., in bronchiectasis, lung abscess) that do not adequately loosen with simpler agents
   May be of value in sinusitis
   May be of value for loosening purulent secretions in surgical infections (e.g., empyema); can cause severe febrile reactions

ADVERSE EFFECTS
   Bronchospasm, coughing, poor deposition
   Irritation of tissues, febrile reactions
   Hypersensitivity reactions

DOSAGE
   50,000–100,000 units in 2 ml N. saline 1–4 times a day, for not more than a few days

PRECAUTIONS
   Prevent bronchospasm by using a bronchodilator
   Add propylene glycol to improve the aerosol properties
   Monitor patient for adverse reactions
   Rinse out mouth and throat after nebulizing drug
   Do not administer to patients allergic to beef protein

Proetz regimen be used, in which the drug is administered as an aerosol with alternating positive and negative pressure. Following administration by aerosol, the patient should, if possible, rinse out the mouth and throat to prevent irritation. The role of dornase in these extrapulmonary conditions requires further evaluation before endorsement can be offered.

The usual dose of dornase is 50,000 to 100,000 units one to four times a day. The powdered drug is dissolved in 2 ml normal saline, and the solution may be diluted further for administration. Some physicians advise the nebulization of dornase intermittently, about one to four times a week for several weeks or months, for patients with chronic purulent sputum. This practice is of doubtful benefit and of undoubted toxic potential.

Availability and Compatibility. Dornase is marketed in the U.S. as Dornavac; in many countries it is called Deanase. It is packaged as the white powder of lyophilized enzyme in a vial containing 100,000 units under a dry inert gas; a vial of 2 ml sterile diluent is provided separately. The drug is compatible with other inhalational drugs, with the exception of soluble forms of penicillin. When mixed with another agent, the combination should be administered without delay.

Recommendations. Since dornase is an expensive drug with a definite toxic potential, its use should be confined to cases in which simpler agents have proved to be inadequate. For most patients, 50,000 units in 2 ml normal saline three times a day is appropriate. In general, the enzyme will only be required when yellow, green, or brown, purulent secretions of marked viscosity persist after several days of optimal inhalation and physical therapy combined with appropriate oral or intravenous antibiotic administration. Such situations are most likely to be found in patients with bronchiectasis or severe pneumonia, and many of these individuals will need to be intubated or tracheotomized. It is rare for dornase to be required by patients with lesser degrees of respiratory involvement, and thus the drug is rarely recommended for nebulization through the oral route.

When dornase is considered, an in vitro attempt to evaluate its effectiveness on the patient's secretions should be made. If the drug is found to be suitable for the situation, a course of not more than about four days should be provided. Prior or simultaneous treatment with a bronchodilator should be given, and the patient should rinse out the mouth and throat after dornase is given via the oral route. In general, dornase aerosolization should be accompanied by an equal volume of 10 per cent propylene glycol, since the latter soothes the mucosa and ensures better deposition of the enzyme.[29]

Trypsin

Trypsin (Tryptar) is a digestive proteolytic enzyme obtained from ox pancreas. It can break down mucoprotein and other proteins, including fibrin, into smaller molecules of polypeptides and amino acids.[13] However, when compared to pancreatic dornase, it has relatively little action on DNA, in part because it is inhibited by this constituent of purulent sputum. Trypsin is less effective than acetylcysteine for general use as a mucolytic agent, but it may be of some value in causing lysis of fibrin and necrotic tissue (Table 3–10). It has also been reported to be effective in the treatment of pulmonary alveolar proteinosis,[25, 30, 31] although it is not successful in most cases. The mucoid sputum from patients with proteinosis may also be dissolved by acetylcysteine, but not by dornase.[5] Trypsin may be considered for use in inhalation therapy to help liquefy obstructing plugs of bloody or fibrinous material in the airways. However, the relatively high incidence of untoward effects has led to a considerable decline in the routine use of this drug.[26, 32]

Untoward Effects. Trypsin is more irritating to mucous membranes than either acetylcysteine or dornase, particularly if large doses or several treatments a day are given. Aerosol therapy may irritate the eye and nose, and may result in glossitis, pharyngitis and laryngitis; severe hoarseness may occur. Severe upper respiratory tract irritation may be treated by irrigating the affected area with 2.5 per cent sodium bicarbonate.

Tracheitis is usually experienced as a retrosternal burning pain, and, occasionally, hemoptysis may occur. Systemic reactions of an allergic nature are liable to occur in 5 to 7 per cent of patients; problems include fever, chills and hives, and some authorities advise giving prophylactic antihistamine therapy before nebulizing trypsin, since the more severe reactions appear to be mediated by the release of histamine. Susceptible patients may develop dyspnea or bronchospasm. The less severe symptoms may tend to diminish with repeated administrations, but since there is a small risk of anaphylactic reactions, it is advisable to discontinue use of the drug if allergic manifestations develop. It is possible to test for sensitivity using intradermal, scratch or patch tests, but since the drug is never an essential medication, this approach cannot be justified.

There is no definite evidence that the enzyme attacks living tissue, but atypical metaplasia of the respiratory mucosa may be caused. The drug should not be given to patients with alpha$_1$-antitrypsin deficiency, even though there is no evidence that trypsin attacks the respiratory tissues of these people. The drug is contraindicated in patients who have hepatic insufficiency.

Dosage and Recommendations. The powdered drug is available as highly purified, lyophilized crystals from bovine pancreas. It is marketed in vials of 250,000 units, which should be dissolved in 5 ml of normal saline for nebulization or instillation. It is known under several brand names, such as Tryptar, Trypure, Trysevac and Parenzyme.

The recommended dosage varies from 25,000 to 125,000 units one to three times a day, although it is advisable not to exceed 50,000 units each time when giving several treatments a day. Large doses may cause coughing, preventing adequate distal deposition in the airways.

There are few situations in which trypsin is indicated, since other agents are safer and

TABLE 3–10. EFFECT OF ENZYMES ON SPUTUM

Enzyme	Substrate Affected			Clinical Value			
	MUCO-PROTEIN	DNA	FIBRIN	MUCOID SPUTUM	PURULENT SPUTUM	CYSTIC FIBROSIS	PROTEINOSIS
Dornase	++*	++++		±	+	±	
Trypsin	+++	+	+++	±		+	+
Chymotrypsin	++	+	+			±	
Streptokinase	±		++++			+	
Streptodornase		+++			+		
Leucine aminopeptidase	+	++			+		

*Activates natural proteases, which depolymerize mucoprotein.

better-tolerated. It could be nebulized in patients with bloody or fibrinous secretions (e.g., consolidation following intrapulmonary hemorrhage), and in the management of pulmonary alveolar proteinosis. For the latter, 100,000 units a day have been given for several weeks. The drug should be given with propylene glycol and a bronchodilator to obtain better effects and less toxicity, and careful watch for toxic effects should be maintained. Trypsin is not compatible with acetylcysteine, and the two should not be administered simultaneously. If it is planned to use trypsin for more than a few days, it should first be determined that the patient does not have deficiency of alpha$_1$-antitrypsin.

Of all proteolytic enzymes, only dornase has established a place in respiratory pharmacology, although a few other enzymes have been considered as possible inhalational mucokinetics (Table 3–10).

Chymotrypsin

Chymotrypsin has been combined with trypsin (e.g., as Chymoral, Chymar and Chymovac), since it is claimed that the combination is similar in effect to trypsin but less irritating to the tissues. However, the drug's value has not been substantiated, and it is not used in inhalation therapy.

Streptodornase and Streptokinase

Streptodornase and streptokinase are proteolytic enzymes derived from the bacterium *Streptococcus hemolyticus*. The two enzymes are usually employed as a combination (2,500 units of streptodornase with 10,000 units of streptokinase, e.g. Varidase), and have actions similar to those of trypsin. However, these enzymes are more irritating than trypsin and are rarely employed in inhalation therapy.[33] They may be injected into empyema cavities to loosen pus, but severe febrile reactions are common and, therefore, such treatment is no longer recommended in empyema management.

Recently, streptokinase has been made available for the treatment of pulmonary embolic disease.

SURFACTANTS

Various mucokinetic agents act like soaps: they have a surface effect that decreases adhesiveness between the mucoid secretions and the epithelium.[8] Although the synthetic surfactants are of disputed value in inhalation therapy, they are still in the mucokinetic armamentarium. Many surfactants used for other purposes in pharmaceutics are not used in inhalation therapy, for example, Tween. The therapeutic agents are often called wetting agents or detergents; they have also been called "mucoevacuants," and although "surfactant" is not an entirely accurate term, it appears to be suitable for the following drugs.

Alevaire

In the early 1950's, Alevaire was introduced into inhalation therapy as a mucolytic detergent aerosol.[34, 35] The active drug in Alevaire is *tyloxapol* (Superinone, Triton-A20, WR-1399); this is a complex polymer capable of lowering the surface tension of mucus, thereby decreasing the viscosity and adhesiveness of sputum. Tyloxapol is nontoxic, and unlike most other detergents, it is well-tolerated by tissues and does not hemolyze red blood cells. Alevaire contains 0.125 per cent tyloxapol, in combination with 2 per cent sodium bicarbonate and 5 per cent glycerin, adjusted to pH 8.2. Since sodium bicarbonate at a pH of 8.2 is also capable of decreasing the viscosity of mucoid secretions, there has been considerable debate as to whether Alevaire is more effective than bicarbonate alone.

No clear, controlled trial has been carried out, and the true value of tyloxapol in inhalational therapeutics remains controversial. Several studies have suggested that Alevaire is no more effective than water, normal saline or 2 per cent sodium bicarbonate.[23, 29, 36, 37] The FDA had sought to have the preparation removed from the market, and during the past several years Alevaire has fallen into relative disuse; although the drug is available, it is no longer promoted. Since convincing proof of the efficacy of the combination in Alevaire has yet to be provided, this controversial preparation cannot be recommended. Hypertonic (2.5 to 5 per cent) sodium bicarbonate can be regarded as a cheap and effective alternative to the combination of sodium bicarbonate, glycerin and tyloxapol, unless new, controlled studies are published that demonstrate additional benefits conferred by the presence of the two latter agents in Alevaire. It is possible that the composition of Alevaire could confer stability on the aerosolized droplets, thereby enhancing their distal deposition. However, there is no definite evidence that any of the theoretic advantages of Alevaire have resulted in any benefits in patients.

Untoward Effects. Adverse effects are rare, and toxic complications have not been a problem with Alevaire. As with many aerosols, nebulization of Alevaire may cause bronchospasm, particularly in asthmatic patients. Some patients complain of irritation to the throat and airways, and occasionally nausea may occur. Prolonged or continuous administration of Alevaire could, theoretically, have an adverse effect on the surfactant produced by the lung, although this has not been demonstrated.[40]

Administration. The following remarks apply to the use of Alevaire, according to the original recommendations of the manufacturer. Undiluted Alevaire can be given by various conventional nebulization devices, although mist tent administration is not recommended. The preparation apparently is a suitable vehicle for small amounts of bronchodilators, decongestants, local anesthetics and antibiotics (excluding tetracyclines); if a drug is added, the combination should be made immediately prior to use. Alevaire should not be overdiluted, nor should it be given as a heated aerosol, since loss of effectiveness will occur. The apparatus should be cleaned after Alevaire has been nebulized to prevent accumulation of sticky residues. Once a bottle is opened, it is advised that it be used within a few days, to prevent contamination of the remaining fluid, since Alevaire does not contain an antiseptic preservative. For dosage, see Table 3–11.

Recommendations. Should Alevaire be marketed again, it would be used only in attempts to loosen sticky secretions when simpler preparations have been found to be less than satisfactory. However, it is probable that sodium bicarbonate, 2 to 5 per cent, will almost always prove to be a simpler and less expensive, yet very adequate, alternative. Varying amounts of Alevaire (0.5 to 10 ml) could be given by nebulization using IPPB or an air compressor, but not by ultrasonic nebulization or mist tent administration. The preparation was alleged to be of particular value when given with drugs such as antibiotics, whose penetration of respiratory secretions may be improved by the surfactant.

Some physicians found Alevaire to be a useful topical debriding adjunct in other situations, such as for the irrigation of sinuses or of surgical or orthopedic wounds that contain sticky secretions. However, its value in such situations has not been substantiated; therefore, it could not be recommended for such usage at present.

Sodium Bicarbonate

Sodium bicarbonate ($NaHCO_3$) has long been used as a topical solution for cleansing wounds, and it has been employed empirically as an irrigating solution for the trachea in tracheotomized patients.[41] There is good evidence that 2 per cent sodium bicarbonate alone is just as effective as Alevaire.[23, 25, 35, 36] There is evidence[25, 41] that mucus is less adhesive in a more alkaline environment, such as that provided by sodium bicarbonate solution, which has a pH of 7.5 to 8.5. The hypertonicity of sodium bicarbonate may account for some of its effectiveness, since hypertonic, topical solutions cause an increase in respiratory tract secretions by virtue of their osmotic effect. It is also known that alkalinization results in the activation of natural proteases that are found particularly in purulent sputum.[42]

It is possible that other electrolyte solutions (such as sodium or potassium carbonate, or sodium phosphate) may have a similar mucus-loosening quality, but these drugs have not been tried in inhalation therapy. The true mucokinetic value of sodium bicarbonate and other inhalational salts remains to be determined by controlled trials. At present, experience justifies the use of sodium bicarbonate as one of the standard mucokinetic agents for mucoid and mucopurulent sputum. However, it is possible that the main value of the agent is to decrease the adhesiveness of sputum rather than its viscosity, although it can undoubtedly decrease viscosity.[23] Its mucokinetic properties are listed in Table 3–12.

Administration. Sodium bicarbonate is usually available in bottles of 1.4, 5 and 7.5 per cent; other concentrations are also marketed. It has been found that both the 5 and 7.5 per cent solutions are usually well-tolerated when given by inhalation, although diluting the 5 per cent solution with an equal volume of sterile water will result in a less irritating product of 2.5 per cent concentration. The 1.4 per cent solution is practically isotonic, and it is not irritating to the respiratory mucosa.

Sodium bicarbonate solution can be prepared by a patient at home simply by stirring the pure powder into sterile (or boiled) cool water; the solution itself should not be

TABLE 3–11. IMPORTANT AEROSOL MUCOKINETIC DRUGS

Trade Name	Main Constituents	Usual Aerosol Dosage	Comments
MUCOMYST	N-acetyl-L-cysteine 10% and 20%	2–5 ml q6h; Range: 1–10 ml q 2–12 hr	Breaks disulfide bonds, causes mucolysis. Malodorous, and may cause bronchospasm. 20% solution should be diluted with equal volume isotonic saline or sodium bicarbonate.
DORNAVAC	Pancreatic dornase (deoxyribonuclease)	100,000 u.tid; Range: 50,000–100,000 u 1–4 times a day	Enzyme: depolymerizes DNA, and is indicated for purulent secretions only. May be irritating; can cause hypersensitivity reactions. Suitable for short-term use only. Dissolve in 1–2 ml normal saline.
TRYPTAR	Trypsin	100,000 u. tid; Range: 25,000–100,000 u 1–3 times a day	Enzyme: digests mucoprotein. May be irritating; can cause hypersensitivity reactions. Suitable for short-term use only. Dissolve in 3 ml normal saline.
ALEVAIRE	Tyloxapol 0.125%, sodium bicarbonate 2%, glycerin 5%	2–5 ml q6h; Range: 0.5–10 ml q 3–8 hr	Wetting agent. Usually given with other medications, (e.g., bronchodilators, antibiotics) to help improve their distal deposition. No longer promoted
	Sodium bicarbonate 1.4–7.5%	2–5 ml q6h; Range: 1–10 ml q 2–8 hr	Wetting agent in low concentrations, bronchomucotropic in higher concentrations. May be combined with other drugs for immediate use.
	Sodium chloride 0.45–15%	2–5 ml q6h; Range: 1–10 ml q 2–8 hr	Hypotonic solution penetrates well, especially when given by ultrasonic nebulization. Hypertonic solutions stimulate cough, and may have mucolytic effect. Normal saline is a standard diluting agent.
	Propylene glycol 2–25%	2–5 ml q4h; Range: 1–10 ml q 1–8 hr	Soothing demulcent for tracheobronchitis (2% solution). Stabilizes droplets; used with medicational aerosols to improve distal deposition. Effective for cough induction (15% or stronger solution).

TABLE 3–12. MUCOKINETIC PROPERTIES OF SODIUM BICARBONATE

Property	Actions*
Alkalinity (pH about 8)	Decreases adhesiveness of mucus Potentiates proteolysis by natural proteases May improve ciliary activity
Hypertonicity (2–7.5% solutions)	Bronchorrheic effect Direct mucolytic effect, e.g., by displacing Ca^{++} from ionic bonds in mucoprotein
Salinity (contributed by sodium)	May dissociate DNA-mucoprotein bonding
Adjuvant (alkaline and saline properties)	May potentiate acetylcysteine
Gastric stimulation (by swallowed solution)	Stimulation of gastropulmonary mucokinetic vagal reflex

*These actions are similar to those of hypertonic sodium chloride (see Table 3–3), but the alkalinity of sodium bicarbonate enhances its mucokinetic effects.

boiled, since it decomposes when heated. Each gram of sodium bicarbonate is equivalent to 12 mEq of sodium (and an equal amount of bicarbonate). To make a 2.5 per cent solution, 25 gm of sodium bicarbonate should be added to 1000 ml of water; this is a suitable concentration for routine nebulization.

The drug can be administered by aerosol (using 1 to 3 ml) or it can be directly instilled into the trachea (2 to 10 ml). Frequent administration does not appear to have any adverse effects, and in usual situations when a mucokinetic effect is wanted, administration every four to eight hours seems to be effective.

Sodium bicarbonate often leaves a deposit in its container after prolonged standing; a small amount of disodium edetate is incorporated in the marketed product to decrease the extent of this precipitation. Sodium bicarbonate appears to be compatible with other mucolytic drugs; indeed, it seems to potentiate the activity of acetylcysteine, which is more effective at an alkaline pH. On the other hand, bronchodilators are inactivated in an alkaline environment, and color changes occur more rapidly because of formation of breakdown products. However, clinical experience shows that sympathomimetics can be added to sodium bicarbonate without loss of effectiveness if the combination is nebulized immediately.

Adverse Effects. The only notable adverse reactions are seen with higher concentrations (greater than 2 per cent). Thus, some patients complain of irritation of the oropharynx and airways when 7.5 or even 5 per cent sodium bicarbonate is nebulized. The amount of bicarbonate given by endotracheal instillation is unlikely to result in any effect on the acid-base balance of the blood, unless large volumes are introduced into the lungs without subsequent removal by coughing, suction or drainage. The administration of large amounts could possibly result in hypernatremia or a metabolic alkalosis.

Recommendations. It is possible that sodium bicarbonate could be regarded as the standard mucolytic drug for all types of sputum, in preference to saline or proprietary drugs. Thus, it is recommended that sodium bicarbonate be used as a diluent for acetylcysteine. It can also be employed as a vehicle for bronchodilators, but the preparation should be freshly constituted immediately prior to use. The dose for nebulization is 2 to 5 ml several times a day; for intratracheal instillation 5 to 10 ml can be used as often as needed, but overuse could produce an alkalosis. Concomitant bronchodilator therapy should be used to prevent reactive bronchospasm.

For routine inhalation therapy, it is practical to use the 30 ml vials of sodium bicarbonate, available in concentrations of 5 to 7.5 per cent. The standard 500 ml bottles can be used on intensive care units where larger volumes of solution are required for periodic instillation into intubated patients' respiratory tracts. Containers of sodium bicarbonate that show cloudiness or particulate deposits should not be used.

When sodium bicarbonate is administered with sympathomimetics, the mixture should always be discarded if not used immediately, and the nebulizer should be cleaned promptly after use. The sodium bicarbonate enhances the natural breakdown of the sympathomimetics into colored products, which may give a red tinge to the subsequently expectorated sputum.

Sodium bicarbonate has other uses in respiratory medicine and critical care. Thus it is used to treat metabolic acidosis, and it is an essential component in the pharmacology of cardiopulmonary resuscitation. A further important use is as an antacid, for the neutralization of gastric acidity and for the treatment of indigestion.

Table 3–11 gives details of sodium bicarbonate and other important mucokinetics that are suitable for aerosolization or instillation.

Ethanol

Ethanol (ethyl alcohol, C_2H_5OH) is a surface active agent, and it has the ability to decrease the surface tension of saline solutions and of respiratory tract secretions. It is remarkably effective at dispersing the bubbles of pulmonary edema foam: this is the value of alcohol in inhalation therapy.[43] Other alcohols, such as octyl alcohol, have a similar antifoaming action, but ethanol is the only alcohol established as an inhalational drug.

The foam produced during acute pulmonary edema is extremely stable; other mucokinetic agents, such as acetylcysteine and electrolyte solutions, do not have an antifoaming action and do not affect the pulmonary edema fluid. Other inhalational surfactants are much less effective than alcohol. The alcohol can be given as an aerosol by nebulization or, more simply, as a vapor, by bubbling oxygen through it.[44]

The stability of the foam in pulmonary edema may be conferred by pulmonary surfactant, which ensures that the smaller the bubbles the more resistant they are to further reduction in size. Alcohol may replace the normal surfactant, thereby leading to loss of stability of the small bubbles. Once the bubbles have been dispersed, the airway obstruction caused by the foam is greatly relieved. However, the true effects of alcohol are undoubtedly more complex than this simplistic explanation. Thus, although alcohol nebulization increases lung compliance in normal subjects, it has no such effect in the presence of pulmonary congestion; its true value and dangers in pulmonary edema have yet to be clearly defined.[43]

Some physicians and therapists believe that giving alcohol and oxygen with IPPB is the treatment of choice for acute pulmonary edema. However, the value of this form of therapy has never been rigorously compared to more conventional treatment with intravenous diuretics, aminophylline and digoxin accompanied by rotating tourniquets, phlebotomy, oxygen and morphine.

Usually, these agents and adjuncts are given concurrently with the alcohol, and it is therefore difficult to establish whether the contribution of the alcohol is a truly useful one. Indeed, most authorities seem to be remarkably unenthused about the inhalational administration of alcohol in their writings on the treatment of pulmonary edema.[45]

Ethyl alcohol appears to have a bronchomucotropic effect (see Chapter 2) in animals, but its clinical value is controversial. Boyd[46] found that when 1 ml/kg of alcohol in water was given by steam inhalation to rabbits, there was no effect, whereas 5 ml/kg increased the volume output and the amount of soluble mucus of respiratory tract fluid. It appeared that the alcohol had a local stimulant effect on the mucosal cells. Much higher concentrations result in an inflammatory reaction in the respiratory mucosa. Whether or not low concentrations of inhaled alcohol can improve mucokinesis *in humans* has not been established. However, it is a common experience that the oral intake of alcoholic beverages results in appreciable amounts of alcohol being excreted into the airways, yet clinical observation of innumerable patients who are partial to such beverages reveals no evidence of a beneficial effect on the respiratory mucosa. Furthermore, relatively high concentrations of alcohol in the airways can be damaging to the respiratory tract and other vital organs. It is, therefore, reasonable to conclude that *ethyl alcohol is not suitable for routine mucokinetic therapy*. If a respiratory patient claims that he obtains benefit from ethanol, then it is cheaper, easier and more pleasurable for him to introduce the alcohol into his body through the gastrointestinal tract, without the respiratory physician or therapist dignifying the experience by suggesting that it serves the mucokinetic cause.

A barely acceptable use of alcohol in routine inhalation therapy (in addition to its possible value in pulmonary edema) is when it is used in low concentration as a vehicle for other mucokinetic drugs, such as lemon oil.[47, 48] Similarly, alcohol may be a constituent of oral medications used in the treatment of respiratory disease, but in such cases it cannot be considered to have a primary action on the respiratory mucosa (See Table 3–13).

Untoward Effects. Many of the properties of ethyl alcohol are clearly harmful to delicate tissues. The drug has a local irritant and astringent effect, and it can cause

TABLE 3–13. ETHYL ALCOHOL AS A RESPIRATORY MEDICATION

Use	Mechanism	Comment
ORAL		
As a solvent, e.g., in elixirs	Many drugs are more soluble in alcohol than in water	Alcoholic content in elixirs may be contraindicated for some patients (e.g., alcoholics).
As a sedative, e.g., a "nightcap".	Central nervous system depressant	Potentiates other depressants; may be dangerous
INHALATIONAL		
As a surfactant (bubble oxygen through alcohol)	Reduces surface tension of mucoid froth	Useful emergency treatment for foaming pulmonary edema
As a bronchorrheic (1–2 ml 30% ethanol in water)	Irritates tracheobronchial mucosa	Should not be employed as a routine mucokinetic agent
As a vehicle for other drugs	Used in low doses as a solvent, e.g., for volatile oils	Should be used only sparingly in this form

vasodilation with exudation of fluid into the mucosa. Alcohol in low concentrations can increase the viscosity of mucus and it can adversely affect the protein content in respiratory secretions. In addition, alcohol has an antiphagocytic effect on polymorphs, and although it also has an antibacterial effect, its overall depression of host defenses tends to favor the development of infections.[49] The imbiber of large amounts of alcohol suffers further disadvantages. The sedative and analgesic effects of the drug decrease ciliary activity and depress the respiratory center and the protective cough reflex. The intoxicated patient sleeps heavily, does not move much, and becomes dehydrated. All these consequences favor the impaction of mucus in the dependent parts of the lungs, and pneumonia readily develops; if the individual also aspirates, then a severe necrotizing pneumonia may result.

Certainly, alcohol in excess is an antimucokinetic agent, and, overall, there are vast numbers of patients who have respiratory disease as a complication of alcoholic intake. In contrast, there is minimal evidence to suggest that alcohol, by any route of administration, offers a mucokinetic benefit to the patient with established respiratory disease. If a mucokinetic effect is seen after inhaling alcohol, it is probable that this is the result of mucosal irritation (such as may be incurred by cigarette smoking); continued inhalation therapy with ethanol may produce bronchitis. However, there is no evidence of a more specific adverse effect, such as surfactant depletion leading to atelectasis.[40]

Recommendations. Ethyl alcohol may be given in the treatment of pulmonary edema, as a vapor or as an aerosol. Oxygen can be bubbled through diluted alcohol, and the vapor inhaled through a face mask or by means of nasal cannula. Alternatively, an alcoholic solution can be nebulized, with or without IPPB. Vodka or a similar strong, clear alcohol can be diluted by an equal amount of water to produce a 50 per cent solution for inhalational use, although a 30 per cent solution is probably adequate. See Table 3–13.

For many reasons, alcohol is not recommended for administration as a routine mucokinetic. One very practical reason for discouraging the use of alcohol as an inhalational agent is that there is a propensity for this liquid to find its way into the gastrointestinal tracts of members of the health team rather than into the respiratory tracts of their patients. Certainly, any respiratory therapy department that orders more than a fifth of vodka a year from the hospital pharmacy should be looked on with suspicion.

Ethasulfate

Ethasulfate (ethylhexyl sulfate, Tergitol) was used as the sodium salt in a 0.125 per cent solution, in combination with 0.1 per cent potassium iodide, in the preparation Tergemist.[50, 51] The product was withdrawn from the market in 1969 after being judged ineffective by the FDA, although favorable reports of its mucolytic properties perhaps outweighed the unfavorable ones. However, the detergent properties of sodium ethasulfate appear to have been of little value in inhalation therapy.[39] Furthermore, in current practice, the administration of potassium iodide is preferred by the oral route. However, since iodides are of accepted mucokinetic value, it may be worth carrying out a controlled investigation into the use of nebulized iodides in the treatment of sputopathies.

Other Inhalational Surfactants

Other proprietary agents with surfactant properties have been tried in inhalation therapy, but none have gained acceptance. Agents reported to have some value include *tacholiquin, polyethylene glycol, sorbitan laureate*[13] and several that have been classified as *cetamacrogols*. At present, the only important drugs of this type are propylene glycol and glycerin.

Glycerin

Glycerin (glycerine, glycerol) is a hygroscopic fluid with a long history of use in inhalation therapy in concentrations of 5 to 50 per cent or more. The principal use of this drug was as a vehicular agent in Alevaire, which contains 5 per cent glycerin. Glycerin is also used in the preparation of some oral mucokinetic agents, including glyceryl guaiacolate and iodinated glycerol. The drug has demulcent, humectant and, possibly, mucolytic properties similar to those of propylene glycol, but it is not a disinfectant. It is said to be more irritating than propylene glycol, with a greater tendency to cause bronchospasm, and it is now rarely employed in inhalation therapy. It will be recalled that propylene glycol has replaced glycerin for most inhalational uses.

Dipalmitoyl Lecithin

Dipalmitoyl lecithin (DPL) is the naturally occuring pulmonary surfactant. It is a phospholipid, and is produced by the alveolar type II cells; it is considered to be the main chemical agent in surfactant, although a number of other subsidiary chemicals have been identified. The name DPL has recently been changed to 1,2-dipalmitoyl-3-phosphatidyl-choline (DPPC).

The functions of natural surfactant are to prevent collapse of the alveoli at small volume, thereby forestalling atelectasis; and to help prevent leakage of capillary fluid into the alveoli, thus protecting the lung from pulmonary edema. At present, surfactant has not been shown to contribute any other important quality to the respiratory tract secretions, nor has it any effect on sputum viscosity, although its presence in pulmonary edema fluid confers exceptional stability to the characteristic foam.

Synthetic DPL has been given by inhalation in experimental subjects, but it has not found a place in therapeutics. It is possible that, in the future, DPL or similar agents will be used in the treatment of various conditions in which alveolar instability is a major pathogenic factor.

VOLATILE MUCOTROPIC INHALANTS
(Table 3–14)

Numerous aromatic, and a few aliphatic, liquids and solids that are readily volatilized have been popular for many years as inhalational mucokinetic agents. Many of these have been studied in detail by Boyd,[48] who uses the term "bronchomucotropic" or, more simply, "mucotropic" to categorize drugs that augment the output of respiratory tract fluid or increase its concentration of mucoproteins. The inhalational mucotropics are usually administered in low concentration in a base of water, and the most popular and simple technique is to add the agents to steaming hot water. The scented fumes certainly have an esthetic appeal (which can be on the negative side, however), and this might account for the popularity of many of these drugs, although actual proof of their effectiveness is far from established. Moreover, some patients find these inhalants irritating, particularly if higher concentrations are used. Many physicians consider that the various scented additives confer no advantage, and that bland cold or hot steam provides the best simple mucokinetic inhalational agent.

Balsams

Perhaps the best known of the mucotropic inhalants are various balsams, which are oxidized volatile oils. They are usually solid or semisolid amorphous products that con-

TABLE 3–14. VOLATILE INHALANTS THAT HAVE BEEN USED AS MUCOKINETICS

Effective	Ineffective
Anisaldehyde	Aloe
Camphene	Anise oil
Cedar leaf oil	Benzoin
Citral	Eucalyptus oil
Ethanol	Friars' balsam
Geraniol	Menthol
Lemon oil	Storax
Limonene	Terpineol
Nutmeg oil	Thymol
Pinene	Tolu

This table rates the effectiveness of some inhalants when given in therapeutic dosage.[46, 48, 53, 54]

sist of mixtures of resin acids, resin alcohols, resinotannols, resenes and esters. Many of them are obtained from oxidation of *terpenes,* which are isometric hydrocarbon compounds with the basic formula $C_{10}H_{16}$. A number of these agents are still available under their traditional names. They are often used by individuals as long-established family remedies, whereas they are less frequently prescribed by physicians.

Friars' Balsam

Friars' balsam is a tincture containing benzoin, aloe, storax and tolu balsam; it is available as the USP preparation "compound benzoin tincture" for dermal purposes. It has long been favored for scenting steam for inhalation, and it has been popular in the inhalational treatment of croup and bronchitis.

Boyd and Sheppard[52] investigated this preparation and concluded that it had no significant effects, unless used in volumes large enough to cause an inflammatory reaction of the respiratory mucosa. This discouraging scientific observation is unlikely to dissuade the enthusiast from employing friars' balsam as an inhalant, or in folk preparations — such as a few drops on a cube of sugar, which is then allowed to dissolve in the mouth.

Tolu Balsam

Tolu balsam is obtained as a resinous exudate from the trunk of *Myroxylon balsamum.* It may have some expectorant action, but is mainly used as a flavor for cough medicines as tolu syrup, and as a constituent of friars' balsam.

Other Volatile Oils

Many naturally occurring fragrant oils (ethereal or essential oils) have been recommended for use as inhalants. The most important of the volatile oils are unoxidized terpenes, which are widely distributed in the plant world. *Turpentine* is the best known of the terpenes, but it is not suitable for inhalational use. *Terpin hydrate* (terpinol) is the main medicinal derivative of turpentine, and it is employed as an oral expectorant; it is discussed later in this chapter.

Eucalyptus is one of the most popular volatile oils, and it is a constituent of many proprietary medications used in the symptomatic treatment of respiratory tract dis-

orders. Eucalyptus contains eucalyptol (cineole), various resins and some tannic acid; its pungent but pleasant odor is credited with remedial qualities. Boyd has shown in controlled studies that eucalyptus has little effect on the respiratory mucosa.[41] Similarly, popular agents like *menthol* and *camphor* have little effect on the respiratory tract[47] and it appears that any response is due to irritation, rather than benign stimulation, of the respiratory tract. Nevertheless, these aromatic agents are used in many cough medications and decongestant mixtures (see Chapter 9).

Most of the available information on volatile mucotropic agents has been published by Boyd,[46-48, 53, 54] who has been the main worker in this area. His animal work suggests that, of the volatile inhalants, alcohol has the greatest mucotropic effect on the trachea of *animals* anesthetized with urethane. Camphanes and pinanes such as *fenchone* (a camphor-like substance), *camphene,* and *pinene* (found in turpentine) have some effect. Other effective terpenes include *citral, citronellal, geraniol, linalyl acetate* and *ionone.* Several substituted phenols also have mucotropic action: *anisaldehyde, anethole, isosafrole* and *eugenol.* Less effect was noted with *p*-menthane derivatives such as carvone, cineole (the main terpene in eucalyptus), dolcymene, limonene, menthol, phellandrene, terpineol and thymol. The agents that are listed as effective, in Table 3-14, may be capable of augmenting respiratory tract fluid secretion when dissolved in alcohol (not more than 1 ml/kg body weight) and added to boiling water in an amount which causes a just perceptible odor. Higher concentrations of these agents actually lose mucotropic activity, probably because such doses inhibit rather than stimulate the secretory cells of the respiratory tract.

Proprietary medications often contain several agents believed to have some mucotropic effect (Table 3-15). *Vicks Vapo Steam* (which is added to steam for inhalational treatment of colds, cough and sputopathies) contains 55 per cent alcohol, 12.4 per cent menthol, 12.4 per cent camphor, 12.4 per cent eucalyptus oil, 5 per cent tincture of benzoin, and 1.8 per cent polyoxyethylene dodecanol as a wetting agent. It is difficult to obtain proof of the active participation of the individual constituents of this popular remedy in the treatment of respiratory tract disorders. The humidifying effect of the steam probably provides the major

**TABLE 3–15. SOME PROPRIETARY
VOLATILE INHALANTS**
(added to steaming hot water)

Product	Main Ingredients
Kaz	camphor 10 mg/ml, methyl-salicylate 4 mg/ml
Steam-Mist	camphor 4 mg/ml, methyl-salicylate 15 mg/ml
Vicks VapoRub	camphor, menthol, turpentine spirits, eucalyptus oil, cedar leaf oil, myristica oil, thymol
Vicks Vapo Steam	polyoxyethylene dodecanol, menthol, camphor, eucalyptus oil, tincture of benzoin, alcohol

therapeutic benefit, but the other agents may contribute some demulcent and mucokinetic qualities, which help provide symptomatic relief, particularly in children, whose relatively narrow airways quickly lose patency in respiratory infections.

ORAL MUCOKINETIC AGENTS

Numerous "expectorant" medications continue to enjoy popular use, although there are but few clinical studies that establish any pharmacologic basis for such use. Boyd terms these drugs "systemic bronchomucotropic agents,"[54] but the term "oral mucokinetic agent" will be used here. Most oral agents are believed to stimulate gastric receptors, thereby initiating the gastropulmonary mucokinetic vagal reflex described in Chapter 2 (see Figs. 2–4 and 2–5). A second mechanism may occur with agents that are absorbed into the blood stream; following absorption they act directly on the bronchial glands or on the secretory mucosa to cause an enhanced output of fluid. These two different mechanisms of action permit the popular expectorants to be classified into two groups: indirect (vagal) mucokinetics and direct mucokinetics.

It is possible that some agents act on medullary centers (including the postulated mucokinetic center) to induce reflex vagal stimulation of the respiratory glands; this mechanism is relatively unimportant in medical practice, although *apomorphine* and, possibly, *carbon dioxide* have such an effect. Direct stimulation of the cholinergic effector fibers in the respiratory tract by parasympathomimetic drugs can result in consider-

able augmentation of respiratory secretions, but such drugs are not of clinical value as mucokinetics, since they are liable to cause bronchospasm.[54] Indeed, spontaneous asthma, which may be mediated by cholinergic mechanisms, is usually associated with an increase in mucus production. An "antimucotropic" pharmacologic effect is produced by anticholinergic drugs (e.g., atropine or hyoscine, as described in Chapter 4). Antihistamines and mucosal constrictant drugs can also result in a decreased mucus production; they are used as "drying agents" (Chapter 9).

VAGAL STIMULANTS

Most oral "cough medications" and "expectorants" belong to this category. These drugs are effective only in animals that have intact vagal afferents from the stomach and duodenum, and efferents to the lungs. This would imply that the vagal mucokinetics could not work in patients who have had surgical vagotomy procedures, but no study along these lines has been carried out.

Salt Solutions

Various salts have long been used for medicinal purposes, and they continue to enjoy the support of large segments of the public who purchase proprietary remedies, drink mineral waters and partake of the assorted benefits offered at bathing spas. Physiologically, most of the salt solutions that are taken orally serve as osmotic stimulants to the bowel, and thereby act as cathartics. The ability of hyperosmolar electrolyte solutions to stimulate receptors in the gastrointestinal mucosa may result in reflex stimulation of the respiratory mucosal glands. Thus, salts used as oral cathartics may also augment the secretion of respiratory tract fluid (see Tables 3–3, 3–16 and 3–17).

The most popular oral mucokinetic salt solutions are ammonium bicarbonate, ammonium chloride, ammonium carbonate, potassium iodide, potassium citrate, sodium chloride, sodium bicarbonate and sodium citrate. However, the true value of such medications remains to be proved, although they are incorporated in numerous "cough medicines," and are readily available in both over-the-counter and prescription preparations (see Chapter 9).

Ammonium Salts

Ammonium chloride and *ammonium carbonate* should be given to adults in a dosage of 0.3 to 1 gm in 5 ml of a suitable, flavored, "expectorant mixture" four times a day. Ammonium chloride preparations are the only salt-type agents described in the section on expectorant agents in AMA Drug Evaluations. The mucokinetic effect would probably not be obtained if enteric-coated preparations were used, since the gastric mucosa is not exposed to the drug. Ammonium salts are rarely used alone, but they are available in many expectorant mixtures, in which the amount is often inadequate (see Table 3–16). Large doses could induce a metabolic acidosis, particularly in patients with hepatic or renal insufficiency, but it is rare to find sufficient enthusiasm for prescribing this expectorant drug in such generous doses.

Other ammonium salts used less commonly as expectorants are ammonium acetate and ammonium bicarbonate.

Potassium Salts

Potassium iodide is considered later (see section on iodides). *Potassium citrate* is generally used to replace potassium in situations of actual or potential hypokalemia. The drug is employed as a mucokinetic in combination mixtures (Tables 3–17, 9–12 and 9–13), although it may produce only a slight action on the respiratory mucosa unless given in a dose of about 0.4 gm/kg body weight.

Sodium Salts

Sodium salts are commonly administered by nebulization or instillation, as already described, but it is probable that subemetic amounts, given orally, may stimulate mucokinesis. Oral expectorants include *sodium citrate,* which is fairly frequently incorporated in cough medicines (see Table 3–17, 9–12 and 9–13). Nebulization of hypertonic salt solutions into the lungs may lead to the swallowing of enough of the drug to activate the gastric mucokinetic reflex: this could be another example of nebulization therapy merely serving as a complex method of delivering an oral expectorant drug.

Other salts that have been used orally include various other citrates and acetates, and *antimony potassium tartrate* (in a dose of 3 mg). The value of these drugs is quite unproved, although there is a lingering clinical impression that oral salt solutions of various kinds are more effective than water alone.

Creosote Derivatives

The tar obtained from various woods, when distilled, yields a number of phenolic compounds. Hard woods such as beech are used as a source of *creosote,* which is a mixture of phenols having a characteristic, not too unpleasant, odor. The most important components are *creosol* (methylguaiacol) and *guaiacol* (Fig. 3–3). Creosote is an antiseptic, once advocated for the treatment of tuberculosis, in which it gained a reputa-

TABLE 3–16. SALTS USED AS ORAL MUCOKINETIC AGENTS

Salt	Examples*	Usual Dose†	Comments
Ammonium carbonate "Sal volatile," $(NH_4)_2CO_3$	–	300–1000 mg	Used in smelling salts; respiratory stimulant; irritating to stomach
Ammonium chloride NH_4Cl	See Tables 3–17 and 3–20	300–1000 mg	Less irritating than ammonium carbonate
Antimony potassium tartrate $C_8H_4K_2Sb_2O_{12}$	Cheralin	2–8 mg	Rarely used emetic; used in treatment of schistosomiasis
Calcium iodide CaI_2	Calcidrine	300–1000 mg	Alternative method for providing iodide
Potassium acetate CH_3COOK		1 gm	Used as an alkalizer, as a diuretic, and as a source of potassium
Potassium citrate $C_6H_5K_3O_7$	Citra	0.4 gm/kg	Used as an alkalizer, as a diuretic, and as a source of potassium
Potassium iodide KI	SSKI, Pima	300–1000 mg	Most effective mucokinetic; used to prevent goiter and in treatment of toxic goiter; antifungal properties
Sodium chloride NaCl	Many	300–1000 mg	Basic mucokinetic and cathartic
Sodium citrate $C_6H_5Na_3O_7$	Codimal Dicoril, Expectico, etc.	1 gm	Used as an alkalizer, and to increase urinary excretion of calcium and lead; anticoagulant for stored blood.

*These examples are "cough medicines" that contain the respective salt and a variety of other constituents.
†Dose can be given up to four times a day.

Brand Name	Basic Dose	Ammonium Chloride mg	Other Mucokinetics	Antihistamines or Decongestants	Antitussive mg	Other
Amonidrin Tablets	1	200	guaifenesin 100 mg			
*Bax Expectorant	5 ml	125	Na citrate 50 mg			alcohol 5%
Baby Cough Syrup	5 ml	13		diphenhydramine 12.5 mg		glycerin 343 mg licorice extract 12 mg
*Benylin Cough Syrup	5 ml	125	Na citrate 50 mg	diphenhydramine 12.5 mg		alcohol 5%
Chlortrimeton Expectorant	5 ml	100	guaifenesin 50 mg Na citrate 50 mg	chlorpheniramine 2 mg phenylephrine 10 mg		alcohol 1%
*Clistin Expectorant	5 ml	120	K guaiacolsulfonate 60 mg Na citrate 120 mg guaifenesin 100 mg	carbinoxamine 2 mg		
Colrex Expectorant	5 ml	50	guaifenesin 50 mg			alcohol 4.7% (sugar-free)
Coricidin Cough Formula	5 ml	100	guaifenesin 50 mg	chlorpheniramine 2 mg phenylpropanolamine 12.5 mg		
DM-4 Children's Cough Control	5 ml	40	K guaiacolsulfonate 38 mg		dextromethorphan 4 mg	glycerin 75 mg alcohol 1.5% lemon flavor
Efricon	5 ml	90	K guaiacolsulfonate 90 mg	chlorpheniramine 2 mg phenylephrine 5 mg pyrilamine 7.5 mg	codeine 11 mg	homatropine 0.25 mg alcohol 5% menthol
Endotussin = NN	5 ml	40	Na citrate 60 mg	methapyrilene 13 mg ephedrine 5 mg	dextromethorphan 10 mg codeine 11 mg	alcohol 4.8% menthol
Histadyl	5 ml	110		methapyrilene 12.5 mg ephedrine 4 mg		
Histovite-D	5 ml	86			dextromethorphan 5 mg.	
Ipsatol Syrup (DM) Noratuss	5 ml 5 ml	22 32.4	ipecac 0.24 mg K guaiacolsulfonate 5.4 mg terpin hydrate 5.4 mg		(dextromethorphan 10 mg) codeine 3.3 mg	tolu balsam cocillana extract 4.4 mg Na benzoate 0.1% cherry flavor alcohol 2%
Quelidrine Syrup	5 ml	40	ipecac 0.005 ml	chlorpheniramine 2 mg phenylephrine 5 mg ephedrine 5 mg	dextromethorphan 10 mg	
Rhinex DM Syrup	5 ml	100	guaifenesin 50 mg	chlorpheniramine 1 mg phenylpropanolamine 12.5 mg	dextromethorphan 7.5 mg	alcohol 5%
Soltice	5 ml	85	Na citrate 85 mg	phenylpropanolamine 12.5 mg		
Triaminicol Cough Syrup	5 ml	90		pheniramine 6.25 mg pyrilamine 6.25 mg phenylpropanolamine 12.5 mg	dextromethorphan 15 mg	cetylpyridinium 0.05 mg
Turpoin Tablets	1	130	K guaiacolsulfonate 130 mg terpin hydrate 65 mg		dextromethorphan 15 mg	

The usual dose of the solution is 2.5–5 ml for infants, 10 ml for children, 5–20 ml for adults, up to four times a day.
*Prescription items.

A) <u>Derivatives of terpene (C_6H_{16})</u>

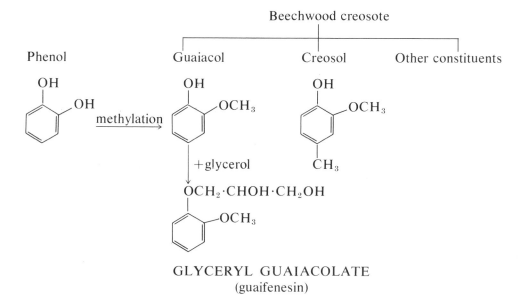

B) <u>Derivatives of phenol (C_6H_5OH)</u>

GLYCERYL GUAIACOLATE
(guaifenesin)

Figure 3–3. Popular oral expectorants

tion of having an expectorant quality (see Chapter 1). When given orally, it may act as a mucokinetic agent, both indirectly, by stimulating the gastric mucosa, and directly, following secretion of the absorbed drug into the tracheobronchial tree. Creosote has been used as an inhalational agent, but administration by aerosol has, not without good reason, fallen into disfavor.

Guaiacol

Guaiacol (o-methoxyphenol) is the monomethyl ether of o-dihydroxybenzene (cat-

echol). It can be obtained from beechwood creosote, by methylation of catechol or by synthesis from o-methoxyaniline. Guaiacol was originally isolated from guaiac resin. Like creosote, guaiacol was once used in the treatment of tuberculosis, and subsequently it also gained favor as an expectorant. Both drugs have also been used as mild topical anesthetics.

Guaiacol derivatives have replaced creosote in mucokinetic pharmacology, since they appear to be less irritating to the bowel and are absorbed more reliably. Various derivatives of guaiacol have been used as

TABLE 3–18. CONTENT OF GUAIFENESIN IN PROPRIETARY COMBINATION PRODUCTS*

	Content of Guaifenesin		For Additional Information See	
	TABLET mg	SOLUTION mg/5 ml	CHAPTER	TABLE
Actifed-C Expectorant		100	9	31
†Actol Expectorant	200	200	9	14
Asbron G Inlay-Tabs/Elixir	100	33	6	16
Brexin Capsules	100			
Broncomar Tablets/Elixir	100	50		
Brondecon Tablets/Elixir	100	50	6	16
†Bronkolixir		50	6	16
†Bronkotabs	100		6	16
†Bronkotabs-HAFS	50			
†Chlortrimeton Expectorant		50	3	16
†Conar Expectorant		100	9	14
†Conar-A Tablets	100		9	14
†Coricidin Cough Relief Formula		50	3	16
†Coryban-D Cough Syrup		50	9	13
Decongest T.D. Tablets	200			
†Dimacol Capsule/Liquid	100	100	9	13
Dimetane Expectorant Liquid		100	9	23
Donatussin Drops		100		
†Dorcol Pediatric Cough Syrup		37.5	9	13
Dyline GG Tablets/Liquid	200	200		
Emfaseem Capsules/Liquid	100	16.7		
Entex Capsules/Liquid	200	100		
Expectico Liquid		100	9	12
†Fedahist Expectorant		100		
†GG-Cen Capsules/Syrup	200	100		
†Glycotuss Tablets/Syrup	100	100		
†Glytuss Tablets	200			
†Guistrey Fortis Tablets	100			
Histalet X Tablets/Syrup	200	200	9	13
Hylate Tablets/Syrup	100	33.3		
†Hytuss Tablets/Capsules	100/200			
Isoclor Expectorant		88.3		
Luffylin-GG Tablet/Elixir	200	33.3	6	12
Mudrane GG Tablets/Elixir	100	26	6	16
Mudrane GG-2 Tablets	100		6	16
Neothylline-G Tablets/Elixir	50	50	6	12
Nilcol Tablets/Elixir	200	33.3	9	13
†Novahistine DMX Liquid		100	9	13
†Novahistine Expectorant		100	9	13
Polaramine Expectorant		100	9	23
Pseudocot-G Laytabs	100			
Pseudo-Hist Expectorant		100		
Quibron Capsules/Elixir	150	50	6	16
Quibron Plus Capsules/Elixir	100	33	6	16
Respinol-G Tablets	200			
†Rhinex-DM Syrup		50	3(9)	16(13)
†Robitussin Lozenges/Syrup	50	100	9	13
†Rhinosyn Pediatric Cough Syrup		100	9	13
Rondec-DM Syrup		100	9	13
Ryna-Cx Syrup		100		
†Ryna = Tussadini Expectorant	100	100		
Slo-phyllin GG Capsules/Syrup	90	30	6	16
†Sorbutuss Syrup		100	3	20
S-T Forte Syrup		80	9	13
Synophylate-GG Tablets/Syrup	100	33.3	6	16
†2/G Syrup		100	9	13
Tedral Expectorant	100		6	16
†Triaminic Expectorant		100	9	12
†Trind Syrup		50	9	13
†Trind-DM Syrup		50	9	13
Tussend Expectorant		200	9	12
Unproco Capsules	200		9	13
†Verequad Tablets/Suspension	100	50	6	16

*Products listed in Physicians' Desk Reference, 1977.

†Available without prescription. For other non-prescription drugs see Cormier, J. F. and Bryant, B. G.: Cold and allergy products. *In Handbook of Nonprescription Drugs.* Washington, American Pharmaceutical Association, 5th ed., 1977. pp. 97–111.

expectorants, but few remain on the market. *Guaiacol carbonate* (Duotal) was formerly recommended but is not used now, whereas *potassium guaiacol sulfonate* (K guaicolsulfonate, thiocol) is still incorporated in some expectorant mixtures. It is claimed that 500 mg is an effective dose, although there is no evidence to support this claim.

Guaifenesin

Guaifenesin (guayanesin, guaianesin, glyceryl guaiacolate) is the most important guaiacol derivative. This drug is the glycerol ether of guaiacol (Fig. 3–3) and it is prepared by condensing glycerol with guaiacol. Glyceryl guaiacolate, as it was formerly called, is the favored derivative for present day use under the name of guaifenesin. It is the main constituent of many expectorant "cough medicines," and it is included in numerous combination products for the treatment of bronchospastic disorders (Table 3–18). Its popularity as an oral expectorant is quite out of proportion to the available scientific evidence of its effectiveness. Claims have been made that the drug has an antitussive action, but no distinct cough suppressant activity has been demonstrated. Moreover, unsubstantiated claims have been made that glycerol is a muscle relaxant, with the implication that glyceryl guaiacolate is a weak bronchodilator (cf. Organidin, i.e. iodinated glycerol).

The true value of guaifenesin remains a source of contentious debate.[55–58a] The drug is certainly a gastric stimulant; excessive dosage results in nausea and vomiting. Subemetic dosages may result in reflex augmentation of respiratory tract fluid secretion, but it is doubtful if the conventional adult dose of 100 to 200 mg, given in chronic bronchitis and similar conditions, is sufficient to cause an appreciable effect.[56] Chodosh, who has been a major supporter of guaifenesin, found that 2400 mg a day had a mucokinetic effect, whereas the more usual dose of 800 mg a day was not distinguishable from a placebo.[59] He postulates that the drug increases the water-bonding in sputum, thereby decreasing its viscosity. Other workers have reported that a single dose of 600 mg of guaifenesin increases mucociliary clearance, but the explanation for this was not elucidated.[58]

Boyd found that large doses of guaifenesin had definite mucokinetic properties in animals, but, as was also found with several other agents, the effectiveness of the drug could be demonstrated only in the autumnal months in Boyd's laboratory in Kingston, Ontario.[47, 54] This remarkable finding leaves open to speculation whether the drug is effective in other regions of the world either during the autumn months or at any other time of the year. The usual recommended dose of 800 to 1600 mg per day has been found to be ineffective by several workers (including a careful study by Hirsch et al.[57] on chronic bronchitics), and it would be straining the spirit of pharmacologic objectivity to suggest that these investigators chose the wrong season in which to conduct their negative studies. On the other hand, there is much favorable testimonial reporting to support the use of guaifenesin as a "cough medicine." It is difficult to determine what would constitute an appropriate dosage, but it is probable that, in relatively large doses, guaifenesin can act as a demulcent agent that enhances mucociliary clearance; however, therapeutic doses may be close to the emetic range. The drug does enter the respiratory tract secretions, but no significant actions on the mucus have been demonstrated; Hirsch has shown that guaifenesin has very little, if any, mucolytic action in vitro.[23]

Adverse Effects. There are few side effects caused by guaifenesin, apart from nausea and vomiting. Excessive dosage can cause drowsiness. The drug can decrease platelet stickiness,[60] suggesting that it should not be given to patients with bleeding problems. The finding that the drug has surface active properties on platelets cannot readily be extended to an interpretation that it has a surfactant effect on mucus, although this has been suggested. Metabolic end-products of guaifenesin excreted in the urine can result in a spurious elevation or a false positive test for 5-hydroxyindoleacetic acid on laboratory testing. Oral guaifenesin has been claimed to cause a positive guaiac test for occult blood in the stool; however, recent studies have negated this claim.[61, 62]

Dosage. The dose that manufacturers recommend in adults is 100 to 200 mg every three to four hours; children are given half this amount, and infants should receive only a quarter of the adult dosage. However, significantly higher doses may be required for definite mucokinesis (e.g., 2400 mg per day), but the risk of causing nausea and vomiting is then much greater. Many combination drug preparations used in the treatment of bronchospastic disease contain guaifenesin in totally inadequate amounts, such as 50 to 100 mg per unit (see Tables

TABLE 3–19. SOME PROPRIETARY COUGH MEDICINES CONTAINING
TRADITIONAL MUCOKINETIC AGENTS*

Preparation	Constituents
COSADEIN	Codeine, chloroform,† eriodictyon, poplar bud, white pine, alcohol, wild cherry, glycerin
CREOMULSION COUGH MEDICINE	Beechwood, creosote, white pine, ipecac, menthol, cascara, wild cherry, alcohol
CREO-TERPIN	Creosote, sodium glycerophosphate, chloroform,† terpin hydrate, alcohol
KIDDIES' PEDIATRIC COUGH SYRUP	Chloroform,† terpin hydrate,† cocillana bark, euphorbia,† wild lettuce,† white squill,† senega root,† potassium guaiacolsulfonate, ammonium chloride, menthol, vitamin C,† wild cherry, alcohol
PINEX REGULAR	Chloroform,† potassium guaiacolsulfonate, oil of pine, oil of eucalyptus, ext. grindelia, alcohol
SEDATOLE	Codeine, squill, sanguinaria, poplar bud, wild cherry, phosphoric acid, menthol, alcohol

*From: Chalmers, R. K. and Cormier, J. F.: Antitussives. *In Handbook of Non-Prescription Drugs*. G. B. Griffenhagen and L. L. Hawkins (Eds.), Washington, American Pharmaceutical Association, 1973, pp. 15–25.
†Constituents removed from preparation after 1973. See Table 3–20 for other examples.

3–16, 3–18, 3–19, 3–20, 6–12, 6–16, 9–12, 9–13, 9–14).

It is recommended that each dose of guaifenesin be followed by a glass of water. Thus, even if the mucokinetic effect of the drug is in doubt, the resulting hydration of the patient by the water may be of great value.

Terpenes

Various volatile oils related to turpentine are incorporated into "cough medicines" for their reputed expectorant effect. Boyd[47, 54] reports that a number of such agents can augment respiratory tract secretions, but only when given in relatively large doses that are poorly tolerated. Such drugs include *anise oil, eucalyptus oil, lemon oil, pine oil, terpin hydrate, terebene, thyme, thymol* and *turpentine oil*. The most popular of these agents is terpin hydrate, although several of the other agents continue to be used for the value of their "medicinal" flavor or odor (Table 3–19).

Terpin Hydrate

This compound is prepared by the hydrating action of strong acids on the pinene in turpentile oil (Fig. 3–3). The dose of the drug as usually given (i.e., 4 to 5 ml) is insufficient to cause any mucokinetic effect, and thus the agent serves mainly as a flavoring vehicle for other active drugs (e.g., elixir of terpin hydrate and codeine, which contains only 85 mg of terpin hydrate per teaspoonful). The recommended adult dose of terpin hydrate is 125 to 300 mg every six hours; although

such a dose is unlikely to have any measurable effect on the respiratory tract, it is well-tolerated, and is usually appreciated. The official terpin hydrate elixir contains only 1.7 per cent weight per volume, providing 85 mg per 5 ml: thus, the minimal dosage should be at least 7.5 ml. Most combination mixtures provide an even smaller dosage of the drug than the recommended suboptimal dose of 125 to 300 mg.

Ipecacuanha

The historical emetic medication ipecacuanha (ipecac) is obtained from the roots of the plant *Cephaelis acuminata*, which was first used by the natives of South and Central America (see Chapter 1). The extract, ipecac, contains several isoquinoline alkaloids, the most important being *emetine* and *cephaeline*. Boyd[54] has shown that subemetic doses of ipecacuanha in animals cause a marked increase in the output of respiratory tract fluid. It is also claimed that the drug can cause some relaxation of respiratory tract muscles Emetine is less toxic, but is probably also less effective, than cephaeline; the related synthetic alkaloid 2-dehydroemetine is similar to emetine.

Ipecac is primarily used as an emetic, but when given in subemetic dose it is a potent stimulator of the gastropulmonary mucokinetic vagal reflex, and it results in increased respiratory gland secretion. A traditional combination, used to treat fevers associated with respiratory tract disease, is Dover's Powder, which contains ipecac and opium powder: this pairing is still found in some proprietary preparations, such as Derfort

TABLE 3–20. EXPECTORANT MIXTURES THAT HAVE CONTAINED IPECACUANHA*

Brand Name	Other Mucokinetic Agents	Antihistamine/ Decongestant	Antitussive	Other
Cerose-DM Elixir	K guaiacolsulfonate 86 mg, Na citrate 195 mg	phenindamine 5 mg, phenylephrine 5 mg	dextromethorphan 10 mg	citric acid 65 mg, alcohol 2.5%, glycerin, (sugar-free)
Cherosed Syrup			dextromethorphan 5 mg	chloroform 15 mg††
Ipaterp (DM) Tablet	ammonium chloride 60 mg, terpin hydrate 120 mg		dextromethorphan 10 mg	licorice extract
Ipsatol Syrup	ammonium chloride 20 mg, tolu balsam 40 mg, squill 17 mg			eucalyptus 17 mg
Mallergan Syrup†	K guaiacolsulfonate 44 mg, Na citrate 197 mg	promethazine 5 mg	codeine 10 mg	citric acid 60 mg, alcohol 7%, chloroform 15 mg
Phenergan VC Expectorant Elixir†	K guaiacolsulfonate 44 mg, Na citrate 197 mg	promethazine 5 mg, phenylephrine 5 mg		citric acid 60 mg, alcohol 7%
Pro-Expectorant Liquid	K guaiacolsulfonate 44 mg	promethazine 5 mg		
Promethazine HCl Expectorant Elixir†	K guaiacolsulfonate 44 mg, Na citrate 197 mg	promethazine 5 mg		citric acid 60 mg, alcohol 7%
Quelidrine Syrup	ammonium chloride 40 mg	chlorpheniramine 2 mg, phenylephrine 5 mg, ephedrine 5 mg	dextromethorphan 10 mg	alcohol 2%
Rem Liquid	ammonium chloride, white pine, tar, horehound, squill, lobelia, sanguinaria, tolu		dextromethorphan 10 mg	menthol, alcohol 1.2%
Romilar CF Syrup		chlorpheniramine	dextromethorphan	acetaminophen, chloroform,†† alcohol
Sorbutuss Syrup	guaifenesin 100 mg, K citrate 85 mg			citric acid 35 mg, menthol, glycerin, sorbital, (sugar-free)
Tusquelin Syrup†	K guaiacolsulfonate 44 mg	chlorpheniramine 5 mg, phenylephrine 5 mg, phenylpropanolamine 5 mg	dextromethorphan 15 mg	alcohol 5%

*The ipecac is present in a wide range of doses, which are usually suboptimal. The basic dose of each mixture is 5 ml, or 1 tablet.
†These products require a prescription. Not all mixtures are currently available.
††Chloroform has been removed in recent years; some other constituents may have been changed also.
See Table 3–19 for other examples.

and Hista-Derfule. Ipecac is also used in a number of "cough medicines" in combination with other, probably less effective, mucokinetics and bronchodilators. It undoubtedly merits more frequent use as a mucokinetic.

It is of interest that a recent study revealed that ipecac is less rapidly effective as an emetic if given with milk rather than with water.[62a] The suggested explanation is that milk coats the gastric mucosa, and renders the vagal receptors less accessible to stimulation by the ipecac. One could utilize this finding to explain a traditional belief that the drinking of milk impairs mucokinesis and increases pulmonary congestion (i.e., retention of sputum) in diseases such as bronchitis. It is possible that milk could serve to reduce the responsiveness of the gastric receptors to the normal stimulation by items such as spices in the diet, thereby impairing the everyday activity of the gastropulmonary mucokinetic vagal re-

flex. Thus, the drinking of milk may interfere with mucokinesis.

Dose. Ipecac syrup (i.e., ipecac, glycerin and syrup) can be given to adults three or four times a day in a dosage of 0.5 to 2 ml, that is, about 0.7 to 3 mg of alkaloids. A dose of 15 to 20 ml of ipecac syrup has a powerful emetic effect, and some patients may develop nausea or vomiting when smaller expectorant doses are given. In children the dose is half that recommended for adults, but some authorities advise giving emetic doses, since vomiting is often followed by expectoration of large amounts of tenacious sputum in children with bronchial infections or asthma.

Syrup of ipecac contains 123 to 157 mg of alkaloids per 100 ml. The fluid extract of ipecac is 14 times more concentrated than the syrup, and it should not be confused with the syrup, since the administration of an equal dose of the extract could cause severe cardiac toxicity: for this reason the fluid extract is no longer available as a single medication. Many combination cough medications have been marketed, but the FDA has ruled that the dosages provided are insufficient to promote mucokinesis. Most manufacturers appear to be removing ipecac from proprietary preparations, whereas the more appropriate response would have been to increase the amount of alkaloids in each standard dose. In Table 3–20, some of the combination preparations that have been available are presented. It is extraordinary to see how manufacturers report the ipecac dosages in very different and confusing units; to avoid confusion the amounts of ipecac are left out of the table.

Recommendations. Ipecac should be considered as a second-line mucokinetic expectorant in patients who cannot tolerate other, more usual expectorants. The appropriate dose would need to be determined in each patient, but 0.5 ml ipecac syrup should be the initial dose in the adult. The fluid extract is available only in combination preparations. The syrup could be given in fruit juice or another beverage, or in a proprietary cough medicine up to four times a day. A major problem to consider is that many respiratory patients are in danger of being made nauseous by drugs such as theophylline, and ipecac may potentiate this liability and result in vomiting.

DIRECT MUCOKINETIC AGENTS

Agents in this group may have some effect through the vagal mechanism, but their main action is believed to be directly on the respiratory mucosa following their absorption from the bowel into the blood stream. Some are secreted into the airways, but others are thought to act mainly on the bronchial glands.

Iodides

Iodine is an essential trace element that does not occur free in nature, although its salts are present in mineral deposits and in sea water. Currently, most iodide salts are obtained from sources such as the brine of oil wells. In the early days of therapeutics, iodine was liberated by burning sponges or seaweeds, as explained in Chapter 1. The important inorganic iodine containing compounds are potassium iodide, sodium iodide, and hydriodic acid.

The long-standing popularity of iodides as oral or intravenous mucokinetic agents persists in spite of the occasional plaintive article suggesting that there is no adequate proof of effectiveness. At present, many clinicians continue to regard the iodides as, possibly, the most effective of the expectorant drugs. Boyd,[54] who has done so much basic work on expectorants found, in animal studies, that a bronchomucotropic effect was obtained only if iodides were given in 20 times the usual dose. However, since he has not carried out adequate studies in humans, the relevance of the animal findings is uncertain.

Mode of Action. At least six mechanisms are postulated as contributing to the favorable action of iodide (I^-) on the respiratory mucosa (see Table 3–21); some of these have been alluded to in Chapter 2.

STIMULATION OF BRONCHIAL GLANDS. There is good evidence that iodide circulating in the blood rapidly enters the bronchial glands of the tracheobronchial mucosa. It is believed that the gland cells are stimulated to secrete the low viscosity, watery mucus that is thought to be the characteristic product of these cells; these secretions[53, 54] have been shown to contain iodide soon after oral administration of the drug. In similar fashion, iodide appears to directly stimulate secretion by the nasal glands and by the salivary glands. Rhinorrhea and ptyalism (salivation) often result from the administration of iodides, and the saliva may develop a characteristic taste because of the presence of the I^- ion. Al-

TABLE 3–21. MUCOKINETIC ACTIONS OF IODIDE*

Bronchomucotropic Action	
ROUTE	EFFECT
Oral	Stimulation of gastropulmonary mucokinetic vagal reflex
Oral or I.V.	Taken up by bronchial glands, which are stimulated to secrete

Action at Mucociliary Level	
SITE OF ACTION	EFFECT
Mucoprotein	Direct mucolytic action, owing to splitting of glycoproteins
	Stimulates digestion by natural proteolytic enzymes in secretions
Inflammatory exudates	Stimulates breakdown of fibrinoid material
Cilia	Causes cilioexcitation
Bronchial muscle	May potentiate bronchodilators by an "antiallergy" effect

*10 to 20 drops (1 to 2 gm) SSKI qid. (oral), or 1 to 3 gm NaI/day (I.V.).

though it has not been clearly proved, it is probable that the watery mucus secretion induced by iodide therapy contributes to the depth of the sol-layer overlying the surface of the tracheobronchial mucosa; some of this fluid can also enter the gel-layer to reduce the viscosity of this material.

STIMULATION OF VAGAL REFLEX. There is evidence that iodides, like many other oral mucokinetic agents, act by stimulating the gastropulmonary mucokinetic vagal reflex through their action on the gastric mucosa. Inorganic preparations are particularly likely to have this effect; larger doses may cause nausea or vomiting.

DIRECT MUCOLYTIC EFFECT. The addition of an iodide (in the form of SSKI or sodium iodide) to sputum in vitro results in a rapid decrease in viscosity. Thus, iodides have a true mucolytic action, although the mechanism by which this occurs is uncertain; the action has been credited to a "lyotropic" effect, in which the iodide alters the macromolecular configuration of mucoprotein strands.[63] The direct mucolytic effect of iodides may be comparable to that of acetylcysteine.[63]

POTENTIATION OF PROTEASES. The normal respiratory tract fluid contains proteases liberated from the polymorphs and other cells present in the fluid. These enzymes are capable of digesting mucoprotein, but it is unlikely that this reaction occurs to any appreciable extent under normal circumstances. The iodide enters the respiratory tract fluid, in which it can potentiate the enzymic activity of the proteases, thereby facilitating the degradation of mucoprotein into less viscous derivatives.

STIMULATION OF CILIARY ACTIVITY. Several drugs have been shown to act directly on the cilia of the respiratory tract. Iodides have been credited with ability to directly stimulate an increase in the rate of ciliary beating.[64]

ANTIINFLAMMATORY EFFECT. Iodides have been used for many years as adjuncts in the treatment of the fibrous lesions of syphilis and other granulomatous diseases, including tuberculosis and fungous infections of the lungs.[65] Iodides were, at one time, thought to be contraindicated in tuberculosis, since it was believed that the ability of the drug to break down granulomas activated the disease; this fear is, of course, no longer a consideration when modern antituberculous chemotherapy is used. The drug is said to be able to bring about resolution and absorption of certain fibrous lesions and inflammatory exudates; a similar property is attributed to streptokinase. Thus, it is possible that iodides may have a favorable effect on partially organized, inspissated mucus lying within a chronically infected respiratory tract; however, there is no evidence to suggest that such an effect occurs in practice.

Iodides have long been recommended for use in sinusitis, asthma and bronchitis, with the expectation that iodotherapy would help reduce the viscosity and tenacity of the mucus in these diseases. There is evidence suggesting that iodotherapy is of particular value in asthmatic children, whose tenacious sputum may be a special problem.[66] There is a possibility that iodides potentiate theophylline and increase its broncholytic effect.[67] Furthermore, it has been claimed (but on dubious grounds) that iodides can have an antiinflammatory or antiallergic effect that may be of therapeutic significance when the drug is given for asthma.[68] For these reasons, iodides are often combined with theophylline in proprietary preparations for the treatment of asthma. Large doses of iodides have been advocated for the treatment of alveolar proteinosis, but there is insufficient evidence to support this advice.

Adverse Effects. Many patients object to iodides because of the metallic taste. This can be reduced by taking the medication in water, milk or juices, but an unpleasant after taste may still occur, presumably because the iodide is secreted in the saliva. Iodides may cause gastric irritation; this can be minimized by taking the drug after meals, or by using one of the organic preparations that are less irritating and less unpleasant tasting. However, about 4 per cent of patients are unwilling to continue iodide therapy because of gastric irritation.[69]

It has been suggested that iodides should not be given in acute inflammatory diseases of the respiratory tract because the irritant effects of the drug may exacerbate the disease. This is not the experience of most physicians, and warnings that iodides can cause laryngitis or bronchitis should be discounted.

Slight rhinitis, causing a "running nose" or nasal stuffiness, is common, and occasionally may be severe. Tearing of the eyes, and even conjunctivitis may also occur. Increased salivation (ptyalism) may be experienced, and the marked salivary gland stimulation that may occur can result in swollen glands and pain around the lower jaw. Occasionally, so much swelling of the parotid glands may occur that mumps may be mimicked;

this is more likely to develop in a dehydrated patient.[70] These reactions are pharmacologic consequences of the ability of an iodide to stimulate the activity of exocrine glands, and this provides indirect evidence that iodides also stimulate increased secretion by the tracheobronchial mucosa. An excessive nasal, lacrimal or salivary reaction may respond to a reduction in iodide dose, but some patients are so hypersensitive that even small dosages can cause the unwanted secretion or the swelling of the salivary glands.

Many patients, particularly adolescents, develop acneiform skin eruptions that can sometimes be severe. Some patients develop an erythematous reaction involving the face, chest, mouth and throat. Very rarely, urticarial, purpuric, hemorrhagic or bullous rashes with fever, malaise and, perhaps, adenopathy occur in hypersensitive subjects. Anaphylaxis, angioneurotic edema and serum sickness reactions occur occasionally following the intravenous administration of an iodide preparation to a hypersensitive patient: very rarely, such reactions may be fatal.

Iodides may suppress thyroid function, and mucokinetic doses may lead to an increase in the serum protein–bound iodine.[71, 72] The uptake of radioactive iodine in thyroid evaluation tests may be depressed for an unpredictable time following iodotherapy. Overall, the effects of iodide on the thyroid gland, and on thyroid diseases, can be quite complex[72]; iodides should not be given to any patient suspected of thyroid disease unless an endocrinologist supervises the management of the patient's thyroid condition. Chronic use of the drug rarely results in hypothyroidism, which may be manifested as myxedema, goiter or both; pseudocretinism has also been described. Very rarely, hyperthyroidism is caused,[72a] but a pregnant woman who takes iodotherapy could give birth to a mentally retarded or hypothyroid baby, or one with a large goiter, or even to a thyrotoxic infant. Thus, iodotherapy is not recommended during pregnancy, and it should be given only for a short time in very young children. However, clinical damage to a child's thyroid gland is unlikely to occur with less than one year of iodotherapy.[73] In Table 3–22, suggestions are offered to reduce the risk of untoward thyroid complications from iodotherapy.

Other side effects attributed to the drug include mental depression, nervousness, in-

TABLE 3–22. GUIDELINES TO FOLLOW IN IODOTHERAPY

1. Do not use in patients with known hypersensitivity to iodide.
2. Do not use in patients with known thyroid disease (unless the condition has been successfully treated).
3. If thyroid status is in doubt, obtain T3, T4 and thyroid-stimulating hormone (TSH) levels before starting iodotherapy.
4. If possible thyroid problems are a concern in iodotherapy, obtain repeat thyroid tests at 6 to 8 week intervals. If no abnormalities appear within six months, further testing is not required.
5. If clinical or laboratory evidence of thyroid abnormality (hypothyroidism, hyperthyroidism or goiter) appears, stop iodotherapy and evaluate thyroid function.
6. If no abnormalities appear, iodine therapy can be continued indefinitely; periodic breaks in iodotherapy are not of proven benefit.
7. Do not administer iodotherapy to pregnant or lactating women.
8. Children can receive iodotherapy, but initial and periodic thyroid function evaluation is advisable; the insidious development of hypothyroidism is a possible complication.
9. Monitor all patients on iodotherapy for other reactions, including adverse dermatologic and salivary gland effects.
10. Start with low dose of iodide, and increase if necessary until a mucokinetic effect is obtained or until intolerance develops.

somnia, parkinsonism, headache and impotence. However, it is fashionable to blame medications for all varieties of bizarre symptomatology, whereas the true causation is far more likely to be coincidental or due to the underlying disease for which therapy is being given.

All side effects subside, without specific measures, if the drug is discontinued. Severe adverse effects are rare, although overdosage can cause extremely unpleasant or even dangerous symptoms (iodism), with life-threatening consequences such as cardiac arrhythmias.[74] Patients, or their health advisers, should always be alert to the possibility of the various complications, since adverse effects can be expected in 10 to 15 per cent of all patients, and as many as 40 per cent of those on large dose therapy.[69] No iodide preparation should be given to a patient who has had an allergic reaction to this group of drugs.

Inorganic Iodides

The simplest and least expensive inorganic iodides are *sodium iodide* and *potassium iodide* (see Table 3–23).

Sodium iodide is most often given by the intravenous route. The standard adult dose is

1 to 3 gm in normal saline by continuous intravenous infusion over 24 hours. This form of therapy appears to be very useful in patients with status asthmaticus.

Potassium iodide is usually administered in the form of drops of a saturated solution of potassium iodide, *SSKI,* which is standardized to contain 1 gm of the drug per ml solution; however, some preparations may contain only about 760 mg per ml.[71] Tablets are available also, but they have been less popular. A standard recommended dose of SSKI is 25 to 35 mg/kg per day in divided doses, but, in practice, most physicians use a greater dose that is measured in drops. The basic single dose for adults is about 10 drops of SSKI (approximately 1.0 ml or 1000 mg, containing 6 milliequivalents of K^+. see Table 3–2); this is given four times a day, but a definite mucokinetic effect may not be produced unless two or three times as much SSKI is given. In alveolar proteinosis, a favorable effect may sometimes be obtained by giving 2 to 3 gm four times a day for a few weeks; larger doses may be required for an effect, but few patients would tolerate this for more than one or two days.

Potassium iodide solutions may liberate some iodine when exposed to light; an alkaline solution is more stable. Proprietary preparations are available, such as Pima, a black raspberry flavored syrup containing 325 mg per teaspoonful. Licorice syrup is often added to compounded solutions to mask the taste and enhance stability. Various other combination products are favored in proprietary mixtures[75] and in foreign formularies.

Iodo-Niacin is an expensive combination tablet of 135 mg potassium iodide with 25 mg niacinamide hydroiodide; there is no evidence that the latter constituent contributes any useful therapeutic effect. Similarly, the combination of sodium iodide and caffeine (*Iodo-caffeine*) has little to recommend it.

Calcium iodide is less frequently used than sodium or potassium iodide, although it has the same effects and side effects. It is available, mainly in combination preparations, as lozenges or syrups (e.g., in combination with codeine and ephedrine as Calcidrine).

Hydriodic acid is available as a syrup, containing approximately 1.4 per cent of the acid. It must be well-diluted for administration to avoid harming the teeth. However, the preparation is relatively unstable and cannot be recommended.

Organic Iodides

The organic preparations are claimed to have a less offensive taste and to cause less gastric irritation and other adverse reactions than do the inorganic iodides; they are also more stable on storage. They are relatively expensive and less readily available. These preparations are indicated only if a patient

TABLE 3–23. IODIDE PREPARATIONS

Preparation	Availability	Amount of Iodide/Unit	Dosage Equivalents
Potassium iodide	Tablets	300 and 325 mg	3 tablets††
	Liquid	500 mg/15 ml	30 ml††
	Saturated solutions (SSKI)	750–1500 mg/ml	10 drops††
	Syrup (e.g., Pima)	325 mg/5 ml	15 ml††
Hydriodic acid†	Syrups	65–75 mg/5 ml	15 ml
Iodinated glycerol (Organidin)	Tablet (30 mg)	15 mg	2 tablets*
	Solution (5%)	25 mg/ml	2 ml*
	Elixirs (1.2%)	30 mg/5 ml	5 ml*
Sodium iodide	Solutions (intravenous)	1 gm/vial	1 gm
Iodo-Niacin	Tablets of potassium iodide and niacinamide hydroiodide	135 mg 25 mg	6 tablets††
Calcidin†	Tablets of iodine with calcium iodate	60, 150 and 300 mg	300 mg

*These doses, which are recommended by the manufacturer, are equivalent to only 50 mg KI: higher doses should probably be used.

†These products are available without prescription; their dosage equivalents compared to KI are uncertain. Doses given are manufacturers' recommendations.

††These dosages are equivalent to about 1 ml SSKI, which contains 6 mEq potassium.

Combination products are marketed that contain in addition one or more of theophylline, chlorpheniramine, codeine or dextromethorphan.

cannot tolerate an inorganic preparation. The most popular organic preparation is iodinated glycerol, which is available in elixir, liquid and tablet preparations (e.g., Organidin). Many authors have claimed that this drug is a useful expectorant, but controlled studies have not been carried out.[76-78] The effectiveness of *Organidin* (iodopropylidene glycerol) must be considered dubious, since the solution contains less than one-thirtieth the iodine content of SSKI (Table 3-23). Organidin is metabolized more slowly, and therefore maintains an effective blood level longer; this is said to be the explanation for its effectiveness in low dosage. However, since iodides are probably picked up by the bronchial glands, which are then stimulated to secrete, a lower total dose would be expected to have a lesser effect.

The low iodide content of Organidin accounts for the fact that it does not interfere with the laboratory determination of serum protein–bound iodine. It has been alleged that the glycerol possesses some muscle relaxing properties,[76, 77] but the significance and value of this possible pharmacologic quality are clinically obscure. Furthermore, Seltzer[76] claims that iodinated glycerol forms stable droplets, and therfore could be a valuable aerosol drug: this suggestion is not unreasonable. The oral dosage for adults recommended by the manufacturer is only 30 to 60 mg four times a day; half as much is given to children. At present, there is insufficient evidence to support the use of Organidin in the low dosages that the manufacturer claims are effective. Perhaps this product has an additional action, similar to that of glyceryl guaiacolate, as well as an iodide effect. Unfortunately, there is inadequate information to explain the actions of Organidin, and all the literature on the product has no more than anecdotal value.

Recommendations. Iodides are probably the best oral mucokinetic agents, and their use is advised in all patients with sputopathies. They seem to be particularly helpful in asthma, and they may be synergistic with theophylline. Iodides are suitable for adults and small children, but are not advisable in infants or pregnant women. In general, they are given by mouth, but in very sick patients, intravenous administration can be used.

The initial oral dose should be relatively small, and if the patient tolerates the drug, the dosage can be increased until a response is obtained or until side effects or intolerance appears. Oral iodide preparations should always be well-diluted, and gastric intol-erance is less a problem if the medication is taken after food, or diluted with water, fruit juice or a beverage. If a patient is unable to tolerate an inorganic iodide, then one of the organic preparations could be tried. However, the benefits of organic iodides have not been adequately proved, and the clinical results may not be sufficiently evident to justify the added expense.

Potassium iodide is available as 300 mg tablets, or as the saturated solution SSKI, which is usually measured out in drops and given in a glass of diluent. Initial therapy in adults should consist of 5 to 10 drops (approximately 0.3 to 1 ml, or 300 to 1000 mg), or even less, given after meals two or three times a day. If the patient tolerates this, then the optimal dosage for adults is probably about 15 drops (i.e., 1 to 1.5 gm) three times a day; half this dosage should be used in children. The full mucokinetic benefit may not appear until after a week or so, and some patients may require much larger doses, for example, up to 2 to 3 gm three times a day. These doses, however, are liable to produce nausea and gastritis. Potassium iodide can be given as a solution, or as tablets or in combination preparations.

Iodide therapy is useful in acute asthmatic attacks. Sodium iodide can be given intravenously for this purpose. In adults, it is recommended that 1 to 3 gm of sodium iodide be added to a liter bottle of intravenous fluid, and administered over 24 hours by continuous drip. The drug is compatible with saline; aminophylline, steroids or antibiotics can be added to the bottle.

Iodide administration can cause a variety of intolerable symptoms, but serious toxicity is rare. In 10 to 15 per cent of patients, side effects may necessitate stopping therapy,[79, 80] but at least 25 per cent of the remaining patients may show obvious mucokinetic benefits,[69, 80] while the others show less definite improvements in mucokinesis. Certainly, there is enough clinical evidence to justify using iodotherapy as a basic form of mucokinetic therapy.

Nebulization of iodide is not currently in favor, although the formerly used detergent preparation Tergemist contained potassium iodide. It is possible that potassium or sodium iodide will return to the inhalation therapy pharmacopeia in the future, since there is enough evidence to suggest that it could be effective. Another possible use of this form of therapy is in the treatment of susceptible fungous diseases of the lung.

However, at present there is an established use for SSKI only as oral therapy for pulmonary sporotrichosis.

Bromhexine

One of the newest and most interesting oral mucokinetic agents is bromhexine (Bisolvon). This agent was introduced in Europe a few years ago, following investigation into an Asian plant, *Adhatoda vasica,* the leaves of which had been used in India for many years as a remedy for cough and asthma (the drug was known as Vasaka).[52] The active constituents were found to be adhatodic acid and the alkaloid compound vasicine (peganine), from which the benzylamine bromhexine was obtained.[54] In recent studies in Germany, a more active metabolite of bromhexine has been found to be superior in effectiveness and tolerance.[83]

A number of investigators have found that bromhexine, when given by mouth, results in an increase in expectoration of sputum in bronchitic patients.[82] Boyd found that the drug augments the output of water and solids into the respiratory tract fluid. There are conflicting reports on whether this effect is inhibited by large doses of atropine.[54, 81] Bronchitic patients who take bromhexine expectorate larger amounts of sputum of decreased viscosity; it appears that depolymerization of the mucopolysaccharides in the mucus is produced by the drug.[84] Bromhexine apparently acts directly on the bronchial glands, and it is believed to bring about liberation of lysosomal enzymes from the lysosomes of the mucus-secreting cells, which digest the mucopolysaccharide fibers. The drug may also act directly on cholinergic receptors, thereby stimulating neurogenic secretion of respiratory tract fluid. Boyd noted that bromhexine is more effective in the autumn months than in springtime.[54]

Although the value of bromhexine is still controversial, it is considered by many physicians in Europe to be useful therapeutic advance.[85] It appears to have definite mucokinetic properties, and it also has been attributed to have some antitussive effect.[82] The drug is relatively well-tolerated, but rarely it causes epigastric discomfort and, more rarely, nausea: it is contraindicated in patients with peptic ulceration. Transient increase in serum aspartate-aminotransferase levels has been reported, but there is no evidence of true liver toxicity.[86] Bromhexine has been shown to increase the secretion of tetracycline into the respiratory tract secretions; because of this it has been compounded with tetracycline for administration as the European proprietary product Bisolvomycin.

Dose. The suggested dosage of bromhexine is 8 to 16 mg three times a day. Bisolvon is available in Europe as a capsule, an elixir and as an ampoule for deep intramuscular or slow intravenous injection. Experimentally, the drug has been found to be safe and effective when given by nebulization in a dosage of 4 ml of the solution.

Carbocysteine

Carbocysteine (S-carboxymethylcysteine, Mucodyne), a derivative of cysteine, is only poorly soluble in water, and therefore is not suitable for topical nebulization therapy. However, it is effective as a mucokinetic when given by mouth. It was introduced in England as a syrup containing 500 mg/5 ml; 500 mg capsules are also available. The drug is known by various names; its chemical name is L-3-[(carboxymethyl)thio]alanine, and its trade names include Mucolytic, Thiodril, Rhinathiol and Rhinothiol.

It is claimed that carbocysteine has an indirect mucolytic action through an effect on the biochemical reactions within the mucus-secreting cells, perhaps resulting in increased secretion of the less viscous sialoglycopeptide and sulfoglycopeptide components of mucus and a decrease in the secretion of the more viscous neutral glycopeptides.[87] Such actions could arise from the activation of sialyltransferase or inhibition of neuraminidase. Moreover, it is claimed that the drug brings about a reduction in the size and number of mucus-producing cells. Since the drug has a blocked thiol group (Figs. 3–2 and 3–4), it may not have the ability to break the disulfide bonds of mucoproteins.

Although carbocysteine has recieved acceptance in the U.K.[88] (where acetylcysteine is not generally accepted), it is part of the

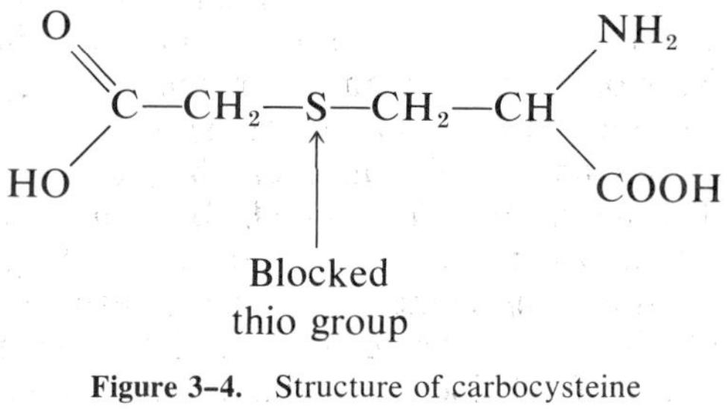

Figure 3–4. Structure of carbocysteine

paradox of practical respiratory pharmacology that this new thiol may fail to become an accepted member of the U.S. expectorant pharmacopeia—both because oral expectorants have been less attractive in the U.S., and because the cost of proving the efficacy of mucokinetic agents is now prohibitive. However, the drug is currently being investigated in the U.S. under the names AHR-3053 and Loviscol.[87]

Miscellaneous

Numerous other drugs, mainly obtained from plants or trees, have been recommended as expectorants, although there is little evidence based on controlled trials to suggest that these agents have anything to offer except placebo value. Their mechanism of action, presuming they work, is uncertain. Some of these agents are listed in Table 3–24.

Licorice (liquorice, glycyrrhiza, glycyrrhizinum, 18β-glycyrrhetinic acid) is a popular component of many cough medicines, and it is credited with some expectorant and antitussive qualities;[82] it also has some laxative, antispasmodic and antigastritic properties. Although its main value is that of a flavorful demulcent, it was used by Greek physicians as long ago as the 3rd century B.C. for the treatment of asthma and dry coughs, and it may have some real mucokinetic value. Licorice has a mineralocorticoid effect, and large doses may cause sodium retention (which may be manifested as edema) and potassium loss (which can cause severe muscle weakness). It may have an antinauseant effect, and it has been used in the treatment of peptic ulcer. It could, therefore, be a useful medication for respiratory patients whose other medications tend to cause nausea, and who are often subject to peptic ulceration.

Paregoric (camphorated tincture of opium) has been reported to have expectorant as well as antitussive properties (see Chapter 9).

Dill oil, anise oil, ajowan fruit extract, Viola odorata (sweet violet), *theaceous plant seeds, Polemonium caeruteum, juniper extract (Junicosan)*, and other plant extracts are noted by Lish and Salem as having some possible effect as oral bronchomucotropics.[82] Boyd lists a number of agents that may augment the output of respiratory tract fluid when given in large and toxic oral doses.[46, 48, 53, 54] These include *cholinergic drugs, saponins* (such as *Guillaia, Grindelia, Sanguinaria, Chionanthus* and *Dioscorea. Senega* and *Squill*), *camphor, chloroform, ethylenediamine dihydroiodide, hexamine tetraiodide, opium, tolu syrup*, and some sulfonamides (*sulfadiazine* and *sulfathiazole*). However, Boyd suggests that animal studies have revealed only four true oral bronchomucotropic drugs: bromhexine and the alkaloids of ipecacuanha—cephaeline, emetine and dehydroemetine.[48]

The British Pharmacopoeia lists additional drugs, obtained from plant sources, that have been credited with expectorant properties.[8] These include the fruits and rhizomes of the plant *Angelica*, the bark of *Guarea* (cocillana, in Cosanyl), the leaves of *Eriodictyon*, the plant *Euphorbia*, and the fresh bulb of *Allium* (garlic, a traditional medication for pulmonary diseases). Other expectorant plants still used in some countries include *Horehound, Primula, Saponaria, Saussurea, Senega* (Seneca snakeroot) and *Urginea*. It is probable that many of these plant products are no less effective than the more familiar expectorant drugs considered to be an indispensable (although unproven) part of the therapeutic regimen in patients with sputopathies. Moreover, some formularies still contain many of these ancient expectorants, for example, the University Hospitals of Iowa "Lung Shrinker".[89] They are incorporated in many of the available over-the-counter, as well as some prescription, cough medicines. Some of the recently available cough medicines containing such traditional agents are listed in Table 3–19.

An additional drug of interest is *pimetine*. This oral medication is related to piperidine, a volatile oil found in black pepper. Cohen has administered pimetine in divided oral doses of 1200 mg per day to chronic bronchitics, and he reported that the drug resulted in a decrease in volume, viscosity and adhesiveness of the sputum.[90] No further mucokinetic studies have been reported on this investigational agent, which is alleged to interfere with the interaction between calcium ions, lipoproteins and mucopolysaccharides; it has been utilized for the prevention of atherosclerotic plaque formation, with dubious benefits.

Any drug with emetic properties can probably serve as an expectorant if given in subemetic dosage. The use of agents such as ipecac, guaifenesin and bromhexine has already been described. Agents such as

TABLE 3–24. SOME TRADITIONAL EXPECTORANTS DERIVED FROM PLANT SOURCES

Agent	Plant Source	Active Components	Biochemical Properties	Physiologic Effects	Comment
Bromhexine	*Adhatoda vasica*	alkaloid derivative of vasicine	depolymerization of mucoprotein; cholinergic stimulation	bronchomucotropic, mucolytic; nauseant and gastric irritant	Available in Europe as mucokinetic drug Bisolvon
Eucalyptus	Myrtaceae	eucalyptol (cineole) and other volatile oils, resins and tannin	mucosal irritant	mucosal irritant	Traditional flavoring and scenting agent
Garlic	*Allium sativum* (garlic bulb)	allyl propyl disulfide, diallyl disulfide	mucosal irritant, possible mucolytic	expectorant, diaphoretic, disinfectant, diuretic	Favored folk remedy, with probable multiple values
Ipecac	*Cephaelis ipecacuanha*, and other varieties	isoquinoline alkaloids	vagal stimulant	emetic, expectorant, diaphoretic, intestinal irritant (causes diarrhea)	Standard emetic, useful expectorant
Licorice	Glycyrrhiza species	glycyrrhiza (a saponin glycoside)	mineralocorticoid effect (causes sodium retention and potassium loss)	demulcent, expectorant, laxative; may cause edema; may improve peptic ulceration	Was formerly used to treat Addison's disease; used in therapy of peptic ulcers
Lobelia (Indian tobacco)	*Lobelia inflata* (lobelia herb)	lobeline and other alkaloids	nicotinic action	respiratory stimulation, bronchodilation; mild expectorant	Old asthma remedy; used to break tobacco habit
Pine tars	Pinus species	phenols, resins, turpentine	mucosal irritants	stimulants of skin and mucous membranes	Used to add flavors or scents to mucokinetic preparations
Squill	*Urginea scilla* (Mediterranean squill) and other species	scillarin A and B and other anthraquinoline glycosides	cardiac glycoside effects	nauseant, expectorant, digitalis-like effect on heart	Traditional drug, potent but dangerous

garlic oil, pine tar and eucalyptus,[91] which have been used as traditional expectorants, probably act as emetics and stimulate the gastropulmonary mucokinetic vagal reflex. *Mustard* has been used as a traditional expectorant: it contains allyl isothiocyanate, which is similar to the active principle in garlic, and it may have bronchomucotropic and mucolytic actions. Other vegetables and spices that could have similar effects[91] include members of the Piperaceae family, such as *cubeb* and *pepper* (which contains piperine and other volatile oils), *chiles*, *horseradish* and other "hot" condiments. A more clearly established emetic drug is the morphine derivative *apomorphine*, usually given subcutaneously in a dosage of 5 mg; a dose of 1 mg is alleged to have an expectorant action. It is probable that apomorphine acts directly on the postulated mucokinetic center in the vicinity of the vomiting center in the brainstem (see Fig. 2–4).

Finally, a few other possible mucokinetic agents have been listed by Lish and Salem.[82] These are *ipedrin (Ipecopan)*, an antitussive and bronchodilator with mucolytic properties; *the para-isomer of aspirin*, which is described as a mild antispasmodic and antiseptic expectorant; *tris(hydroxyethyl)amine HCl*, which is similar to but less toxic than ammonium chloride; *asverin (AT-327, 1-methyl-3-(di-2-thienylmethylene) piperidine citrate)*, described as an excellent expectorant with almost no side effects; *R-522*, a complex molecule, which is alleged to have antitussive and expectorant properties; *Hederix*, a sedative, antitussive and expectorant drug; *Biotussal (580)*, which may cause an increase in secretion production; *Sinecod (HH-197)*, an antitussive with bronchomucotropic effects; Acussan, an expectorant. There is no recent information on any of these drugs; in practice, they should probably be allowed to rest in peaceful neglect.

SECONDARY AGENTS USED IN MUCOKINETIC THERAPY

A large variety of pharmaceutic agents are used clinically in "expectorant" or "cough" mixtures, although their true contributions are rarely known. Among these are the additives and synergists, some of which have been discussed already in Chapter 1. A summary of the various classes of such agents will be presented in this section.

Additives. These are simple pharmacologics, used in a fairly nonspecific way, to improve the formulation, preservation or patient acceptance of the primary drug.

HUMECTANTS. These are hygroscopic agents, such as glycols, that improve the ability of the mixture to retain water.

DEMULCENTS. These agents are similar to humectants, but essentially they are compounds of high molecular weight that dissolve to form syrupy fluids. These drugs are able to soothe inflamed mucosal surfaces by directly coating the irritated epithelium. Most of the agents are gums, mucilages and starches; in oral mixtures they help mask unpleasant tastes of other constituents.

Demulcents are useful components of cough preparations, particularly lozenges or pastilles, that soothe the pharynx when allowed to dissolve in the mouth. It is difficult to visualize such a function in fluid medications that are taken by mouth with rapid passage through the oropharynx to enter the gastrointestinal tract; the claim that such medications possess a demulcent effect is, therefore, not valid in practice. Demulcents that are frequently used include acacia, agar, glycerin, glycyrrhiza, methylcellulose, propyelene glycol and tragacanth; popular domestic agents include honey and syrup.

FLAVORS. These are added to most expectorant or cough medicines. Usually, a plant product with a pungent taste or odor is welcomed by most patients who readily accept the notion that such medicaments have a beneficial action on the respiratory tract. Although some drugs, such as licorice, may, in fact, possess some mucokinetic properties, most flavoring agents (such as quinine, eriodictyon, and cherry syrup) are of less than proven value.

IRRITANTS. Strong smelling drugs (such as ammonia, menthol, camphor, etc.) are incorporated in mixtures, but they are unlikely to be of value to the lungs when given orally. Although irritants may have a slight expectorant effect, they are also liable to cause severe bronchospasm in susceptible individuals, since their main action is nonspecific mucosal irritation.

LOCAL ANESTHETICS. The addition of local anesthetics to pastilles or lozenges that are dissolved in the mouth offers a reasonable form of topical therapy for the symptoms of oropharyngeal inflammation. However, it is unlikely that the respiratory tract is benefited once these agents (such as phenol or benzocaine) are swallowed. The use of these agents is considered further in Chapter 9.

TABLE 3–25.   MAIN MUCOKINETIC DRUGS

Drugs That Act Mainly on Sol-Layer

CLASS OF DRUG	EXAMPLES	ORAL	I.V.	TOPICAL	HYDRATION, DILUTIONAL	VAGAL STIMULATION	STIMULATION OF BRONCHIAL GLANDS	DIRECT ACTION ON MUCUS
Water	Steam, mist			+	+			
	Plain water	+		+	+			
Electrolyte	Ammonium salts	+				+		(+)
	Sodium salts	+	+	+	+	+	(+)	+
Creosote derivatives	Glyceryl guaiacolate (guaifenesin),	+				+	(+)	(+)
	Terpin hydrate	+				+	(+)	
Ipecacuanha	Emetine, cephaeline, etc.	+				+		
Iodide	SSKI,	+		(+)		+	+	+
	Sodium iodide		+	(+)		+	+	+
Alkaloid	Bromhexine	+				(+)	+	+
Thiol	Carbocysteine	+					+	+

Drugs that Act Mainly on Gel-Layer

CLASS OF DRUG	EXAMPLES	ORAL	I.V.	TOPICAL	SPLIT DISULFIDE BONDS	PROTEOLYSIS	FIBRINOLYSIS	MUCOSAL IRRITANT
Thiol	Acetylcysteine	(+)	(+)	+	+			+
Enzyme	Deoxyribonuclease			+		+		(+)
	Trypsin			+		+		(+)
	Streptodornase			+		+		(+)
	Streptokinase			+			+	(+)
Iodide	SSKI, sodium iodide	+	+	+		+	+	
Electrolyte	Hyperosmolar NaCl			+		+		+
Oxidizing agent	Ascorbic acid + O_2			+		+		(+)
Amide	Urea			+		+		(+)

Drugs that Decrease Adhesiveness of Mucus

CLASS OF DRUG	EXAMPLES	ORAL	I.V.	TOPICAL	DETERGENT OR WETTING ACTION	INCREASE IN MUCUS pH	MUCOSAL IRRITANT
Surfactant	Tyloxapol			+	+		
	Ethasulfate			+	+		
	Ethyl alcohol	(+)	(+)	+	+		+
Alkali	Sodium bicarbonate	(+)		+	(+)	+	+
Hygroscopic	Propylene glycol			+	(+)		+
	Glycerin			+	(+)		+

Drugs that Stimulate Cilia
(See Table 2–6).

+ = usual route or effect.
(+) = unestablished route or effect.

PRESERVATIVES. Many medications contain methyl and propyl parabens, which are alleged to be inert antibacterial agents that prevent contamination by microorganism. Some recent work suggests that the parabens could have bronchodilator effect (see Chapter 4); general experience, however, does not support this suggestion.

pH ADJUSTERS. Frequently, manufacturers add acids or alkalis to adjust the pH of the mixture to discourage deterioration of the drug. Surprisingly little consideration is given to the pH of the various inhalational drugs, although this factor is of importance in normal mucokinesis. Thus, the usual pH of nasal secretions is 7.0, and the activity of the cilia ceases at a pH of 6.4, whereas it is vigorous at 8.5.[92]

ANTIOXIDANTS. Antioxidants such as EDTA (ethylene-diaminetetraacetate) are often added to drugs to prevent oxidation by air or metals. The antioxidants are present in such small amounts that they are unlikely to have any pharmacologic effect on the respiratory tract, although they might have mucokinetic effects if given in higher concentrations.

While pharmacologically unproven components can be accepted in oral medications, it is important that all inhalational drugs should be of demonstrated value and safety. It would be regrettable if those very patients who have respiratory disease as a consequence of having exposed themselves to the numerous, harmful inhalational agents in cigarette smoke were to be treated with inhalation of "medications" that might be equally harmful. Thus, there is need for careful scientific consideration before any new drug is introduced as an inhalational mucokinetic; equal thought and continuing review should certainly be directed at old drugs.

Synergists. Although water and various drugs undoubtedly increase the amount of respiratory tract secretions or alter their viscosity, other drugs may help improve mucokinesis by other means (see Table 3–25).

CILIARY STIMULANTS. Various agents can increase ciliary activity, thereby aiding in the movement of secretions up the repiratory tree. Sympathomimetics, iodide and alkaline solutions are among the most useful ciliary stimulants (see Chapter 2).

COUGH STIMULANTS. Few drugs stimulate cough, other than by causing nonspecific irritation (see Chapter 9). Mechanical and psychic stimuli are extremely valuable, and,

indeed, if these are not provided, then pharmacologic mucokinetics may have a deleterious action on the patient, since loosened secretions may move downward into the dependent parts of the lung.

Encouraging the patient to cough is the most important requirement; IPPB, ultrasonic aerosols, catheter stimulation, and other similar modalities of respiratory therapy are essential parts of the mucokinetic effort. There is little need for irritants, such as cigarette smoke, although many patients provide a self-serving justification of the synergistic benefits of their inhalational habit.

AIRWAY DILATORS. Agents that increase the diameter of the bronchial lumen allow more rapid airflow, resulting in improvement in cough effectiveness. Thus, bronchodilators and mucosal vasoconstrictors are synergistic. Similarly, the antiinflammatory effect of corticosteroid therapy on allergic airways results in improved mucokinesis. Antihistamines, however, because of their drying action on the respiratory mucosa, do not provide a mucokinetic benefit. Similarly, atropine and other anticholinergic agents that can decrease bronchospasm also inhibit bronchial gland secretion, and therefore have an antimucokinetic effect. On the other hand, *tolazoline hydrochloride,* which is a vasodilator (with an opposite effect to that of the mucosal vasoconstrictors) has been credited with improving airflow and expectoration, although more careful studies in patients with cystic fibrosis have failed to show any effect of the drug on sputum viscosity or mucokinesis (see Chapter 4).

ANTIBIOTICS. In general, antibiotics and chemotherapeutic substances do not have any mucokinetic properties. However, it is claimed that aerosolized *kanamycin sulfate* has a mucolytic effect.[93] Some *sulfonamides* may also have mucolytic properties;[48] thus, *sulfanilamide* increased output of respiratory tract fluid by 55 per cent, *sulfathiazole* up to 650 per cent, and *sulfadiazine* up to 216 per cent.

PARASYMPATHOMIMETIC STIMULANTS. Boyd has shown in animal studies that various parasympathomimetic drugs are powerful augmentors of respiratory tract fluid secretion.[94] Whereas most expectorants appear to augment output by 100 to 200 per cent, several parasympathomimetic agents have been shown to increase output by 1000 to 1500 per cent. Animal studies have shown marked mucokinesis following subcutaneous injections of the following drugs: *acetylcho-*

line, mecholyl, carbachol, urecholine, furmethide, physostigmine, prostigmine, pilocarpine, arecoline and others. All these agents are believed to act directly on the secretory cells of the respiratory tract, and their effect is blocked by atropine. Similar effects are produced by direct stimulation of the vagal efferent supply to the lungs.

Unfortunately, no parasympathomimetic agent is specific enough to be of value as a therapeutic mucokinetic. These drugs produce a wide variety of cholinergic effects throughout the body, including contraction of the pupil, increased peristalsis, cardiovascular effects, salivation and sweating. They may also produce bronchospasm, and therefore they are contraindicated in respiratory patients. However, it is possible that specific mucokinetic parasympathomimetic drugs might be produced in the future.

CONCLUSION

An attempt has been made to detail the structure, production and movement of the respiratory tract secretions in health and in disease, and to describe the effect of pharmacologic agents on these secretions. Rational drug therapy can be employed to improve the consistency of abnormal sputum and to increase the effectiveness of expectoration.

The various pharmacologic and mechanical factors that improve and increase removal of respiratory tract secretions have been enumerated. The phenomenon encompassed by the various mechanisms has been termed "mucokinesis." This word implies more than expectoration (removal of respiratory secretions by coughing), since it incorporates all the phenomena involved in increasing the overall excretion of respiratory tract secretions, through changes in secretion, alterations in consistency and improvement in elimination of the mucoid material that lines the respiratory tract mucosa.[94] The main mucokinetic drugs are summarized in Table 3-25.

Further understanding of the basic pharmacology of respiratory tract fluid and mucokinesis will occur, and drug therapy will become more rational as our understanding increases. New drugs will appear, and some of the established and traditional expectorants and nostrums will be retired from the respiratory pharmacopeia. We are now entering the era of scientific inhalation therapy, and the relatively neglected area of mucokinetic pharmacology will be one of the beneficiaries of this new interest.

REFERENCES

1. Dulfano, M. J., Adler, K. and Wooten, O.: Physical properties of sputum. Effects of 100 per cent humidity and water mist. Am. Rev. Respir. Dis. 107:130–132, 1972.
2. Gibson, L. E.: Use of water vapor in the treatment of lower respiratory disease. Am. Rev. Respir. Dis. 110 #6 Pt. 2:100–103, 1974.
3. Richards, J. H. and Marriott, C.: Effect of relative humidity on the rheologic properties of bronchial mucus. Am. Rev. Respir. Dis. 109:484–486, 1974.
4. Sadove, M. S., Miller, C. E. and Shima, A. T.: Postoperative aerosol therapy. J.A.M.A. 156:759–763, 1954.
5. Muir, D. C. F.: Clinical Aspects Of Inhaled Particles. Philadelphia, F. A. Davis Company, 1972. Chs. 1 and 9.
6. Morrow, P. E.: Aerosol characterization and deposition. Am. Rev. Respir. Dis. 110 #6 Pt. 2:88–99, 1974.
7. Graff, T. D.: Humidification: indications and hazards in respiratory therapy. Anesth. Analg. 54:444–448, 1975.
8. Martindale: The Extra Pharmacoepia. London, The Pharmaceutical Press, 27th ed., 1977. pp. 596–606.
9. Bickerman, H. A., Sproul, E. E. and Barach, A. L.: An aerosol method of producing bronchial secretions in human subjects. Dis. Chest 33:347–362, 1958.
10. Barton, A. D. and Lourenco, R. V.: Bronchial secretions and mucociliary clearance. Arch. Intern. Med. 131:140–144, 1973.
10a. Dautrebande, L.: Microaerosols: Physiology, Pharmacology, Therapeutics. New York, Academic Press, 1962.
11. DiSant'Agnese, P. A.: Cystic fibrosis (mucoviscidosis). Amer. Fam. Phys. 7:102–111, March, 1973.
12. Webb, W. R.: New mucolytic agents for sputum liquefaction. Postgrad. Med. 36:449–453, 1964.
12a. Cato, A. E., Scott, J. A. and Sisson, A. M.: The Clinical significance of the hypertonicity of acetylcysteine preparations. Respir. Care 22:731–735, 1977.
13. Sheffner, A. L. and Lish, P. M.: Acetylcysteine and other mucolytic agents. In International Encyclopedia Of Pharmacology And Therapeutics, Vol. III, Section 27. Antitussive Agents. H. Salem and D. M. Ariado (Eds.), New York, Pergamon Press, 1970, Chap. 15.
14. Hirsch, S. R., Viernes, P. F. and Kory, R. C.: Clinical and physiological evaluation of mucolytic agents nebulized with isoproterenol: 10% N-acetylcysteine versus 10% 2-mercaptoethane sulfonate. Thorax 25:737–743, 1970.
15. Hirsch, S. R. and Kory, R. C.: An evaluation of the effect of nebulized N-acetylcysteine on sputum consistency. J. Allergy 39:265–273, 1967.

16. Tecklin, I. S. and Holsclaw, D. S.: Bronchial drainage with aerosol medications in cystic fibrosis. Phys. Ther. 56:999–1003, 1976.

17. Wood, R. E., Boat, T. F. and Doershuk, C. F.: Cystic fibrosis. Am. Rev. Respir. Dis. 113: 833–878, 1976.

18. Chodosh, S., Baigelman, W., Medici, T. C. and Enslein, K.: Long-term use of acetylcysteine in chronic bronchitis. Curr. Ther. Res. 17:319–334, 1975.

19. Barton, A. D.: Aerosolized detergents and mucolytic agents in the treatment of stable chronic obstructive pulmonary disease. Am. Rev. Respir. Dis. 110 #6 Pt. 2:104–110, 1974.

20. Piperino, E. and Berssenbruegge, D. A.: Reversal of experimental paracetamol toxicosis with N-acetylcysteine. Lancet 2:738–739, 1976.

21. Lyons, L., Studdiford, J. S. and Sommaripa, A. M.: Treatment of acetaminophen overdosage with N-acetylcysteine. N. Engl. J. Med. 296:174, 1977.

21a. Peterson, R. G. and Rumach, B. H.: Treating acute acetaminophen poisoning with acetylcysteine. J.A.M.A. 237:2406–2407, 1977.

22. DeTemmerman, P.: Sodium 2-mercaptoethane sulfonate (MESNA) in respiratory resuscitation. Acta Anaesth. Belg. 2:115–126, 1971.

23. Hirsch, S. R.: In vitro evaluation of expectorant and mucolytic agents. Bull. Physiopathol. Respir. 9:435–438, 1973.

24. Steen, S. N., Ziment, I., Freeman, D. S. and Thomas, J. S.: Evaluation of a new mucolytic drug. Clin. Pharmacol. Ther. 16:58–62, 1974.

25. Lieberman, J.: Measurement of sputum viscosity in a cone-plate viscometer. An evaluation of mucolytic agents in vitro. Am. Rev. Respir. Dis. 97:662–672, 1968.

26. Lieberman, J.: The appropriate use of mucolytic agents. Am. J. Med. 49:1–4, 1970.

27. Spier, R., Witebsky, E. and Paine, J. R.: Aerosolized pancreatic dornase and antibiotics in pulmonary infections. J.A.M.A. 178:878–886, 1961.

28. Levine, E. R.: Inhalation therapy—aerosols and intermittent positive pressure breathing. Med. Clin. N. Amer. 51:307–321, 1967.

29. Benjamin, C.: The use and efficacy of mucolytic agents. S. Afr. Med. J. 45:948–952, 1971.

30. Arora, P. L., Rogers, L. M. and Mayock, R. L.: Alveolar proteinosis: experience with trypsin therapy. Am. J. Med. 48:889–899, 1968.

31. Riker, J. B. and Wolinsky, H.: Trypsin and aerosol treatment of pulmonary alveolar proteinosis. Am. Rev. Respir. Dis. 108:108–113, 1973.

32. Anon: Today's drugs: mucolytic agents. Br. Med. J. 2:581–582, June, 1971.

33. Huang, N. N.: Aerosol therapy: principles, intermittent aerosol, continuous aerosol. In Guide To Drug Therapy In Patients With Cystic Fibrosis. The National Cystic Fibrosis Research Foundation, 1972. pp. 26–43.

34. Miller, J. B. and Boyer, E. H.: A nontoxic detergent for aerosol use in dissolving viscid bronchopulmonary secretions. J. Pediatr. 40:767–771, 1952.

35. Tainter, M. L., Nachod, F. C. and Bird, J. A.: Alevaire as a mucolytic agent. N. Engl. J. Med. 253:764–767, 1955.

36. Palmer, K. N. V.: Reduction of sputum viscosity by a water aerosol in chronic bronchitis. Lancet 1:91, 1960.

37. Alevaire: Notice of withdrawal of approval of new drug application. Fed. Reg. 38:6305–6309, 1973.

38. Miller, J. B.: Detergent aerosol therapy: a 15-year review of laboratory and clinical tolerance. Clin. Med. 74:37–40, 1967.

39. Paez, P. N. and Miller, W. F.: Surface active agents in sputum evacuation: a blind comparison with normal saline solution and distilled water. Chest 60:312–317, 1971.

40. Modell, J. H., Heinitsh, H. and Giammona, S. T.: The effects of wetting and antifoaming agents on pulmonary surfactant. Anesthesiology 30: 164–173, 1969.

41. Feldman, S. A. and Crawley, B. E.: Tracheostomy And Artificial Ventilation. Baltimore, Williams and Wilkins Company, 2nd ed., 1972. p 66.

42. Lieberman, J.: Inhibition of protease activity in purulent sputum by DNA. J. Lab. Clin. Med. 70:595–605, 1967.

43. Obenour, R. A., Saltzman, H. A., Seiker, H. O. and Green, J. L.: Effects of surface-active aerosols and pulmonary congestion on lung compliance and resistance. Circulation 27:888–892, 1963.

44. Luisada, A. A., Goldman, M. A. and Weyl, R.: Alcohol vapor by inhalation in the treatment of acute pulmonary edema. Circulation 5:363–369, 1952.

45. Ziment, I.: Why are they saying bad things about IPPB? Respir. Care 18:677–689, 1973.

46. Boyd, E. M.: A review of studies on the pharmacology of expectorants and inhalants. Int. J. Clin. Pharmacol. 3:55–60, 1970.

47. Boyd, E. M.: Studies on respiratory tract fluid. Arzneim. Forsch. 22:612–616, 1972.

48. Boyd, E. M.: Pharmacological agents and respiratory tract fluid. In Sputum: Fundamentals And Clinical Pathology. M. J. Dulfano (Ed.), Springfield, Ill., Charles C Thomas, 1973, Chap. 15.

49. Brayton, R. G., Stokes, P. E., Schwartz, M. S. and Louria, D. B.: Effect of alcohol and various diseases on leucocyte mobilization, phagocytosis and intracellular bacterial killing. N. Engl. J. Med. 282:123–128, 1970.

50. Levine, E. R.: A more direct liquefaction of bronchial secretion by aerosol therapy. Dis. Chest 31:155–168, 1957.

51. Miller, W. F.: Fundamental principles of aerosol therapy. Respir. Care 17:295–306, 1972.

52. Boyd, E. M. and Sheppard, E. P.: Friar's balsam and respiratory tract fluid. Am. J. Dis. Child. 111:630–634, 1966.

53. Boyd, E. M.: Expectorants and respiratory tract fluid. Pharmacol. Rev. 6:521–542, 1954.

54. Boyd, E. M.: Respiratory Tract Fluid, Springfield, Ill., Charles C Thomas, 1972.

55. Chodosh, S. and Medici, T. C.: Expectorant effect of glyceryl guaiacolate. Chest 64:543–544, 1973.

56. Hirsch, S. R. and Kory, R. C.: Expectorant effect of glyceryl guaiacolate. Chest 64:544–545, 1973.

57. Hirsch, S. R., Viernes, P. F., and Kory, R. C.: The expectorant effect of glyceryl guaiacolate in patients with chronic bronchitis. Chest 63:9–14, 1973.

58. Thomson, M. L., Pavia, D. and McNichol, M. W.: A preliminary study of the effect of guaiphenesin on mucociliary clearance from the human lung. Thorax 28:742–747, 1973.

58a. Robinson, R. E., Cummings, W. B. and Deffenbaugh, E. R.: Effectiveness of guaifenesin as an expectorant: a cooperative double-blind study. Curr. Ther. Res. 22:284–296, 1977.

59. Chodosh, S.: Objective sputum changes associated with glyceryl guaiacolate in chronic bronchial diseases. Bull. Physiopathol. Respir. 9:452–456, 1973.

60. Wurzel, H. A.: Effects of glyceryl guaiacolate on function of platelets. Bulletin of Pathology 9:150, Aug., 1968.

61. Brown, J. R., Self, T. H., Taylor, W. J., Stargel, W. W., and Boswell, R. L.: Guaifenesin effects on guaiac test for occult blood. J.A.M.A. 236:1881, 1976.

62. Ogburn, R. M. and Craner, G. E.: Negative guaiac after glyceryl guaiacolate. N. Engl. J. Med. 293:1267, 1975.

62a. Varipapa, R. J. and Oderda, G. M.: Effect of milk on ipecac-induced emesis. N. Engl. J. Med. 296:112–113, 1977.

63. Marriott, C. and Richards, J. H.: The effects of storage and of potassium iodide, urea, N-acetylcysteine and Triton X-100 on the viscosity of bronchial mucus. Brit. J. Dis. Chest. 68:171–182, 1974.

64. Carson, S., Goldhamer, R. and Carpenter, R.: Mucus transport in the respiratory tract. Am. Rev. Respir. Dis. 93 Suppl.:86–92, March, 1966.

65. Kremer, W. F.: Current uses of iodides in therapy. Clin. Pharmacol. Ther. 1:advertising pp. 5–8, May, 1960.

66. Falliers, C. J., McCann, W. P., Chai, H., Ellis, E. F. and Yazdi, N.: Controlled study of iodotherapy for childhood asthma. J. Allergy 38:183–192, 1966.

67. Salem, H. and Jackson, R. H.: Oral theophylline preparations — a review of their clinical efficacy in the treatment of bronchial asthma. Ann. Allergy 32:189–199, 1974.

68. Siegal, S.: The asthma-suppressive action of potassium iodide. J. Allergy 35:252–270, 1964.

69. Bernecker, C.: Potassium iodide in bronchial asthma. Br. Med. J. 4:236, 1969.

70. Dworetzky, M.: The dangers of therapeutic agents used in the treatment of asthma. South. Med. J. 62:649–654, 1969.

71. Friend, D. G.: Iodide therapy and the importance of quantitating the dose. N. Engl. J. Med. 263:1358–1360, 1960.

72. Vagenakis, A. G. and Braverman, L. E.: Adverse effects of iodides on thyroid function. Med. Clin. N. Amer. 59:1075–1088, 1975.

73. Martin, M. M. and Rento, R. D.: Iodine goiter with hypothyroidism in two newborn infants. J. Pediatr. 61:94–99, 1962.

73a. Gutknecht, D. R.: Asthma complicated by iodine-induced thyrotoxicosis. N. Engl. J. Med. 296:1236, 1977.

74. Tresch, D. D., Sweet, D. L., Keelan, M. H. and Lange, R. L.: Acute iodide intoxication with cardiac instability. Arch. Intern. Med. 134:760–762, 1974.

75. Seltzer, A.: The use of iodides in asthma. Med. Ann. D. C. 26:17–19, 1957.

76. Seltzer, A.: A superior iodide preparation for respiratory tract diseases, iodopropylidene glycerol (Organidin). Med. Ann. D. C. 30:130–132, 1961.

77. Segal, M. S.: Comments on Organidin (iodinated glycerol). Int. Correspondence Soc. Allergists Series 23, 1960. pp. 205–206.

78. Nemoitin, B. O. and Lazo-Wasem, E. A.: Bioavailability of organically bound iodine. J. Pharm. Sci. 63:1323–1325, 1974.

79. Bickerman, H. A.: Antitussive drugs. In Drugs of Choice 1976–1977. W. Modell (Ed.), Saint Louis, The C. V. Mosby Company, 1976. Chap. 28.

80. Leonardy, J. G.: The use of iodides in bronchial asthma. South. Med. J. 61:959–962, 1968.

81. Anon.: Today's drugs. Br. Med. J. 2:581–582, June 1971.

82. Lish, P. M. and Salem, H.: Expectorants. In International Encyclopedia Of Pharmacology And Therapeutics, Volume III. Section 27. Antitussive Agents. H. Salem and D. M. Aviado (Eds.), New York, Pergamon Press, 1970. Chap. 14.

83. Zeth, K.: Investigations for reduction of surgical risks due to pulmonary diseases during planned secretolysis. (In German). Med. Mschr. 27:226–229, 1973.

84. Hamilton, W. F. D., Palmer, K. N. V. and Gent, M.: Expectorant action of bromhexine in chronic obstructive bronchitis. Br. Med. J. 3:260–261, Aug., 1970.

85. Lal, S. and Bhalla, K. K.: A controlled trial of bromhexine ('Bisolvon') in out-patients with chronic bronchitis. Curr. Med. Res. Opin. 3:63–67, 1975.

86. Editorial: Bromhexine. Lancet, 1:1058, 1971.

87. Information on file with A. H. Robins Company.

88. Edwards, G. F., Steel, A. E., Knott, J. K. and Jordan, J. W.: S-carboxymethylcysteine in the fluidification of sputum and treatment of chronic airway obstruction. Chest 70:506–513, 1976.

89. Richerson, H. B.: Expectorants. Hosp. Formulary Management, Sept., 1967.

90. Cohen, B. M.: Bronchoperviant effects of pimetine. J. New Drugs 6:162–173, 1966.

91. Claus, E. P., Tyler, V. E. and Brady, L. R.: Pharmacognosy. Philadelphia, Lea and Febiger, 5th ed., 1970.

92. Negus, V.: The Biology Of Respiration. London, E. S. Livingstone, 1965, p. 82.

93. Lifschitz, M. I. and Denning, C. R.: Safety of kanamycin aerosol. Clin. Pharmacol. Ther. 12:91–95, 1971.

94. Boyd, E. M. and Lapp, M. S.: On the expectorant action of parasympathomimetic drugs. J. Pharmacol. Exp. Ther. 87:24–32, 1946.

95. Ziment, I.: On first looking into Dulfano's sputum. Respir. Care 19:620–623, 1974.

4

BRONCHOSPASM

The airways of the human lung are endowed with a spiral covering of involuntary muscle, which probably causes more harm than benefit. It is unfortunate that these muscle fibers undergo inappropriately severe constriction in reaction to various types of irritation; the consequent bronchospasm is a major problem in most chronic obstructive pulmonary diseases. In the following sections, the anatomy, physiology and biochemistry of bronchospasm will be discussed.

MECHANISMS

ANATOMY

The most important anatomic structures in the airways, from the pharmacologic viewpoint, are the smooth muscle, the ciliated epithelium and the bronchial glands, with their vascular and nerve supplies[1, 1a] (Table 4-1).

Smooth Muscle

The tubular airways of the tracheobronchial tree present regional differences in structure. The trachea is semirigid, because of its incomplete rings of cartilage; the more distal bronchi contain only plates of cartilage, which disappear once the level of the bronchioles is reached. The amount of smooth muscle[2, 2a] that envelops the tubular airways is almost inversely proportional to the amount of cartilage; thus, the muscle fibers are most prolific in the distal bronchioles, and they extend down as far as the alveolar ducts. The fibers are arranged in a geodesic lattice formation, which enables

them to have a profound regulatory effect on the diameter of the lumen of the airways.

Epithelial Layer

The epithelium lining the mucosa of the airways is pseudostratified in the trachea and bronchi, and becomes columnar and then cuboid as it progresses down the bronchioles. The alveoli consist of specialized epithelial cells that are flat and thin. The epithelial cells from the nose to the terminal bronchi are ciliated, but the alveolar ducts and alveoli are devoid of cilia.

Goblet cells, which are large, nonciliated cells packed with mucus granules, are scattered throughout the epithelial layer. At the level of the respiratory bronchioles, goblet cells are no longer present in normal airways. The goblet cells, and the cilia, are not supplied by efferent nerves; nevertheless, they function in an intricately coordinated fashion.[3]

Submucosa

The vascular connective tissue layer beneath the epithelium contains specialized bronchial glands, the cells of which produce seromucous secretions that are carried to the surface of the ciliated epithelium by ciliated excretory ducts. The bronchial glands are similar to other exocrine glands, such as sweat glands, lacrimal glands, nasal glands and salivary glands, in structure, anatomic arrangement and function. The bronchial glands contain both mucous and serous secretory cells; the relative proportion of each type of secretion varies with the state of hydration and with different types of nervous and pharmacologic stimulation. In general, it

TABLE 4–1. ANATOMY OF ASTHMA

Structure	Sympathetic Innervation	Parasympathetic Innervation	Role in Asthma
Airway smooth muscle	Causes broncho-dilation	Involved in bronchospasm	Bronchospasm as a result of parasympathetic predominance
Goblet cells	No control	No control	Secretion occurs as a direct result of irritant stimulation
Bronchial glands	No control	Stimulation causes secretion	Secretions are more viscous during asthma attack
Mucosal blood vessels	Causes vasodilation	Effect is uncertain	Vasodilation is common in asthma attack; results in mucosal congestion
Lymphatics	No control	No control	Uncertain
Mast cells	Indirectly inhibits	Indirectly stimulates	Stimulation results in release of mediators that cause asthmatic response

appears that bronchial glands produce secretions that are more fluid than the viscous mucoid product of the goblet cells (see Chapter 2).

The bronchial glands are found mainly in the trachea and bronchi; there is a marked decrease in their presence more distally, and it is unusual for them to be found in the respiratory bronchioles. In patients with chronic obstructive airway disease, both the bronchial gland cells and the goblet cells hypertrophy; the glands increase in size and number, and they appear more distally in the bronchioles. The ratio of the diameter of bronchial gland tissue to the diameter of the bronchial wall is known as the Reid index; this ratio is usually 0.25 to 0.35, whereas in bronchitis the ratio is often in the range of 0.40 to 0.80. Chronic sputum producers usually are found to have an increase in goblet cells and in bronchial glands, and an elevated Reid index is found in tissue removed at surgery or autopsy.

Nerve Supply

The airways of the lung are innervated by the autonomic nervous system. Both afferent and efferent fibers are present; probably, each type is mixed, with sympathetic and parasympathetic components (Table 4–2).

Sympathetic Nerves. Efferent sympathetic fibers arise from the spinal cord from T1 to T5 and, possibly, from some of the subsequent thoracic levels. The post-ganglionic fibers that arise from the pulmonary plexuses supply the muscles and blood vessels in the large airways, but there is no supply to the alveoli. There is no evidence to suggest that there is an efferent sympathetic supply to the bronchial glands that are found in the trachea, bronchi and bronchioles.

It is thought that some afferent sympathetic nerves originate in the parenchyma of the lungs, but knowledge as to their course and function is quite obscure, and it is probable that the main receptor functions of the lung are subserved by parasympathetic afferent nerves.

Parasympathetic Nerves. Efferent parasympathetic fibers originating in the vagus nerves form the major part of the pulmonary plexuses, which lie in the hilar areas of the lungs. Parasympathetic nerves spread from here along the blood vessels to the bronchi, but are absent from bronchioles and alveolar ducts. There is a rich and widely dispersed

TABLE 4–2. NERVES SUPPLYING THE LUNGS

	Sympathetic*	Parasympathetic
EFFERENT COMPONENT	T_1-T_5 give rise to pulmonary plexuses	Vagus nerve supplies pulmonary plexuses
TRANSMITTERS	Epinephrine, norepinephrine	Acetylcholine
EFFECTOR RESPONSES	Bronchial muscle relaxation; mucosal blood vessel vasodilation	Bronchial gland secretion; bronchial muscle constriction
AFFERENT COMPONENT	None identified	Irritant, cough, and other receptors in airways
MIMETIC AGENTS	Catecholamines and derivatives	Cholinergic drugs, histamine
BLOCKING AGENTS	Antisympathomimetic agents, e.g., beta-blockers such as propranolol	Anticholinergic agents, e.g., atropine

*Sympathetic responses are mixed (see Tables 4–5, 4–6). Predominant effect is listed.

network throughout all the layers of the airway walls. Sympathetic nerve fibers commingle with the parasympathetic fibers, and it is difficult to separate these two components of the autonomic nerve supply. However, the parasympathetic differ from the sympathetic fibers in that they supply the bronchial glands, as well as the bronchial muscles and the blood vessels.[4]

Most of the afferent fibers originating in the airways and the pulmonary parenchyma are thought to be parasympathetic, and they run to the brain in the vagus nerves.[5] They arise from a variety of afferent receptors, the most important being the "irritant" or "cough" receptors.[6] The afferent nerve fibers are responsible for many different and complex reflexes that affect breathing, and they provide the afferent limb input into the complicated neurogenic regulation of bronchomotor tone.[7, 7a]

The complete story of the nerve supply to the lungs has not yet been worked out. The current state of rather confusing anatomic knowledge is analyzed in detail by Nagaishi in his outstanding book on the functional anatomy of the lung.[1]

Blood Vessels

The respiratory submucosa is well-supplied with blood vessels that originate from the bronchial arteries. The alveoli are supplied by branches of the pulmonary artery; connections between the two vascular systems do exist. The vessels are supplied by sympathetic and parasympathetic fibers, and they are markedly affected by inflammatory processes. Dilation of the mucosal vasculature increases the permeability of these vessels, and can be followed by leakage of fluid, resulting in edema of the submucosal layer. In such circumstances, leucocytes usually enter the edematous interstitium, resulting in the pathologic state of inflammation.

Lymphatics

Drainage of interstitial fluid from the lungs depends largely on the functioning of parenchymal lymphatic vessels. There is an extensive lymphatic network throughout the lungs, and generalized damage to the lymphatic vessels or nodes by inflammatory disease, malignant disease or fibrosis may result in interstitial edema with increased airway resistance. The exact function and control of the lymphatics is poorly understood, but there is no doubt as to their importance.

Mast Cells

In close association with the bronchial musculature are the mast cells,[8] which are most prevalent in the peripheral airways than in the proximal airways.[6] These secretory cells possess surface receptors that can be stimulated by antigens, messengers, hormones and drugs. The cells are packed with granules, which store heparin as well as histamine and other mediators, the release of which affects the adjacent muscle cells and results in bronchospasm.[9]

Mast cells are the subject of a great deal of research interest, since they play a key role in asthma, and many pharmacologic antiasthma agents apparently act at the level of the connective tissue mast cells of the lungs. Although the basophils circulating in the blood stream store and release similar mediators, the presence of the mast cells in the pulmonary parenchyma establishes these cells as the most important source of allergic responses in asthma. Mast cells are present, to an equal extent, in the lungs of both asthmatic and nonasthmatic individuals, and the mechanism by which these cells become converted into explosive devices primed to liberate the mediators of bronchospasm is not completely understood.[10]

PHYSIOLOGY, IMMUNOLOGY AND BIOCHEMISTRY

The characteristic findings in acute bronchospasm are bronchoconstriction and mucus production, with some vascular engorgement and inflammatory edema in the submucosa. The mechanism of bronchoconstriction is extremely complex and is incompletely worked out, although tremendous gains in knowledge have been made in the past decade.[11] Asthma and other serious forms of pathologic bronchoconstriction are very common in humans, but are relatively rare in most other mammals. Several species, such as the guinea pig, are notoriously susceptible to severe asthma, but most of the usual laboratory animals are relatively poor models for study of this human problem.[12] There is no good explanation of why man should have evolved such a high prevalence of hyperreactive airways throughout the populations of the world, and there is no satisfactory answer to the philosophic, teleologic question of whether mankind would, as a species, be better off without the unstriped muscle layer in his respiratory tree.

Bronchomotor Tone

Reisseisen, in 1882, made some of the earliest detailed studies of the bronchial musculature.[2] He thought that the muscles played an important role in the rhythmic alteration in airway caliber that occurs during the phases of the normal respiratory cycle. On bronchoscopy, one can readily see the dilation of the larger airways during inspiration, and their narrowing during expiration, but it is far from certain that active bronchial muscular relaxation and contraction are required for this rhythm. Variations in airway diameter are caused mainly by the changes in intrathoracic pressure during the respiratory cycle, and alterations in caliber occur even when the bronchial musculature has been pharmacologically "paralyzed" by local anesthetics and bronchodilators. Bouhuys[13] points out that, in healthy persons, the airway smooth muscle may be concerned with functions such as regulation of gas distribution, but that this role is "probably of marginal significance." Airway muscle may be a "phylogenetic remainder of an important functional tissue in lower animals"— such as the lungfish, in which the muscle is essential.

The normal respiratory tree is maintained in a state of slight bronchoconstriction, which provides a resting bronchomotor tone to the airways. Widdicombe[14] suggests that the tonic airway resistance undergoes regulation to provide the most advantageous ventilatory adaptation to variations in anatomic dead space. The changes in this resting tone and the effects of various maneuvers and irritants are very actively and finely adjusted in the normal lung, whereas, in the diseased lung, detrimental bronchospasm replaces the normal advantages that might be conferred by the phenomenon of bronchomotor tone.[2]

The control of bronchomotor tone and bronchial muscle responses is extremely complex, and involves afferent input from chemoreceptors, irritant receptors, J-receptors, stretch receptors, and so forth, which activate a variety of reflex breathing responses.[15-17] It is thought that the asthmatic has an inherent or acquired increase in bronchomotor tone and a heightened susceptibility to reflex bronchospastic responses to numerous and variable stimuli.[18, 18a] Many workers consider that the basic defect in asthma is an abnormal balance between the sympathetic and parasympathetic systems innervating the lungs, a concept known as the autonomic imbalance theory.[19, 20]

Receptor Theory

All muscle fibers and secretory cells can be affected by natural hormones or messengers, and by a variety of administered drugs. The particular effect produced depends on the characteristic relationship between the stimulating molecule and the intrinsic organization of the cell. A specific agent may cause a precisely determined reaction by activating a series of events in specialized cells of certain organs. Most of these findings can be explained by assuming that the cells possess specific receptor sites to which activating messenger molecules with the appropriate configuration can become fixed, much as a key fits in a lock.[21]

It has been proved possible to satisfactorily explain the characteristic effects of autonomic nervous system stimulation by the receptor theory (Table 4–3). The sympathetic nerve fibers are known to release the natural hormone transmitters, norepinephrine and epinephrine, whereas the parasympathetic fibers release acetylcholine. Concerning the action of these agents on bronchial muscle fibers, epinephrine causes relaxation, while acetycholine causes contraction; norepinephrine itself has a minor bronchodilator effect. These findings are correlated with the receptor theory by ascribing the presence of both adrenergic and cholinergic receptors in the bronchial muscular tissue. The complex nature of the response of the adrenergic receptors to stimulation by epinephrine and similar adrenergic (sympathomimetic) agents has led to the recognition that these receptors can be subclassified into at least three categories:[22] alpha, beta-1 and beta-2. The cholinergic receptor is stimulated by acetylcholine and other parasympathomimetic agents, and the variation in responses allows further categorization into subclasses of receptors, for example, nicotinic and muscarinic—the bronchial muscle receptors being classified as muscarinic.

In addition to alpha, beta and cholinergic receptors, bronchial muscle tissue provides specific receptors for other mediators, such as histamine (histaminergic receptors) and

TABLE 4–3. CLASSIFICATION OF AUTONOMIC RECEPTORS INVOLVED IN ASTHMA

Type of Receptor	Category of Receptor	Examples of Stimulators (Agonists)	Examples of Blockers (Antagonists)	Effect of Stimulation
Adrenergic (Sympathomimetic)	Alpha (α) Beta-1 ($\beta1$) Beta-2 ($\beta2$)	Phenylephrine Methamphetamine Terbutaline	Phentolamine Tolamolol Butoxamine	Mucosal constriction Cardiac excitation Bronchodilation
Cholinergic (Parasympathomimetic)	Muscarinic	Acetylcholine, methacholine, muscarine	Atropine, ipratropium	Bronchospasm
	Nicotinic	Acetylcholine, nicotine	Curare	Contraction of respiratory muscles
Histaminergic	H1 H2	Histamine Histamine	Diphenhydramine Burimamide, cimetidine	Bronchospasm (?) Inflammatory reaction
Serotoninergic	M D	Serotonin Serotonin	Atropine Dibenzyline	May be involved in asthmatic response
Prostaglandin	A, E, F, etc.	PGE $PGF_{2\alpha}$	SC-19220 Fenamates	Bronchodilation Bronchoconstriction

serotonin (serotoninergic receptors).[23] The most important of the various receptors in the pharmacologic treatment of bronchospasm are the adrenergic receptors (Table 4–4); these are found in most tissues of the body as well as in bronchial muscle; therefore, drugs used in the treatment of bronchospasm usually have numerous side effects in other tissues.[22]

Adrenergic Receptors. Pharmacologic investigations have yielded results that suggest that bronchial muscle has two different types of adrenergic receptors, alpha and beta-2. These receptors also exist in other tissues: alpha-receptors are found particularly in mucosal blood vessels, and also occur in bronchial muscle; beta-2 receptors are distributed principally in bronchial muscle, peripheral blood vessels, peripheral limb muscles, other smooth muscle and the central nervous system. A similar class of receptors is found principally in heart muscle

TABLE 4–4. DISTRIBUTION OF ADRENERGIC RECEPTORS

Tissue	Alpha	Beta-1	Beta-2
Bronchial muscle	Yes	No	Yes
Bronchial blood vessels	Yes	Yes(?)	Yes(?)
Heart	Yes	Yes	No
Systemic blood vessels	Yes	No(?)	Yes
Skeletal muscle	No(?)	No(?)	Yes
C.N.S.	?	?	Yes(?)

The adrenergic receptors supply many other tissues, but the ones listed are of importance in the pharmacology of asthma.

and in adipose tissue; these are beta-1 receptors. The alpha receptors, in general, mediate excitatory effects, whereas the beta receptors mediate inhibitory effects, except in the myocardium.[20]

ALPHA-RECEPTORS. Alpha receptors are stimulated by a variety of agents generally classified as mucosal vasoconstrictants, since their principal effect is on the alpha receptors located on the blood vessels of mucous membranes. Bronchial muscle contains a relatively sparse supply of alpha receptors,[23] and their stimulation can result in only mild bronchoconstriction.[24]

BETA-1 RECEPTORS. Beta-1 receptors in the heart are stimulated by many agents including drugs used principally as bronchodilators; the effects on the heart in such circumstances constitute unwanted side effects. Stimulation of the cardiac beta-1 receptors results in chronotropic and inotropic effects, characterized by increased cardiac output, tachycardia and a tendency to arrhythmias.

BETA-2 RECEPTORS. Beta-2 receptors in the lung mediate bronchial muscle relaxation. Stimulation of the other beta-2 receptors in mucosal and peripheral blood vessels results in vasodilation. Beta-2 receptor stimulators also affect the nervous system and peripheral muscles, resulting in anxiety, nervousness, insomnia and tremor. The metabolic effects of stimulation of beta-2 receptors in muscle and liver include glycogenolysis, by which glycogen is converted to glucose and energy is made available.

A drug such as epinephrine stimulates all

three types of adrenergic receptors (alpha, beta-1 and beta-2), and thus causes a considerable number of reactions besides bronchial muscle relaxation. The actual effects measured in an individual patient, however, are influenced by many factors, such as the dose of the drug, the route of administration, prior exposure to adrenergic agents, individual variation and reflex responses. The search for new pharmacologic bronchodilators has been directed at the development of potent and selective beta-2 stimulators;[25] further attempts are being made to exclude the unwanted beta-2 effects on blood vessels and the nervous system.

Cholinergic Receptors. More attention has been directed at cholinergic pharmacology in recent years, and the important role of the vagus in mediating both normal bronchomotor tone and bronchospasm has been clarified.[7a, 26, 26a] There is now evidence that many of the allergic and other reactions in the lung that cause bronchospasm do so by stimulating the mast cells to induce the release of mediators such as histamine. These molecules then act on muscle cells to cause a minor degree of bronchospasm; however, the major bronchospastic response is indirect, resulting from the effect of the mediators on parasympathetic afferent receptors, which cause vagal stimulation.[26] The ensuing reflex results in a release of acetylcholine at the neuromuscular junction, and this transmitter acts on the muscle cells to cause a more profound degree of contraction (Figure 4–1). This bronchoconstrictive reflex can be blocked by anticholinergic drugs, such as atropine, which thus potentiate bronchial muscle relaxation—or, at least, cause inhibition of bronchial muscle contraction.

Other Receptors. It is probable that many

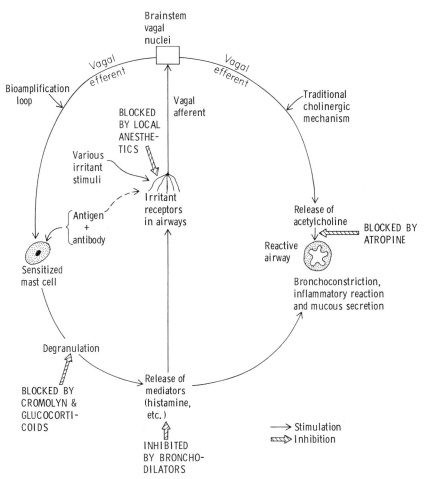

Figure 4–1. Stimulation of irritant receptors in the airways results in reflex bronchoconstriction through the vagal efferents to the airways. Further amplification of the bronchospastic process results from vagally-induced release of mast cell mediators. Bronchodilators, cromolyn, glucocorticoids, atropine and local anesthetics may each help relieve reflex bronchospasm by their actions at different sites.

TABLE 4–5. EFFECTS OF STIMULATION OF ADRENERGIC RECEPTORS

Tissue	Alpha	Beta-1	Beta-2
Bronchial muscle	Weak contraction	No effect	Relaxation
Bronchial glands	Inhibition(?)	?	Stimulation(?)
Cilia	?	?	Stimulation
Bronchial blood vessels	Constriction	Uncertain	Dilation
Systemic blood vessels	Constriction	?	Dilation
Cardiac muscle	Excitation	Stimulation	No effect
Skeletal muscles	?	?	Excitation
C.N.S.	?	?	Excitation

receptors in lung tissue (such as the histaminergic and serotoninergic receptors, and also prostaglandin receptors)[23] play a role in bronchospasm, but the full significance of the overall mechanism awaits clarification. However, it is known that drugs with antihistamine or antiserotin actions are of little value in the prevention or treatment of most types of pathologic bronchospasm.

Table 4–4 classifies the different types of receptors that may be involved with bronchial muscle, and Table 4–5 summarizes current knowledge of the relevant changes of significance in asthma that occur with stimulation of the adrenergic receptors. The corresponding physiologic effects of importance are listed in Table 4–6. Stimulation of beta-2 receptors results in relaxation of bronchial muscles, and drugs used in the treatment of asthma and other forms of bronchospasm that are beta-2 stimulators are classified as sympathomimetic or adrenergic agents. Stimulation of alpha-receptors can cause contraction of bronchial muscles, but since there are few alpha-adrenergic receptors in normal airways, these drugs have comparatively little bronchoconstricting effect.

Mediators of Bronchospasm

Asthma has an allergic basis in many patients; this implies that a particular antigen to which the patient has been sensitized (such as pollen components) reacts with a specific antibody.[27] The main class of antibody (immunoglobulin or Ig) that participates in the allergic reaction, in most cases, appears to be IgE (reagin). Allergic subjects produce a specific IgE, which then becomes attached to the surface of tissue mast cells; in the asthmatic, large numbers of primed cells are located in the immediate proximity of bronchial muscle cells. The importance of IgE in allergic asthma is suggested by the fact that such patients often have a serum concentration of reagin five to seven times the normal level. Very few normal people have elevated IgE levels, and not all asthmatics have increased levels.

When an inhaled or blood-borne antigen reacts with the specific fixed antibody, the process results in a series of reactions, including a cation-dependent activation of a serine esterase, that results in breakdown of the mast cell granules and the release of the extremely potent chemical mediators.[9] These molecules diffuse into the surrounding tissues, activating the responsive tissue cells and evoking the vagal reflex[28] (Figure 4–1). The result is the characteristic combination of reactions seen in asthma: namely, bronchospasm, viscous mucus secretion, eosinophilia, vasodilation and edema of the airways. Mediator release, causing similar

TABLE 4–6. PHYSIOLOGIC EFFECTS OF ADRENERGIC STIMULATION

	Alpha	Beta-1	Beta-2
Bronchospasm	Slight increase	?	Decrease
Respiratory secretions	Slight decrease	?	Slight increase
Cough	?	?	Decrease
Airway resistance	Decrease	?	Decrease
Heart rate	Reflex slowing (ectopy)	Increase (ectopy)	No effect
Mean blood pressure			
-weak stimulus	May increase	Varies	Varies
-strong stimulus	Increase	May decrease	May decrease
Skeletal muscle	No effect(?)	No effect(?)	Tremor
C.N.S.	?	?	Agitation, etc.

TABLE 4–7.   HYPERSENSITIVITY REACTIONS IN ASTHMA

Type of Reaction	Descriptive Names	Antibodies Involved	Nature of Reaction	Clinical Result
I.	Anaphylactic, immediate, reagin(IgE)-mediated, atopic	IgE (reagin, long-term homocytotropic antibody), and IgG (short-term homocytotropic antibody).	Antibodies sensitize mast cells and basophils, which then react with antigen to release mediators.	Mediators produce "early" bronchospastic response within 10–20 minutes, lasting 1–2 hours; reaction involved in "allergic" asthma and in hay fever.
II.	Cytotoxic	IgG and IgM (±complement).	Autoantibodies result in lytic damage to target cells.	Probably not involved in most hypersensitivity lung diseases.
III.	Toxic complex, intermediate, antigen-antibody complex, precipitin-mediated, Arthus type	IgG and IgM ("precipitating antibodies"), react with excess antigen and complement to form precipitin and anaphylotoxin complexes.	Complexes attract and break down polymorphonuclear leucocytes, which release lysosomal enzymes.	Liberated enzymes cause inflammatory reaction in bronchial walls, and act on mast cells to release mediators; results in "delayed" bronchospastic response in 4–8 hours, lasting 24–96 hours; involved in asthma and in hypersensitivity pneumonitis.
IV.	Delayed, tuberculin, cell-mediated, lymphocyte-mediated	No antibody identified; reaction involves sensitized T-lymphocytes.	Attracts lymphocytes, which become transformed; they then liberate lymphokines.	Lymphokines may induce inflammatory reactions in some hypersensitivity lung diseases; can result in asthmatic component and granulomatous reaction; reaction involved in hay fever.

TABLE 4–8.   HUMORAL MEDIATORS IN HYPERSENSITIVITY REACTIONS

Mediators	Source
PRIMARY	
Histamine	Preformed; stored in granules of mast cells, basophils and platelets; present in many tissues
Slow reacting substance of anaphylaxis (SRS-A)	Produced by mast cells and basophils following immunologic stimulation
Eosinophil chemotactic factor of anaphylaxis (ECF-A)	Preformed; stored in mast cells and basophils
Neutrophil chemotactic factor of anaphylaxis (NCF-A)	Preformed; released by basophils and mast cells
Platelet activating factor (PAF)	Released from basophils and mast cells
Kallikrein	Formed from precursor, prekallikrein, which is found in granulocytes and in plasma
SECONDARY	
Prostaglandins	Synthesized and stored by many different cell types in lung and elsewhere
Serotonin (5-hydroxytryptamine, 5-HT)	Released from storage in platelets and other tissue cells
Bradykinin	Derived from plasma kininogen by action of kallikrein.
Other vasoactive amines	Kinins, etc.; similar to bradykinin

TABLE 4–9. SOURCES AND ACTIONS OF MEDIATORS INVOLVED IN ASTHMA

Mediator	Source					Actions			
	MAST CELLS	BASO-PHILS	NEUTRO-PHILS	PLATE-LETS	OTHER	BRONCHO-SPASM	INFLAMMATION (EDEMA, ETC.)	MUCUS SECRETION	OTHER
PRIMARY									
Histamine	+	+		+	+	+(reflex)	+	+	
SRS-A	+	+				+(slow)	+		
ECF-A	+	+							Attracts and deactivates eosinophils
NCF-A	+								Attracts neutrophils, which liberate enzymes
PAF	+	+							Attracts and degranulates platelets
Kallikrein		+	+		+				Involved in formation of bradykinin
SECONDARY									
Prostaglandins					+	+			Regulate pulmonary vascular resistance
Serotonin				+	+	?		+	Stimulates pulmonary chemoreflexes
Bradykinin					+	+	+		Stimulates irritant receptors

reactions, may also occur from other tissue cells that participate in immunologic reactions, such as the granule-containing basophils and eosinophils, but the role of these blood cells has not been clearly established in the sequence of events leading to bronchospasm.

This complex process resulting in mediator release may occur in as many as 50 per cent of patients who have asthma, and it appears that the mechanism accounts for the most important forms of allergic asthma.[29] The hypersensitivity reaction is classified by allergists as Type I, immediate hypersensitivity reaction, accounting for extrinsic asthma.[30, 31] Other stimuli, such as trauma, cold and hypoxia can also result in a Type I reaction, because mast cell breakdown is readily induced by a variety of factors.

In some asthmatics, a delayed reaction may occur several hours after exposure to an allergen; this reaction may also be involved in some nonatopic asthmatics. This delayed reaction also seems to involve the release of the same or similar mediators (particularly slow-reacting substance of anaphylaxis, SRS-A), and is considered to be a major factor in extrinsic, nonatopic, Type III asthma. Allergists also recognize Type II

and Type IV allergic reactions (see Table 4–7), but these play a minor role, at most, in inducing bronchospasm.[30] Type IV reactions are mediated by soluble substances, termed lymphokines, which are liberated by sensitized lymphocytes.

The important chemical mediators in the asthmatic response are histamine, slow-reacting substance of anaphylaxis, eosinophil chemotactic factor of anaphylaxis, prostaglandins, kallikrein, bradykinin, serotonin and platelet activating factor.[32] Each of these appears to act through a distinct receptor mechanism, and some cells are thought to have as many as nine separate receptors that can participate in reactions with individual mediators.[33] A discussion of the best known of these mediators follows, but it should be realized that this information will require continuing modification, since there is a very rapid growth of knowledge in this extremely active field of immunology[33-35] (Table 4–8). Primary mediators are those released from mast cells and basophils, which then invoke the release of secondary mediators (Table 4–9).

Histamine. This substance is preformed, and is stored in the granules of mast cells, in particular, and also in basophils and platelets. Its release is associated with the development of bronchial muscle contraction, increased bronchial gland secretion (and, possibly, goblet cell secretion) and increased vascular permeability, with edema of the bronchial submucosa.[29] Inhalation of histamine produces only slight bronchospasm in normal individuals, but there is a markedly hyperreactive response in asthmatic subjects. The response to aerosolized histamine is only partly blocked by giving atropine,[35a] or by vagotomy, since this mediator works largely by stimulating a pulmonary vagal reflex initiated at airway irritant receptors[6, 36] (Figure 4–1).

The lungs have the highest histamine concentration of any organ in the body, and although an allergen may produce widespread reactions involving many tissues, the lungs of the allergic individual have the greatest susceptibility to the histaminergic response. Asthmatics who die in status asthmaticus characteristically show depletion of mast-cell granules; the same phenomenon is found in nonallergic asthma and in atopic asthma.[8] Basophilic degranulation may also be found in the same circumstance.

Slow-Reacting Substance of Anaphylaxis (SRS-A). Unlike histamine, the formation of SRS-A seems to occur only after the immunologic reaction has occurred, and its release is therefore delayed.[28] It is not certain where SRS-A is formed, but most appears to be produced by mast cells and basophils; eosinophils also may release SRS-A. SRS-A results in a direct, profound, slow and prolonged contraction of bronchial muscle, and it increases vascular permeability. Moreover, SRS-A appears to potentiate the action of histamine, and it may have other specific effects, such as impairing ciliary activity.

Eosinophil Chemotactic Factor of Anaphylaxis (ECF-A). This substance is preformed, and is stored in the granules of mast cells and basophils. When released, ECF-A attracts circulating eosinophils to the site of the immunologic reaction. The significance of this response is uncertain, although it is a hallmark of allergic reactions.[9, 27] It is possible that eosinophils serve to inactivate SRS-A, perhaps by means of the enzyme arylsulfatase, which is liberated; also, eosinophils produce histaminase, which inactivates histamine[27] (Figure 4–2).

Prostaglandins. The lung produces a number of extremely potent hormonal sub-

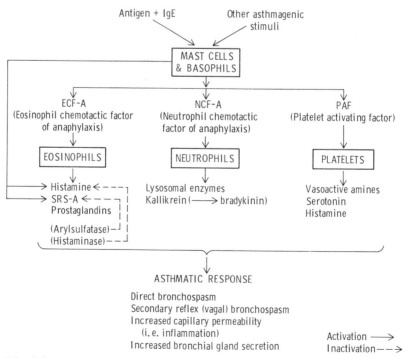

Figure 4–2. Stimulation of mast cells and basophils results in the release of mediators, some of which cause secondary mediator release from the eosinophils, neutrophils and platelets. The primary and secondary mediators participate in the complex asthmatic response. The eosinophilic enzymes, arylsulfatase and histaminase, serve to metabolize SRS-A and histamine, respectively.

stances, which are also found in many other tissues, including the prostate glands. These prostaglandins have profound effects on bronchial muscle: some of them cause bronchoconstriction, others cause bronchodilation. Prostaglandins of the F series ($PFG_{2\alpha}$) are powerful bronchoconstrictors; aerosolization of this agent causes much more pronounced bronchial muscle constriction than does histamine, particularly in asthmatics. Thus, $PGF_{2\alpha}$ is 8000 times more reactive in the lung of the asthmatic than in the nonasthmatic, whereas histamine is only 10 times more reactive in the asthmatic than in the nonasthmatic.[39] The exact role of this prostaglandin in the bronchospastic response of disease remains to be elucidated, but it probably augments its effect by causing reflex stimulation of airway irritant receptors. However, $PGF_{2\alpha}$ plays a complex role in bronchospasm, with several different effects.[38] There is evidence that $PGF_{2\alpha}$ is released during exercise, and may play a role in post-exercise bronchospasm.

The effects of prostaglandins can be variable; thus PGE_2 and PGA have been shown to have both relaxant and constrictive effects.[33] Only one prostaglandin, PGE_1, seems to have no bronchoconstrictor activity; this agent is, in fact, a powerful bronchodilator.

Other Mediators. A variety of other chemical mediators have been implicated in allergic reactions, such as those occurring in atopic asthma; the number of mediators is constantly increasing as new ones are discovered.[12, 27, 28, 40]

Serotonin (5-hydroxytryptamine), *bradykinin* (which is formed from plasma kallikrein) and other kinins may participate as mediators in various animals, although their role in asthma in man is far less certain. *Platelet activating factor* (PAF) is released by mast cells and basophils; it causes platelets to release histamine and serotonin. Another recently discovered mediator is *neutrophil chemotactic factor of anaphylaxis,* which serves to activate neutrophil accumulation and breakdown, with release of lysosomal enzymes. Each of these agents may act as a potent bronchoconstrictor in experimental circumstances, but they play, at most, a subsidiary role as mediators in bronchospasm in man. It is certain that more mediators will be identified in the future, and their interaction will undoubtedly provide the opportunity for the development of complex flow diagrams demonstrating the multifactorial mechanism of bronchospasm, a phenomenon that is duplicated in many other biologic processes, such as the clotting cascade in the blood. *Calcium ions* and, perhaps, *magnesium ions* are involved in some of these reactions in the immunologic cascade and in the clotting mechanism.[35, 40a]

Interaction of Mediators and Vagus

It has long been known that various forms of stimulation of the lungs cause release of the mediators; more recently it has become clear, as explained earlier, that the mediators can stimulate vagal activity. Thus, Gold[26, 36] has shown that antigen-antibody reactions in asthmatics result in the release of mediators, which in turn stimulate irritant receptors in the lung, which trigger a vagal reflex (Figure 4–1). This results in bronchoconstriction, which is produced by the action of acetylcholine on the muscle cells. Furthermore, vagal stimulation of the mast cells in the presence of antigen potentiates the release of more histamine and other mediators. Thus there is a closed-loop bioamplification system, which accounts for the progressive and dramatic increase in bronchomotor tone in the hyperreactive lungs of the asthmatic.[41]

Although this mechanism may explain the development of acute, progressive asthma in response to an allergen, it does not explain chronic asthma, nonallergic asthma or other forms of bronchospasm. Obviously, the mechanism is extremely complex, but it is important to realize that multiple interreactions are probably involved in all forms of bronchial muscle overactivity. Equally important, it appears that even the asthmatic who has a very specific allergy (for example, to ragweed) is primed to react to a large variety of other provocative factors should the stimulus be sufficient to activate the highly volatile system that underlies the bronchospastic response.[12]

The Role of Cyclic 3',5'-AMP

Autonomic impulses, mediators and drugs act directly or indirectly on airways to affect the state of contraction of bronchial muscle. The mechanism that is activated or inhibited within the cells involves a series of biochemical reactions in which the nucleotide *cyclic 3',5'-adenosine monophosphate* (c-AMP) is pivotal.[42, 43]

It is known that the mast cells associated with muscle fibers have surface beta-2 receptors, which are specific for adrenergic agents. The adrenergic molecules involved are either the natural transmitter epinephrine, which is released by sympathetic postganglionic fibers supplying the mast cells and the muscle cells, or circulating epinephrine, liberated as a hormone from the adrenal gland. This "first messenger" can be given as a therapeutic drug, either systemically or by aerosol, to produce the same effects. Other synthetic sympathomimetic drugs will also combine with and stimulate the beta-2 receptor, if they have the appropriate molecular configuration.

The beta-2 receptor on the surface of the cells is the site of an enzyme, formerly called adenyl cyclase, and now *adenylate cyclase.* It is activated when the beta-2 receptor is stimulated, and, in the presence of magnesium ions, it catalyzes the conversion of the ubiquitous intracellular molecule adenosine triphosphate (ATP), into cyclic 3',5'-AMP (Figures 4–3).

Cyclic AMP has been called the "second messenger," since, once it has been produced as a result of the stimulatory effect of the first messenger, it, in turn, affects the activities of enzymes in a large variety of cells.[44] In the mast cell and muscle cells, c-AMP converts inactive protein kinase to the active form; then this enzyme catalyzes the phosphorylation of functional proteins, which then interact with the contractile mechanism of the adjacent muscle cell to inhibit muscle contraction.[45] It appears that c-AMP in the muscle cell also counteracts the effect of or inhibits the generation and release of the bronchoconstrictive mediators in the asthmatic response. The net effect of the accumulation of intracellular c-AMP is bronchial muscle relaxation, although the exact mechanism by which this is brought about is unclear.

Normally, c-AMP undergoes fairly rapid

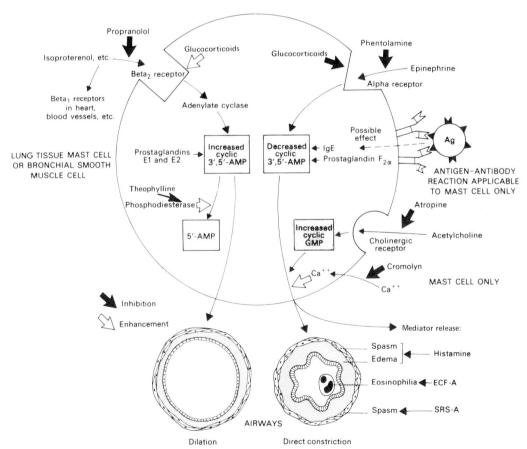

Figure 4–3. Schematic representation of the pharmacologic control of bronchial tone and allergen-induced release of chemical mediators. Cholinergic or alpha-adrenergic stimulation in the presence of beta-adrenergic blockade results in bronchial constriction directly, as well as enhanced release of mediators from lung tissue. This may result in an amplification phenomenon since there is both enhanced release of mediators as a result of allergens reacting with IgE, and an enhanced bronchoconstricting effect of such mediators on the bronchi. (Adapted from Townley, R. G.: Pharmacologic blocks to mediator release: clinical applications. Adv. Asthma Allergy, *2*(3):7, 1975)

TABLE 4–10. PHARMACOLOGY OF CYCLIC NUCLEOTIDE CONTROL

Agent	Sites of Action	Effect on Cyclic Nucleotides	Mast Cell Mediators	Effect
Beta-2 stimulator (e.g. terbutaline)	Beta receptor-adenylate cyclase stimulation	↑ c-AMP	Inhibited	Bronchodilation, mucosal vasodilation
Alpha stimulator (e.g., phenylephrine)	Alpha receptor (ATPase ?)	↓ c-AMP	Enhanced	Bronchoconstriction, mucosal vasoconstriction
Methylxanthine (e.g., theophylline)	Phosphodiesterase inhibition	↑ c-AMP	Inhibited	Bronchodilation, pulmonary vasodilation
Acetylcholine	Cholinergic receptor	↑ c-GMP	Enhanced	Bronchoconstriction, mucus secretion
Prostaglandins E_1, E_2	Uncertain	↑ c-AMP	Inhibited(?)	Bronchodilation
Prostaglandin $F_{2\alpha}$	Various	↓ c-AMP, ↑ c-GMP	Enhanced	Bronchoconstriction
Glucocorticoid	Various	↑ c-AMP	Inhibited	Bronchodilation

breakdown to the inactive nucleotide 5'-adenosine monophospate (5'-AMP) by the intracellular enzyme *phosphodiesterase*. Inhibition of this enzyme greatly prolongs the activity of c-AMP. Thus phosphodiesterase inhibitors may be more effective bronchodilators than are the sympathomimetic drugs that act on the beta-2 receptor to induce a transient increase in intracellular c-AMP. However, phosphodiesterase inhibitors alone do not always increase the intracellular level of c-AMP; thus, these drugs serve best as potentiators of the beta-2 stimulating drugs.

A second, complementary, system exists in the cells, that counteracts the effect of cyclic 3',5'-AMP, in a yin-yang fashion.[44] The cholinergic receptors are believed to be associated with the cell-wall enzyme *guanylate cyclase*. When stimulated, this enzyme catalyzes the conversion of the nucleotide guanosine triphosphate to *cyclic 3',5'-guanosine monophosphate* (cyclic 3'5'-GMP), which is structurally similar to cyclic 3',5'-AMP.[42] It appears that cyclic 3',5'-GMP acts through a separate protein kinase system to produce the opposite physiologic effects to those induced by c-AMP.[46] Cyclic GMP is also broken down by a specific phosphodiesterase system. There appears to be less c-GMP than c-AMP in muscle cells, and thus the c-GMP system is less powerful, and less important in therapeutics.

It is probable, though unproved,[21] that the alpha-receptor modulates both a decrease in cyclic 3',5'-AMP and an increase in cyclic 3',5'-GMP.[20, 47] Membrane-bound ATPase is thought to be activated by agents that stimulate the alpha-receptor; this can result in the biochemical events leading to bronchospasm. Blockade of the alpha-receptors of the lung, by agents such as aerosolized phentolamine, may result in an improvement in asthma in certain cases.[20]

There is confusion about whether the cyclic nucleotide messengers play their roles in the muscle cell, the mast cell or both. The evidence is that the mechanism occurs in both types of cell (as well as in many other types of tissue cells in the body). In the mast cell, increased c-AMP levels result in inhibition of mediator production and release, and the adrenergic system or sympathomimetic drugs may act in this way to influence the asthmatic response (Table 4–10). However, it is probable that c-AMP and c-GMP have a more important role within the muscle cell, where they participate in the reactions that control muscle tone. Thus, bronchodilator drugs (sympathomimetics and phosphodiesterase inhibitors) appear to act directly on the muscle cell, whereas other drugs, such as corticosteroids, have more effect on the mast cells.[33]

SUMMARY OF THE MECHANISMS OF BRONCHOSPASM

Mast cells affect the contraction of bronchial muscle through the release of mediators such as histamine, SRS-A and other molecules. The surface of the sensitized mast cell contains fixed IgE antibody receptors, activation of which can stimulate or inhibit the release of mediators. The mediators leave the mast cell and cause bronchospasm directly, but more importantly, they also do so indirectly by stimulating a vagal reflex, thereby causing bioamplification of the bronchospastic process. Stimulation of the cholinergic receptors on the muscle cell activates the cyclic-GMP system, thereby inducing bronchospasm.

The sympathetic nervous system and sympathomimetic drugs activate an adrenergic, beta-2 receptor, apparently both in mast cells and in muscle cells. The beta-2 receptor stimulation activates the cell-wall enzyme adenylate cyclase, which catalyzes the conversion of ATP to cyclic 3',5'-AMP; accumulation of this second messenger leads to processes in the mast cell that inhibit mediator release. The same process occurs in the muscle cell, and thereby brings about relaxation of constricted bronchial muscle. Cyclic 3',5'-AMP is readily broken down by phosphodiesterase, but this enzyme is inactivated by phosphodiesterase inhibitors, which are thus able to enhance the relaxation process in bronchial muscles.

The two main classes of therapeutic agents acting through the c-AMP system to cause bronchodilation are, therefore, (1) sympathomimetic, adrenergic agents that are beta-2 receptor stimulators and (2) phosphodiesterase inhibitors. Anticholinergic drugs and, perhaps, antihistamines and other antimediator drugs potentiate these primary bronchodilators. It is believed that other hormones and drugs such as certain prostaglandins and corticosteroids, can enhance cyclic 3',5'-AMP production. Thus, the most important drugs in the treatment of bronchospasm act by increasing the production and accumulation of lung tissue cyclic 3',5'-adenosine monophosphate.

The yin-yang balance involved in the complex process of bronchospasm is emphasized by the fact that bronchoconstriction through cholinergic and antigen-antibody reactions involves an additional messenger system, which is complementary to mediator release. The first messenger of this system, acetylcholine, activates the cell-wall enzyme guanylate cyclase, which catalyzes the conversion of GTP to cyclic 3',5'-GMP; the accumulation of this second messenger favors the development of bronchial muscle contraction.

Attempts have been made to classify the mechanistic imbalance that underlies the bronchial muscle hyperactive contraction seen in patients with bronchospastic diseases. Although it has been thought that the abnormality exists at the level of the beta-2 receptor, which has diminished responsiveness to stimulation, this beta-adrenergic blockade theory is not entirely satisfactory. Thus, beta-blocking drugs do cause bronchospasm in asthmatics, but not in normal persons. Therefore, it seems that beta-receptor hyporesponsiveness exacerbates the asthmatic process but does not account for its presence. Other workers consider that the asthmatic suffers from autonomic imbalance, with hyperresponsiveness or hyperreactivity of the cholinergic mechanism, and relative underresponsiveness of the sympathetic mechanism. Reed[48] considers that asthma is a result of antagonism between cholinergic and adrenergic responses, and between alpha and beta adrenergic responses, with the probability that the interaction centers on the flux of ionized calcium, which is critical to smooth muscle contraction. Whatever the true explanation may prove to be, the complexity of the processes involved will ensure that therapy will have to be directed at multiple points in the chain of events that cause bronchial muscle to go into spasm.

PHARMACOLOGY OF BRONCHIAL MUSCLE RELAXATION

Many agents have been used over the years in the treatment of asthma and similar disorders. Some of the traditional remedies are as simple as steam, others are complex mixtures of drugs that have individual qualities ranging from the dubious to the excellent. In recent years, more specific drugs have been developed, and the modes of action of the various agents have been used as a basis for tailoring molecules in the laboratory to achieve more powerful and specific antiasthma drug therapy. The detailed understanding of the processes involved in asthma and other forms of bronchospasm should result in a more rational use of established drugs and will lead to the introduction of new, specific agents designed to exert an effect at particular links in the chain of biochemical events that bring about bronchial obstruction.

Drugs used in the treatment of asthma can be classified in various ways, but the following groups of agents are readily identified:

1. Bronchodilators
   A. Beta-2 adrenergic receptor stimulators
   B. Phosphodiesterase inhibitors
   C. Anticholinergic drugs
   D. Prostaglandins
   E. Other bronchial muscle relaxants
2. Antimediator drugs
   A. Corticosteroids
   B. Antihistamines
   C. Bischromones
   D. Immunosuppressive drugs

E. Antiinflammatory agents and analgesics
F. Diethylcarbamazine
3. Agents affecting alpha receptors
  A. Alpha-adrenergic receptor stimulators
  B. Alpha-adrenergic receptor blockers
4. Miscellaneous drugs
  A. Mucokinetic agents
  B. Antimicrobial agents
  C. Cough medications
  D. Tranquillizers
  E. Anesthetics
    (1) local
    (2) general
  F. Narcotic analgesics
  G. Gases
    (1) carbon dioxide
    (2) helium
  H. Others
    (1) Phenytoin
    (2) Alcohol

The treatment of asthma includes, of course, many other approaches besides drug therapy. The range of methods advocated for prophylaxis or management is extraordinary and includes control of allergy (hyposensitization immunotherapy, and adjustment of climate, environment and diet); biofeedback, hypnotism and other forms of individual or group psychotherapy; acupuncture; carotid body resection and other lung denervation procedures; lung lavage; special regional procedures (for example, spa therapy, salt-mine environmental therapy); massage, spinal manipulation, and so forth.

The range of available treatments can be attributed to the fact that asthma and other bronchospastic diseases undergo natural exacerbations and remissions, which are often responsive to the complex interaction of physical and psychic factors. As a result, much of the published work on the pharmacology of drugs used in the treatment of asthma shows conflicting information, which makes it particularly difficult to compare the numerous drugs with one another. Furthermore, dosages, preparations and means of administering drugs are other variables that have to be taken into account.[49] For these reasons, it is difficult to answer questions such as: Is inhalation therapy better than oral therapy? Is epinephrine a stronger drug than racemic epinephrine? What is the correct dose of oral ephedrine? And so on. Thus, whatever information is provided on individual agents may require considerable revision as new and better controlled data

become available. It is hoped that future comparative studies on bronchodilator drugs will compare "matched doses," using appropriate amounts to produce the same peak responses, as described by Freedman.[49] Furthermore, there is still a need for improved criteria in the laboratory assessment of clinical responsiveness to bronchodilator drugs.[49a]

BRONCHODILATORS

Since bronchodilators are of major importance in respiratory pharmacology, they will be discussed at length in this chapter, and will be viewed in respect to their chemical and physiologic interrelationships. Those agents of use in clinical therapeutics will be considered in greater detail in Chapter 5. Most of the bronchodilator drugs in use are either beta-2 stimulators or phosphodiesterase inhibitors. The anticholinergic agents, prostaglandins and other bronchial muscle relaxants are of much less practical importance.

Beta-2 Adrenergic Receptor Stimulators

The prototype drug is the natural hormone and first messenger, epinephrine. This molecule is classified as a *catecholamine* (Figure 4-4), since it is a derivative of catechol. Other class names are used for epinephrine and related drugs; any of the following terms may be found in the literature: catecholamines; hydroxyphenylethylamines; sympathomimetics; beta-2 adrenergic receptor (or adrenoreceptor) stimulators. The non-chemical terms are the most suitable, since some of the related bronchodilating drugs are neither catecholamines nor simple derivatives of phenylethylamine.

The benzene ring with hydroxyl groups at positions 3 and 4 is catechol (o-dihydroxybenzene), and this configuration results in beta-2 (and also beta-1) activity (Table 4-11). Separation of the catechol from the amino group by two carbon atoms in the side chain confers the greatest possible sympathomimetic properties on the molecule.

The side chain of the two carbon atoms (α and β) terminating in an amino group constitutes an ethylamine chain. The amino group controls the degree of specificity that the molecule possesses as an adrenoreceptor stimulator.[50] The substitution of appropriate radicals in the amino group results in an alteration in the balance of alpha, beta-1 and

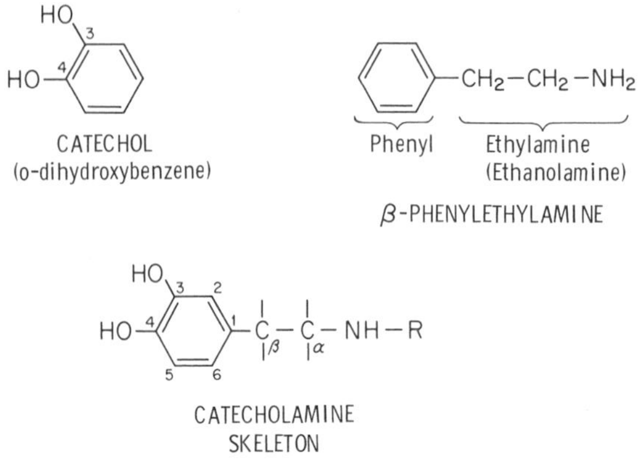

Figure 4–4. The catecholamine molecule is made up by combining catechol to an ethylamine (ethanolamine) chain. Sympathomimetics, which do not possess the hydroxy-group configuration of catechol, are known as β-phenylethylamine derivatives.

beta-2 properties; the more the $-NH_2$ group is substituted, the greater beta-2 specificity becomes, with a corresponding decrease in alpha and beta-1 activity. If no radicals are substituted in the $-NH_2$ group (as is the case of norepinephrine) the molecule has considerable alpha and some beta-1 receptor activity, with correspondingly little beta-2 activity. The addition of one methyl (CH_3-) group to the amino group (as in phenylephrine) may actually result in maximal alpha activity.

The 3,4 hydroxy structure of the catechol nucleus is characteristic of the earlier sympathomimetic drugs. If only one of these two hydroxy groups is present, much of the activity may be lost, unless other substituents take the place of the missing group. Absence of both hydroxy groups, such as with ephedrine and amphetamine, results in compounds with relatively less peripheral alpha and beta activity, and comparatively greater stimulatory action on the central nervous system.

The 3,4 hydroxy configuration allows the molecule to be metabolized by two different enzymes (Figure 4–5): catechol-O-methyltransferase and sulfatase.

Catechol-O-methyltransferase (COMT). This enzyme is widely distributed throughout the body and is present in the blood and in lung tissue. COMT catalyzes the

TABLE 4–11. EFFECTS OF SUBSTITUENTS IN CATECHOLAMINE MOLECULE

Benzene Nucleus   Ethylamine Chain

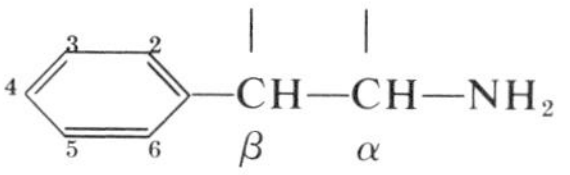

Modification	Effect
—OH GROUPS IN BENZENE NUCLEUS	
No -OH	Results in greater central nervous system stimulation
-OH at 3 or 4	Results in α activity
-OH at 3 and 4	Results in α and β activity
-OH at 3 and 5	Associated with selective β_2 activity, orally effective
Loss of -OH at 3 or 4	Results in reduction in β activity
Replacement for -OH at 3 or 4	Results in orally effective drug
Certain substituents at 2, 3, 4 or 5	Results in β-receptor blockers
—C—C GROUP IN ETHYLAMINE CHAIN	
2 carbon chain	Results in maximal sympathomimetic activity
Substituent on αC	Results in protection from MAO (and therefore drug has longer action)
Presence of -OH on βC	Results in decreased central nervous system stimulation, and may increase other α and β effects
SUBSTITUENTS IN THE TERMINAL —NH$_2$ GROUP	
Addition of -CH$_3$ groups, etc.	Increases β_2 activity and decreases α and β_1 activity
Minimal substitution	Results in greatest α activity

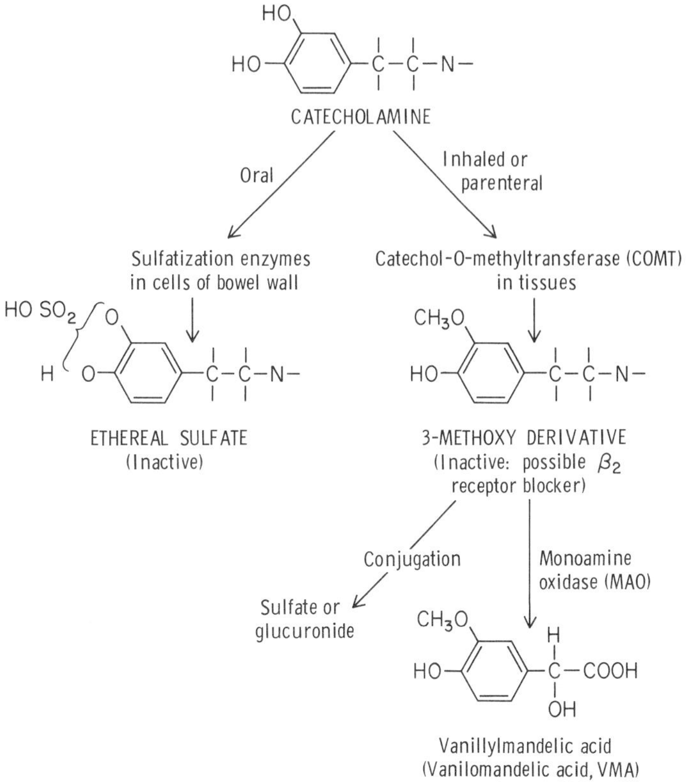

Figure 4-5.

This outline presents a simplified metabolic pathway showing the possible breakdown of a basic catecholamine such as epinephrine.

conversion of the hydroxy group into the inactive 3 O-methyl (3-methoxy) derivative at position 3 in the benzene nucleus of the active sympathomimetic drug. The derivative does not appear to have bronchodilator properties; in fact, it may compete with sympathomimetic agents for the beta-2 receptor sites, whereby it could cause beta-2 blockade.[51] Certain beta-blocking drugs have been synthesized by incorporating methoxy substituents into the benzene nucleus. It is possible that overuse of a catecholamine bronchodilator leads to the induction of COMT, with consequent increase in enzymic conversion to the 3-methoxy derivative, thus causing more blockade of the beta-2 receptor. This could account for the phenomenon of tachyphylaxis, or refractoriness, whereby excessive use of a bronchodilator leads to a loss of effectiveness of the agent with the possible development of a paradoxic, bronchoconstrictor response. Agents that act as substrates for COMT have relatively short half-lives of activity, since enzymic breakdown by the ubiquitous COMT occurs fairly rapidly. For these reasons, efforts have been made to develop bronchodilator drugs that are not susceptible to metabolic degradation by COMT.

Sulfatase. This enzyme is found mainly in the wall of the bowel, where it brings about the conversion of catecholamines to inactive ethereal phenolic sulfates. For this reason, sympathomimetic agents that have a 3,4 hydroxy configuration in the benzene nucleus are relatively ineffective when administered orally, since the drug undergoes a considerable amount of sulfatization when it is absorbed and passes through the cells of the wall of the gut. Drugs such as salicylamide deplete these cells of sulfatase,[51, 52] but it is not known if this property can be used therapeutically to improve the absorption of catecholamines.

Enzymic degradation of the ethylamine side chain occurs along the metabolic pathway of catecholamine breakdown (Figure 4-5). Monoamine oxidase (MAO) has its action on the α-carbon atom and the amino group. Protection against oxidation by this enzyme is provided by adding a side radical to the α-carbon atom:[50] for this reason, ephedrine, which possesses such a structure, has a longer half-life than epinephrine. MAO inhibitors do not appear to prolong the action of sympathomimetic bronchodilators, although the related tricyclic antidepressant drug, amitriptyline, has been found to have an antiasthma effect, which, however, is thought to result from an antimediator action, similar to that of cromolyn.[53] Alternative conversion steps (for example, by conjugation, to form glucuronides) and other poorly understood metabolic pathways are also involved in the breakdown of bronchodilators.[54] The complete series of events leading to inactivation of the various sympathomimetics has not been fully worked out as yet; further enzyme conversions may eventually be demonstrated.[55]

The newer sympathomimetics are not susceptible to the action of either COMT or sulfatase: this immunity has been achieved by effecting alterations of the 3,4 hydroxy substitution in the benzene nucleus which characterizes catecholamines. One of the important new agents, salbutamol, contains a CH_2OH- radical at position 3, which means it is a saligenin and not a catecholamine: this drug can be given by the oral route, and it has a longer half-life than the catecholamine derivatives. Other long-acting sympathomimetics that are effective when administered orally, such as terbutaline and metaproterenol, owe these properties to the fact that they are not catecholamines; these agents are resorcinols, since they have a 3,5-hydroxy (rather than a 3,4-hydroxy) configuration in the benzene nucleus. The resorcinol configuration results in greater beta-2 selectivity when there is also a large substituent present in the amino group.

Various other adrenergic stimulators are currently available. They differ structurally from the epinephrine-like catecholamines either because of changes in the 3,4-hydroxy configuration or because of substitutions in the ethylamine chain that affect either the α and β carbon atoms or the amino group. Some of the new agents (such as rimiterol) differ considerably from the former simple catecholamine derivatives, since large radicals have been added to the ethylamine chain.

Phosphodiesterase Inhibitors

The second messenger, cyclic $3',5'$-AMP, undergoes enzymic breakdown by phosphodiesterase to the inactive $5'$-AMP. Thus, the intracellular level of c-AMP can be maintained by interfering with the inactivation process. The most important of the pharmacologic agents that can be used to inhibit

phosphodiesterase are the methylxanthines, which occur in a number of important plants.

There are three natural methylxanthine alkaloids that enjoy popular and widespread use. *Caffeine* is found mainly in coffee beans, tea leaves, and kola nuts; *theobromine* is a major constituent of cocoa; *theophylline* is found mainly in tea leaves. Theobromine is a word of Greek derivation, meaning "divine food"; its linguistic origin is similar to that of theophylline, which means "divine leaf." The methylxanthines are phosphodiesterase inhibitors, and they have long been used in therapeutics for the treatment of asthma and similar conditions. While coffee and tea and, perhaps, to some extent, cocoa and cola, do have mild bronchodilating properties, only theophylline is powerful enough to be of pharmacologic significance as a phosphodiesterase inhibitor (PDI).

Although theophylline is a powerful inhibitor of phosphodiesterase, it is difficult to use the drug optimally: first, because it is relatively insoluble in water (1:120); second, because the therapeutic serum level required is close to the toxic range. Various derivatives of theophylline have been prepared in an effort to improve solubility and acceptability and to decrease toxicity; however, none of the products available offers substantial practical advantages, and the PDIs of the future will probably differ more radically from theophylline.

At present, the only other important PDI is papaverine (see Table 6–17), but this drug (an alkaloid derived from opium) is mainly of value as a weak relaxer of the smooth muscles of blood vessels walls. Although papaverine is used in England as a component of antiasthmatic mixtures, it is, at best, a very weak bronchodilator. A related drug, quazodine (MJ 1988), has been shown to be 18 times as active as theophylline.[56] Other investigational PDIs[56] (Table 4–12) include ICI 58301, which is related to, and is more potent than, theophylline; ICI 30966 is a similar agent with therapeutic potential. Several other groups of promising investigational agents have been reported, including the imidazopyrazines (such as CEIP and CDIP), the pyrazole pyridine compounds (such as SQ 20009) and imidazolidinones (such as I_{MM} and I_{BM}).[58] The compound I_{BM} is 5000 times more potent than theophylline. A class of compounds known as substituted 6-thioxanthines also has been reported to have bronchodilator properties.[59]

An important consideration is that the

TABLE 4–12. PHOSPHODIESTERASE INHIBITORS

Compounds	Classification
Theophylline and derivatives	Methylxanthines
Papaverine	Opium alkaloid
Quazodine (MJ 1988)	Related to papaverine
ICI 58301	Triazolopyrimidine
CEIP, CDIP	Imidazopyrazines
SQ 20009	Pyrazole pyridine
I_{MM}, I_{BM}	Imidazolidinones
Various	Substituted 6-thioxanthines

PDIs may inhibit the phosphodiesterase system which catalyzes the breakdown of the cholinergic second messenger, cyclic 3'5'-GMP. This messenger mediates the bronchoconstrictive response; a PDI that inhibits its breakdown would potentiate the bronchoconstriction caused by this system. Although there is insufficient knowledge about cyclic GMP phosphodiesterase, it appears that the c-AMP PDIs have relatively less effect on the c-GMP system.[58] However, there is a need for further research to elucidate the role of cyclic GMP and the effect of various phosphodiesterase inhibitors on its degradation.

Anticholinergic Drugs

Some of the earliest drugs used in inhalation therapy for the treatment of asthma were the anticholinergic drugs related to *atropine*.[59a] There is evidence that an extract of the plant *Atropa belladonna* (deadly nightshade), which was called belladonna, was used in the 16th century in the treatment of asthma. The chief constituent of belladonna is atropine. This drug was widely used in the 18th century and was given to asthmatic patients by various routes.

Atropine is a plant alkaloid; its chemical name is dl-hyoscyamine or dl-trophyl tropate. Besides being found in belladonna, atropine is also in stramonium, which is obtained from *Datura stramonium* (Jamestown weed, Jimson weed, and so forth). For many years, Asthmador cigarettes have been made from these two plant sources of atropine; when the material is burned, the smoke liberates belladonna and stramonium, and inhalation of these compounds can result in some alleviation of bronchospasm.

Although the roles of various older remedies remain equivocal, it is worth pondering the possible pharmacologic rationale underlying the following advice, taken from a medical textbook published in 1944:[68] "A mixture containing equal parts of the leaves of stramonium, lobelia, black tea, and potassium nitrate is burnt in a tin plate, and the fumes inhaled; relief is thus sometimes afforded. Various other preparations, in the form of cigarettes of stramonium, potassium nitrate, and belladonna are used, but should be discouraged, as their frequent use tends to produce chronic bronchitis."

Atropine is an important parasympatholytic drug that is particularly effective as a muscarinic blocker of neurotransmission by acetylcholine to smooth muscle. Thus, bronchodilation is one of the many possible effects of systemic administration of atropine and similar drugs. Therapeutic selectivity is obtained by local application of the drug; thus, inhibition of bronchospasm can be effectively achieved by nebulization of atropine. Moreover, aerosol (or smoke) administration of atropine does not seem to affect the bronchial glands, whereas systemic administration causes vagal inhibition with a resulting decrease in secretion by these glands, and consequent "drying" of the respiratory mucosa.

The effect of atropine as a pulmonary parasympatholytic drug illustrates two important, discrete functions of the vagal supply to the lungs. The first function, affecting bronchial muscles, is demonstrated by the effects of smaller doses of atropine given topically, and by larger systemic doses; the drug interferes with the cyclic-GMP mediated bronchospasm initiated by cholinergic receptor stimulation.[60] Moreover, atropine markedly prolongs the effect of cyclic-AMP stimulators such as isoproterenol. By these means, atropine is of value in the treatment of bronchospasm. The second vagal function affects mucus secretion by the bronchial gland; however, the vagal supply to the bronchial gland is blocked only by larger doses of atropine, such as the systemic doses given before anesthesia to keep the lungs dry. Thus, there are two different vagal efferent systems in the lungs that may be inactivated selectively by the appropriate use of atropine. It is of great interest that atropine has been shown to reverse asthmatic bronchospasm induced by drugs that block the beta receptors (such as propranolol)[19, 61]; this suggests that in at least these patients the bronchoconstriction is due to unopposed cholinergic activity, and that atropine may obviate the well-known danger involved in giving beta blockers to asthmatics. Excessive mucus production, as is seen in bronchorrhea, may be inhibited by aerosolized atropine.[62]

There has been a recent renewal of interest in the rise of atropine as a research tool in the laboratory for studying bronchospasm, and as an aerosol for the treatment of asthma. However, it is unlikely that atropine itself will become an important antiasthma drug, since newer aerosol anticholinergic agents (such as N-isopropyl-nortropine tropic acid ester, also known as *ipratropium bromide, Sch 1000* and Atrovent) are much more powerful bronchodilators,[62a, 62b] Ipratropium, like atropine, is a more effective bronchodilator in bronchitics than in asthmatics.[62c] Bronchitics may obtain equivalent bronchodilatation from ipratropium as can be obtained with a selective beta-2 adrenergic stimulating agents.[63] Ipratropium, like atropine, potentiates the bronchodilator effects of beta-adrenergic drugs and may decrease the side effects.[62b, 62c] Studies of ipratropium have shown that the aerosol is effective and well-tolerated in the treatment of asthma, in which it appears to have its major effect on the larger airways;[64] an equal bronchodilator effect to that of isoproterenol can be achieved, but the effect of the anticholinergic drug may persist for a longer time (up to four hours).[64-66] The effective inhalational dose of ipratropium lies between 10 and 80 μg; this range does not cause atropine-like side effects.[67]

Atropine is classified as an antimuscarinic, anticholinergic agent; it competitively antagonizes the muscarinic actions of acetylcholine (ACh) on exocrine glands, and on smooth and cardiac muscles. Atropine seems to be relatively more potent as an antagonist of ACh against bronchial muscles when

TABLE 4–13. ATROPINE

	Effects		
	TOPICAL	LOW SYSTEMIC DOSE	HIGH SYSTEMIC DOSE
BRONCHIAL MUSCLE	Bronchodilation	Brochodilation	
RESPIRATORY SECRETIONS	No effect	Decreases and thickens	
MOUTH	Dries mucosa	Decreases and thickens saliva	Very dry mouth
BOWEL MUSCLE		Decreases spasm	
GASTROINTESTINAL EXOCRINE GLANDS		Reduces secretions	
EYES	Mydriatic, paralyses accommodation	Blurs vision	Blurs vision
NOSE	Reduces rhinorrhea	Reduces rhinorrhea	
SKIN	Inhibits sweating	Inhibits sweating	Skin becomes hot and dry; patient develops hyperpyrexia
NERVOUS SYSTEM		Antiparkinsonism	Ataxia
BRAIN		Dizziness, fatigue, sedation	Delirium and hallucinations, leading to coma
HEART		Slight slowing	Tachycardia
BLADDER		Relief of spasm	Urinary retention

	Uses
PREANESTHESIA	To prevent cardiac slowing, bronchospasm and any increase in respiratory secretions
ANTIPARKINSONISM	Atropine is no longer used.
GASTROINTESTINAL SEDATIVE	For treatment of spasm, and functional bowel syndromes
OPHTHALMIC	To relax pupil (mydriasis)
ASTHMA	Inhalation helps alleviate bronchospasm (potentiates beta-2 stimulators, and prevents exercise-induced asthma); topical administration does not adversely affect secretions
ALLERGIC RHINITIS	Atropine may help

Preparations

Antiasthma cigarettes and powders contain atropine-like drugs, e.g. Asthmador.
Dylephrin: combination of epinephrine and atropine (formerly marketed in the U.S., but no longer available); was given by aerosolization
Atropine sulfate solutions: various concentrations are available, e.g. 0.03%–4%
Atropine methonitrate: used in combination aerosol preparations in United Kingdom; less toxic than atropine sulfate

Use in Asthma
(Not Approved in U.S.)
Aerosol: use atropine sulfate 1% solution in a diluent; give about 1 mg every 4–6 hours
Combination aerosols of atropine with epinephrine or isoproterenol are available in United Kingdom.

compared to similar agents, such as scopola-mine. The pharmacologic actions of atropine include central excitation, respiratory depression, suppression of certain forms of tremor (particularly Parkinsonism), dilation of the pupil (mydriasis), paralysis of accommodation (cycloplegia, which can result in photophobia and glaucoma), slowing of heart rate (small doses), tachycardia (large doses), slight increase in blood pressure, decreased sweating, decreased salivary and gastric secretion, and decrease of gastrointestinal motility. The drug decreases excessive nasal and respiratory tract secretions when given systemically; for these reasons atropine is used in the treatment of rhinitis and in the preparation of patients for general anesthesia (Table 4–13).

Although it is often stated that atropine increases the viscosity of bronchial secretions and impairs ciliary clearance, there is little evidence that such effects occur. More recent studies suggest that the drying effect of asthma is found only in a certain subgroup of patients with excessive airway secretions.[70] While the available information is relatively scanty, there is adequate evidence that giving several inhalations a day of atropine does not have a drying effect on bronchial secretions in patients with chronic obstructive airway disease.[71] The drying properties of atropine are probably dose-dependent, since systemic doses can cause a decrease in volume and an increase in viscosity of bronchial secretions.

In the treatment of bronchospasm, it is suggested that atropine sulfate be given by inhalation as a 1 per cent solution in a dosage of 0.05–0.1 mg per kg up to four times a day.[72] In the United Kingdom, atropine (in various forms) has, for many years, been a standard component of compound inhalational solutions with epinephrine or isoproterenol for the treatment of asthma.[73] Atropine is usually employed as the sulfate, although the methonitrate may be more active. (See Table 6–17).

The results of comparative studies reveal that nebulized atropine sulfate or methonitrate may be as effective as isoproterenol, but with fewer chronotropic side effects on the heart and a longer duration of action.[72] Although atropine is not approved for inhalational use in the U.S., there appears to be no valid contraindication to its use by knowledgeable clinicians and therapists as a secondary drug in the treatment or prophylaxis of bronchospasm.

It is possible that atropine aerosol is more effective in bronchitis than in asthma,[73] but the drug can be very successful for the prevention and alleviation of asthma induced by exercise.[74] A further use of atropine has been described in asthmatics: those patients who have a greater response to atropine than to isoproterenol are less likely to respond to glucocorticoid therapy than subjects who have a lesser response to atropine.[73] The role of atropine in the management of asthma due to irritants or allergies requires further clarification.[60, 73] However, it is clear that atropine, or newer anticholinergic agents, do have a definite therapeutic role in various forms of asthma, particularly in those patients who are not controlled by maximal dosages of, or who suffer unacceptable side effects from, sympathomimetics.[75]

In addition to atropine and ipratropium, various other anticholinergic agents have been successfully used in the treatment of bronchospasm over the years. These include hyoscyamine, scopolamine (hyoscine), banthine, epoxytropine tropate and methoscopolamine (Pamine).[69] At present, atropine is the only generally available anticholinergic drug that has established its value in asthma.

Prostaglandins

These hormonal agents are unsaturated fatty acids synthesized from precursors such as arachidonic acid. The prostaglandins occur widely in nature, and they are present in most body secretions.[76] It is not certain where the lung prostaglandins originate, but they may be formed by mast cells and eosinophils, the granules of which contain arachidonic acid. Synthesis of prostaglandins by microsomal prostaglandin synthetase can be inhibited by various antiinflammatory drugs, including aspirin, indomethacin, phenylbutazone and fenamates. These agents can cause asthma in susceptible subjects, whereas in other adult patients aspirin, in particular, may have a beneficial effect on chronic asthma.[77, 77a]

Several different classes of prostaglandins have been identified; they are PGA, PGE and PGF. Most knowledge has been accumulated on prostaglandins of the E and F series; both of these groups occur in human lung tissue. The most important prostaglandins in the pathophysiology of asthma are PGE_1, PGE_2 and $PGF_{2\alpha}$ (Table 4–14). PGE_2 is the most abundant subgroup of the E series, and is found particularly in bronchial tissue, whereas $PGF_{2\alpha}$ (the main PGF)

Table 4–14. PROSTAGLANDINS INVOLVED IN ASTHMA

	PGE_1	PGE_2	$PGF_{2\alpha}$
DISTRIBUTION	Not found in human lung	Found mainly in bronchial tissue	Found mainly in pulmonary parenchyma
RECEPTOR SITES ACTIONS	(?) Adenylate cyclase Increases c-AMP	Adenylate cyclase Increases c-AMP	Phosphodiesterase, and others Increases c-GMP, decreases c-AMP
AEROSOL EFFECT — overall	Bronchodilator	Bronchoconstrictor → bronchodilator	Bronchoconstrictor
NORMAL LUNG— low dose	No effect	Irritative; may cause bronchospasm	May cause cough and some bronchospasm
—high dose	May cause some bronchodilation	May cause some bronchodilation	Usually causes some bronchospasm
ASTHMATIC LUNG—low dose	Slight bronchodilation	Bronchoconstriction or bronchodilation	Marked bronchospasm
—high dose	Moderate bronchodilation	Marked bronchodilation usually (initially may cause severe cough, mucus production and wheezing)	Severe bronchospasm
DURATION OF ACTION	Less than 1 hour	About 1 hour	1 hour, or longer
EFFECT ON PULMONARY VASCULATURE	May decrease vascular resistance	Decreases vascular resistance	Increases vascular resistance
EFFECT ON RESPIRATORY CENTER	May stimulate	May stimulate	May stimulate
EFFECT OF ANTICHOLINERGIC DRUGS	No effect	No effect	Partially block late bronchoconstriction
RECEPTOR BLOCKERS	None identified	None identified	Aspirin, fenamates, etc.

is concentrated in the pulmonary parenchyma, which contains 20 times as much $PGF_{2\alpha}$ as PGE_2.[78]

The actions of the prostaglandins can be variable, since they may have different initial and late effects.[39, 79] They are very potent when given by aerosol, but they have little bronchodilator effect on the lungs when given systemically, presumably because they are rapidly inactivated by pulmonary enzymes unless administered topically.[80] However, when given intravenously, prostaglandins may cause slight bronchospasm. At present, it appears that if prostaglandins enter the therapeutic armamentarium they will be strictly inhalational drugs.[38]

Prostaglandin F. Members of this class are found to cause bronchoconstriction, and they may play a role in the pathophysiology of asthma. The only important prostaglandin in this class with regard to bronchospasm is $PGF_{2\alpha}$. It is thought that $PGF_{2\alpha}$ is a mediator of bronchospasm that is released when an antigen acts upon IGE-sensitized lungs. Extraordinarily small, aerosolized amounts of this prostaglandin cause bronchospasm in asthmatic patients, but not in normal lungs.[39] Various evidence suggests that $PGF_{2\alpha}$ decreases the amount of cyclic 3',5'-AMP in bronchial muscle cells, while stimulating guanyl cyclase, thus leading to an increase in the level of cyclic 3',5'-GMP.[81] Furthermore, $PGF_{2\alpha}$ may alter muscle cell membrane permeability to calcium, thereby permitting this ion to enter the cell and cause contraction.[82] Administration of $PGF_{2\alpha}$ causes an early bronchoconstriction, which may be a direct effect; this is followed, after a few minutes, by an additional constriction of the large airways, which can be inhibited (at least partially) by atropine.[83] This suggests that part of the bronchoconstrictor effect of $PGF_{2\alpha}$ is mediated through tracheobronchial cholinergic receptors.[81, 84] There is also evidence that $PGF_{2\alpha}$ activates phosphodiesterase, thereby leading to the breakdown of c-AMP; it is possible that this enzyme serves as a receptor site for $PGF_{2\alpha}$.[33]

It is postulated that drugs such as fenamates and polyphloretin phosphate, which may prevent bronchospasm in some circumstances, act by blocking the prostaglandin F receptors.[85, 86] Asthmatics demonstrate an abnormally enhanced response to the bronchoconstrictive properties of $PGF_{2\alpha}$; they show up to 8000 times as much reactivity to an aerosolized dose as do normal subjects.[79] The levels of serum prostaglandins are elevated in asthmatics, with a proportionally greater increase in $PGF_{2\alpha}$.[87] Although all these findings suggest multiple opportunities for $PGF_{2\alpha}$ to affect bronchial tone, the exact role of PGF in normal lungs and in asthma requires further clarification.

Prostaglandin E. There are two important members of this class: PGE_2, which is found in the human lung, and PGE, which is not. Both these prostaglandins can cause marked bronchodilation. In aerosol studies, PGE_1 usually causes relaxation of bronchial muscle; in contrast, PGE_2 can also cause bronchoconstriction.[33] Low doses of PGE_2 appear to be irritative to the airways and cause bronchospasm, whereas higher doses cause bronchodilation; intravenous administration is liable to cause bronchospasm rather than bronchodilation.[88] The liability of PGE_2 to cause bronchospasm is greatly enhanced in asthmatic subjects.[39, 79] Asthmatic patients may develop bronchospasm during the administration of intravenous PGE_2, which is sometimes used to produce a therapeutic abortion.[88] In some asthmatics PGE_1 given as an aerosol can also cause bronchospasm. There may be subsets of asthmatics who are extremely sensitive to the undoubted irritant properties of aerosolized prostaglandins.[79]

When prostaglandins of the E series cause bronchodilation in asthmatics, they appear to be at least as potent as isoproterenol.[89] Some reports suggest that they are much more powerful than isoproterenol, with PGE_2 appearing to be more potent than PGE_1.[80, 86] In addition to their effects on bronchial muscle, the prostaglandins, in common with other bronchodilator drugs, may have potent effects on the pulmonary circulation (Table 4–14) and other autonomic activities in the lung.[90]

There is evidence that the bronchodilator properties of the PGEs are related to their ability to increase intracellular cyclic 3'5'-AMP.[9, 91, 92] It is possible that the receptors for the PGEs are related to cellular adenylate cyclase;[33] thus, the prostaglandin E receptor may be closely associated with the beta-2 receptor. However, the prostaglandins may be able to cause bronchial muscle relaxation when sympathomimetic drugs are not successful. The mechanism by which the PGEs cause coughing and mucus production is not certain, but it may be a result of direct mucosal irritation.

The bronchodilation produced by aerosolized PGE_1 or PGE_2 lasts only about one hour; these agents are thus not longer-lasting than isoproterenol, and they have a much shorter duration of action than the newer sympathomimetic bronchodilators or the effective anticholinergic aerosols. The marked tracheobronchial irritation that the prostaglandins cause is a further severe disadvantage.

Prostaglandins A. Prostaglandins A are of little significance in bronchospasm.[86] This series of prostaglandins does not have a primary effect on the lung; most work has suggested that PGA has a major effect on blood pressure and sodium excretion.[38, 91] However, aerosolized PGA can cause both bronchodilation and bronchoconstriction.[33] Higher concentrations of PGA than of PGE_2 are required to produce these airway reactions. There is evidence that PGE_2 is about twice as potent a bronchoconstrictor as PGA.[88]

Prostaglandins B. Prostaglandins B have recently been shown to have some bronchoconstrictor properties, and in some laboratory studies they have been shown to have weak bronchodilator activity.[88]

The diverse effects on the respiratory tract and on breathing in man and in animals have been recently reviewed in detail.[88, 90] The potent and varied properties of these agents suggest that they will have a future role in the management of asthma, but it is difficult to predict what this role will be.

Other Bronchial Muscle Relaxants

A number of interesting drugs merit consideration, either because they have been used in the past in the treatment of asthma, or because they have recently gained attention as investigational agents (Table 4–15). These agents appear to act as bronchial muscle relaxants.

Khellin. One of the oldest known bronchodilator preparations has been obtained as an extract from the fruit of an umbelliferous plant, *Ammi visnaga,* which is found in some Mediterranean countries. The main pharmacologically active constituent in the extract is *khellin;* other identified drugs include *khelloside* and *visnagin.* Khellin has been used as a traditional remedy, with reputed value as a mild, smooth muscle relaxant, in the management of ureteric colic and cholecystitis, and as a coronary vasodilator. It had also been advocated in the treatment of asthma; this led the British pharmaceutical firm Fisons to embark on a laboratory research program that culminated in the serendipitous discovery of *cromolyn sodium* (known in Britain as disodium cromoglycate). Cromolyn is discussed in detail in Chapter 8.

Khellin is classified as a bischromone. Since it is too nauseating and causes other

TABLE 4–15. MINOR BRONCHIAL MUSCLE RELAXANTS

Drugs	Site of Action	Comments
BISCHROMONES Khellin, khelloside, visnagin	Unknown; potentiate c-AMP mechanism	These traditional muscle relaxants are too toxic for use in asthma.
MARIJUANA DERIVATIVES Tetrahydrocannabinol	Vagolytic effect; acts proximal to muscarinic receptor site	Aerosolized derivatives reduce bronchomotor tone, and decrease bronchospasm
PITUITARY EXTRACTS Anterior lobe extract, posterior lobe extract	No information	Although used in aerosol form, there is no evidence as to effectiveness
DOPAMINERGICS Levodopa, bromocriptine, apomorphine	Metabolic derivatives are beta-2 adrenergic stimulators	May be of some value as bronchodilators; nauseating effect may contribute to reflex mucokinesis
GANGLION-BLOCKERS Hexamethonium	Competes with acetylcholine for receptor site	Hypotensive effect precludes use as a bronchodilator
CORONARY VASODILATORS Amyl nitrite, sodium nitrite	Unknown mechanisms; act mainly on smooth muscle of blood vessels	Vasodilators, used in the treatment of angina; inhalation of amyl nitrite may be of some value in asthma

disagreeable side effects, it had been hoped that a modified chromone might be more effective and less toxic. Although this reasoning led to the development of cromolyn, this derivative is not a muscle relaxant, and it is not of value as a bronchodilator. It is a curious coincidence that cromolyn turned out to be a potent prophylactic drug that interferes with the antigen-antibody reaction that releases the mediators of bronchospasm. It is not known how khellin itself causes muscle relaxation, but it presumably acts through the cyclic-AMP mechanism.

Marijuana. Several recent studies have confirmed the long-standing and half-forgotten value of marijuana for the relief of bronchospasm. Tashkin and coworkers[93, 94] found that both smoked marijuana and oral Δ^9-THC (tetrahydrocannabinol — the major active ingredient) relax the bronchomotor tone in normal airways, and also can cause bronchodilation in asthmatic lungs.[93] Although the effect is not as great as that of isoproterenol, bronchodilatation can last longer when marijuana is used: oral Δ^9-THC relaxes airways for up to six hours, whereas inhaled marijuana smoke is more like isoproterenol in that it causes bronchodilatation for about one hour. In asthmatics, smoked marijuana results in bronchodilatation for as long as two hours; oral Δ^9-THC has an effect for up to four hours. Smoked marijuana appears to be more effective than oral ingestion of the drug or its derivatives; recently, microaerosolized Δ^9-THC has been found to be an effective bronchodilator.[95]

The exact mechanism by which marijuana acts on bronchial muscle is uncertain, but it does not appear to be a central effect;[96] in this regard, marijuana has a different action from that of other narcotic drugs, which depress the respiratory center. It is thought that the drug may have a vagolytic action[94] that is exerted proximal to the muscarinic receptor site; it does not inhibit these receptors, and does not cause beta-adrenergic stimulation.[97] The various side effects of marijuana and its derivatives preclude it from clinical use in the treatment of asthma. Those who smoke the drug in the belief that it could benefit their lungs should be informed that this practice could, in fact, cause bronchitis. Aerosolized Δ^9-THC is also irritating to the airways.[97a] However, there is a possibility that a derivative of marijuana may eventually be accepted as a suitable drug for use in the management of bronchospasm.[97b]

Pituitary Extracts. The pituitary gland is packed with powerful hormones that have multiple effects, controlling various functions in all parts of the body. It is, therefore, not surprising that the pituitary has been considered to participate in the control of bronchospasm, although there is little information regarding any primary role. However, it is surprising to find that this limited understanding has not inhibited pharmaceutic manufacturers from utilizing extracts of pituitary in the treatment of asthma. Although there is virtually no acceptable published evidence to suggest that these hormonal extracts are of value in the control of bronchospasm, the encyclopedic British publication Martindale's Extra Pharmacopoeia, lists at least seven proprietary inhalational products containing pituitary extract that are marketed in Britain (see Table 6-17). All these commercial concoctions contain epinephrine, and a seemingly random variety of other drugs. The "synergistic" agents that are chosen include atropine, papaverine, hyoscine and amethocaine, as well as extracts of both the anterior lobe and the posterior lobe of the pituitary gland.

At present, there is little reason to believe that the pituitary components are of relevance in the mixtures that also use epinephrine, although the gland extracts have been used for many years.[98] It would be interesting to know the data on which the various manufacturers base their selection of agents and that which determine the absolute amount of each in an inhalational dose of the product. Detailed information is not currently available; therefore this curious use of pituitary derivatives in polypharmaceutic combinations must be viewed with skepticism.

L-dopa. Anticholinergic drugs have long had a role in the treatment of the neurologic disease parkinsonism, just as they have had a long history of value in the treatment of asthma. In the past few years, a new, more effective antiparkinsonism drug has virtually replaced anticholinergic drugs as the agent of choice for the management of this disorder of the corpus striatum of the brain. The new agent, L-dopa (lévodopa, Dopar, Larodopa, Levopa), is a precursor of dopamine, to which it is converted by tissue enzymes. Dopamine is a catecholamine, 3,4-dehydroxyphenylethylamine; this compound is a precursor of the adrenergic transmitter norepinephrine. Dopamine itself has direct and indirect adrenergic activity and is an important neurotransmitter. There are specific dopaminergic receptors in various tissues, particularly in the brain and

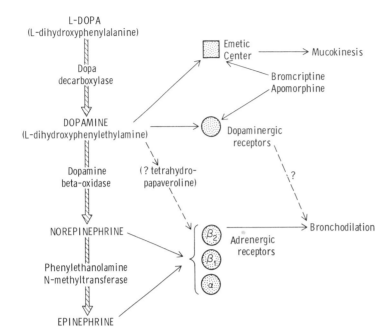

Figure 4–6. The drug L-dopa is converted to dopamine, which is a precursor of norepinephrine and epinephrine. Dopamine acts on dopaminergic receptors, which may facilitate bronchodilation; dopamine may also be converted to the bronchodilator, tetrahydropapaveroline. A further action of dopamine is on the emetic center, thereby causing vomiting and stimulating mucokinesis. Apomorphine and bromocriptine may have similar actions.

kidney; the administration of oral levodopa can result in enhanced neurologic transmission at these receptor sites. This is believed to be the mechanism by which the drug alleviates the tremulousness and rigidity that characterize Parkinson's disease.

A number of observers have noted that some bronchitic patients who receive levodopa for management of concurrent parkinsonism apparently experience some bronchodilation, which may be attributable to the drug. Although this observation requires further substantiation, it has been suggested that the bronchodilation is in large measure attributable to the metabolic conversion of levodopa to tetrahydropapaveroline, which is an effective beta-2 adrenergic stimulator.[99] (Fig. 4–6).

More recently, there have been reports that *bromocriptine* (2-bromo-α-ergocryptine, CB-154) can help in intractable asthma as a result of its ability to induce bronchodilation.[100] This investigational agent is a powerful dopaminergic agonist, which has a somewhat similar effect to that of levodopa. Other agents that may also have a dopaminergic effect include *apomorphine* and the investigational agent *piribedil*. At present, there is no clear role for any of these drugs in the management of bronchospasm, though their possible adjuvant value deserves consideration. It is of interest that all these agents stimulate the emetic center in the hindbrain, and may cause nausea and vomiting; this would suggest that these dopaminergic drugs may also have a mucokinetic effect.

Glucagon. Glucagon, a pancreatic hormone having powerful effects on glucose metabolism, opposite to those of insulin, acts by stimulating the synthesis of cyclic AMP. It has recently been demonstrated[101] that aerosolized glucagon may decrease airway resistance in asthmatics. However, the evidence at present does not suggest that this hormone has an important future in bronchodilator pharmacology.

Hexamethonium. Hexamethonium is a ganglion-blocking agent that competes with acetylcholine and prevents this transmitter from acting on postganglionic receptors. It has been shown in the laboratory that hexamethonium can antagonize the bronchoconstrictor effect of nicotine in guinea pigs. Several investigators have shown that this ganglion-blocker can antagonize bronchoconstriction in humans,[102] but, since the drug has a potent hypotensive effect, it is not of practical value in the treatment of bronchospasm. Certainly, atropine is more effective and much safer, and therefore is a preferable anticholinergic for use in asthma.

ANTIMEDIATOR DRUGS

Many cases of asthma are clearly related to the actions on bronchial muscle of mediators that are released from mast cells and basophils. It is disappointing to find that

TABLE 4–16. ANTIMEDIATOR DRUGS USED IN ASTHMA

Drugs	Site of Action	Comment
GLUCOCORTICOIDS Prednisone	Various actions on mast cells, beta-2 receptors, and at other sites	Established value in acute therapy and in prophylaxis
ANTIHISTAMINES Heparin, ascorbic acid	Interfere with histamine release or action; other actions depend on specific agent	Minor value in allergic asthma; further studies required for evaluation of these agents, which have multiple sites of action.
BISCHROMONES Cromolyn	Stabilize mast cell surface	Established value in prophylaxis of allergic asthma and exercise-induced asthma
IMMUNOSUPPRESSIVES Azathioprine, 6-mercaptopurine, thioguanosine	Antimetabolic effect on immunocompetent cells	No established value in any form of asthma
ANTIINFLAMMATORY AGENTS Aspirin, aminophenazone, dipyrone, flufenamic acid, phenylbutazone	Interfere with $PGF_{2\alpha}$	May be of prophylactic value in some patients; may cause asthma in hypersensitive patients.
ANTIFILARIAL AGENT Diethylcarbamazine	Inhibits release of mediators	May be of value in tropical asthma. Aerosol may prevent exercise-induced asthma.

pharmacologic agents that are specific antagonists of individual mediators are of relatively little value in asthma.[103] In contrast, nonspecific agents, such as corticosteroids and cromolyn, may be spectacularly successful in the management of various types of asthma, particularly those cases with an allergic etiology.

A number of potent agents can be regarded as having antagonistic effects against several of the mediators, whereas others have more specific actions against one or two of the mediators. In many cases, the documentation of efficacy is inadequate, particularly with respect to asthma. Thus, it is possible that some metabolic inhibitors, some enzyme poisons (such as colchicine) and some centrally acting muscle relaxants (such as chlorphenesin) may have a significant antimediator effect, but they have not been shown to be effective in the treatment of asthma. The following agents vary in value from excellent to dubious (see Table 4–16).

Glucocorticoids

The antiinflammatory corticosteroid drugs have multiple, nonspecific sites of action, and they intercede in the asthmatic pathophysiologic mechanism at several points. As a consequence, these powerful agents are particularly effective in the prophylaxis of asthma, and they also provide a potent therapeutic weapon in the treatment of acute asthmatic bronchospasm. The glucocorticoids are discussed in detail in Chapter 7.

Antihistamines

Although histamine is one of the most important mediators of asthma, it is disappointing to find that none of the large number of antihistamine drugs has proved to be of great value in the prophylaxis or management of asthma. It is probable that the available drugs do not reach the part of the lung mast cell where the release of histamine occurs; these agents do not interfere with the action of histamine in the lungs once it is released. On the other hand, antihistamines often have an anticholinergic effect, which can result in a decrease in mucous gland secretory activity. The resulting drying effect is generally undesirable in the lungs, whereas this action is therapeutically appreciated in the upper respiratory tract. The antihistamines are therefore of value in allergic rhinitis and conjunctivitis, but are of little benefit in allergic asthma (see Chapter 9).

Heparin. Heparin is a natural anticoagulant produced by mammalian tissues, including mast cells. It has some antiserotonin action, and is claimed to possess marked antihistaminic potency. Heparin has been reported to be of value in a variety of allergic conditions, including eczema and hay fever. Intravenous heparin has been observed to decrease the wheezing that sometimes accompanies pulmonary embolus. Such observations have led to heparin being given by aerosol to patients with chronic obstructive pulmonary disease, and a decrease in airway resistance has been reported.[104] However, other studies have cast doubt on the use of heparin in the treatment of bronchospasm. The evidence suggest that intravenous administration is not beneficial in asthma.[105] Further studies using aerosolized heparin in asthma may be justified, to determine whether any important therapeutic effect can be attributed to the antimediator properties of this drug.

Ascorbic Acid. Ascorbic acid has gained notoriety as a controversial drug for the prevention and treatment of the common cold. Ascorbic acid does have some antihistaminic properties, and it can inhibit histamine-induced airway constriction.[106] However, these findings cannot be used to endorse the use of ascorbic acid as an antihistamine, or to suggest that it is of value in asthma. Nevertheless, the drug may have a role in the respiratory tract, since it also has some mucokinetic properties (see Chapters 3 and 9).

Bischromones

As described earlier in this chapter, the bischromones include the traditional drug khellin; new pharmacologic derivatives of this ancient drug have been developed in recent years. The most important bischromone is cromolyn, which interferes with the release of the various asthmagenic mediators from mast cells, and thereby provides for effective prophylactic therapy for many patients with allergic asthma. *Cromolyn* is discussed in detail in Chapter 8.

Immunosuppressive Drugs

A number of cytotoxic drugs are of value in the treatment of immunologic diseases and in the prevention of rejection of a transplanted donated organ by the host's body. Some workers have employed immunosuppressives in the treatment of asthma, with varying results.[103] Drugs that have attained some success include the purine analogues *azathioprine* (imuran), *6-mercaptopurine,* and *thioguanosine*.[103, 107] At present, however, there is little to suggest that agents of this type have any practical role in the treatment of asthma.

Antiinflammatory Agents and Analgesics

A number of drugs that have been useful in the treatment of rheumatologic disorders have been reported to have some success in the treatment of asthma. However, the results are variable, and usually the benefits are minor. Nevertheless, these agents are worth considering, since they, or related drugs, may become more significant in this respect in the future.

Aspirin. Although aspirin (acetylsalicylic acid) and related analgesic agents have achieved notoriety as etiologic agents in some forms of hypersensitivity asthma, there are asthmatic patients who appear to benefit from the prophylactic use of aspirin.[86] Since salicylates have profound effect on immunologic processes and interfere with prostaglandin production,[108] it is conceivable that, in some patients, aspirin has relatively more effect on the activity of $PGF_{2\alpha}$, and thereby interferes with the prostaglandin-induced bronchospastic process. However, it must be emphasized that salicylates and related antiinflammatory analgesics should be regarded with great suspicion in the therapy of asthma, since these drugs are notorious for their ability to cause severe asthma in those patients who suffer from aspirin hypersensitivity.[109] In addition to aspirin, the following analgesics may cause hypersensitivity asthma in susceptible patients: acetaminophen, aminopyrine, indomethacin and mefenamic acid; tartrazine, a chemically related dye, can also share this asthmagenic property; this is unfortunate, since the dye is used in many pharmaceutic products, including some antiasthma drugs.

A number of analgesic, antirheumatic agents have been reported to be beneficial in asthma.[102] These include phenazone (antipyrine), aminophenazone (aminopyrine), phenylbutazone, flufenamic acid and dipyrone.[110] However, all these agents can cause serious side effects, such as agranulocytosis, and they cannot be recommended. Moreover, there is a possibility that any of these drugs could cause severe bronchospasm in a hypersensitive patient; such reactions may be unpredictable. Thus, further studies are required before any antiinflammatory or analgesic drug can be regarded as suitable for therapeutic trial in asthma.

Chloroquine. Chloroquine is a drug with multiple antiinflammatory effects. It is used mainly as an antimalarial, but it is also of value in selected patients with rheumatic diseases, such as rheumatoid arthritis and discoid lupus erythematosus. Since it has antianaphylactic properties, and it antagonizes histamine as well as other mediators, chloroquine has been investigated for its value in the treatment of asthma. Although some workers were impressed with the effectiveness of chloroquine, the overall conclusion must be unfavorable.[111]

Diethylcarbamazine.

Diethylcarbamazine (Hetrazan) is an antihelminthic drug that is related to piperazine. It is used in the treatment of some forms of filariasis, although it may cause severe allergic reactions in such cases. Filarial infection is often accompanied by eosinophilia and asthma, and it has long been known that the syndrome of tropical eosinophilic pneumonia accompanied by asthma responds rapidly to treatment with diethylcarbamazine. Studies have shown that this drug inhibits the release of mediators, such as SRS-A, in certain animals, and it also has been found to inhibit $PGF_{2\alpha}$-induced bronchospasm.[103, 112] Diethylcarbamazine citrate has been given orally with varying results in the treatment of asthma, but the overall impression has not been favorable.[113] More recently, the almost insoluble diethylcarbamazine pamoate, as an aerosol, has been reported to provide useful protection against exercise-induced asthma in children.[114] Thus, in several respects, the drug appears to be comparable to cromolyn, both in its clinical effectiveness and in its mechanism of action as an anti-mediator. At present, however, diethylcarbamazine cannot be regarded as useful in asthma, but if it were to be tried, the drug should probably be investigated in cases of asthma with marked eosinophilia or, perhaps, in children with poorly controlled exercise-induced asthma.

If diethylcarbamazine is administered orally, the dose should presumably be that recommended for the treatment of tropical eosinophilia, that is, 2 to 4 mg/kg three times a day after food for one to three weeks. The drug may cause side effects such as malaise, headaches, weakness, arthralgias, anorexia, nausea and vomiting. Patients infected with filaria may experience a more violent reaction, with fever, tachycardia, urticaria, rash, skin edema and lymphadenopathy. The drug should, therefore, always be given cautiously, under close medical supervision.

AGENTS AFFECTING ALPHA RECEPTORS

Alpha receptors are widely distributed in the lungs, and a wide variety of results can be obtained by using drugs that are alpha-adrenergic agonists or antagonists. The mast cells and bronchial muscle cells have a sparse supply of alpha receptors compared to beta-2 receptors. Stimulation of the alpha receptors activates cyclic-AMP production; the end result is bronchospasm, with an increase in airway resistance. However, stimulation of the alpha receptors supplying pulmonary blood vessels results in vasoconstriction; if the mucosa is inflamed and boggy, the resulting mucosal shrinkage may outweigh the alpha adrenergic bronchospasm, and result in a balance that decreases airway resistance. Thus alpha receptor stimulators may actually improve airway dynamics in bronchial asthma, as discussed in Chapter 5. Since alpha receptor stimulating drugs are mainly of benefit in the treatment of the upper respiratory tract mucosa, further consideration of these agents is provided in Chapter 9.

Alpha-adrenergic Receptor Blockers. Alpha-adrenergic receptor blockers have been used by investigators for the treatment of asthma. The blockers result in a decrease of alpha-adrenergic tone in bronchial muscle, and thereby can result in a decrease in airway resistance.

It has been shown that ATPase activity is increased in the leucocytes of asthmatics.[115] This suggests that the mechanism favoring cyclic-GMP production is enhanced; one may then conjecture that decreasing ATPase activity by using an alpha-adrenergic blocking drug could reduce the tendency to bronchospasm. Recent work has shown a complex relationship between c-AMP and c-GMP and the adrenergic blocking agents in asthmatic subjects.[116, 117] Several studies have indicated that suitable alpha-blocking drugs can, in fact, relieve asthma that is resistant to conventional therapy (Table 4-17).

Thymoxamine. Thymoxamine is one of the most specific alpha-receptor blocking drugs. Inhalation of 1 ml of a 1.5 per cent solution of this agent by asthmatic patients can result in a marked potentiation of the bronchospasmolytic effect of beta-2 stimulating drugs.[117, 118] The introduction of thymoxamine into the armamentarium for the

TABLE 4–17. ALPHA-BLOCKING AGENTS IN ASTHMA

Agents	Administration*	Comments
AVAILABLE AGENTS		
Phentolamine (Regitine)	Inhalation: 5 mg in 1 ml; oral: 50–100 mg tid	Reported to be useful for preventing exercise-induced asthma, and for intractable asthma
Phenoxybenzamine (Dibenzyline)		Similar to phentolamine, but has not been adequately studied
Tolazoline (Priscoline)	Oral: 2 mg/kg	Has not been adequately evaluated in asthma
INVESTIGATIONAL AGENTS		
Ibidomide(AH5158)	I.V.: 20 mg	This agent combines α, β_1 and β_2 blocking properties. The alpha blockade may override the beta-2 blocking effect.
Indoramin	Oral: 20–70 mg	Reported to be useful for preventing exercise-induced asthma
Practolol	I.V.: 5 mg (+ isoproterenol)	Reported to be effective in status asthmaticus
Thymoxamine	Inhalation: 15 mg in 1 ml; I.V.: 0.1–0.2 mg/kg	Aerosol is too irritating; effect of intravenous dose is short-lasting

*The listed dosages are those that have been used by investigators. Since the administration of the alpha-blocking agents in asthma is not an approved use, the above dosage cannot be regarded as recommendations.

treatment of asthma cannot be expected, however, since thymoxamine has only a short duration of action when given intravenously, and it is too irritating when given by inhalation. It has other disadvantages, in that it is expensive and can cause headaches.[118a]

Phentolamine. Phentolamine (Regitine) is a less-specific, but well-established, alpha blocking drug, which also has some beta-adrenergic, antihistaminic, antiserotonin and parasympatholytic activity. It is used successfully in the management of certain types of hypertension and for relieving arteriolar spasm. It has been reported[119] to be of value in the treatment of exercise-induced asthma when given by inhalation in a dose of 5 mg; or as long-term oral therapy, 50 to 100 mg three times a day, in intractable asthma. Phentolamine, like thymoxamine, can also potentiate the bronchodilator effect of simultaneously nebulized isoproterenol.[118]

Phenoxybenzamine. Phenoxybenzamine (Dibenzyline) resembles phentolamine, but it is a longer-acting drug. It may have a similar beneficial effect when administered to asthmatics.[119] However, no relevant studies in humans have been reported.

Tolazoline. Tolazoline (Priscoline) has less potent alpha-receptor blocking effects than phentolamine, and is less likely to be of value in asthma. It had been suggested that tolazoline could be of value as a mucokinetic agent in cystic fibrosis, but a controlled study did not corroborate this claim.[120] There is no available information relating to the effects of other alpha-blocking agents on mucokinesis, and it is unlikely that they would offer any therapeutic advantages in the various sputopathies.

Indoramin. Indoramin is an alpha-adrenergic blocking agent with useful antihypertensive properties. It has also been found to have antihistamine and antiserotonin actions, and it is preferentially concentrated in the lung.[121] This constellation of qualities has led to investigations into its use in asthma, and some studies do suggest that it is of value in preventing exercise-induced asthma.[121, 122] Although there is some controversy regarding the effect of indoramin,[122, 123] the agent may still prove to be of value in certain types of asthma.

Other alpha-adrenergic blockers have also been shown to possess useful bronchodilator qualities. Among these agents are *ibidomide* (AH5188)[124] and *practolol.*[125] Both of these investigational drugs also have beta-adrenergic blocking effects that might be expected to result in bronchospastic properties. Nevertheless, the alpha-blocking effect may override the adverse action on the beta-2 receptors, thereby permitting the drug to produce significant bronchodilation in suitable subjects. At present, neither of these agents can be considered to have a role in asthma, although they may be useful in asthmatics who require therapy with a beta-1 blocker for the management of concurrent angina or hypertension.

Further studies are now required to establish what the role of alpha-adrenergic blocking drugs might be in asthma. It can be projected that the pharmaceutic industry will eventually synthesize an adrenergic drug that has potent beta-2 activity, negligible beta-1 properties and marked alpha-blocking activity; an anticholinergic effect might also be usefully incorporated! Such a combination of properties might be very valuable in the treatment of forms of asthma that are clearly correlated with imbalance of autonomic function.

MISCELLANEOUS DRUGS USED IN TREATING BRONCHOSPASM

A large variety of drugs are given to patients with respiratory disease, whose primary purpose may be aimed at the nonbronchospastic components of the pulmonary problem. Nevertheless, some of these agents may have a direct, beneficial effect in asthma, and they can be used as adjuvants in the management of many patients with bronchospasm (Table 4–18).

Mucokinetic Agents

The drugs that are used to improve respiratory tract secretion clearance are considered in detail in Chapters 2 and 3. Most of these agents probably have no direct effect on the bronchial muscles, but those oral medications that act through the gastro-pulmonary mucokinetic vagal reflex could possibly cause vagally-induced broncho-spasm if given in markedly excessive dosage (see Figure 2–4). Some mucokinetic agents administered by aerosol can also induce bronchospasm as a consequence of direct irritation of the respiratory mucosa.

Iodides. Iodides are believed to be powerful mucokinetic agents; some workers consider these drugs also to have an antiasthma effect.[126, 127] Indeed, William Osler,

the great medical teacher of the late 1800s, considered potassium iodide to have a specific value in preventing asthma attacks.[127] Although the asthma-suppressive effect of potassium iodide has been attested to by a few enthusiasts, there is no recent, controlled data to support their claims. Nevertheless, potassium iodide may provide useful chronic therapy for asthmatics who have problems clearing their sputum.[126] In acute asthma, sodium iodide can be given intravenously 1 to 3 grams per day. In chronic therapy a saturated solution of potassium iodide (SSKI) can be given in a dose of 24 mg/kg per day or more.

Antimicrobial Agents

The use of antimicrobial drugs in chronic bronchitis has long been recommended, although recent work casts doubt on the value of prophylactic administration of antibiotics to prevent exacerbations of the respiratory problem.[128] Infection can act as a nonspecific irritant, and thereby trigger bronchospasm; antibiotic therapy can eliminate this etiologic factor. However, there is evidence that some antibiotics have a more specific pharmacologic effect that appears to increase the threshold of the susceptible lung to bronchospastic reactions.

The particular antibiotics reported to have an antibronchospastic effect are the macrolide agents, *troleandomycin* (Triacetyl-oleandomycin TAO), and *erythromycin*. It has been reported that TAO, when given in a daily dosage of 250 to 500 mg per day to asthmatic or bronchitic patients who require steroid therapy, results in an improvement in the bronchospasm.[129, 130] The steroid dose should be reduced, or the patient will be more likely to develop Cushing's syndrome.

TABLE 4–18. MISCELLANEOUS MINOR ANTIASTHMA DRUGS

Drug	Class	Mechanism of Action	Comments
IODIDE e.g., SSKI or sodium iodide	Mucokinetic	Nonspecific antiasthma effect	Useful agent for treatment of acute asthma with sputum retention
MACROLIDE e.g., erythromycin, TAO	Antibiotic	Potentiates glucocorticoid activity, as well as anti-microbial effect	Can be given to treat susceptible infection in asthmatic requiring concomitant steroid therapy
HYDROXYZINE	Ataractic	Tranquilizer, antihistamine, bronchodilator (possible antimediator effect)	Useful synergistic agent in the treatment of asthma; can be used for preoperative preparation of patient with bronchospastic disorders

This suggests that TAO has a steroid-sparing effect, the nature of which is not understood. However, it is possible that the macrolides affect steroid metabolism; they may also have a stimulating effect on the adrenal cortex.[129] These antibiotics also potentiate the effect of theophylline (see Chapter 6).

Although TAO is rarely used, erythromycin is a valuable antibiotic for the treatment of many pulmonary infections. Not all preparations of erythromycin have the macrolide steroid-sparing effect, but erythromycin estolate (Ilosone) does seem to offer this advantage. This drug should, therefore, be considered for administration to an asthmatic patient requiring glucocorticoids, if there is evidence of a nonspecific or mixed bacterial or myoplasmal pulmonary infection. The approximate oral dose for an adult is 250 to 500 mg six hourly for up to 10 days; in children 30 to 50 mg/kg per day should be given in divided doses.

No other antimicrobial agent has been credited with specific properties that render it valuable in the management of bronchospasm. On the contrary, several antibiotics have the potential to cause bronchospasm in allergic subjects, and most antimicrobial agents can induce bronchospasm when given by aerosol. Further discussion of antibiotic drugs is provided in Chapter 10.

Cough Medications

Many agents are thought of as being cough medications. These are considered in detail in Chapter 9. Although some of these drugs might have some bronchodilator effect (for example, benzonatate), none has been found to offer a major, direct contribution to the management of bronchospasm.

Tranquillizers

Acute asthma is usually accompanied by severe anxiety. Correction of this factor can result in a physiologic improvement in airway mechanics. Anxiety is usually assuaged, to a considerable degree, by the simple reassurance provided by the competent physician, nurse or therapist. However, physicians are often tempted to prescribe pharmacologic reassurance in the form of a tranquillizer. The very emotional, panic-stricken asthmatic who is hyperventilating may improve considerably following the administration of a tranquillizing drug, but there is no reason to believe that the various agents that are commonly used offer any direct bronchospasmolytic effect.

Diazepam. Diazepam (Valium) is a very popular tranquillizer. In common with other potent agents of this type, diazepam can cause depression of the respiratory center,[131] which would be particularly disadvantageous if the patient is hypoventilating. Although some workers have suggested that diazepam can be dangerous when administered to the anxious respiratory patient with hypercapnia, at least one study has shown that oral administration of 5 to 10 mg four times a day may be safe and beneficial in such cases.[132] It has also been shown that intravenous diazepam can be given to patients with obstructive lung disease without depressing respiration.[133] However, there is no evidence to suggest that the drug has any bronchodilator effect. Further discussion is provided in Chapter 11.

Hydroxyzine. Hydrozyzine (Atarax, Vistaril) is the one tranquillizer that has been claimed to have a definite bronchodilator effect.[134] This drug has a number of useful properties in addition to its antianxiety (or "ataractic") effect. Hydroxyzine has anticholinergic, antihistaminic and antiserotonic properties with both central and peripheral sites of action. It is an effective antiemetic as well. Hydroxyzine has been used in combination bronchodilator preparations with ephedrine and theophylline (as Marax); its ataractic properties counteract the central side effects of the other bronchodilator components.[135] Several studies have shown that oral or intramuscular administration of hydroxyzine alone can can cause useful bronchodilation.[134-136] The main side effect is drowsiness; some patients may also develop dry mouth, tremulousness, headache and even nausea. The drug does not produce respiratory depression, and it is therefore a particularly valuable preoperative sedative for patients with respiratory diseases.

Hydroxyzine is available as the hydrochloride and as the pamoate; these are equivalent preparations. It is marketed for both oral and intramuscular administration (Table 4–19). The appropriate adult dose is 25 mg three or four times a day, but up to 100 mg can be given as often as every four hours to patients who require an ataractic for severe emotional disturbance. An aerosol form is being evaluated for use in the treatment of asthma. Hydroxyzine is discussed further in Chapter 9.

Barbiturates. Barbiturates are sedative drugs that are frequently used as adjunctive therapy in the management of asthma, but this use is not based on any bronchospas-

TABLE 4-19. HYDROXYZINE

Product	Availability	Dosage	Uses
ATARAX (Hydroxyzine hydrochloride) VISTARIL (Hydroxyzine hydrochloride) VISTARIL (Hydroxyzine pamoate)	Tablets: 10, 25, 50, 100 mg; syrup: 10 mg/5 ml Ampoules for I.M. use: 25 mg/ml, 50 mg/ml Capsules: 25, 50, 100 mg; oral suspension: 25 mg/5 ml	Under 6 years of age: 50 mg/day in divided doses; over 6 years of age: 25-100 mg every 4-8 hours	1. Tranquilizer (ataractic) 2. Preoperative preparation 3. Antiemetic 4. Antihistamine 5. For alcoholism 6. Bronchodilator (alone or in combination preparations) 7. Antispasmodic

molytic properties. Perhaps the most commonly used agent is phenobarbital, which is combined with ephedrine and theophylline in proprietary products such as Tedral. The barbiturates may affect the respiratory system adversely, since they can cause respiratory depression by their central action (Chapter 11). Barbiturates such as *thiopental* (Pentothal) can actually potentiate bronchospasm; therefore, intravenous anesthesia with this agent should be avoided in asthmatics. In spite of these considerations, aerosolized barbiturates have, in the past, been credited with bronchodilator properties. No acceptable evidence to support such claims is available.

A further problem with barbiturates is that they induce the formation of microsomal enzymes in the liver that hydrolyze corticosteroids.[137] Thus, the concomitant administration of a barbiturate (as in Tedral) to a steroid-dependent asthmatic may reduce the therapeutic effect of the glucocorticoid, an additional reason for avoiding the use of barbiturates in patients with severe asthma.

Anesthetics

Both local and general anesthesia have been reported to be effective in reversing some forms of bronchospasm.

Local Anesthetics. In recent years, local anesthetics have been administered into tracheobronchial airways with increasing frequency as fiberoptic bronchoscopy has gained in popularity. There is no doubt that these anesthetics reduce airway reactivity and serve to prevent coughing and bronchospasm during instrumentation. Their value in the treatment of asthma is less certain, although cocaine, procaine and lidocaine have each been reported to be capable of reversing bronchospasm. Moreover, recent work has shown that aerosolized local anesthetics may cause mild bronchoconstriction in patients with reactive airways.[138] Nevertheless, the commonly used local anesthetics

may be of use in the prophylaxis of irritative bronchospasm, and they can be helpful in eliminating persistent coughing secondary to tracheobronchial irritation.

COCAINE. Cocaine is one of the most potent local anesthetics. It is a useful anesthetizing agent for mucosal surfaces, since it interferes with the uptake of norepinephrine by adrenergic nerve terminals, and thereby results in mucosal vasoconstriction. It can be used to facilitate bronchoscopy; 5 ml of a 10 per cent solution can be diluted to a 4 per cent solution, which is usually effective. Cocaine has been used as a bronchodilator, and was the active principle in a former proprietary product, "Tucker's Asthma Specific."[139] However, the drug is addictive, and it has no place in the present day management of bronchospastic disorders.

LIDOCAINE. Lidocaine (lignocaine, Xylocaine) is probably the most popular agent for topical anesthesia of the tracheobronchial tree, and is usually given in concentrations of 4 to 10 per cent. Although lidocaine aerosol can cause a nonspecific nociceptive bronchospasm in reactive airways,[138] this effect is not usually clinically detrimental. In fact, it is a common experience during bronchoscopy to find that the administration of topical lidocaine serves to reverse bronchospasm. Recent laboratory studies have shown that the drug can reverse spasm of guinea pig tracheal muscle;[140] at least one clinical study has shown that topical (aerosolized) 2 per cent lidocaine both prevents and reverses bronchospasm in anesthetized patients.[141] This study found that intravenous lidocaine was ineffective in bronchospasm, in a dose of 1 mg/kg followed by 1 to 2 mg per minute. It has also been reported that both intravenous and aerosolized lidocaine can alleviate persistent irritating cough.[142, 143] The role of lidocaine in the management of bronchospasm obviously merits further careful study.[144, 144a]

TABLE 4–20. GENERAL ANESTHETICS—EFFECTS ON ASTHMATIC LUNG

Agent	Strength*	Effect in Light Anesthesia On			Comments
		RESPIRATION	RESPIRATORY SECRETIONS	BRONCHIAL MUSCLE	
LIQUID INHALATIONAL AGENTS					
Chloroform	0.25–1%	Depresses	May increase	Relaxes	No longer used; powerful, but dangerous; has been used as an oral bronchodilator
Ether (diethyl ether)	5–30%	Stimulates	Increases	Relaxes	Rectal enema may relax bronchospasm; has been used as an oral bronchodilator; intravenous bolus stimulates coughing
Halothane (Fluothane)	1–6%	Depresses	No effect	Relaxes	Most useful general anesthetic for asthmatics
Methoxyflurane (Penthrane)	0.2–3%	Depresses	No effect	Relaxes	Similar to halothane, but more potent, with slow induction and slow recovery
Trichlorethylene (Trilene, Trimar)	1–2.5%	Stimulates	No effect	May relax	Reported to stimulate lung stretch receptors
Vinyl ether (Vinethene)	3–6%	Stimulates	May increase	Relaxes	Similar to ether, but more potent and less irritating
GASEOUS INHALATIONAL AGENTS					
Cyclopropane	10–50%	May depress	May increase	Relaxes	Powerful anesthetic; poor relaxant; explosive
Nitrous oxide	50–70%	Slight depression	No effect	No effect	Weak but safe; can result in severe hypoxemia
INTRAVENOUS AGENTS					
Ketamine (Ketaject, Ketalar)	1–10 mg/kg	May depress	No effect	May relax	Powerful analgesia with little anesthetic effect; for short procedures
Thiopental (Pentothal)	2.5–5%	Depresses	No effect	May constrict	Short-acting anesthetic with little analgesic effect

*The greater strength is required for induction of anesthesia; the lower strength may suffice for maintenance. Total dose depends upon individual patient factors.

PROCAINE.   Procaine (Novocain) is used less commonly at present, but was favored by Dautrebande as a bronchodilator;[145] he advocated its incorporation with isoproterenol and other synergistic agents in the original form of Aerolone. Dautrebande claimed that aerosolized procaine potentiated the bronchodilator effect of agents such as isoproterenol. Other workers have reported that the drug is of value in severe asthma when administered intravenously as a 0.1 per cent solution in a dosage of 4 mg/kg over the course of 20 minutes. The question of the effectiveness of procaine as a bronchodilator is discussed further in Chapter 12.

General Anesthetics.   Years ago it was found that status asthmaticus could sometimes be alleviated by giving the patient a general anesthetic. Such treatment is rarely used currently, but should be considered when a patient fails to respond to more conventional therapy or if the continued distress that the status occasions demands dramatic intervention. The main general anesthetics are presented in Table 4–20; the more important ones are discussed in the following section.

CHLOROFORM.   Chloroform is one of the earliest general anesthetics to have been introduced, although currently it is rarely employed. It has also had a long history of use in the treatment of respiratory diseases:[139] early work led to the belief that chloroform can relax bronchial muscle. Until recently, it was used in a number of proprietary cough medications, both for the management of bronchospasm and to improve expectoration. There is little investigational evidence to suggest that the drug is of significant value in either respect, whether given orally or by inhalation. For further discussion, see Chapter 3.

CYCLOPROPANE.   Cyclopropane was formerly regarded as a suitable general anesthetic, but the gas is explosive and difficult to use safely, and is therefore no longer in favor. Furthermore, cyclopropane is a marked respiratory depressant, it increases tracheobronchial secretion and may exacerbate bronchospasm.[146] The combination of sympathomimetic drug therapy and cyclopropane anesthesia acts synergistically on the heart and predisposes it to arrhythmias. For all these reasons, this anesthetic is particularly contraindicated in patients with respiratory disorders.

DIETHYL ETHER.   Diethyl ether is a valuable inhalational anesthetic, but it has the disadvantage of being a tracheobronchial tree irritant. However, this agent can produce relaxation of constricted bronchial muscle. Ether has been given over the years, either by inhalation, subcutaneous injection or rectal instillation as a therapeutic measure for the treatment of severe asthma.[141] For many years, rectal administration was enthusiastically advocated:[139] a 60 per cent solution was obtained by adding 60 ml ether to 120 ml olive oil, and the warm solution was given by rectal tube every 12 to 24 hours in a dosage of about 1 ml solution per pound body weight. An alternative and probably safer approach would be to induce general anesthesia in a patient with status asthmaticus, and to maintain this state for 30 minutes, during which time bronchial tone might diminish, with consequent release of inspissated respiratory secretions.

HALOTHANE.   Halothane (Fluothane) is currently considered to be one of the general anesthetics of choice for asthmatic patients who require anesthesia. This inhalational agent can relax bronchial muscle, and, unlike ether, it does not irritate the respiratory mucosa, and therefore does not cause an increased output of respiratory tract secretions. Halothane's ability to cause bronchial relaxation is not consistent: it has been claimed that it exerts its bronchodilator effect only in the presence of hypocapnia.[147]

METHOXYFLURANE.   Methoxyflurane (Penthrane) is the most potent of the inhalational anesthetic agents. Although this is not a particularly safe drug, it is sometimes used as a self-administered analgesic during childbirth. However, methoxyflurane has been reported to have bronchodilating properties, similar to those of halothane.[148] Whether this agent could be of therapeutic value in intractable asthma when administered in a subanesthetic dosage remains to be determined.

NITROUS OXIDE.   Nitrous oxide was the first general anesthetic to be introduced into modern anesthesia. The gas is a useful analgesic with relatively weak anesthetizing capability. The release of inhibitions that can occur during induction resulted in the drug's common name, "laughing gas." Relatively high concentrations (50 to 80 per cent) of the gas are required to produce anesthesia; oxygen is added in a concentration of 20 to 50 per cent. If high concentrations of nitrous oxide are given, the patient is liable to become hypoxic. Thus, although nitrous oxide is sometimes used in intensive care units to induce mild anesthesia in patients who are required to submit to painful procedures, this anesthetic is relatively unsuitable for most patients with respiratory diseases. Nitrous oxide has not been shown to be of value in patients with bronchospasm.

TRIBROMOETHANOL. Tribromoethanol (Avertin) was formerly used to induce basal narcosis. When the drug was in favor it was recommended for the treatment of status asthmaticus by rectal enema, in similar fashion to the rectal use of ether.[141]

Other inhalational general anesthetics are less likely to be of value in asthma. Overall, anesthetic agents in the treatment of asthma are falling into disuse; the patient with severe asthma that does not respond to conventional therapy is usually intubated and given respiratory assistance for a few hours or days. This procedure may necessitate providing sedation for the patient rather than anesthesia. In certain patients with status asthmaticus or severe bronchitis, it is worth inducing anesthesia to allow bronchopulmonary lavage as a means of removing inspissated secretions.[149] The choice of the appropriate anesthetic (for example, ether or halothane) will improve the chances of success.

Narcotic Analgesics. Unlike the simple analgesics, such as aspirin, the narcotic analgesics have a poorly-defined role in bronchospasm; in general, they are of little value, and they are often contraindicated. Many of these agents are useful cough suppressants, but they also depress the respiratory center. They may cause a dangerous decrease in respiratory drive, particularly in hypoventilating patients with slight hypercarbia. See Chapter 9 for a detailed discussion.

MORPHINE. Morphine (and the related narcotic, *opium*) has, at times, been advocated for use in bronchial asthma; however, it is a powerful respiratory depressant and is therefore potentially dangerous in this condition. In contrast, it may be very valuable in the treatment of cardiac asthma, in which left ventricular failure causes pulmonary edema and bronchospasm. Some younger adults and children with a moderate asthma attack may appear to benefit from morphine, particularly when the bronchospasm is emotional in origin and is accompanied by hyperventilation. However, since morphine can cause tissues to release histamine, there are good theoretical grounds for avoiding the use of this narcotic in most asthmatics.[150]

MEPERIDINE. Meperidine (Demerol) is generally believed to be a safer narcotic to administer to bronchospastic patients who require a potent analgesic. However, recent work[150] suggests that this agent may also cause bronchoconstriction, although some older studies suggested that it could cause bronchodilation.

Gases

OXYGEN. Although oxygen is often required by bronchospastic patients for relief of the symptoms caused by hypoxemia, it does not appear to be a bronchodilator. Patients who develop reactive airway spasm on rapid breathing may experience a decrease in airway resistance when given oxygen, which can be attributed to the decreased need to hyperventilate. The relief of bronchospasm that may be noted is an indirect consequence of oxygen therapy in these patients.

HELIUM. Helium is an inert gas that has been reported to have uniquely valuable properties that help relieve severe bronchospasm. Barach[151] has consistently claimed that a mixture of 80 per cent helium and 20 per cent oxygen is of value in asthma; further improvement in bronchospasm was achieved by providing the gaseous mixture with a continuous positive pressure breathing arrangement. The theorized basis for the improvement has been related to the relatively low density of helium: since the pressure required to move a gaseous mixture through a restricted orifice is inversely proportioned to its density, the bronchoconstricted patient may find it easier to breathe in the helium-oxygen mixture. Barach implies that the mixture is not only easier to breathe, but that inhalation of the gases for 10 minutes every two to three hours results in progressive relaxation of the bronchi. This claim is difficult to correlate with the persuasive physiologic argument of Comroe:[152] a gaseous mixture of decreased density should be of significant value only when airflow is turbulent; this does not pertain in the distal airways of a bronchoconstricted lung, where airflow is streamlined. Inhalation of a helium-oxygen mixture could result in a decreased ventilatory effort when there is partial obstruction in the upper airways, since rapid flow with eddy currents causes turbulence. Thus, Comroe's argument suggests that the mixture could be of value in upper airway narrowing, but may actually be disadvantageous in asthma when the greater viscosity of helium-oxygen compared to air would necessitate a greater driving pressure (and therefore more patient effort) to achieve streamlined flow through the small airways.

Thus, the use of helium in the treatment of asthma is somewhat controversial, although it is clear that very few clinicians use this form of therapy. Motley[153] has a uniquely personal regard for helium, and uses 40 per cent oxygen with 60 per cent helium in some routine IPPB therapies. He claims that the mixture results in a more uniform alveolar ventilation, with more effective removal of carbon dioxide from hypoventilating lungs; moreover, it is claimed that aerosols are distributed more effectively in the lungs. Since helium is a relatively expensive gas, it is unlikely that the advocates of helium-oxygen therapy will persuade physicians to use this modality in the treatment of bronchospasm in the current era of sophisticated drug availability. See also Chapter 13.

CARBON DIOXIDE. Carbon dioxide has, at various times, been recommended as a bronchodilator. It is known that accumulation of carbon dioxide in the body can result in dilation of the muscular vessels in many organs, although the pulmonary vasculature probably is not affected.[154] There is little information to suggest that carbon dioxide has any definite effect on muscle contractibility other than in the systemic blood vessels, and the long-standing concept of using the gas as a bronchodilator had not been subjected to careful evaluation in the past. Recently, however, a careful study, using body plethysmography, revealed that the inhalation of 6 per cent carbon dioxide can cause relaxation of peripheral and central airways in young asthmatic adults.[155] It is speculated that inhalation of this gas causes changes in intracellular pH that alter calcium binding, and that this influences bronchomotor tone. However, more studies are required to determine under what circumstances inhalation of carbon dioxide can cause bronchodilation, particularly since the gas will stimulate hyperventilation initially and this can result in the induction of bronchospasm.

Although carbon dioxide is not generally thought of as a bronchodilator, it is of use in other areas of clinical medicine.[156] Thus, inhalation of 5 to 10 per cent carbon dioxide can be given for a few minutes to stimulate deep breathing, and thereby prevent or correct post-operative atelectasis. The gas can also be given in 5 per cent admixture with oxygen for about 10 minutes as a treatment for hiccuping (singultation). Rela-

TABLE 4–21. ADDITIONAL AGENTS THAT HAVE BEEN CREDITED WITH BRONCHODILATOR PROPERTIES WHEN GIVEN BY INHALATION

Drug	Actions
4-Aminoheptane	Unexplained effect
Ammonium chloride	Mucokinetic
Barbiturates	Sedatives
Calcium chloride	May have "antiallergic" properties
Calcium levulinate	Unexplained effect
Dibenzylmethylamine	Unexplained effect
Histamine (low concentrations)	Unexplained effect
Lobeline	Respiratory stimulant
Methapyrilene (Histadyl)	Antihistamine
Para-aminobenzoic acid	Unexplained effect
Pentamethylenetetrazol	Respiratory stimulant
Phenisonone (Dapanone)	Listed as a bronchodilator
Phenylpropanolamine	Mucosal decongestant
Picrotoxin	Respiratory stimulant
Propylene glycol	Mucokinetic; unexplained effect
Pyrilamine	Antihistamine
Quazodine	Antiasthmatic
Sodium acid phosphate	Unexplained effect
Strychnine	Respiratory stimulant
Triethylene glycol	Possible mucokinetic (cf. propylene glycol)

tively few physicians use carbon dioxide inhalation as a means of increasing cerebral circulation for impending or developing stroke, although this form of treatment does have advocates. Whenever inhalational carbon dioxide is administered, the patient must be monitored for the development of complications, which include respiratory depression and central nervous system narcosis.

Possible Bronchodilators. A review of the literature, and particularly the older books on the treatment of respiratory diseases, unearths a plethora of possible remedies that have been advocated for the relief of bronchospasm. Most of those tabulated in Table 4–21 have been favorably reported on by reputable workers, although documentation of their effectiveness is generally inadequate. Of particular interest are two of the more recently endorsed agents.

PHENYTOIN. Phenytoin (diphenylhydantoin, Dilantin) is used mainly in the treatment of epilepsy, and it is of therapeutic value in a number of other recurrent, spasmodic disorders that have a neurologic basis. In recent years, the drug has been proposed as suitable therapy for a bewildering variety of diseases,[157] and at least one investigator has found it to be useful in the management of asthma.[158] At present, there are no controlled studies available on which to base a scientific judgment about the value of this latter-day panacea in the treatment of bronchospastic disorders.

ALCOHOL. Alcohol has a dubious value in asthma, with some enthusiastic claims that particular individual beverages are beneficial.[102, 139] However, such beverages have also been authoritatively reported to cause bronchospasm.[159] Thus, the role of alcohol in the treatment of asthma remains controversial. This unsatisfactory evaluation of alcohol applies to its use in many other areas of medicine, and a similar degree of ambiguity must also be attached to many of the drugs that have been purported to act as bronchodilators.

The major drugs that are of proven benefit in asthma have established indubitable credentials, and they will be discussed in detail in the following chapters. There are numerous unproved and doubtful remedies that appear to have little to offer in modern therapeutics. Many of the agents that were given brief consideration in the present chapter have been presented as material for speculation rather than as medications that should be prescribed to asthmatic patients. Some additional agents, culled from several sources, are catalogued in Table 4–21. Few of these are of any practical significance, but they serve to demonstrate the wide variety of possible bronchodilators. There are other agents that are occasionally proposed on an anecdotal basis (for example, Vitamin B_{16}), but there is no basis for examining all these dubious bronchodilators in any scientific fashion. Furthermore, it is evident from this Chapter and from Chapters 5 and 6 that there is already a surfeit of minor bronchodilators that have little to offer in practical therapeutics.

REFERENCES

1. Nagaishi, C.: Functional Anatomy and Histology of the Lung. Baltimore, University Park Press, 1972.
1a. Staub, N. C.: Some aspects of airways structure and function. Postgrad. Med. J. 51 (Suppl. 7):21–34, 1975.
2. Ellul-Micallef, R.: Airway smooth muscle in health and in asthma. Brit. J. Dis. Chest 67:107–113, 1973.
2a. El-Naggar, M.: Smooth muscles of the airway in asthma: recent advances in anatomy, physiology and biochemistry. Resuscitation 5:31–41, 1976.
3. Ziment, I.: Mucokinesis—the methodology of moving mucus. Respir. Therapy 4:15–20, Mar./Apr., 1974.
4. El-Bermani, A. W. I. and Grant, M.: Acetylcho-

linesterase-positive nerves of the rhesus monkey bronchial tree. Thorax 30:162–170, 1975.
5. Nadel, J. A.: Neurophysiologic aspects of asthma. In Asthma: Physiology, Immunopharmacology and Treatment. K. F. Austen and L. M. Lichtenstein (Eds.). New York, Academic Press, 1973.
6. Nadel, J. A.: Factors influencing airway smooth muscle. In Evaluation of Bronchodilator Drugs. D. M. Burley, et al. (Eds.). The Trust for Education and Research in Therapeutics, England, 1974, pp. 11–15.
7. Aviado, D. M.: Regulation of bronchomotor tone during anesthesia. Anesthesiology 42:68–80, 1975.
7a. Nadel, J. A.: Parasympathetic regulation of lungs and airways. Postgrad. Med. J. 51 (Suppl. 7): 86–90, 1975.
8. Orr, T. S. C.: Mast cells and allergic asthma. Brit. J. Dis. Chest 67:87–106, 1973.
9. Bowers, G. A. and Orange, R. P.: Mediator release from human lung. In Asthma. C. E. Reed and S. C. Siegel (Eds.). Published by Medcom, Inc., New York, for Syntex Laboratories, Inc., 1974. pp. 25–31.
10. Lichtenstein, L. M.: Mediator release from basophils. In Asthma. C. E. Reed and S. C. Siegel (Eds.). Published by Medcom, Inc., New York, for Syntex Laboratories, Inc. 1974, pp. 19–23.
11. Wilson, A. F. and Galant, S. P.: Recent advances in the pathophysiology of asthma. West. J. Med. 120:463–470, 1974.
12. Assem, E. S. K.: Models for the study of release of mediators of anaphylaxis. In Evaluation of Bronchodilator Drugs. D. M. Burley et al. (Eds.). The Trust for Education and Research in Therapeutics, England, 1974, pp. 29–50.
13. Bouhuys, A.: Breathing—Physiology, Environment and Lung Disease. New York, Grune and Stratton, 1974. p. 457.
14. Widdicombe, J. G.: The regulation of bronchial calibre. In Advances in Respiratory Physiology. C. G. Caro (Ed.). London, Edward Arnold and Company, 1966.
15. Casden, R. and Beall, G. N.: Control of airway resistance. Respir. Therapy 3:49–52, May/June, 1973.
16. Cohen, A. B., and Gold, W. M.: Defense mechanisms of the lungs. Ann. Rev. Physiol. 37:325–350, 1975.
17. Guz, A.: Regulation of respiration in man. Ann. Rev. Physiol. 37:303–323, 1975.
18. Reed, C. E.: The pathogenesis of asthma. Med. Clin. N. Amer. 58:55–63, 1974.
18a. Gayrard, P., Orehek, J., Grimaud, C. and Charpin, J.: Beta-adrenergic function in airways of healthy and asthmatic subjects. Thorax 30: 657–662, 1975.
19. Grieco, M. H. and Pierson, R. N.: Mechanism of bronchoconstriction due to beta adrenergic blockade. J. Allergy Clin. Immunol. 48:143–152, 1971.
20. Middleton, E.: Autonomic imbalance in asthma with special reference to beta adrenergic blockade. Adv. Intern. Med. 18:177–197, 1972.
21. Lefkowitz, R. J.: β-Adrenergic receptors: recognition and regulation. N. Engl. J. Med. 295:323–328, 1976.

22. Ziment, I.: The pharmacology of airway dilators. Respir. Therapy 4:51–55, May/June, 1974.

23. Fleisch, J. H., Kent, K. M. and Cooper, T.: Drug receptors in smooth muscle. *In* Asthma: Physiology, Immunopharmacology and Treatment. K. F. Austen and L. M. Lichtenstein (Eds.). New York, Academic Press Inc., 1973.

24. Patel, K. R. and Kerr, J. W.: The airways response to phenylephrine after blockade of alpha and beta receptors in extrinsic bronchial asthma. Clin. Allergy 3:439–448, 1973.

25. Jack, D.: Selective drug treatments for bronchial asthma. J. Canad. Med. Assoc. 110:436–441, 1974.

26. Gold, W. M.: Cholinergic pharmacology in asthma. *In* Asthma: Physiology, Immunopharmacology and Treatment. K. F. Austen and L. M. Lichtenstein (Eds.). New York, Academic Press Inc., 1973.

26a. Koelle, G. B.: Cholinergic and non-cholinergic pharmacology of the bronchioles. Postgrad. Med. J. 51 (Suppl. 7):63–66, 1975.

27. Austen, K. F. and Orange, R. P.: Bronchial asthma: the possible role of the chemical mediators of immediate hypersensitivity in the pathogenesis of subacute chronic disease. Am. Rev. Respir. Dis. 112:423–436, 1975.

28. Kaliner, M.: Immunologic mechanisms for release of chemical mediators of anaphylaxis from human lung tissue. J. Canad. Med. Assoc. 110:431–435, 1974.

29. Mathison, D. A. and Stevenson, D. D.: Bronchopulmonary diseases: immunologic perspectives. Postgrad. Med. 54:105–111, 1973.

30. Pepys, J.: Immunological mechanisms in asthma. *In* Identification of Asthma (Ciba Foundation Study Group No. 38), Edinburgh, Churchill Livingstone, 1971, pp. 86–98.

31. Patterson, R., Zeiss, C. R. and Kelly, J. F.: Classification of hypersensitivity reactions. N. Engl. J. Med. 295:277–279, 1976.

32. Austen, K. F., Lewis, R. A., Wasserman, S. I. and Goetzl, E. J.: Generation and release of chemical mediators of immediate hypersensitivity in human cells. *In* New Directions in Asthma. M. Stein (Ed.). Park Ridge, Illinois, American College of Chest Physicians, 1975.

33. Collier, H. O. J. and Gardiner, P. J.: Pharmacology of airways smooth muscle. *In* Evaluation of Bronchodilator Drugs. D. M. Burley, et al. (Eds.). The Trust for Education and Research in Therapeutics, England, 1974, pp. 17–27.

34. Rebuck, A. S.: Antiasthmatic drugs: pathophysiological and clinical pharmacological aspects. Drugs 7:344–369, 1974.

35. Said, S. I.: Humoral mediators in bronchial asthma—implications for therapy. *In* New Directions in Asthma. M. Stein (Ed.). Park Ridge, Illinois, American College of Chest Physicians, 1975.

35a. Casterline, C. L., Evans, R. and Ward, G. W.: The effect of atropine and albuterol aerosols on the human bronchial response to histamine. J. Allergy Clin. Immunol. 58:607–613, 1976.

36. Gold, W. M.: Experimental models of asthma. *In* New Directions in Asthma. M. Stein (Ed.). Park Ridge, Illinois, American College of Chest Physicians, 1975.

37. Brocklehurst, W. E.: SRS-A anonymous and disreputable. Proc. Roy. Soc. Med. 66:1198–1199, 1973.

38. Shaw, J. O. and Moser, K. M.: The current status of prostaglandins and the lungs. Chest 68:75–80, 1975.

39. Mathé, A. A., Hedqvist, P., Holmgren, A. and Svanborg, N.: Bronchial hyperreactivity to prostaglandin $F_{2\alpha}$ and histamine in patients with asthma. Br. Med. J. 1:193–196, Jan., 1973.

40. Kaliner, M. and Austen, K. F.: Immunologic release of chemical mediators from human tissue. Ann. Rev. Pharmacol. 15:177–189, 1975.

40a. Steer, M. L., Atlas, D. and Levitzki, A.: Interrelations between β-adrenergic receptors, adenylate cyclase and calcium. N. Engl. J. Med. 292:409–414, 1975.

41. Reed, C. E.: Abnormal autonomic mechanisms in asthma. J. Allergy Clin. Immunol. 53:34–41, 1974.

42. Sutherland, E. W.: On the biological role of cyclic AMP. J.A.M.A. 214:1281–1288, 1970.

43. Jard, S.: What cyclic AMP is all about. Res. Staff Phys. June 1975, pp. 49–66.

44. Goldberg, N. G.: Cyclic nucleotides and cell function. Hosp. Practice, May 1974, pp. 127–142.

45. Wiklund, R. A.: Cyclic nucleotides. Anesthesiology 41:490–500, 1974.

46. Murad, F.: Mechanism of action of some bronchodilators. Am. Rev. Respir. Dis. 110#6 Pt. 2:111–118, 1974.

47. Townley, R. G.: Pharmacologic blocks to mediator release: clinical applications. Adv. Asthma Allergy. 2:7–16, Fall, 1975. (Published by Fisons Corporation).

48. Reed, C. E.: The pathogenesis of asthma. Med. Clin. N. Amer. 58:55–63, 1974.

49. Freedman, B. J.: Principles of comparative drug trials with special reference to bronchodilators. *In* Evaluation of Bronchodilator Drugs. D. M. Burley et al. (Eds.). The Trust for Education and Research in Therapeutics, England. 1974, pp. 219–237.

49a. Tinkelman, D. G., Avner, S. E., and Cooper, D. M.: Assessing bronchodilator responsiveness. J. Allergy Clin. Immunol. 59:109–114, 1977.

50. Innes, I. R. and Nickerson, M.: Norepinephrine, epinephrine, and the sympathomimetic amines. *In* The Pharmacological Basis of Therapeutics, L. S. Goodman and A. Gilman (Eds.). New York, McMillan Publishing Co., Inc., 5th ed. 1975.

51. Davies, D. S.: Metabolism of isoprenaline and other bronchodilator drugs in man and dog. Bull. Physiopathol. Respir. 8:679–683, 1972.

52. George, C. F., Blackwell, E. W. and Davies, D. S.: Metabolism of isoprenaline in the intestine. J. Pharm. Pharmacol. 26:265–267, 1974.

53. Meares, R. A., Mills, J. E., Horvath, T. B., Atkinson, J. M., Pun, L., and Rand, M. J.: Amitriptyline and asthma. Med. J. Aust. 2:25–28, July 1971.

54. Evans, M. E., Walker, S. R., Brittain, R. T. and Paterson, J. W.: The metabolism of salbutamol in man. Xenobiotica 3:113–120, 1973.

55. Sharman, D. F.: The catabolism of catecholamines. Br. Med. Bull. 29:110–115, 1973.

56. Van den Brink, F. G.: The pharmacology of bronchiolar muscle relaxation. Bull. Physiopathol. Respir. 8:475–486, 1972.

57. Davies, G. E., Rose, F. L. and Somerville, A. R.: New inhibitor of phosphodiesterase with anti-bronchoconstrictor properties. Nature (New Biol.) 234:50–51, 1971.

58. Sheppard, H.: Phosphodiesterase inhibitors and analogs of cyclic AMP as potential agents for the treatment of asthma. In Asthma: Physiology, Immunopharmacology and Treatment. K. F. Austen and L. M. Lichtenstein (Eds.). New York, Academic Press Inc., 1973.

59. Bowden, K. and Wooldridge, K. R. H.: Structure-activity relations-III. Bronchodilator activity of substituted 6-thioxanthines. Biochem. Pharmacol. 22:1015–1021, 1973.

59a. Gandevia, B.: Historical review of the use of parasympatholytic agents in the treatment of respiratory disorders. Postgrad. Med. J. 51 (Suppl. 7):13–20, 1975.

60. Yu, D. Y. C., Galant, S. P. and Gold, W. M.: Inhibition of antigen-induced bronchoconstriction by atropine in asthmatic subjects. J. Appl. Physiol. 32:823–828, 1972.

61. Reed, C. E.: Abnormal autonomic mechanisms in asthma. J. Allergy Clin. Immunol. 55:34–41, 1974.

62. Wick, M. M. and Ingram, R. H.: Bronchorrhea responsive to aerosolized atropine. J.A.M.A. 235:1356, 1976.

62a. Chervinsky, P.: Double-blind study of ipratropium bromide, a new anticholinergic bronchodilator. J. Allergy Clin. Immunol. 59:22–30, 1977.

62b. Ruffin, R. E., Fitzgerald, J. D. and Rebuck, A. S.: A comparison of the bronchodilator activity of Sch 1000 and salbutamol. J. Allergy Clin. Immunol. 59:136–141, 1977.

62c. Herzog, H.: Comparison of anticholinergic agents other than bronchodilators and the effect of combining these drugs. Postgrad. Med. J. 51 (Suppl. 7):146–148, 1975.

63. Petrie, G. R. and Palmer, K. N. V.: Comparison of aerosol ipratropium bromide and salbutamol in chronic bronchitis and asthma. Br. Med. J. 1:430–432, Feb., 1975.

64. Hoffbrand, B. I., et al. (Eds.): The place of parasympatholytic drugs in the management of chronic obstructive airways disease (Proceedings of an International Symposium). Postgrad. Med. J. 51 (Suppl. 7):1–161, 1975.

65. Emirgil, C., Dwyer, K., Baskette, P. and Sobol, B. J.: A new parasympatholytic bronchodilator: a study of its onset of effect after inhalation. Curr. Ther. Res. 17:215–224, 1975.

66. Yeager, H., Weinberg, R. M., Kaufman, L. V. and Katz, S.: Asthma: comparative bronchodilator effects of ipratropium bromide and isoproternol. J. Clin. Pharmacol. 16:198–204, 1976.

67. Gross, N. J.: Sch 1000: a new anticholinergic bronchodilator. Am. Rev. Respir. Dis. 112:823–828, 1975.

68. Warner, E. C. (Ed.): Savill's System of Clinical Medicine. London, Edward Arnold and Co., 1944, 12th ed., p. 187.

69. Segal, M. S.: Sch 1000: a new anticholinergic bronchodilator. Amer. Rev. Respir. Dis. 113:893, 1976.

70. Lopez-Vidriero, M. T., Costello, J., Clark, T. J. H., Das, I., Keal, E. E. and Reid, L.: Effect of atropine on sputum production. Thorax 30:543–547, 1975.

71. Klock, L. E., Miller, T. D., Morris, A. H., Watanabe, S. and Dickman, M.: A comparative study of atropine sulfate and isoproterenol hydrochloride in chronic bronchitis. Am. Rev. Respir. Dis. 112:371–376, 1975.

72. Cavanaugh, M. J. and Cooper, D. M.: Inhaled atropine sulfate: dose response characteristics. Amer. Rev. Respir. Dis. 114:517–524, 1976.

73. Paterson, J. W. and Shenfield, G. M.: Bronchodilators Part I. BTTA Review (Tubercle). 4:25–40, 1974.

74. Godfrey, S.: Exercise-induced asthma – clinical, physiological and therapeutic implications. J. Allergy Clin. Immunol. 56:1–17, 1975.

75. Editorial: Bronchodilators, new and old. Br. Med. J. 2:387–388, Aug., 1976.

76. Andersen, N. H. and Ramwell, P. W.: Biological aspects of prostaglandins. Arch. Intern. Med. 133:30–50, 1974.

77. Szczeklik, A., Gryglewski, R. J. and Czerniawska-Mysik, G.: Relationship of inhibition of prostaglandin biosynthesis by analgesics to asthma attacks in aspirin-sensitive patients. Br. Med. J. 1:67–69, Jan. 1975.

77a. Mathé, A. A., Hedqvist, P., Strandberg, K. and Leslie, C. A.: Aspects of prostaglandin function in the lung. N. Engl. J. Med. 296:850–855, 910–914, 1977.

78. Smith, A. P.: Lungs. In The Prostaglandins, Vol. 1. P. W. Ramwell (Ed.) New York, Plenum Press, 1973.

79. Mathé, A. A. and Hedqvist, P.: Effect of prostaglandins $F_{2\alpha}$ and E_2 on airway conductance in healthy subjects and asthmatic patients. Am. Rev. Respir. Dis. 111:313–320, 1975.

80. Parker, C. W. and Snider, D. E.: Prostaglandins and asthma. Ann. Intern. Med. 78:963–965, 1973.

81. Patel, K. R.: Atropine, sodium cromoglycate, and thymoxamine in $PGF_{2\alpha}$ induced bronchoconstriction in extrinsic asthma. Br. Med. J. 2:360–362, May, 1975.

82. Fanburg, B. L.: Prostaglandins and the lung. Am. Rev. Respir. Dis. 108:482–489, 1973.

83. Drazen, J. M.: In vivo effects of humoral mediators. In New Directions in Asthma. M. Stein (Ed.). Park Ridge, Illinois, American College of Chest Physicians, 1975.

84. Alanko, K. and Poppius, H.: Anticholinergic blocking of prostaglandin-induced bronchoconstriction. Br. Med. J. 1:294, Feb., 1973.

85. Sanner, J. H.: Substances that inhibit the action of prostaglandins. Arch. Intern. Med. 133:133–146, 1974.

86. Smith, A. P.: Role of prostaglandins in the pathogenesis and treatment of asthma. In Asthma: Physiology, Immunopharmacology and Treatment. K. F. Austen and L. M. Lichtenstein (Eds.). New York, Academic Press, 1973.

87. Nemoto, T., Aoki, H., Ike, A., Yamada, K. et al.: Serum prostaglandin levels in asthmatic patients. J. Allergy Clin. Immunol. 57:89–94, 1976.

88. Smith, A. P.: Prostaglandins and the respiratory system. In Prostaglandins: Physiological,

Pharmacological and Pathological Aspects. S. M. M. Karim (Ed.). Baltimore, University Park Press, 1976.

89. Smith, A. P.: Prostaglandins and asthma. Br. Med. J. 2:613, June, 1975.

90. Kadowitz, P. J., Joiner, P. D. and Hyman, A. L.: Physiological and pharmacological roles of prostaglandins. Annu. Rev. Pharmacol. 15: 285–306, 1975.

91. Nakano, J.: The prostaglandins: their effect on 14 clinical conditions. Res. Staff Phys., Oct., 1973, pp. 93–106.

92. Zurier, R. B.: Prostaglandins, inflammation, and asthma. Arch. Intern. Med. 133:101–110, 1974.

93. Tashkin, D. P., Shapiro, B. J. and Frank, I. M.: Acute effects of smoked marijuana and oral Δ^9-tetrahydrocannabinol on specific airway conductance in asthmatic subjects. Am. Rev. Respir. Dis. 109:420–428, 1974.

94. Tashkin, D. P., Shapiro, B. J., Lee, Y. E. and Harper, C. E.: Effects of smoked marijuana in experimentally induced asthma. Am. Rev. Respir. Dis. 112:377–386, 1975.

95. Vachon, L., Robins, A. G. and Gaensler, E. A.: Airways response to microaerosolized delta-9-tetrahydrocannabinol. Chest 70:444, 1976.

96. Vachon, L., Fitzgerald, M. X., Solliday, N. H., Gould, I. A. and Gaensler, E. A.: Single dose effect of marijuana smoke: bronchial dynamics and respiratory-center sensitivity in normal subjects. New Engl. J. Med. 288:985–989, 1973.

97. Abboud, R. T. and Sanders, H. D.: Effect of oral administration of delta^9-tetrahydrocannabinol on airway mechanics in normal and asthmatic subjects. Chest 70:480–485, 1976.

97a. Tashkin, D. P., Reiss, S., Shapiro, B. J., Calvarese, B., Olsen, J. L., and Lodge, J. W.: Bronchial effects of aerosolized Δ^9-tetrahydrocannabinol in healthy and asthmatic subjects. Am. Rev. Respir. Dis. 115:57–65, 1977.

97b. Shapiro, B. J., Tashkin, D. P. and Vachon, L.: Tetrahydrocannabinol as a bronchodilator. Why bother? Chest 71:558–559, 1977.

98. Brown, O. H.: Asthma—Presenting an Exposition of the Nonpassive Expiration Theory. St. Louis, The C. V. Mosby Co., 1917.

99. Sandler, M.: Levodopa and chronic bronchitis. Brit. Med. J.:1:642, Mar., 1974.

100. Taylor, A. J. N., Soutar, C., Shneerson, J. and Turner-Warwick, M.: Bromocriptine in the treatment of intractable asthma. Thorax 31: 488, 1976.

101. Imbruce, R., Goldfedder, A., Maguire, W., Briscoe, W. and Nair, S.: The effect of glucagon on airway resistance. J. Clin. Pharmacol. 15:680–684, 1975.

102. Herxheimer, H.: A Guide to Bronchial Asthma. London, Academic Press, 1975.

103. McCombs, R. P.: Diseases due to immunologic reactions in the lungs. New Engl. J. Med. 286:1186–1194, 1972.

104. Youngchaiyud, P., Kettel, L. J. and Cugell, D. W.: The effect of heparin aerosols on airway conductance in patients with chronic obstructive pulmonary disease. Am. Rev. Respir. Dis. 99:449–452, 1969.

105. Fine, N. L., Shim, C. and Williams, M. H.: Objective evaluation of heparin in the treatment of asthma. Am. Rev. Respir. Dis. 98:886–887, 1968.

106. Zuskin, E., Lewis, A. J. and Bouhuys, A.: Inhibition of histamine induced airway constriction by ascorbic acid. J. Allergy Clin. Immunol. 51:218–226, 1973.

107. Arkins, J. A., Gotway, C. A., Hogan, M. R. and Fink, J. N.: The effect of 6-mercaptopurine on spontaneous canine asthma. J. Allergy 44: 108–112, 1969.

108. Vane, J. R.: Prostaglandins and the aspirin-like drugs. Hosp. Practice, March 1972, pp. 61–71.

109. McDonald, J. R., Mathison, D. A. and Stevenson, D. D.: Aspirin intolerance in asthma. J. Allergy Clin. Immunol. 50:198–207, 1972.

110. Hady, S.: Dipyrone in bronchial asthma. Br. Med. J. 1:744, Mar., 1973.

111. Isomaki, H. and Kreus, K. E.: Chloroquine in the treatment of bronchial asthma. Ann. Allergy 26:61–65, 1968.

112. Abaitey, A. K. and Parratt, J. R.: Cardiovascular effects of diethylcarbamazine citrate. Br. J. Pharmac. 56:219–227, 1976.

113. Benner, M. and Lowell, F. C.: Failure of diethyl-carbamazine citrate (Hetrazan) in the treatment of asthma. J. Allergy 46:29–31, 1970.

114. Sly, R. M. and Matzen, K.: Effect of diethylcarbamazine pamoate upon exercise-induced obstruction in asthmatic children. Ann. Allergy 33:138–144, 1974.

115. Logsdon, P. J., Carnright, D. V., Middleton, E. and Coffey, R. G.: Alpha blockade in treatment of asthma. Lancet 2:232, 1972.

116. Alston, W. C., Patel, K. R. and Kerr, J. W.: Response of leucocyte adenyl cyclase to isoprenaline and effect of alpha-blocking drugs in extrinsic bronchial asthma. Br. Med. J. 1:90–93, Jan., 1974.

117. Haddock, A. M., Patel, K. R., Alston, W. C. and Kerr, J. W.: Response of lymphocyte guanyl cyclase to propranolol, noradrenaline, thymoxamine, and acetylcholine in extrinsic bronchial asthma. Br. Med. J. 2:357–359, May, 1975.

118. Patel, K. R. and Kerr, J. W.: Alpha-receptor-blocking drugs in bronchial asthma. Lancet 1:348–349, 1975.

118a. Wardle, E. N.: Atropine or thymoxamine for chronic asthma. Br. Med. J. 1:1085, April, 1977.

119. Gross, G. N., Souhrada, J. F. and Farr, R. S.: The longterm treatment of an asthmatic patient using phentolamine. Chest 66:397–401, 1974.

120. Feather, E. A. and Russel, G.: Effect of tolazoline hydrochloride on sputum viscosity in cystic fibrosis. Thorax 25:732–736, 1970.

121. Bianco, S., Griffin, J. P., Kamburoff, P. L. and Prime, F. J.: Prevention of exercise-induced asthma by indoramin. Br. Med. J. 4:18–20, Oct., 1974.

122. Prime, F. J.: Prevention of exercise-induced asthma by indoramin. Br. Med. J. 4:770, Dec., 1974.

123. Godfrey, S.: Prevention of exercise-induced asthma by indoramin. Br. Med. J. 4:469, Nov., 1974.

124. Skinner, C., Gaddie, J. and Palmer, K. N. V.: Comparison of intravenous AH 5158 (ibidomide) and propranolol in asthma. Br. Med. J.:2:59–61, April, 1975.

125. Howard, J. C., Cochrane, P. and Conway, M.: Practolol and isoprenaline in status asthmaticus. Lancet 2:47–48, 1972.

126. Falliers, C. J., McCann, W. P., Chai, H., Ellis, E. F. and Yazdi, N.: Controlled study of iodotherapy for childhood asthma. J. Allergy 38:183–192, 1966.

127. Siegel, S.: The asthma-suppressive action of postassium iodide. J. Allergy 35:253–270, 1964.

128. Tager, I. and Speizer, F. E.: Role of infection in chronic bronchitis. New Engl. J. Med. 292:563–571, 1975.

129. Itkin, I. H. and Menzel, M. L.: The use of macrolide antibiotic substances in the treatment of asthma. J. Allergy 45:146–162, 1970.

130. Spector, S. L., Katz, F. H. and Farr, R. S.: Troleandomycin: effectiveness in steroid-dependent asthma and bronchitis. J. Allergy Clin. Immunol. 54:367–379, 1974.

131. Lakshminarayan, S., Sahn, S. A., Hudson, L. D. and Weil, J. V.: Effect of diazepam on ventilatory responses. Clin. Pharmacol. Therap. 20:178–183, 1976.

132. Kronenberg, R. S., Cosco, M. G., Stevenson, J. E. and Drage, C. W.: The use of oral diazepam in patients with obstructive lung disease and hypercapnia. Ann. Intern. Med. 83:83–84, 1975.

133. Zsigmond, E. K., Shiveley, J. G. and Flynn, K.: Diazepam and meperidine on arterial blood gases in patients with chronic obstructive pulmonary disease. J. Clin. Pharmacol. 15:464–469, 1975.

134. Heurich, A., Sousa-Poza, M. and Lyons, H. A.: Bronchodilator effects of hydroxyzine hydrochloride. Respiration 29:135–138, 1972.

135. Bierman, C. W., Pierson, W. E. and Shapiro, G. G.: Exercise-induced asthma: pharmacological assessment of single drugs and drug combinations. J.A.M.A. 234:295–298, 1975.

136. Muittari, A. and Mattila, M. J.: Bronchodilator action of drug combinations is asthmatic patients: ephedrine, theophylline and tranquilizing drugs. Curr. Ther. Res. 13:374–385, 1971.

137. Editorial: Barbiturates in asthma. Br. Med. J. 3:490, Aug., 1972.

138. Miller, W. C. and Awe, R.: Effect of nebulized lidocaine on reactive airways. Am. Rev. Respir. Dis. 111:739–741, 1975.

139. Unger, L.: Bronchial Asthma. Springfield, Ill. Charles C Thomas, 1945.

140. Weiss, E. B., Anderson, W. H. and O'Brien, K. P.: The effect of a local anesthetic, lidocaine, on guinea pig trachealis muscle in vitro. Am. Rev. Respir. Dis. 112:393–400, 1975.

141. Loehning, R. W., Waltemath, C. L. and Bergman, N. A.: Lidocaine and increased respiratory resistance produced by ultrasonic aerosols, Anesthesiology 44:306–310, 1976.

142. Smith, F. R. and Kundahl, P. C.: Intravenously administered lidocaine as cough depressant during general anesthesia for bronchography. Chest 63:427–429, 1973.

143. Howard, P., Brennan, S. R., Anderson, P. B. and Cayton, R. M.: Aerosolized lignocaine and irritable airways. Thorax 31:242, 1976.

144. Manheim, A.: Lidocaine in obstructive pulmonary disease. J.A.M.A. 220:1500, 1972.

144a. Weiss, E. B. and Patwardhan, A. V.: The response to lidocaine in bronchial asthma. Chest 72:429–438, 1977.

145. Dautrebande, L.: Microaerosols: Physiology, Pharmacology, Therapeutics. New York, Academic Press, 1962.

146. Collins, V. J.: Principles of Anesthesiology. Philadelphia, Lea and Febiger, 1966.

147. Deutsch, S. and Vandam, L. D.: General anesthesia I: Volatile agents. In Drill's Pharmacology in Medicine, J. R. DiPalma (Ed.). New York, McGraw-Hill Book Company, 4th ed., 1971, p. 155.

148. Douglas, R. B. and Forsey, S. M.: Bronchodilation induced by methoxyflurane. Br. Med. J. 4:106, Oct. 1973.

149. Ramirez-R, J. and Obenour, W. H.: Bronchopulmonary lavage in asthma and chronic bronchitis: clinical and physiologic observations. Chest 59:146–152, 1971.

150. Douglas, R. B., Bidgood, K., Buxbaum, M. and Wagon, R.: Effects of pethidine on the bronchi. Br. Med. J. 4:880, Oct., 1976.

151. Barach, A. L.: Helium-oxygen therapy: historical aspects and recent developments. Respir. Care 19:599–602, 1974.

152. Comroe, J. H.: Physiology of Respiration. Chicago, Year Book Medical Publishers Incorporated, 2nd ed., 1974, p. 283.

153. Motley, H. L.: Helium-oxygen therapy. Respir. Care 18:668–670, 1973.

154. Murray, J. F.: The Normal Lung. Philadelphia, W. B. Saunders Company, 1976, Ch. 5.

155. Fisher, H. K. and Hansen, T. A.: Site of action of inhaled six per cent carbon dioxide in the lungs of asthmatic subjects before and after exercise. Am. Rev. Respir. Dis. 114:861–870, 1976.

156. Egan, D. F.: Fundamentals of Respiratory Therapy. St. Louis, The C. V. Mosby Company, 2nd ed., 1973, pp. 298–301.

157. Bogoch, S. and Dreyfus, J.: The Broad Range of Use of Diphenylhydantoin: Bibliography and Review. New York, The Dreyfus Medical Foundation, 1970.

158. Winter, B.: Bilateral carotid body resection for asthma and emphysema. Int. Surg. 57:455–466, 1972.

159. Pepys, J.: In Asthma: Physiology, Immunopharmacology and Treatment, K. F. Austen and L. M. Lichtenstein (Eds.). New York, Academic Press, 1973, p. 10.

PHARMACOLOGY OF SYMPATHOMIMETIC AGENTS

All the important sympathomimetic bronchodilators are either catecholamines or related compounds. The natural adrenal gland hormone and neurotransmitter, epinephrine, is the prototype drug. However, it is customary to compare the various bronchodilator agents with isoproterenol, which can be regarded as the standard bronchodilator.

GENERAL PHARMACOLOGY OF SYMPATHOMIMETICS

Bronchodilator drugs related to the catecholamines continue to proliferate in number. Unfortunately, it is difficult to compare one agent with another, although there are a number of recent reviews that provide useful information on the numerous drugs currently in use around the world.[1-11] Many reports of comparison use poor criteria, so that an analysis of the available literature results in numerous conflicting conclusions regarding the potency and specificity of these drugs. Although it is important to try to compare the properties of the bronchodilators, the information that will be provided will undoubtedly require modification when new information from carefully designed trials becomes available.

The following section describes general pharmacologic principles concerning the use of the beta-2 adrenergic receptor stimulating drugs.

Classification

The sympathomimetic bronchodilators can be classified in many ways, none of which is entirely satisfactory (Table 5–1). They can be categorized on the basis of chemical structure into catecholamines (such as epinephrine, isoproterenol and isoetharine), resorcinol derivatives (such as metaproterenol and terbutaline), saligenins (such as salbutamol) and so forth.[12] However, this method of subdividing the agents is not helpful to those who use the drugs clinically. The receptor activity of drugs allows their breakdown into categories according to selectivity; thus, some drugs are highly selective beta-2 stimulators, whereas others have potent beta-1 properties or alpha effects.[12] The mode of usual administration allows a classification into inhalational, oral and parenteral agents; most agents can be given by several routes, even though one route is usually strongly favored for each drug. Perhaps the most useful classification subdivides the drugs into short- and long-acting categories, even though such categorization cannot be considered cut and dried, since variations occur, depending on the route of administration, dose given, prior exposure to the drug, severity of the bronchospasm and so forth. The short-acting agents are those that are generally given by aerosol; the long-acting drugs can usually be given orally as well as by aerosol. Some short-acting drugs can have their activity prolonged by

TABLE 5–1. CLASSIFICATIONS OF SYMPATHOMIMETIC BRONCHODILATORS

CHEMICAL	Catecholamines, resorcinols, saligenins, etc.
ACTION	Direct, indirect, mixed
POTENCY	Short-acting, intermediate, long-acting
DELIVERY	Oral, inhalational, parenteral (injection)
SELECTIVITY	Beta-2, beta-1, alpha
MARKETING	Tablets, oral solutions, injectable solutions, inhalational solutions, inhalational powders, metered aerosols

preparing them as slow-release formulations, whereas a long-acting drug can have a relatively short half-life in an individual patient.

Freedman[13] points out that a rational comparison of bronchodilators can be made by considering the biologic half-life, which is the time taken for the increase in a flow-rate parameter (such as forced expired volume in one second, FEV_1), to fall to half the maximum value attained after giving the drug. Such studies should utilize matched doses, using the appropriate dose of each agent to produce the same maximum FEV_1; thus weight-for-weight equivalence must be determined from dose-response curves to establish equipotentiality for peak effect. A sensible alternative would be to compare equimolar doses of different agents, using amounts in proportion to their molecular weights.[14] All the factors listed in Table 5–2 may have to be taken into consideration when comparing the effectiveness of different bronchodilators. Unfortunately, these variables have not been standardized, and the various individual studies do not permit easy comparison. Thus, the following discussion is derived from imprecise data, and will undoubtedly require revision when more rigorously determined comparisons become available.

Chemical Structure and Formulation

Apart from differences in the internal configuration of the molecular formula of each bronchodilator, the marketed products are made available as different salts, such as hydrochlorides, sulfates and bitartrates. There is little significant difference between them, but it is important to compare the amount of base in each product when dosages of these drugs are considered.

The various drugs can be packaged in different ways to facilitate their delivery.[15] Thus, aerosol formulations can consist of solutions in water or in alcohol, or they can be given as powders. Oral forms can be given as tablets or elixirs, and intramuscular preparations can be formulated for rapid action, or as slow-release depot products, for example, by suspending the drug in oil. Table 5–3 contrasts the various components that accompany isoproterenol in different manufacturers' formulations of this drug in their marketed products.

There is probably little to choose between the various aerosol preparations of isoproterenol, but powders are less desirable, because they can irritate the airways. The different oral formulations are apparently very similar, although there may be different absorption rates, attributable to such factors as whether the drug is given as a tablet or as a solution.

Dosage and Mode of Administration

Surprisingly, dosages of bronchodilator drugs are poorly established, particularly when they are to be given by inhalation. Oral drugs tend to be given according to a more rigorous convention, such as one tablet three or four times a day, and a physician can prescribe precise daily dosages. The more common bronchodilators, such as isoproterenol, epinephrine and isoetharine, are unsuitable for oral administration because they are metabolized in the cells of the bowel

TABLE 5–2. VARIABLES IN COMPARISON OF BRONCHODILATOR DRUG EFFECTIVENESS

Physical	Pharmacokinetic	Physiologic
Molecular weight	Plasma half-life	Increase in FEV_1
Formulation and packaging	Onset of action	Increase in specific airway conductance
Route of administration	Persistence of any measurable effect	Changes in cardiovascular parameters
Effect of adjuvants	Cumulative effect	
	Development of resistance	

TABLE 5-3. CONSTITUENTS OF MARKETED ISOPROTERENOL PRODUCTS

	Isuprel Mistometer	Isuprel 1:5000	Isuprel 1:200	Isuprel 1:100	Medihaler-Iso	Norisodrine
MANUFACTURER	Winthrop	Winthrop	Winthrop	Winthrop	Riker	Abbott
PREPARATION	hydrochloride	hydrochloride	hydrochloride	hydrochloride	sulfate	hydrochloride
SOLVENT	alcohol	water	water	water	(suspension)	water, alcohol
BUFFER	sodium lactate lactic acid	sodium lactate lactic acid sodium chloride hydrochloric acid	sodium chloride sodium citrate	sodium chloride sodium citrate citric acid		
PRESERVATIVE	ascorbic acid	sodium bisulfite	chlorbutanol sodium bisulfite	chlorbutanol sodium bisulfite		
STABILIZER		glycerin	glycerin			ascorbyl palmitate
FLAVOR	aromatic flavor			saccharin		saccharin
PROPELLANT	F 12, F 114				fluorochloro- hydrocarbons	fluorochloro- hydrocarbons
ADMINISTRATION	metered aerosol	parenteral injection	nebulization	nebulization	metered aerosol	metered aerosol

TABLE 5–4. FACTORS CAUSING
IMPRECISION IN BRONCHODILATOR
AEROSOL DOSAGE

PRESCRIPTION	Imprecise and inaccurate ordering
PREPARATIONS	Different concentrations of base in various marketed preparations
PACKAGING	Varying amounts of drug delivered by different metered inhaler products
EQUIPMENT	Malfunction of equipment resulting in variations in amounts nebulized
MEASUREMENT	Inaccurate measurement of solutions into nebulizer
PATIENTS	Variations in technique, co-operation and reliability when taking treatments
DISEASE	Inability to breathe deeply and to hold breath, or coughing on inhalation, reduce deposition of aerosol in airways.
DRUG RELIABILITY	Shelf-life stability is limited, and old products lose effectiveness

wall; absorption is erratic, and a relatively high incidence of side effects is produced as a result of systemic absorption.

With the inhalational agents, precision in dosage cannot be obtained, for many reasons, as categorized in Table 5–4. In general, milligram doses are not prescribed. It is usual to recommend a number of puffs from a simple nebulizer or of a metered product several times a day; alternatively, physicians order administration by IPPB of a number of drops or ml, diluted or nondiluted, for a number of minutes, to be repeated every few hours. There is obviously tremendous variation in different patients' abilities to use inhalational devices;[16] the amount of drug deposited in the lung will vary considerably. Similarly, the amount deposited in the oropharynx and then absorbed systemically is very variable, since the quantity of aerosol per puff varies,[17] and there are individual variations in each patient's technique.[18] (See Tables 1–26, 1–30 and 5–5.)

Aerosol Therapy. Aerosols are very popular, because smaller doses can be administered with a consequent decrease in systemic side effects, and the onset of action appears within seconds or minutes. When metered aerosols are used, it should be realized that each manufacturer's product provides a different dose per puff, and the total number of doses in each cartridge varies.[18a] Patients should, therefore, be advised to cautiously experiment with the aerosol to determine the appropriate dosage, as long as the recom-

mended maximum is not exceeded. Thus, initially, one or two puffs should be used, and if the bronchodilatation is suboptimal, a further one or two puffs may be taken 10 minutes later; in this way, a patient can establish whether one puff is enough or whether four puffs are needed. For short-acting agents, repeat treatment may be required every three or four hours, whereas with a long-acting drug, treatments every six to eight hours could suffice. Patients should be instructed how to keep the nebulizer clean, and they should be asked to demonstrate their technique periodically to ensure that correct usage is employed.

If a hand-bulb nebulizer is used, the same approach should be taken to establish the appropriate dosage. If extrapulmonary side effects develop in a patient who uses the nebulizer correctly, then instructions to follow treatments with a mouth rinse may lead to a reduction in the systemic absorption through the oral mucosa. The fact that substantial systemic absorption does occur in the mouth can be utilized when treating young children, who do not cooperate with the synchronized deep breath followed by the inspiratory pause that is required for effective aerosol therapy. If the aerosol is nebulized beneath the tongue, effective bronchodilation can be achieved.[19]

When IPPB or an air compressor is used to deliver the aerosol, probably not more than 10 per cent of the amount put in the nebulizer is eventually deposited in the lungs;[18, 20] with a cooperative patient, a metered aerosol may deliver a higher percentage into the airways (Table 1–30). It is conventional to dilute a drug when it is given by positive pressure and to deliver the aerosol during each inspiration for 10 to 20 minutes, but it should be recognized that adequate therapy can be attained by nebulizing an undiluted bronchodilator for not more than 2 to 3 minutes;[21] indeed, four breaths of undiluted drug, using the IPPB to provide long, deep inhalations, may well suffice for many patients. The actual dose delivered by an IPPB treatment is extremely variable, and it may be necessary to experiment with each patient to determine the optimal dosage that should be put in the nebulizer. Moreover, in patients with small airway obstruction (such as may be demonstrated by the flow-volume curve or by frequency dependence of compliance), an aerosol may fail to reach the diseased sites; in such circumstances, oral or parenteral therapy may be far more effective.

TABLE 5–5. METHODS OF ADMINISTRATION FOR BRONCHODILATORS

Route	Forms	Example	Comment
Oral	Tablets	Metaproterenol	Most convenient
	Solutions	Metaproterenol	For children
Sublingual	Tablets	Isoproterenol	For occasional patient
	Aerosols	Isoproterenol	For infants
Inhalational	Solutions	Many products	With IPPB, etc.
	Metered solutions	Many products	Very convenient
	Metered powders	Norisodrine Aerohalor	Causes irritation
Rectal	Suppositories	Isuprel Glossets	Rarely used
Intramuscular	Solutions	Ethylnorepinephrine	For occasional patient
	Slow-release solutions	Epinephrine in oil	For prolonged effect
Subcutaneous	Solutions	Terbutaline	For severe bronchospasm
	Slow-release solutions	Sus-Phrine	For prolonged effect
Intravenous	Solutions	Isoproterenol	For status asthmaticus

The manufacturers' recommendations for aerosol dosages of various drugs should be taken as a guide, but should not be followed slavishly. When a patient has an endotracheal tube in place, a higher percentage of the drug will be deposited in the lung, and the dosage may need to be adjusted accordingly to avoid overdosage; although in these circumstances the drug will not enter the mouth, systemic absorption can probably occur almost as effectively from the lung as it can through the oral mucosa and stomach.[18] This topic is discussed in greater detail in Chapter 1.

Although IPPB is now regarded as a controversial therapeutic modality, it can be of great value in the administration of the various aerosol bronchodilators in asthmatics, particularly those with obstruction of large airways, who cannot take a deep enough breath to obtain effective relief from simpler methods of nebulization.[20, 21] It is inappropriate for any asthmatic to rely only on IPPB aerosolization of a bronchodilator, since oral preparations should always provide the basic form of management.

Oral Therapy. Until recently, there has been a relative dearth of suitable oral sympathomimetic bronchodilator drugs: ephedrine has been the traditional mainstay, and a few minor agents such as protokylol and methoxamine have been used to a much lesser degree. The development of new drugs, such as metaproterenol, terbutaline, salbutamol and fenoterol, offers the opportunity to provide effective, long-acting, relatively well-tolerated bronchodilator therapy in the form of tablets, capsules and liquids. In all bronchospastic patients, except those

with the mildest degrees of obstruction, oral administration should be considered as the basic route for bronchodilator therapy. The method is easy, does not necessitate complex apparatus or trained personnel, and requires little cooperation or skill; moreover, when compared to aerosol therapy, oral preparations are less expensive for the majority of patients. Also, the attainment of a therapeutic blood level results in the bronchodilator being available to all parts of the respiratory tree, whereas an aerosol reaches only the least obstructed areas. For this reason, oral therapy can be more effective in the treatment of small airway obstruction, such as characterizes many forms of asthma. It has been shown[21a] that after sufficient aerosolized bronchodilator has been given to produce maximal bronchodilatation in a patient, further airway opening can then be obtained by giving the drug by the oral route; in contrast, aerosolization is less likely to produce additional bronchodilatation after maximal airway opening has been attained by oral therapy.

The main disadvantage of oral therapy is that the therapeutic blood level required for bronchodilatation is usually sufficient to produce stimulation of receptors at other sites. Side effects are, therefore, much more common with oral bronchodilator therapy than with aerosol administration. However, the development of more effective and specific oral beta-2 bronchodilators will tend to make aerosolization a less attractive alternative.

Parenteral Therapy. Most bronchodilators are given by mouth or by aerosol, but several can be given by subcutaneous or intramuscular injection. However, the parenteral route is preferred only for emergency treatment, and is particularly useful when a patient is too dyspneic to take a deep breath or too nauseated to take oral medications. Undoubtedly, certain patients obtain added psychologic benefit when a drug is given by injection; in some circumstances it may be advisable to allow a cooperative, trained patient to have an injectable drug for home use in emergencies. Occasionally, a patient whose bronchospasm cannot be controlled by oral or inhalation therapy may respond to daily injections of a delayed-release formulation of epinephrine.

Intravenous Therapy. Sympathomimetic bronchodilators are rarely given intravenously, since profound systemic effects may result, with the danger of cardiac stimulation being a major problem. Children seem to tolerate intravenous bronchodilator therapy fairly well, and adults with status asthmaticus have been successfully managed with intravenous isoproterenol or metaproterenol, although salbutamol is safer. However, the hazards associated with carelessness in this form of therapy are so great that it should be undertaken only in an intensive care unit with electrocardiographic and blood pressure monitoring.

The various sympathomimetic drugs can be used intravenously for their cardiovascular properties, and, of course, they are valuable agents for the treatment of cardiac failure and shock.[22] Isoproterenol is one of the most valuable pressor agents for use in the management of septic shock, since its powerful beta-2 properties result in marked peripheral vasodilation and improved tissue perfusion. Epinephrine is used rarely as a pressor agent, but, in the treatment of cardiac arrest, an intracardiac injection of this drug

may reestablish the heartbeat. More recently, salbutamol has been reported to be particularly useful when given intravenously in the treatment of shock.[23] Other roles for selective beta-2 stimulants include their use, by intravenous administration, to delay the progress of premature labor occurring near the termination of pregnancy.[24] In general, it is inadvisable to treat bronchospasm with an intravenous infusion of a sympathomimetic; intravenous therapy should be reserved for the management of cardiovascular emergencies, until the role of this form of therapy in asthma has become better established.

Side Effects (See Table 5–6)

All sympathomimetic bronchodilators cause specific and nonspecific side effects, many of which can be explained by the actions of these agents on adrenergic receptors (Table 5–7). The more potent and selective beta-2 stimulating agents, which cause less overall unwanted side effects, nevertheless do result in prominent vascular and neuromuscular side effects, and this unfortunate quality may limit the success that can be expected from newer derivatives of the catecholamines. When the drugs are given by inhalation, bronchodilatation is attained with proportionally fewer side effects, but adequate treatment of bronchospasm with aerosol therapy tends to result in neuromuscular symptoms also.

Beta-2 side effects with oral or parenteral therapy can be annoying, especially in older patients, resulting in nervousness, agitation, hand tremors, poor sleep and (mainly in the case of ephedrine) difficulties in micturition in men who have prostatic enlargement. Fortunately, tolerance to the side effects

---

TABLE 5–6. POSSIBLE SIDE EFFECTS OF SYMPATHOMIMETIC BRONCHODILATORS

NERVOUS SYSTEM	Excitation, agitation, anxiety, tremulousness, insomnia, faintness, dizziness, sweating, psychosis
CARDIOVASCULAR	Tachycardia, changes in blood pressure, palpitations, arrhythmias, vasoconstriction or vasodilation, angina, myocardial necrosis
ALIMENTARY	Dry mouth, gagging, nausea, vomiting
GENITOURINARY	Urinary retention (in men with prostatic hypertrophy)
OPHTHALMIC	Glaucoma
METABOLIC	Hyperglycemia, hyperthyroidism
BLOOD GASES	Decrease in PaO_2
RESPIRATORY	Tracheal irritation, bronchial irritation, chest discomfort, bronchospasm
PREGNANCY	Inhibition of premature labor
INTERACTION WITH OTHER DRUGS	E.g., other bronchodilators, monoamine oxidase inhibitors, general anesthetics, hypotensive agents, pressor agents, thyroid hormones, insulin, oral hypoglycemics
OTHER	Tachyphylaxis, paradoxic response (bronchospasm)

**TABLE 5–7. POSTULATED CLINICAL EFFECTS OF STIMULATION OF
ADRENERGIC RECEPTORS**

	Alpha	Beta-1	Beta-2
Bronchospasm	Slight increase	No effect	Marked decrease
Respiratory tract secretions	Slight decrease	No effect	Slight increase(?)
Airway resistance	Decrease(?)	No effect	Decrease
Cough	No definite effect	No effect	Decrease
Heart rate	Reflex slowing (ectopy?)	Increase, ectopy	No effect
Blood pressure			
weak stimulus	May increase	Varies	Varies
strong stimulus	Increase	May increase	May decrease
Skeletal muscle	No effect	No effect	Tremor
C.N.S.	?	?	Anxiety, insomnia, etc.

tends to occur; tremor, for instance, may decrease markedly after two or three weeks of therapy.[25]

Beta-1 Side Effects. Beta-1 side effects are a particular problem with bronchodilator therapy. Aerosolization of those sympathomimetic agents that also act on the beta-1 receptors usually causes some increase in the heart rate, although this is minor when small dosages are given correctly, particularly if the patient rinses out the mouth. With larger inhalational doses (such as may be obtained with IPPB), and with oral or parenteral therapy, tachycardia and extrasystolic beats are frequent, particularly if the the patient has an irritable myocardium and is hypoxic. For this reason, to avoid the possibility of arrhythmia, drugs with marked beta-1 properties (such as isoproterenol) should be given with oxygen supplementation, unless the patient is known to be well-oxygenated and to have a healthy myocardium.[26] Unfortunately, even the more selective beta-2 stimulators can cause cardiovascular changes in sensitive patients, and palpitations may be experienced with larger doses. Comparisons of the ratio of beta-1 to beta-2 effects of various agents have been made, but the information currently available allows only an approximate analysis.[5, 7, 11, 27, 28]

The effects of the sympathomimetics on blood pressure are variable, and are related to the amount of the drug that enters the bloodstream. With a minimal aerosolized dose, there may be no significant changes, but with larger doses and with oral therapy the blood pressure may be affected.[22] In the case of a beta-receptor stimulator, the mean blood pressure may decrease, and lightheadedness, dizziness and fainting can occur. If the drug has alpha-stimulating properties, there may be an increase in blood pressure. Many of the sympathomimetic effects are magnified in patients with hyperthyroidism, and they may be more serious if the patient has vascular disease, particularly coronary artery disease. Individuals with arrhythmias or chronic ischemic heart disease may develop anginal-type pain when given excessive bronchodilator therapy. Intravenous sympathomimetic therapy is especially hazardous in patients with these problems. Headache is an ominous side effect, since intracerebral hemorrhage can follow in susceptible patients with cerebrovascular disease.

Nonspecific Side Effects. Nonspecific side effects (Table 5–6) can occur with all the sympathomimetic drugs. Headache, dizziness, faintness and sweating may be related to cardiovascular effects. Nausea and, occasionally, vomiting may follow administration of these agents by any route. Inhalation therapy may produce oropharyngeal symptoms, such as dry mouth, gagging, irritation of the mucosa and unpleasant taste; sublingual isoproterenol can damage the teeth if given in this fashion on a chronic basis.

Aerosol therapy can result in irritation of the tracheobronchial tree, and may even induce tracheobronchitis;[29] this problem may be worse with preparations that contain alcohol. Sensitive patients with very reactive airways ("twitchy lungs") may develop initial bronchospasm, particularly if a powdered preparation is inhaled. There have been occasional reports of paradoxic responses to the bronchodilator,[29-31] and although this phenomenon appears to be rare, the physician should be alert to the possibility and should discontinue the drug if the patient shows evidence of increasing problems with bronchospasm while on daily therapy. Many patients appear to develop tachyphylaxis, particularly with oral drugs; ephedrine seems to be the worst offender in this respect, but it has been suggested that

TABLE 5–8. MECHANISMS FOR BRONCHOCONSTRICTION CAUSED BY BRONCHODILATOR AEROSOLS

1. Tachyphylaxis to beta-2 effect, with persistence of alpha effect (e.g. epinephrine)

2. Beta-2 receptor blockade, caused by breakdown products or metabolites of sympathomimetic agents (e.g. 3-methoxy-isoproterenol), results in bronchospasm

3. Irritation of reactive airways caused by components in bronchodilator aerosol

4. Adverse reaction to a nonsympathomimetic component in bronchodilator preparation

5. Bronchospasm caused by exaggerated inhalational maneuver when attempting to use aerosol

6. Overdosage, causing symptoms of an anxiety response, which may trigger bronchospastic reflex

7. Rebound phenomenon, similar to that occurring with mucosal constrictor aerosols

8. Over-reliance on ineffective bronchodilators allows asthmatic attack to progress unchecked

9. Faulty aerosol dispensers may not deliver effective dose of drugs

10. Improper use of IPPB may irritate airways and cause a bronchospastic reaction

continued administration of long-acting drugs will, in general, tend to produce a state of diminished responsiveness.[32] The factors that could result in a patient developing bronchospasm after using a sympathomimetic aerosol are presented in Table 5–8.

Tachyphylaxis. The problem of tachyphylaxis is not yet understood,[33] but in this situation a patient may develop tolerance or refractoriness to a bronchodilator and to its beta-1 side effects. This complication should be suspected in a patient for whom a bronchodilator drug results in progressively less bronchodilation with a need for an increase of the dosage at shorter and shorter intervals. Although the phenomenon of resistance or tolerance to the drug differs from the paradoxic response, in which the drug actually causes bronchospasm (directly or as a rebound phenomenon),[30, 30a] management is the same—the drug should be discontinued. Various factors, including paradoxic response and tachyphylaxis as well as excessive dosage, have been invoked to explain deaths in patients who may have used excessive amounts of bronchodilator in aerosol form.[34] The possible sequences of events leading to fatalities from isoproterenol are diagrammed in Figure 5–1. Fortunately, there is considerable evidence

to suggest that the overall incidence of tolerance, resistance or paradoxic response to chronic treatment with beta-stimulants is very low.[6]

Hypoxemia. Hypoxemia has been described as a complication of sympathomimetic therapy, in that the arterial oxygen tension (PaO_2) may decrease. This problem has also followed the therapeutic administration of atropine and aminophylline to asthmatics, and appears to result from the drug-induced increase in pulmonary blood flow to areas that are poorly ventilated because of bronchospasm or retention of secretions that exacerbates the ventilation-perfusion imbalance (see Figure 5–2). There is a considerable literature on this subject, and the evidence suggests that a variable, but usually slight, fall in PaO_2 may occur following the administration of any bronchodilator drug by aerosol or by other routes.[6] Particular care is therefore required when giving a sympathomimetic (or a theophylline) drug to a patient with airway obstruction whose PaO_2 is less than 60 mm Hg: in such cases it is wise to administer oxygen with the bronchodilator. There may be a particular danger in using beta-adrenergic drugs such as isoproterenol in patients with severe pulmonary insufficiency, since the resulting increase in shunting may worsen the respiratory distress syndrome.[34a]

Management Problems

When a sympathomimetic agent loses effectiveness or produces untoward effects in a patient who relies on medications for relief of bronchospasm, the physician may be put into a dilemma about what alternative treatment can be offered. If severe complications, such as tachyphylaxis, develop to one drug, then it is possible that none of the related sympathomimetic agents will be any better, since cross-reactivity may occur,[34b] although this does not always happen.[30a] Under such circumstances, it may be necessary to rely on another class of drug, such as theophylline, or to use corticosteroid therapy; once control is reestablished, it may be possible to return to the sympathomimetic agent, but minimal dosages should be used. Some patients may fare remarkably better if an aerosol is simply withdrawn, and no other drug substituted.[31] Certain conditions, such as age, or cardiovascular or nervous system instability, necessitate particular caution, since adverse effects may be more common,

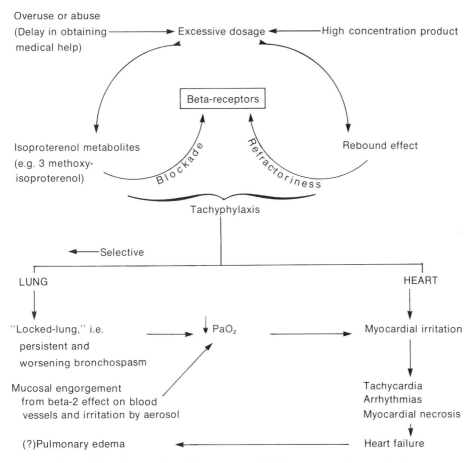

Figure 5–1.   Causes of Fatalities Associated With Isoproterenol Aerosolization.

MECHANISM BY WHICH BETA-2 STIMULATORS CAN CAUSE HYPOXEMIA

Figure 5–2. Bronchodilator aerosols may cause hypoxemia by their systemically mediated vasodilator effect on the vasculature in poorly ventilated lung units. The drugs serve to cause a shunt-like effect.

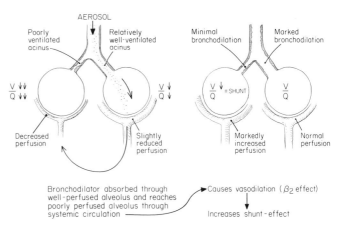

TABLE 5–9. CONDITIONS DEMANDING PARTICULAR CARE WHEN
ADMINISTERING BRONCHODILATOR THERAPY

AGE	Very young, very old
CARDIAC	Tachycardia, arrhythmia, unstable angina, recent myocardial infarction
CARDIOVASCULAR	Hypotension, hypertension, labile blood pressure
NERVOUS SYSTEM	Anxiety, mania, insomnia, tremulousness, headache
OPHTHALMIC	Narrow angle glaucoma
ENDOCRINE	Unstable diabetes, hyperthyroidism
PULMONARY	Hypoxemia, hyperreactive airways
PHARMACOLOGIC	Treatment with other sympathomimetic drugs, theophylline derivatives, monoamine oxidase inhibitors, tricyclic antidepressants, general anesthetics, thyroid replacement, antidiabetic agents
GENERAL	Nausea, vomiting, any known adverse response to bronchodilator therapy
SPECIAL CONDITIONS	Pregnancy, prostatic hypertrophy (ephedrine)

and are certainly more hazardous, in these circumstances (Table 5–9).

It is intriguing to speculate whether a patient whose asthma is "brittle" would obtain better results if different bronchodilators were used in rotation; one drug could be used on odd days or during odd weeks, and another on even days or during even weeks, or each of several drugs could be used for a month in sequence. It may be advisable to use two different drugs alternately on an everyday basis, or even to change the drug used for each successive treatment. Certainly, the unstable asthmatic is likely to benefit psychologically from such a rigorously formulated approach to bronchodilation therapy, but there is no practical information to attest to the validity of such regimens. Manufacturers claim that the use of two different aerosol bronchodilators in sequence may have an adverse result due to apparent potentiating of the side effects. Therefore, any rotation regimen should allow enough time between doses of the different agents to avoid summation of the extrapulmonary reactions.

Precautions

Solutions of sympathomimetic drugs are unstable and are readily oxidized, particularly in the presence of oxygen, sunlight, alkalis and metals. The drugs should be stored in dark bottles and should be reasonably fresh; if a solution becomes discolored with a pink or brown tinge (caused by oxidation products, such as adrenochromes), it should be discarded. Various additives are incorporated in the solution (Table 1–9) to keep the drug acidic and to inhibit oxidation.[15] In practice, a bronchodilator is often nebulized with other alkaline drugs (such as acetylcysteine and sodium bicarbonate), or by using oxygen to produce the aerosol; however, the medication can be given immediately under such circumstances, before substantial oxidative breakdown occurs, and then adequate bronchodilatation is generally attained. The drug remaining in the nebulizer or tubing at the end of the treatment may show a pink tinge, and the respiratory and salivary secretions may be markedly pink. In fact, the physician who is unaware of this phenomenon may be inclined to embark on a misdirected work-up for the apparent hemoptysis that is witnessed. Although there are fears that breakdown products, such as the adrenochromes, could be competitive beta-blockers,[32, 35] experience suggests that no adverse effects are produced in the average patient.

When a sympathomimetic is given by inhalation, the therapist should always be alert to the possible development of adverse effects. The patient should be evaluated initially with simple pulmonary function tests; the pulse rate, heart rhythm and blood pressure should also be checked. Additional care should be taken when the patient has tachycardia, arrhythmias, hypertension, hypotension, severe anxiety, tremulousness, nausea, unstable diabetes, hyperthyroidism or a known hypersensitivity to bronchodilators (Table 5–9). If the patient is hypoxic, oxygen will usually be necessary, but this may require careful supervision to avoid depressing respiration in a patient who has a hypoxic drive. During initial therapy, the patient should be constantly monitored to ensure that no adverse changes occur in any of the monitored parameters. At the end of the treatment, the pulse, blood pressure and pulmonary function values should be recorded, and any adverse effects should be noted. Once the patient's response to a drug has been carefully evaluated, subsequent treatments can be given with less worry, although IPPB sessions for the acutely ill patient should always be supervised and monitored.

A particular precaution is required if a patient is on an antidepressant drug, such as a monoamine oxidase inhibitor or a tricyclic compound. These drugs may potentiate the sympathomimetics and cause serious changes in blood pressure, such as a hypertensive crisis. Patients on digitalis preparations are more susceptible to arrhythmias when sympathomimetic agents are also given. Epinephrine and other bronchodilators can cause problems in diabetics if given in large amounts, since these agents may antagonize the actions of insulin or hypoglycemic drugs. Caution is needed when an asthmatic patient is about to undergo anesthesia, since the sympathomimetic agents have a greater tendency to cause myocardial irritation in the presence of a general anesthetic. If the patient requires a bronchodilator before surgery, a short-acting aerosol should be used rather than a long-acting oral drug. A further contraindication is the presence of narrow-angle glaucoma.

If a patient self-administers treatment with a metered cartridge, clear instructions on its

TABLE 5-10. PRECAUTIONS WHEN USING METERED SYMPATHOMIMETIC BRONCHODILATORS

1. Shake cartridge before use; use in inverted position.
2. Keep delivery port clean; rinse in water periodically.
3. Do periodic visual checks on quality of the spray.
4. Store in cool place.
5. Avoid overuse, e.g., use maximum of four puffs every three hours of isoproterenol or epinephrine, and maximum of four puffs every six hours of metaproterenol or terbutaline.
6. Keep port of nebulizer about one inch from open mouth for optimal delivery of aerosol.
7. Proper inhalational technique must be used, i.e., exhale air, take in a deep breath of the aerosol, hold breath, breathe out; take a few normal breaths, and repeat process if necessary. In some patients, inhalation of aerosol from the point of resting tidal volume may produce more effective drug deposition.
8. If patient is unable to take an effective breath, delivery of the aerosol beneath the tongue may provide some bronchodilation.
9. To prevent oropharyngeal irritation or adverse side effects, gargling and mouth rinsing with a glass of water after each treatment may help.
10. Physicians should monitor how many puffs a day a patient uses; thus, a cartridge with 300 doses should last at least 15 days for isoproterenol or epinephrine, and longer for other agents.

TABLE 5-11. MANAGEMENT OF PATIENT WHO REACTS ADVERSELY TO BRONCHODILATORS

Problem	Corrective Action
Overfrequent use of aerosol	Educate patient or withdraw aerosol.
Incorrect use of aerosol	Educate patient, or use a different mode of administration.
Tachycardia after aerosol use	Decrease dose, use a gargle after each treatment.
Tachyphylaxis	Discontinue preparation, use another bronchodilator (either a sympathomimetic or some other class of drug).
Increased hypoxemia	Administer aerosol with oxygen.

use and cautions to avoid abuse must be brought to the patient's attention (Table 5-10). The physician should be particularly alert to the possibility that many anxious or immature patients might overuse these preparations. Counselling will be required if an asthmatic is clearly using excessive amounts for therapeutic, psychologic or sociologic reasons. Thus, some patients conspicuously display their frequent "need" for aerosol therapy to elicit sympathy or to provide a medical basis for avoiding responsibility. Undoubtedly, some patients become virtually addicted to their aerosols, since they appreciate the central nervous system stimulation that is obtained. Such individuals are at particular risk of developing tachyphylaxis and adverse reactions. If a patient appears to be doing poorly with aerosol therapy, certain measures can be taken, such as reeducating the patient in the proper use of the drug or, in some cases, withdrawal of the aerosol from the treatment plan (Table 5-11).

When aerosol therapy is correctly used, the incidence of adverse effects and potentiation of other drugs is minimized. In all circumstances, it is important to establish the minimal effective dosage (number of puffs and frequency of use) of the bronchodilator; when such a regimen is used the majority of patients will experience no serious complications. Added precautions should be taken when giving the drug to the very young, or to the elderly patient with multiple organ dysfunction, since unusual and adverse effects are more likely to occur in such subjects. Pregnant women may be given these drugs during the first trimester after due consideration of the very small possibility that they could have an adverse effect on the fetus or the pregnancy. At present, however, there is no evidence that the sympathomimetics are teratogenic.

General Observations

In general, an oral bronchodilator should be preferred to an aerosol for basic therapy. The oral preparations are easier to administer and are often long-acting. Aerosols should be used for "fine-tuning," for management of mild bronchospasm requiring only occasional treatment and for very dyspneic patients who may require aerosol delivery by IPPB.

If a patient does not respond appropriately to a sympathomimetic, tachyphylaxis or a paradoxic response could be at fault. It may be necessary to withdraw the agent and to reevaluate the overall drug regimen. Careful questioning and observation will frequently reveal that the patient is using the drug incorrectly or inappropriately. In such circumstances, it may be possible to reinstitute the drug and to ensure its correct administration.

In acutely ill patients, the sympathomimetic agents may no longer be effective enough to justify their use; a theophylline, corticosteroid or both may be indicated. If the patient has an acute acidosis, this should be corrected, since catecholamines and derivatives are less effective when the arterial pH is less than 7.24.

Careful attention to the choice and dosage of the drug, and a knowledgeable consideration of other factors involved in the pharmacology of bronchospasm, should enable the physician to tailor the therapy of the individual patient with considerable success in the majority of cases.

In the following sections, the sympathomimetics that are available to the physician will be described in detail. For the sake of convenience, they will be classified as shorter-acting or longer-acting drugs. These agents are compared in Tables 5–12 and 5–13, which are derived from numerous sources of published information. There is lack of unanimity of agreement about individual properties, and the information should be read with this in mind.

INDIVIDUAL SYMPATHOMIMETIC BRONCHODILATORS

SHORTER-ACTING SYMPATHOMIMETIC BRONCHODILATORS

Isoproterenol

Isoproterenol is isopropylnorepinephrine (see Figure 5–3); in England, the drug is called isoprenaline. It is marketed by various manufacturers. In the U.S., the best-known trade name is Isuprel, but it is also known as Medihaler-Iso, Aludrine, Norisodrine and so forth. In England, the main additional proprietary names are Aleudrin and Prenomiser. Isoproterenol was introduced into medicine in the 1940s, and although it is still a widely-used aerosol bronchodilator, its value in asthma has become controversial.[36]

Structure and Metabolism. Isoproterenol is a catecholamine; therefore, it is deactivated by catechol-O-methyltransferase in the tissues and by sulfatization in the bowel.[35] The structure of the molecule endows it with powerful beta-2 properties; it has virtually no alpha-adrenergic activity, but it does have marked beta-1 effects.

The drug is one of the most powerful bronchodilators, and has a rapid onset of effect. Its bronchodilator action following administration by aerosol can persist for as short a time as 20 minutes, although it often is effective for 90 to 120 minutes. The drug is rapidly metabolized by the intracellular enzyme catechol-O-methyl transferase (COMT) to 3-methoxy-isoproterenol, an agent that can cause weak blockade of the beta-2 receptor sites.[32, 35] However, this theoretic disadvantage of isoproterenol does not cause any problem in the average asthmatic, and the short half-life may be an advantage, since toxic drug accumulation does not occur. After an intravenous dose, over 50 per cent of the isoproterenol is excreted unchanged in the urine, whereas following aerosol administration 90 per cent of the excreted drug is in the conjugated form.[7]

Since isoproterenol has strong beta-1 effects, it is also used in the treatment of cardiovascular diseases. Its main use is to stimulate the heart, and it can be given by mouth for the treatment of Stokes-Adams attacks and other forms of heart block. However, absorption from the bowel is very erratic, since much of the drug is conjugated to form the inactive sulfate. The drug is of value for intravenous use in the treatment of septic shock, where its powerful peripheral vasodilator action can result in improvement of venous return to the heart.

Actions. When isoproterenol is given by aerosol in the management of bronchospasm, small doses (for example 200 mcg) can result in bronchodilatation, within one minute, without causing any significant side effects.[37] If larger or more frequent doses are given, cardiac and nervous system problems may

TABLE 5–12. STRUCTURE AND ACTIONS OF SYMPATHOMIMETIC BRONCHODILATORS

Structure:
$$\text{ring (positions 2,3,4,5,6)} - CH_\beta - CH_\alpha - NH-$$

	1	2	3	4	5	6	β	α	NH-	Vasoconstriction Alpha	Cardiac Stimulation Beta₁	Bronchodilation, Nervous System Stimulation, Vasodilation Beta₂	Persistence of Effect of Aerosol
EPINEPHRINE	H	H	OH	OH	H	H	OH	H	CH_3	+++	++++	+++	Short
R-EPINEPHRINE	H	H	OH	OH	H	H	OH	H	CH_3	++(+)	+++(+)	++(+)	Short
ISOPROTERENOL	H	H	OH	OH	H	H	OH	H	$CH(CH_3)_2$	(+)	++++	++++	Short
RIMITEROL	H	H	OH	OH	H	H	OH	H	C_5H_{10}		(+)	++++	Short
ISOETHARINE	H	H	OH	OH	H	H	OH	C_2H_5	$CH(CH_3)_2$		+(+)	+++	Medium
ETHYLNOREPINEPHRINE	H	H	OH	OH	H	H	OH	C_2H_5	H	++	++	++(+)	Medium
EPHEDRINE	H	H	H	H	H	H	OH	CH_3	CH_3	++	++	+++	Long
METHOXYPHENAMINE	H	OCH_3	H	H	H	H	H	CH_3	CH_3		++	+(+)	Long
PROTOKYLOL	H	H	OH	OH	H	H	OH	H	$(C_{10}H_{12}ClNO_2)$		++(+)	++(+)	Long
METAPROTERENOL	H	H	OH	H	OH	H	OH	H	$CH(CH_3)_2$		+(+)	++(+)	Long
SALBUTAMOL	H	H	CH_2OH	OH	H	H	OH	H	$C(CH_3)_3$		+(+)	++++	Long
TERBUTALINE	H	H	OH	H	OH	H	OH	H	$C(CH_3)_3$		+(+)	+++(+)	Long
FENOTEROL	H	H	OH	H	OH	H	OH	H	$CH(CH_3) \cdot CH_2 \cdot C_8H_4OH$		+(+)	++++	Long

The relative effects on adrenergic receptors have not been established with accuracy; the above information will require revision when reliable information becomes available.

TABLE 5-13. COMPARISON OF MAIN SYMPATHOMIMETIC BRONCHODILATORS*

	Epinephrine	Isoproterenol	Isoetharine	Ephedrine	Metaproterenol	Terbutaline	Salbutamol
Chemical category	Catecholamine	Catecholamine	Catecholamine	Phenylalkylamine	Resorcinol	Resorcinol	Saligenin
Receptor action	Direct	Direct	Direct	Indirect and direct	Direct	Direct	Direct
Mucosal vessels	Constrictor	Dilator	Dilator	Constrictor	Dilator	Dilator	Dilator
Heart rate	Marked ↑	Marked ↑	Slight ↑	Moderate ↑	Marked ↑	Slight ↑	Varies
Peripheral resistance	↓ or ↑	→	→	Varies	→	→	→
Blood pressure: Small dose							
mean	N or ↑	Varies	Varies	Varies	Varies	N or →	N or →
systolic	← ↑	N or ↑	Varies	↑	N or ↑	N or →	N or →
diastolic	N or ↓	→	Varies	↑	→	N or →	N or →
Large dose							
mean	Varies	N or →	→	← →	N or →	N or →	N or →
systolic	← or ↑	← →	→	← ↑	← →	← →	→ or →
diastolic				N			N or →
Tachyphylaxis	May occur	May occur	May occur	Readily occurs	May occur	May occur	May occur
Onset of aerosol action	Rapid	Rapid	Rapid		Rapid	Slow	Slow
Significant effect (hrs)	1–1½	1–2	1½–2½	4–6(?)	3–5	3–7	4–6
Comparative oral dose (mg)		10(?)	(20)	25	20	5	4
Comparative aerosol dose (mg)	0.20	0.10	0.35		0.65	0.25	0.10

N = no change, ↑ = increase, ↓ = decrease
*This information is derived from many sources, and the data must be regarded as approximations, which require further evaluation.

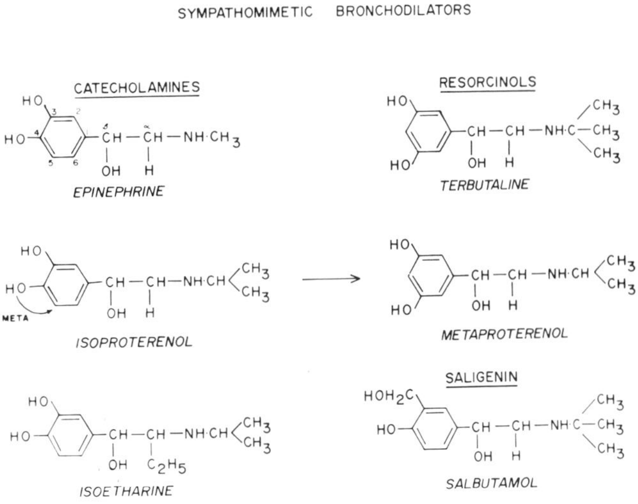

SYMPATHOMIMETIC BRONCHODILATORS

Figure 5–3. The important sympathomimetic bronchodilators are not all catecholamines. The related resorcinol and saligenin derivatives are not susceptible to enzymic degradation of the dihydroxy groupings of the catechol molecule. They are therefore effective when given by mouth, and their effects are long lasting.

arise. Nervousness, tremors, headache, nausea, sweating, flushed skin and hypotension may occur, but are rarely severe. Tachycardia and palpitations are common after large aerosol doses, and various arrhythmias or anginal pain may be produced. Case reports reveal that if comparatively huge doses are taken (for example 675 mg in 3 days, about 18 times the usual dose), myocardial necrosis may result,[38] although the more usual outcome might be the development of one of the life-threatening arrhythmias. Cardiac arrest may be a potentially higher risk when the drug is given to patients with heart failure.[39] Although isoproterenol is used as a pressor agent in the management of hypotension, its main action is to cause peripheral vasodilation. This can result in a fall in the mean pressure; if intravenous fluids are also given, a pressor effect may result. In general, the diastolic pressure is decreased, while the systolic pressure is usually increased; small doses have a variable effect on mean pressure, whereas large doses may have little effect or cause a slight fall (see Table 5–13).

In the 1960s, the introduction in the United Kingdom of a metered preparation of isoproterenol (Medihaler-Iso Forte) that was five times as concentrated as the one now available, was associated with a dramatic sevenfold increase in the number of deaths from asthma.[40] Although there is still debate as to what caused these deaths,[34] it is possible that over-use of the aerosol (particularly by children) contributed to a fatal arrhythmia. Alternative explanations include the suggestion that a paradoxic response can occur with large doses, due to the induction of more COMT, which metabolizes isopro-

terenol to 3-methoxyisoproterenol, which is a weak beta-blocker[32, 35] (see Fig. 5–4). There is little evidence to suggest that this is an important factor in practice, since well-documented paradoxic responses are extremely rare.[29] The Freon propellant used in metered aerosols has been blamed, but it is unlikely that this could reach a high enough blood level to be fatal.[41]

A further concern about isoproterenol is that the more it is used, the less effective it might become as a bronchodilator;[30] patients then use excessive doses in an effort to obtain relief. However, tolerance to the beta-1 effects also develops, suggesting that overuse of the nebulizer is unlikely to be the only explanation of the excessive number of deaths.[42] Although the whole phenomenon of tachyphylaxis is poorly understood, it is important that a bronchodilator drug be discarded from the regimen of a patient who finds that larger and more frequent treatments are required. The deaths in the 1960s may have reflected the fact that patients developed too great a reliance on the aerosol, so that medical advice was not sought early enough when a severe exacerbation of the asthma developed; the patients continued to use isoproterenol with its disadvantages, rather than being hospitalized for more appropriate treatment with aminophylline and corticosteroids[34] (see discussion in Chapter 1).

The major features of isoproterenol are summarized in Table 5–14.

Dosages and Recommendations. Isoproterenol can be given by aerosol, by oral administration, sublingually[19] or intravenously. Oral therapy produces a variable response[43] and is rarely used. Both aerosol

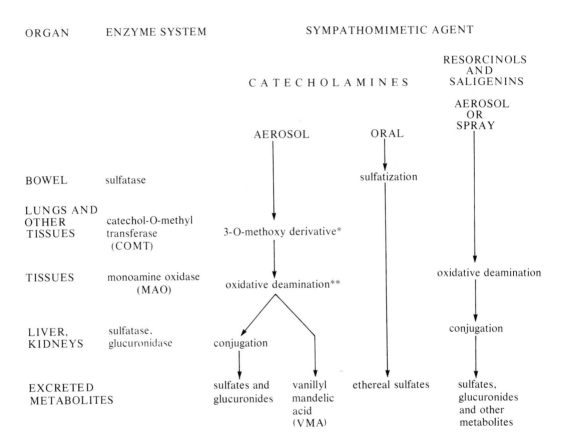

*This metabolite may be a competitive blocker at beta-2 receptor sites.

**This conversion is blocked by monoamine oxidase inhibitors.

Figure 5–4 Metabolic breakdown of sympathomimetic agents.

TABLE 5–14.   ISOPROTERENOL

CHEMICAL NAME	Isopropylnorepinephrine
OTHER NAMES	Isoprenaline (in the United Kingdom)
BRAND NAMES	Aludrine, Isuprel, etc.
USES	Bronchodilator
	Pressor agent, useful in septic shock
	Cardiac stimulant, used in treatment of Stokes-Adams attacks (heart block)
	Pulmonary vasodilator (may reduce pulmonary hypertension)
PROBLEMS	Relatively high incidence of tachyarrhythmias, which could be life-threatening
	May cause fall in PaO_2
	Relatively short acting; may need to be administered every 1–2 hours in acute asthma
	Overfrequent use can cause tachyphylaxis, and may result in paradoxic bronchospasm
	Metered product could be overused by anxious patient, with adverse results including myocardial necrosis and fatal tachyarrhythmias
	Not reliable when given by mouth
	Hazardous when given intravenously
PREPARATIONS	Marketed as chloride and as sulfate

therapy[44, 45] and intravenous delivery[46, 47] can cause dangerous side effects, although appropriately used aerosols are very safe in practice.

AEROSOL. Isoproterenol is available both as a solution and as a powder; it is packaged in metered aerosols and as solutions for administration by nebulizers, with or without positive pressure. Metered aerosols deliver from 0.04 to 0.125 mg per puff, depending on the preparation used (see Table 5–15). In general, one puff every three to six hours may suffice, but up to four puffs can be allowed. Patients who develop side effects should be advised to rinse out the oropharynx so as to limit systemic absorption; this also decreases throat irritation. If more frequent dosing is required to control bronchospasm, use of a different drug should be considered. It is possible that smaller dosages, such as 20 mcg (0.02 mg) might produce a maximal response in some patients,[48] but it is conventional to use the larger, metered dosages. Physicians should recognize that the dose liberated by one puff of a commercial preparation (for example Norisodrine Aerohaler 10%) may be less than one-third the dose of a competing aerosol (such as Isuprel Mistometer).

The drug is often given by IPPB, using 0.5 ml of a 1:200 solution. Although this could be given undiluted, it is conventional to add 2 ml of water or normal saline to provide enough solution for 7 to 15 minutes of nebulization. For patients who obtain a suboptimal response, 1 ml of the 1:200 solution could be used, or 0.5 ml of a 1:100 solution. The same amounts of isoproterenol can be used, undiluted, in a hand-bulb or air-compressor nebulizer; most patients require 2 to 15 puffs for optimal therapy, and the appropriate dose must be established by careful trial, hopefully without error. A powder preparation is available for inhalation, but it is not recommended, since it tends to cause more airway irritation.

The majority of patients do well with a simple hand-bulb or a metered preparation; IPPB should be used only if the simpler methods are shown to be less effective in a particular patient. In all cases, overuse of the drug must be thoroughly discouraged, but a routine prophylactic puff or two by an asthmatic, every morning, or every night or before exercise, may be justified to help keep the patient relatively comfortable. Prolonged use of metered aerosol preparations of isoproterenol, in a dose of 1 to 4 puffs four times a day, provides safe and effective routine therapy for the average patient with chronic bronchospastic disease,[49] and one to three inhalations can be safely given as often as every four hours in subacute asthma.[50]

ORAL (Table 5–16). Tablets of isoproterenol are used in the treatment of Stokes-Adams attacks, and they can also be used for the treatment of asthma, although oral and sublingual administration are less satisfactory alternatives to aerosols. For the occasional adult patient who may prefer the sublingual route (for example the elderly, dyspneic patient who is unable to use aerosols correctly) a 10 or 15 mg tablet is placed beneath the tongue and allowed to dissolve and be absorbed until an effect is produced; then, the rest of the tablet can be discarded. Oral or sublingual dosages in adults range from 5 to 20 mg every four to six hours. The oral elixir that is available tends to result in unreliable therapy, since gastric absorption is erratic, but it is useful for young children who cannot use aerosols. Combined prepa-

TABLE 5–15. ISOPROTERENOL PRODUCTS FOR AEROSOL THERAPY

Product	Constituents	Strength	Approx. Dose of Drug Per Puff mg.	Administration
METERED AEROSOLS				
Isuprel Mistometer (15 ml)	Isoproterenol hydrochloride solution (in alcohol)	2.8 mg/ml	0.125	1–4 inhalations 4–8 times a day. Up to 8 inhalations may be taken over course of 1 hour in an emergency.
Luf-Iso (15 ml)	Isoproterenol sulfate suspension	2 mg/ml	0.075	
Medihaler-Iso (15 and 22.5 ml)	Isoproterenol sulfate suspension	2 mg/ml	0.06	
Norisodrine Aerohaler 10%	Isoproterenol sulfate powder	10 mg	0.04	Use smaller dose in children. Individual patient tolerance varies widely.
Norisodrine Aerohaler 25%	Isoproterenol sulfate powder	25 mg	0.11	
Norisodrine Aerotrol (15 ml)	Isoproterenol hydrochloride solution (in alcohol)	2.8 mg/ml	0.12	
*Vapo-N-Iso Metermatic (15 ml)	Isoproterenol sulfate suspension	2 mg/ml	0.06	
METERED COMBINATION AEROSOLS				
Duohaler (7.5 ml)	Isoproterenol hydrochloride } suspension Phenylephrine bitartrate }	4 mg/ml 6 mg/ml	0.137 0.126	1–3 inhalations 4–6 times a day. Effect is longer-lasting than that from isoproterenol alone.
Duo-Medihaler (15 and 22.5 ml) *Nebair (10 ml)	Isoproterenol hydrochloride Thonzonium bromide	1 mg/ml 1.5 mg/ml	0.063 0.095	
SOLUTIONS FOR AEROSOLIZATION				
Iprenol (1:100, 1:200)	Isoproterenol hydrochloride	10 mg/ml, 5 mg/ml		2–7 inhalations of 1:100 solution 4–6 times a day 2–15 inhalations of 1:200 solution 4–6 times a day. IPPB: 0.1–0.5 ml 1:100 solution 0.2–1.0 ml 1:200 solution } 4–6 times a day with or without 2–3 ml diluent
Isoproterenol USP (1:100, 1:200)	Isoproterenol hydrochloride	10 mg/ml, 5 mg/ml		
Isuprel (1:100, 1:200, 1:400)	Isoproterenol hydrochloride	10 mg/ml, 5 mg/ml		
Vapo-Iso (1:200)	Isoproterenol hydrochloride	5 mg/ml		
COMBINATION SOLUTION FOR AEROSOLIZATION				
Aerolone	Isoproterenol hydrochloride 2.5 mg. Cyclopentamine hydrochloride 5 mg. } in 1 ml Propylene glycol 80%			6–12 inhalations 4–6 times a day or 0.5–1.0 ml with or without 2–3 ml diluent

*No longer marketed.

Maximum dosage should be discouraged. The use of a mouthwash following inhalational administration may decrease incidence of systemic side effects. With IPPB, supplemental O_2 may be needed to prevent the development of hypoxemia.

Metered cartridges contain about 100 doses/5 ml.

The most potent metered aerosol preparations deliver more than three times the amount of isoproterenol base as does the least potent preparation. All isoproterenol products require a prescription.

TABLET 5–16. NONINHALATIONAL ADMINISTRATION OF ISOPROTERENOL

Preparation	Availability	Dosage	
		ADULTS	CHILDREN
SUBLINGUAL OR ORAL TABLET			
Isoproterenol USP	10, 15 mg	5–20 mg 3–6 times a	5–10 mg, up to maxi-
Isuprel (glosset)*	10, 15 mg	day, up to maximum of 60 mg/day	mum of 30 mg/day
SUSTAINED ACTION TABLET			
Proterenol	15, 30 mg	Not advised for bronchospasm	
ELIXIR OR SYRUP			
Isuprel Compound†	Isoproterenol HCl 2.5 mg Ephedrine 12 mg Phenobarbital 6 mg } per Potassium iodide 150 mg } 15 Theophylline 45 mg } ml Alcohol 19%	5–30 ml up to 4 times a day	Not recommended
Norisodrine	Isoproterenol sulfate 3 mg } per Calcium iodide 150 mg } 5 Alcohol 6% } ml	2.5–10 ml q3–4h	2.5–5 ml q3–6h
INTRAVENOUS SOLUTION			
Iprenol, Isuprel	1:5000 (200 mcg/ml)	0.03–0.2 mcg/kg/ minute; or 0.01–0.02 mg (0.5–1 ml of 1:50,000 solution); repeat if necessary	0.1–0.8 mcg/kg/ minute

*Glosset can be administered by rectal route.
†This preparation is not recommended.

rations with other bronchodilators are not recommended.

PARENTERAL. Intravenous therapy with isoproterenol has been used for asthmatic children in a dosage of 0.8 mcg/kg per minute; this can be tolerated for many hours. It is suggested that, initially, the isoproterenol be infused at a rate of 0.1 mcg/kg per minute with increments of 0.1 mcg/kg per minute every 10 to 15 minutes until a response or adverse effects occur.[51] In adults with very severe status asthmaticus, the aerosol will not reach the site of the most severe obstruction, and intravenous therapy may be valuable: the appropriate dosage is 0.03 to 0.2 mcg/kg per minute,[47] and a response should occur within minutes. Intravenous administration is more likely to cause a fall in PaO_2 by increasing the shunt through poorly ventilated lung areas; furthermore, arrhythmias and blood pressure changes may occur. However, the half-life of the beta-1 effects lasts only one minute, and the blood level only four minutes (compared to a blood level half-life for aminophylline of about three hours).[46] Thus, although this form of therapy is not yet standard practice, it can be effective, and the risk is unlikely to be great if the patient is carefully monitored in an intensive care setting with the isoproterenol delivery being controlled by use of a constant-infusion pump. Intravenous isoproterenol can also be given to treat bronchospasm during anesthesia (provided cyclopropane is not being used): 1 ml of the 1:5000 solution is added to 10 ml saline and 0.5 to 1 ml of the diluted solution (containing 0.01 to 0.02 mg isoproterenol) is carefully administered, and can be repeated if necessary.

Precautions. Although isoproterenol has theoretic disadvantages because it is a powerful beta-1 stimulator, the drug is well-established, it is relatively inexpensive, and it is quite safe when used correctly in aerosol form in the vast majority of patients.[37, 41] The physiologic ratio of bronchodilator potency to cardiostimulatory effect is markedly affected by the route of administration, and may differ considerably when the drug is given by other than the inhalational route. Cardiac arrhythmias may be produced following aerosolization, but in most stable patients with chronic obstructive airway disease no significant cardiac side effects are produced.[41] As a precautionary measure, when the drug is given by IPPB, slight oxygen enrichment could be provided to counteract the fall in PaO_2 that may occur.[52] However, a fall in PaO_2 does not always occur; indeed, the PaO_2 may be increased by aerosol therapy with isoproterenol in low dosage.[53] As long as physicians, nurses, respiratory therapists and patients are knowledgeable about the drug and monitor its use, isoproterenol will continue to be a favored bronchodilator for routine administration.[36] In general, bronchospastic patients feel better when using regular isoproterenol therapy, even though there may be no progressive improvement in pulmonary function; in most cases, the development of refractoriness does not become a problem.[49]

There is a danger if isoproterenol is given to patients who are being treated with monoamine oxidase (MAO) inhibitor antidepressant drugs, since these agents may delay the metabolic breakdown of isoproterenol. Severe hypertensive reactions can occur in these circumstances. Caution is needed when a patient who uses isoproterenol requires a general anesthetic, since many of these agents potentiate the effect of the sympathomimetic drug on the heart, and arrhythmias may result. If a patient develops bronchospasm after receiving a beta-blocker drug, careful administration of large doses of isoproterenol may relieve the condition, whereas epinephrine and other preparations with alpha-adrenergic activity may increase the bronchospasm and airway resistance.

Availability. Isoproterenol is available as the hydrochloride and sulfate for nebulization (see Table 5–15); and as noninhalational preparations (Table 5–16), i.e. as sublingual tablets and in oral combination products, which are of limited value. Isoproterenol is also available for intravenous administration, and is used in this form mainly as a pressor agent. Discolored or cloudy solutions of isoproterenol should not be used, although they are unlikely to cause significant harm.

Isoproterenol in Combination

Isoproterenol with Phenylephrine. Several studies[52, 54, 55-57] have shown that the addition of phenylephrine to isoproterenol in a metered aerosol dispenser results in a more effective bronchodilator that produces a longer persistence of bronchodilatation. Although these claims were not corroborated in a more recent study,[58] there are pharmacologic grounds for expecting the combination product to have a more prolonged effect. Similarly, there is a basis for explaining the reported decreased possibility for a fall in PaO_2 after nebulization of the combination[52] (see Fig. 5–5); indeed, the combination of isoproterenol with phenylephrine may result in an improvement in PaO_2.[59]

Theoretically, the addition of phenylephrine would lead to a prolongation of the beta-2 effect of isoproterenol in the lungs, since the powerful alpha-activity of phenylephrine should counteract the beta-1 effect of isoproterenol on the mucosal vessels. The resulting tendency to mucosal constriction should decrease blood flow, and thereby

ADVANTAGES OF ADDING AN ALPHA-STIMULATOR TO A BETA-2 STIMULATOR AEROSOL DRUG

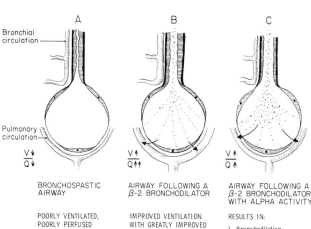

Figure 5–5. The addition of an alpha-receptor stimulator to a beta-2 stimulator theoretically results in a prolongation of the bronchodilator effect and a decrease in side-effects. A further advantage is that the increased shunt-like effect caused by beta-2 drugs is prevented by the alpha-agent, and the PaO_2 may rise rather than fall. These theoretical advantages are not always seen, however.

decrease the rate of removal of the isoproterenol. Rebound vasodilation, which occurs after initial mucosal decongestion in the nose, does not appear to be a problem in the lung. The systemic effects of any circulating isoproterenol (cardiac stimulation and shunting through the lungs) would be expected to be decreased as a result of the mucosal vasoconstriction caused by the addition of phenylephrine. At present, more facts are needed to support the conventional belief that phenylephrine is of value, in the light of the negative findings.

The combination aerosol product is marketed in two similar forms, as Duo-Medihaler and as Duohaler; each releases 137 mcg of isoproterenol and 126 mcg of phenylephrine per puff (Table 5–15). The aerosol is used in the same manner as are other metered isoproterenol products. At present, the combination should be considered as a possible improvement over isoproterenol alone, and can be regarded as particularly suitable for hypoxemic asthmatics who obtain only short-lived relief from isoproterenol on its own. The combination aerosol should not need to be used as frequently as isoproterenol alone, and dosage administration every four to six hours usually suffices.

Isoproterenol with Cyclopentamine. The great aerosol innovator, Dautrebande, devised a combination of drugs for the rational, pharmacologic treatment of bronchospasm.[11] He recommended isoproterenol in combination with cyclopentamine (Clopane, a mucosal decongestant, which has mainly alpha-adrenergic activity), procaine hydrochloride (for local anesthesia), atropine (to potentiate the bronchodilator effects by its anticholinergic action) and propylene glycol (a hygroscopic substance that stabilizes aerosol droplets). A diminished variation of his recommendation is currently marketed as Aerolone, which contains only isoproterenol and cyclopentamine (Table 5–15).

Aerolone is administered as is isoproterenol, either in a hand-bulb nebulizer, with an air compressor or by IPPB. The present formulation is comparable to Duo-Medihaler but, unlike the latter, it is not available as a metered product. Aerolone is rarely used, but perhaps deserves greater popularity. Dautrebande's original formulation may have greater merit, and it is rather regrettable that this interesting combination of products is not marketed.

A similar combination of isoproterenol and thonzonium was marketed as a metered product (Nebair), but is no longer available (Table 5–15).

Epinephrine

Epinephrine was discovered in 1897, and was introduced into medicine in the early 1900s. Thus, it was used in the treatment of asthma long before isoproterenol became available; it was first used as an aerosol in 1937. The drug is called adrenaline in England, and it is marketed throughout the world under a variety of commercial names. The base is relatively insoluble in water, but the hydrochloride and bitartrate salts are water-soluble. The bitartrate salt is said to be more stable and less irritating than the hydrochloride. The various preparations are relatively unstable and are prepared as acid solutions for optimal stability; they readily oxidize when exposed to air or alkalinity.

The naturally occurring drug is the levorotatory isomer l-epinephrine. When the drug is synthesized, an equal amount of the dextrorotatory isomer is also produced, and the mixture is called racemic epinephrine. The properties of the racemic mixture differ from those of l-epinephrine, and will be considered later; d-epinephrine has only about one-fifteenth the activity of the l-isomer, and it is not used on its own in clinical medicine.

Structure and Metabolism. Epinephrine is a catecholamine (Figure 5–3) and is extremely susceptible to enzymic breakdown by COMT and sulfatization. The structure of the molecule endows it with a mixture of alpha, beta-1 and beta-2 stimulatory properties. The alpha-adrenergic properties are potent, and epinephrine constricts mucosal and skin arterioles, while the beta-2 properties result in vasodilation, particularly affecting the skeletal muscle vessels.

Most of the epinephrine that is administered is inactivated in the liver, and the products are excreted in the urine. Only about 10 per cent is excreted by the kidney in its original form.

Actions. Epinephrine has had a long history of usefulness in the treatment of acute bronchospasm. For many years, it has been given subcutaneously as an agent of choice for status asthmaticus. At present, however, newer agents may be displacing epinephrine in acute asthma. Epinephrine has also been given by aerosol, but it is less satisfactory than other agents, although proprietary, metered products of epinephrine can be purchased without prescription, such as Primatene. Other metered bronchodilators, such as isoproterenol, cannot be obtained without a prescription; this presents a curious anomaly, since epinephrine has probably more potential for serious side effects than many other sympathomimetic bronchodilator agents.

The alpha-adrenergic properties can be utilized in many ways. The drug is used topically to arrest surface bleeding, and it can be given by injection to reduce blood flow in that area in order to help hemostasis or to limit removal of a primary drug (such as a local anesthetic) with which it is given simultaneously. An injection of intracardiac epinephrine can be used to resuscitate a patient with cardiac arrest. Another important use of the drug is in the acute management of allergic emergencies. It can also be used in the emergency treatment of hypoglycemia, since it causes glycogenolysis, whereby liver and muscle glycogen are converted to glucose; for this reason, it can cause marked changes in the blood sugar of diabetic patients.

When large parenteral doses of the drug are given, the blood pressure may initially rise, and then it may fall—presumably because the beta-2 effect (vasodilation) appears after the initial alpha effect (vasoconstriction). Vasodilation occurs mainly in the skeletal muscle mass, whereas vasoconstriction occurs in the skin vessels. Large doses of epinephrine usually result in an increase in systolic and a decrease in diastolic blood pressure with a variable effect on the mean, whereas small doses have less effect on the diastolic pressure and tend to result in an increase in the mean pressure (see Table 5–13); thus, the drug has a variable effect on blood pressure, although systolic pressure usually increases. When aerosol therapy is used, the blood pressure is usually unaffected, but subcutaneous administration can have marked pressor effects.

Epinephrine is not effective when given by mouth and has too much cardiovascular activity when given intravenously. Therefore, when used for bronchodilation, it is usually given subcutaneously or, more often, as an aerosol. Rebound effects may occur, with worsening of bronchospasm, but are rare in practice. The important features of epinephrine are summarized in Table 5–17.

Dosages and Recommendations. Various formulations of epinephrine are available, and different strengths are marketed for administration by various routes (Table 5–18).

SUBCUTANEOUS. Usually, a 1:1000 solution is used. The appropriate dose is 0.1 to 0.5 mg; the injection should be given very slowly over the course of a few minutes, and administration should be stopped if adverse symptoms develop. The injected area should be massaged, to facilitate absorption of the drug. If necessary, a further injection can be given after about half an hour, to a maximum of 1 mg; this total dose may be repeated, if needed, every four to six hours. It is rarely necessary or desirable to use more than two injections in this fashion; if the response is suboptimal, another drug should be used. Repeated doses of epinephrine should not be used as the basic treatment in most asthmatics, although there are some patients who appear to do well with this drug; in some cases, it may even be appropriate to prescribe this form of therapy for domiciliary use. However, any patient who routinely uses subcutaneous epinephrine should be suspected of a psychologic dependency on this exaggerated method of control of bronchospasm.

There are patients who are very tolerant of

TABLE 5–17.   EPINEPHRINE

OFFICIAL NAME	l-epinephrine; l-3,4-dihydroxyphenylethanolamine
OTHER NAMES	Adrenaline, suprarenin
CLINICAL USES	Bronchodilator, topical vasoconstrictor, for various allergic reactions, vasopressor, intracardiac stimulant, to increase blood sugar
AVAILABILITY	Aqueous solutions (for inhalation and parenteral use); suspensions in oil (for intramuscular use)
CONCENTRATIONS	1:100 (1%) for inhalation; 1:200 (0.5%) to 1:1,000 (0.1%) for parenteral administration
ADVERSE REACTIONS	Agitation, restlessness, palpitations, tachyarrhythmias, sweating, headache, pallor, nausea, angina, euphoria, psychosis, urinary retention, bronchial irritation
DISADVANTAGES	Frequency of disturbing side effects; short-lasting effect when given by aerosol; availability of different concentrations can result in errors in dosing

TABLE 5-18. EPINEPHRINE PRODUCTS

Product	Constituents	Strength	Availability	Dosage Adult	Child
METERED AEROSOLS					
*Asmatane Mist	Epinephrine bitartrate suspension	7 mg/ml	0.16 mg base/puff	1-4 inhalations 4-6 times/day; up to 8 inhalations in an emergency	1-3 inhalations 4-6 times/day
Asthmahaler (15 ml)	Epinephrine bitartrate suspension	5.5 mg/ml	0.20 mg base/puff		
Asthma Meter Mist (15 ml)	Epinephrine solution	4 mg/ml	0.20 mg/puff		
Asthma Nephrin	Racemic epinephrine HCl	8.3 mg/ml	0.30 mg/puff		
Bronitin Mist (20 ml)	Epinephrine bitartrate suspension	7 mg/ml	0.16 mg base/puff		
Bronkaid Mist (15 and 22.5 ml)	Epinephrine solution	4 mg/ml	0.20 mg/puff		
Epinephrine (various)	Epinephrine hydrochloride	5.5 mg/ml	0.20 mg base/puff		
Medihaler-Epi (15 ml)	Epinephrine bitartrate suspension	7 mg/ml	0.16 mg base/puff		
Primatene Mist (15 and 22.5 ml)	Epinephrine	5 mg/ml	0.20 mg/puff		
Primatene Mist Suspension (10 ml)	Epinephrine bitartrate suspension	7 mg/ml	0.16 mg base/puff		
*Vaponephrin Metermatic	Racemic epinephrine HCl	8.3 mg/ml	0.30 mg/puff		
SOLUTIONS FOR INHALATION					
Adrenalin	Epinephrine hydrochloride	1% (1:100)	10 mg/ml	Hand bulb: 2-6 inhalations 4-6 times a day. IPPB: 0.3-1 ml diluted or undiluted every 2-4 hours	Hand bulb: 2-4 inhalations 4-6 times a day. IPPB: 0.3-0.6 ml diluted or undiluted every 2-4 hours
Asthma Nephrin	Racemic epinephrine HCl	2.25%	22.5 mg/ml		
Breatheasy	Epinephrine hydrochloride	2.20%	22 mg/ml		
Epinephrine USP	Epinephrine hydrochloride	1% (1:100)	10 mg/ml		
†Micronephrin	Racemic epinephrine HCl	2.25%	22.5 mg/ml		
Vaponephrin	Racemic epinephrine HCl	2.25%	22.5 mg/ml		
NASAL TOPICAL SOLUTIONS					
Adrenalin	Epinephrine hydrochloride	1:1000	1 mg/ml	Use as needed.	Use as needed.
Epinephrine (various)	Epinephrine hydrochloride	1:1000	1 mg/ml		
SUBCUTANEOUS PREPARATIONS					
†Adrenalin	Epinephrine hydrochloride	1:1000	1 mg/ml	0.1-1 ml q4-6h	0.01 ml/kg q4h
†Asmolin	Epinephrine (aqueous suspension)	1:400	2.5 mg/ml	0.05-0.4 ml q4-6h	0.004 ml/kg q4h
†Epinephrine USP	Epinephrine (HCl or bitartrate)	1:1000	1 mg/ml	0.1-1 ml q4-6h	0.01 ml/kg q4h
†Sus-Phrine	Epinephrine (aqueous suspension)	1:200	5 mg/ml	0.05-0.3 ml q4-6h	0.004 ml/kg q8-12h
INTRAMUSCULAR PREPARATIONS					
†Asmolin	Epinephrine (aqueous + glycerin)	1:400	2.5 mg/ml	0.05-0.6 ml q4-8h	0.008 ml/kg q8h
†Adrenalin in oil	Epinephrine (in oil)	1:500	2 mg/ml	0.2-1 ml q8-16h	0.01-0.02 ml/kg q12-24h
†Epinephrine in oil (various)	Epinephrine (in oil)	1:500	2 mg/ml	0.2-1 ml q8-16h	0.01-0.02 ml/kg q12-24h
INTRAVENOUS PREPARATIONS					
†Various	Epinephrine hydrochloride	1:1000	1 mg/ml	Up to 0.25 ml, slowly	Not recommended

*No longer marketed
†Requires a prescription; other listed products are available without prescription.
The formerly marketed more potent metered aerosol preparations delivered almost twice the amount of epinephrine base as does the least potent preparations.

epinephrine; for these asthmatics, a more concentrated preparation (1:400) can be used. An aqueous 1:200 suspension of epinephrine is marketed as Sus-Phrine, in which the drug is present both as a solution and as a crystalline suspension. This formulation exerts a prolonged effect, which may persist for as long as 8 to 10 hours, and it may be useful to prevent frequent or recurring attacks of severe asthma, since it provides both immediate and sustained bronchospasmolytic effects. An initial test dose should not exceed 0.1 ml in adults or 0.005 ml/kg in children. Care should be taken to ensure that the injection is not made intravenously. The maximum dose for adults is 0.3 ml every four hours; for children, no more than 0.15 ml every eight hours is advised.

INTRAMUSCULAR. Several long-acting preparations are marketed that are suitable for intramuscular administration. These preparations include epinephrine-in-oil 1:500; the bronchodilator effect may persist for up to 16 hours after one dose. These preparations are similar to subcutaneous Sus-Phrine; appropriate dosages should be given, observing similar precautions to those discussed above. Intramuscular injections should not be given into the buttocks, which are susceptible to subcutaneous infection. In general, the use of epinephrine-in-oil is no longer favored because of the possibility of sterile abscesses and other tissue complications

INTRAVENOUS. Epinephrine is rarely given intravenously in the management of asthma, although the 1:1000 aqueous preparation could be used, cautiously, in adults. The same preparation, diluted to 1:10,000, can be given by intracardiac injection as a resuscitative measure during the management of a cardiac arrest.

AEROSOL. The much more concentrated 1:100 solution is used for nebulization: solutions are available as metered products and as preparations for aerosolization with various nebulizers or IPPB. Although most antiasthma products are available only with a physician's prescription, there are many patients who do well enough with the over-the-counter preparations of metered epinephrine; physicians should be willing to endorse these products. Epinephrine is less commonly given by IPPB, since racemic epinephrine is generally preferred. If given by IPPB, it should be diluted in the manner advised for racemic epinephrine. An aerosol preparation may offer a useful emergency standby for very allergic patients, such as those who develop serious reactions to insect stings: the aerosol drug may permit easy, rapid emergency treatment by nebulization into the oropharynx and lungs. However, this form of therapy is not regarded as optimal, and the susceptible allergic patient should prefer the use of subcutaneous epinephrine in such emergencies.

No solution of epinephrine should be used if it has developed a brown color, since the responsible adrenochromes have been reported to cause adverse reactions (such as hallucinations); however, beta-blockade has not been observed.

Care must always be taken to ensure that the appropriate concentration of epinephrine is given. The risk of an inappropriate selection causing a serious misadventure is sufficiently great to further detract from the popularity of epinephrine as a bronchodilator.

Racemic Epinephrine

The combined mixture of d- and l-epinephrine is currently favored for aerosol therapy in place of l-epinephrine. The racemic mixture is available for nebulization as 2.25 per cent solution forms of the hydrochloride, and as metered preparations containing 8.3 mg/ml (see Table 5–18).

The levo-form is 15 times more active than the dextro-form, but one manufacturer claims that the racemic preparation offers the advantages of the potent beta-2 properties of the levo-isomer combined with the lessened beta-1 and alpha activity conferred by the dextro-isomer. This claim is difficult to accept on theoretic grounds, and no adequate controlled trial has been conducted to establish the superiority of racemic epinephrine. The racemic mixture probably has only half the activity of l-epinephrine; nevertheless, clinical experience has led to the racemic drug being used as much as the levo-isomer as an aerosol bronchodilator.

Racemic epinephrine currently appears to be less popular than isoproterenol, both for metered aerosol use and for nebulization with IPPB. However, it may have real advantages over isoproterenol, since the alpha-adrenergic effect of racemic epinephrine results in mucosal vasoconstriction, with the attendant benefits of prolongation of bronchodilator action, lessened risk of hypoxemia, and reduction of mucosal engorgement.

One important disadvantage of the epinephrine drugs compared with isoproterenol should be kept in mind. If an asthmatic patient is given a beta-blocking agent and develops bronchospasm as a result, treatment with isoproterenol may reverse the spasm, whereas epinephrine may worsen the condition, since the combination of the alpha-adrenergic effect of the epinephrine with the beta blockade potentiates the bronchospastic mechanism.

Dosages and Recommendations. The two available solutions for aerosolization are administered according to the manufacturers' recommendations (Table 5-18). The metered product (Vaponefrin Metermatic) is no longer marketed. The drug is an effective, inexpensive alternative to isoproterenol for routine use. It is recommended for the treatment of laryngotracheobronchitis,[59a] since its alpha-adrenergic effect results in decongestion of the inflamed mucosa. It may be of particular value in the treatment of croup in children, although this has not been clearly established.[60] Further studies are also required to confirm the claim that it is useful in patients who have been intubated: it may help reduce the mucosal swelling found in post-intubation laryngotracheitis.

After nebulization therapy, a warm, alkaline mouthwash or gargle can be used to remove excessive drug, and to prevent drying and irritation of the oropharynx, which can be a problem with both forms of epinephrine. Patients should be cautioned to avoid breathing the aerosol through the nose, in order to avoid causing irritation of the nasal mucosa.

Ethylnorepinephrine

Ethylnorepinephrine has been available since the 1930s; it was introduced as a bronchodilator in 1944 but has never become popular. The drug is marketed as the hydrochloride, as Butanefrine and, more commonly, as Bronkephrine (Table 5-19). It is similar to epinephrine (Figure 5-3) but

TABLE 5-19.   ETHYLNOREPINEPHRINE

BRAND NAMES	Bronkephrine, Butanephrine
PROPERTIES	Similar to epinephrine; has less pressor effect, causes less central nervous system excitation and has less effect on blood sugar
AVAILABILITY	For intramuscular and subcutaneous injection as a 0.2% solution
DOSAGE	Child 0.1–0.5 ml, adult 0.3–1.0 ml; every 3–4 hours

with less effect on blood pressure; however, it is alleged to have much less bronchodilator activity than isoproterenol. It is claimed to cause less central nervous system excitation than does epinephrine, and it may, therefore, be more acceptable for children. Indeed, it has been recommended as a drug of choice for home administration for asthma.[61]

Ethylnorepinephrine is available only as an aqueous 0.2 per cent solution for injection, and can be given by either the intramuscular or the subcutaneous route, in a dosage of 0.1 to 0.5 ml (0.2 to 1 mg) in children, and 0.3 to 1.0 ml (0.6 to 2 mg) in adults. It is used mainly in the treatment of status asthmaticus, particularly in patients who develop adverse blood pressure responses to an injection of epinephrine. Diabetics with asthma find the drug of value since it is less likely to cause an increase in the blood sugar. Ethylnorepinephrine could also be given by inhalation, but it does not appear to have been used in this fashion. Although it can also be given intravenously, this route is not recommended, since experience with this form of therapy is lacking.

Isoetharine

Isoetharine (Dilabron) resembles isoproterenol in structure, except that it has an ethyl group on the α-carbon atom (Fig. 5-3); it is, in fact, the N-isopropyl analogue of ethylnorepinephrine (Table 5-12); it can be called isopropylethylnorepinephrine. The drug was introduced in 1950. It is made available as isoetharine mesylate and isoetharine hydrochloride for aerosol therapy; an oral product, isoetharine methanesulfonate, has not been marketed in the U.S., although it also is an effective bronchodilator.[62]

Actions. It has been shown that isoetharine has relatively little beta-1 activity and negligible alpha activity (Table 5-12). The evidence suggests that it is less potent than isoproterenol as a bronchodilator, since, weight for weight, it has only one-third to one-half the potency.[56] Although aerosol administration of isoetharine causes markedly less cardiac stimulation than does isoproterenol, there is ample evidence to show that isoetharine does cause some beta-1 adrenergic stimulation;[63] thus, the drug is not truly a selective beta-2 stimulator, as is often implied. Moreover, when given orally it can affect blood pressure, resulting in a gradual fall in both systolic and diastolic values.[64]

Isoetharine is made available in the U.S.

TABLE 5–20. ISOETHARINE*

OFFICIAL NAME	N-isopropylnorepinephrine (Dilabron)
AVAILABILITY	In U.S., available for aerosol use only in combination with phenylephrine (Bronkometer and Bronkosol). In some other countries, it is available as oral tablets.
ADVANTAGES	The aerosol preparations are effective as medium-acting bronchodilators, of moderate potency, with relatively low potential for side-effects.
DISADVANTAGES	The aerosol preparations can cause significant cardiac stimulation if used in large doses; may cause a slight fall in blood pressure.
USES	One of the standard aerosol bronchodilator preparations, mainly of use in patients with liability to cardiac arrhythmias

*Recently, the FDA required that phenylephrine be removed from the marketed combination products of isoetharine.

only as combination aerosol products (Bronkosol and Bronkometer), which contain isoetharine and phenylephrine (Table 5–20). The addition of the phenylephrine is supposed to decrease some of the side effects and prolong the action of the isoetharine, in similar fashion to its role in combination with isoproterenol in Duo-Medihaler. However, a recent study, in which Bronkosol was compared with isoetharine alone, throws doubt on the benefit of the added phenylephrine.[64a] In the study, the combination had no more potent or persistent bronchodilator effects, nor did it result in less side effects; furthermore, the addition of the phenylephrine did not have any beneficial effect on oxygen saturation. In spite of these discouraging observations, Bronkosol enjoys considerable popularity, and in many hospitals it is the bronchodilator of choice. Bronkosol is undoubtedly relatively potent, and the recommended dosage produces significant bronchodilatation for three to four hours. The product is safe, and in usual inhalational

doses it has little cardiovascular side effects; the blood pressure may be decreased slightly, and the pulse may be insignificantly altered. Central nervous system stimulation is unlikely to be a problem, and tremulousness is rarely caused. Rebound problems do not appear to occur following the usual dosage of the combination preparation.

A formerly marketed preparation also contained thenyldiamine, which is an antihistamine. In general, this class of drugs has not been found to be of value in inhalation therapy. Thenyldiamine could not be demonstrated to add any benefit to the combination of isoetharine and phenylephrine and was therefore removed from the formulation. Whether the manufacturer will be required by the FDA to remove phenylephrine remains to be seen. Although the combination is well-established, such a bureacratic requirement is not unlikely.†

Oral and intravenous preparations of isoetharine would probably be of value in the treatment of bronchospasm,[63] but these formulations have never been made available in the U.S. Although the aerosol product is extremely popular in the U.S., it is much less popular in Great Britain (where Bronkosol aerosol is named Bronchilator, and 10 mg tablets are available as Numotac). It is curious that an oral form of isoetharine is not available in the U.S., since there is evidence to suggest that it would be very useful.[4]

Dosages and Recommendations (Table 5–21). The metered aerosol Bronkometer should be used in similar fashion to metered preparations of other bronchodilators. Generally, one or two puffs every four hours suffice, but some patients need four puffs for an adequate effect and they may find that repeat treatments are required more often than every four hours. The half-life varies in different patients, and it decreases following intensive use; for most patients, the bronchodilator effect probably lasts one to three hours.

TABLE 5–21. ISOETHARINE PREPARATIONS*

Brand Name	Constituents†		Availability	Dose/Puff	Dosage
Bronkosol	Isoetharine hydrochloride	1%	Aqueous glycerin solution		3–7 inhalations undiluted, or 0.25–1 ml diluted (using IPPB)
	Phenylephrine hydrochloride	0.25%			
Bronkometer	Isoetharine mesylate	0.61%	Metered alcoholic solution	340 mcg	1–4 puffs q3–6 hr; maximum 12 puffs a day
	Phenylephrine hydrochloride	0.125%		70 mcg	

*Oral preparations are not available in U.S.A. The available products require a prescription.
†Thenyldiamine hydrochloride, an original constituent, is no longer included and phenylephrine was recently withdrawn from these preparations.

When the drug is administered, as Bronkosol solution, by a hand nebulizer or a simple air compressor, three to seven inhalations are recommended. If the preparation is delivered by IPPB, it is usual to dilute 0.5 ml of Bronkosol with 1.5 ml of water or saline; as much as 1 ml of the drug may be needed for maximal effect when using IPPB. Thus, the optimal dose and concentration is usually established by cautiously increasing the amount of the bronchodilator, or perhaps by decreasing the amount of diluent.

Although an oral preparation is not marketed, appropriate dosages of tablets or syrup have been recommended, with a range between 2 and 10 mg four times a day.[64, 65] The response to oral isoetharine is not known with certainty, but it may be similar to the effect produced by the same dosage of metaproterenol. A slow-release oral tablet has been shown to be comparable in bronchodilator potency and in persistence of effect to an equal dose of metaproterenol.[66]

The main value of Bronkosol is in providing frequent bronchodilator therapy in patients who do not tolerate the less expensive isoproterenol or epinephrine; such patients are, particularly, those with cardiac irritability. Since elderly patients with myocardial ischemia are frequently in need of bronchodilator therapy in intensive care unit settings, Bronkosol often becomes a standard drug on such units. Fewer patients need Bronkometer, since isoproterenol products are less expensive and are safe alternatives, but if isoproteronol causes unpleasant symptoms, Bronkometer or Bronkosol (with a hand-bulb nebulizer) should be tried instead. Many physicians alternate their patients' therapy using isoproterenol, racemic epinephrine and Bronkosol on a rotational basis. It should be recognized that the marketed products of isoetharine are probably very comparable in efficacy and in side effects to the aerosolizable combination of isoproterenol with phenylephrine. However, Bronkometer does not appear to have been studied in comparison with Duo-Medihaler.

Rimiterol

The latest bronchodilator to be marketed in England is rimiterol (WG 253, R798, Pulmadil). This compound is a catecholamine derivative, and it is classified as one of the aryl-2-piperidyl carbinol series of sympathomimetic amines, in which the side chain is cyclized about the α-carbon atom to form a piperidyl ring. It is comparable to isoetharine, whose substituent at the α-atom can be regarded as an uncyclized side chain[67] (Table 5–12).

Rimiterol is a selective beta-2 adrenergic stimulator, as may be expected, since it lacks the terminal ethanolamine chain configuration that is usual in alpha and beta-1 stimulating drugs. However, it is susceptible to sulfatization, and it is, therefore, unsuitable for oral administration. The drug can be given by metered aerosol or by IPPB; it has also been shown to be safe when given intravenously.[68]

Rimiterol has bronchodilating properties similar to those of isoproterenol, and it is a potent short-acting drug, but produces no significant extrapulmonary cardiovascular effects. Thus, when compared with the long-acting agent salbutamol, rimiterol had a similar but shorter bronchodilator effect, and much less beta-1 stimulant activity, when given as a 0.5 per cent solution.[67] Rimiterol is the only bronchodilator that is a potent, short-acting selective stimulator of the beta-2 receptors of bronchial muscle. Its bronchodilator effect lasts about two hours, which is comparable to the persistence of bronchodilatation following isoproterenol. When given by aerosol, beta-1 reactions such as tachycardia are minimal, and nervous system side effects are not a problem.[69] This drug has qualities that should make it popular for the aerosol management of mild to moderate bronchospasm; it could contend as a drug of choice for administration by IPPB.[67, 68] However, at present there appear to be no plans to introduce rimiterol into the U.S.

LONGER-ACTING SYMPATHOMIMETIC BRONCHODILATORS

Ephedrine

This drug has a history as a medicinal of over 5000 years. It is obtained from the shrub *Ephedra sinica*. The Chinese used its sympathomimetic properties in their ancient preparation Ma Huang (yellow astringent). It was not until 1923 that the drug entered Western medicine, and it has become a favorite oral bronchodilator since then. Ephedrine is sometimes known as Ephetonin.

Structure and Metabolism. The ephedrine that is available is, chemically, phenylisopropanolmethylamine; it is produced by synthesis, and the product is the levorotatory isomer l-ephedrine. Five other isomeric forms exist; none of these preparations are regarded as bronchodilators. The drug is not a catecholamine, since it has no hydroxy groupings in the benzene nucleus; chemically, it is classified as a phenylalkylamine alkaloid (Tables 5–12 and 5–14). It resembles epinephrine, in that it has a single methyl substitute group in the amine group of the ethanolamine side chain; this configuration might be expected to confer moderately strong beta-2 properties, in association with some alpha-adrenergic activity and marked beta-1 effectiveness. However, since ephedrine lacks hydroxy groups in the benzene nucleus (Table 5–12), it is only a moderately strong direct stimulator of beta-2 receptors. Ephedrine also has an indirect bronchodilator effect, and it is sometimes classified pharmaceutically as an indirectly acting phenylisopropylamine; this class of drugs releases the sympathetic neurotransmitter norepinephrine from storage granules in adrenergic nerve endings, which, in turn, stimulates the adrenergic receptors.

Ephedrine differs from most alkaloids in being water soluble; it dissolves to form a very alkaline solution. The drug is usually employed in the form of either its hydrochloride or its sulfate. The sulfate contains less ephedrine base, but it causes less tissue irritation than the hydrochloride and is, therefore, preferred for the injectable preparation.

Since the drug is not a substrate for sulfatization, it can be given by mouth. The methyl group on the alpha carbon atom renders it resistant to the enzyme MAO. Its main metabolite is norephedrine, formed by demethylation, but 40 per cent or more of the drug is excreted unchanged in the urine.[70] It is well-absorbed when given by mouth, and it has a plasma half-life of about three to twelve hours, with a mean of about five to seven hours;[70a] the half-life becomes shorter following repeated administration of the drug. After an oral dose of 25 mg, the onset of action occurs slowly over the next hour; significant bronchodilatation may persist for about four hours.[71] The rate of excretion is affected by the pH of the urine, with more rapid excretion in an acid urine; the effect of the acid-base balance on the half-life of ephedrine has not been studied, but it may be significant.[5] The drug is effective when given as a 2 per cent solution by aerosolization, but, in practice, it is not given by this route.[5] It is suitable for intravenous and subcutaneous use, although it is not administered by injection in the treatment of bronchospasm.

Actions. Ephedrine is a moderately effective bronchodilator, but has become less popular for this purpose. Although it is still of value in the prophylactic management of mild asthma,[72] recent reports have suggested that the drug is of little value either therapeutically[73, 74] or as a preventative[75] in various forms of asthma. A major problem is that much of its action appears to depend upon the drug liberating catecholamine from storage granules; with prolonged administration or large dosages, these granules in the nerve endings seem to become gradually depleted. Thus, the rapid development of tachyphylaxis is a characteristic problem accompanying the use of ephedrine. The bronchodilator effect of ephedrine can diminish significantly within a few days of initiating the drug, using three or four times a

TABLE 5–22. EPHEDRINE

OFFICIAL NAME	Phenylisopropanolmethylamine, or L-α-[1-(methylamino) ethyl] benzyl alcohol; the levo-isomer of ephedrine is used
CLINICAL USES	Minor bronchodilator, pressor agent, mucosal constrictor, cardiac stimulant, central nervous system stimulant, mydriatic; also used in treatment of myasthenia gravis, narcolepsy and enuresis
INDICATIONS	Minor bronchospasm, especially in younger patients
DISADVANTAGES	Annoying side effects (including nervousness, insomnia, tremor, cardiac irritation, urinary retention in elderly men); may aggravate diabetes mellitus, hyperthyroidism and glaucoma (this is unconfirmed)
CONTRAINDICATIONS	Moderate or severe bronchospasm; hypertension or cardiac disease; anxiety, agitation, poor sleep; concomitant use of MAO inhibitor or hypertensive agents; glaucoma
AVAILABILITY	Mainly as sulfate, but also as hydrochloride; generally used in combination preparations with theophylline and a tranquilizer
DOSAGE	Adults: 15–50 mg 4–6 times a day; children aged 6–12: 6.25–12.5 mg 4–6 times a day; children aged 2–6: 0.3–0.5 mg/kg 4–6 times a day

day dosage. As a result, some patients require progressively larger doses, and they may become habituated to the drug.

Ephedrine is used occasionally for other purposes, such as the treatment of heart block, as a pressor agent, as a mucosal decongestant for the treatment of nasal allergies, as a central nervous system stimulant, as an agent in the treatment of myasthenia gravis and as a mydriatic (although it is less effective in darkly pigmented eyes); it is also used in treating enuresis and narcolepsy by preventing deep sleep (see Table 5–22). These central properties are a problem when the drug is used in the treatment of asthma, since it causes nervousness, marked anxiety and insomnia; in older men, it causes relaxation of bladder musculature and may result in the development of urinary retention. Because of its annoying central stimulating qualities, the drug is often given in suboptimal dosage in combination with theophylline; however, it probably does not confer any useful bronchodilator action in such reduced dosage, although the central nervous system is still stimulated.[76] Usually, a tranquilizer is incorporated in these combination tablets, such as Marax, Tedral and so forth (see Table 6–16). Other preparations of ephedrine combined with a barbiturate are marketed; some brands also contain an antihistamine, a mjcokinetic or a cough suppressant (Table 5–23). In these preparations, ephedrine is usually present as the hydrochloride, whereas the sulfate is used both on its own and in combination preparations.

Dosage and Recommendations. When used alone, ephedrine sulfate is preferred to the hydrochloride (Table 5–24); the usual dose is 15 to 50 mg four times a day in adults. More often, proprietary combination products (Table 5–23) are used, and one or two tablets (or the equivalent of an alternative preparation) are administered three or four times a day. The recent spate of criticisms of combination products containing theophylline and ephedrine is based on the fact that many are no more effective than the same dose of theophylline given alone. Although doctors and patients are often satisfied with the combination products, it is recommended that initial consideration be given to using single drug therapy. However, it is clear that not all authorities accept the criticisms of combination preparations containing ephedrine.[72]

The dosage for children has been a subject of contention. Recently it has been recommended that older children can receive 6.25 to 12.5 mg, not more often than every four hours, up to a maximum of 75 mg a day. For children aged 2 to 6, the appropriate dose is 0.3 to 0.5 mg per kg., which can be given every four hours up to a maximum of 2 mg per kg per day.

Since the drug is an inferior agent, the recent availability of newer oral sympathomimetics makes ephedrine a poor choice for the management of bronchospasm, except in milder cases that respond to the drug[70]. Not only is ephedrine unreliable in its effect, with a marked tendency to lose effectiveness due to tolerance, it also has too many side effects. The drug is contraindicated in hypertension and in cardiac disease (since it has alpha and beta-1 adrenergic effects), and it should not be used in nervous or agitated people, or in those who sleep poorly. If a depressed patient is treated with a monoamine oxidase inhibitor antidepressant, then the action of ephedrine will be potentiated, and the resulting marked rise in blood pressure could cause a subarachnoid hemorrhage.

Unfortunately, many patients with bronchospastic disease are elderly men who are hypertensive and have cardiac disease, and who are also agitated, sleep poorly and have prostatic hypertrophy; some may even be on monoamine oxidase inhibitor drugs for depression. Under these circumstances, it is surprising that such patients can tolerate ephedrine-containing bronchodilators, which are often prescribed with relative disregard for the side effects; although patients may tolerate such therapy, it would be prudent to avoid the use of ephedrine in the face of such contraindications.

Pseudoephedrine

The *dextro-stereoisomer* of ephedrine, called pseudoephedrine or isoephedrine, is the only isomeric form of ephedrine used to any extent in therapeutics. Racemic ephedrine (a combination of dextro- and levoephedrine, also known as *racephedrine*) is virtually the same as l-ephedrine. Levo- and racemic-pseudoephedrine, although closely related to d-pseudoephedrine, are not of medical value.

TABLE 5–23. PROPRIETARY BRONCHODILATOR COMBINATIONS CONTAINING EPHEDRINE*

Brand Name	Basic Dosage Form	Ephedrine	Antihistamine	Barbiturate	Mucokinetic	Other
Benadryl with Ephedrine	Capsule	25 mg	Diphenhydramine 50 mg			
Calcidrine	Elixir, 5 ml	4.2 mg			Calcium iodide 152 mg	Codeine 8.4 mg Alcohol 6%
Ephed-Organidin	Tablet	24 mg	Methapyrilene 70 mg		Iodinated glycerol 60 mg	
Ephedrine and Nembutal 25	Capsule	25 mg		Pentobarbital 25 mg		
Ephedrine and Amytal	Pulvule	25 mg		Amobarbital 50 mg		
Ectasule Sr	Capsule†	60 mg		Amobarbital 30 mg		
Ectasule Jr	Capsule†	30 mg		Amobarbital 15 mg		
Ectasule III	Capsule†	15 mg		Amobarbital 8 mg		
Ephedrine and Seconal	Pulvule	25 mg		Secobarbital 50 mg		
KIE	Syrup, 15 ml / Tablet	24 mg / 24 mg			KI 450 mg / KI 400 mg	
Novalene	Tablet	24 mg		Phenobarbital 16 mg	KI 162 mg	Calcium lactate 162 mg
Pyribenzamine with Ephedrine	Tablet	12 mg	Tripelennamine 25 mg			
Pyribenzamine Expectorant	Solution, 4 ml	10 mg	Tripelennamine 20 mg		Ammonium chloride 80 mg	(±Codeine 8 mg)
Slo-Fedrin A 30 / A 60	Capsule† / Capsule†	30 mg / 60 mg		Amobarbital 15 mg / Amobarbital 30 mg		
Rynatuss	Tablet	10 mg	Chlorpheniramine 5 mg			Carbetapentane 60 mg Phenylephrine 10 mg
	Suspension, 5 ml	5 mg	Chlorpheniramine 4 mg			Carbetapentane 30 mg Phenylephrine 5 mg

*Other combination preparations that also contain a theophylline are listed in Table 6–17.
†Time-release preparation.
Note: These preparations usually require a prescription; some are controlled substances, in Schedules 4 and 5.

TABLE 5–24. EPHEDRINE AND PSEUDOEPHEDRINE*

Brands	Capsules or Tablets (mg)	Slow-Release Capsules (mg)	Elixirs/Syrups (mg/5 ml)	Injections (mg/ml)	Nasal Solutions (Per Cent)
EPHEDRINE SULFATE					
Ectasule Minus		15,30,60			
Slo-Fedrin		30,60			
Various	25†,30,50	25,50	4.5,10†,20†	25,50	1,3
PSEUDOEPHEDRINE HYDROCHLORIDE					
D-Feda		60	30†		
Neofed		60			
Novafed		120	30†		
Pseudo-Bid		120			
Sudabid		120			
Sudadrine			30†		
Sudafed	30†,60†		30†		
Sudecon	60		30†		
Various products	30†, 60				

*Numerous combination products of these drugs are available. These products are listed in Facts and Comparisons.
†Available without prescription.

Pseudoephedrine is used mainly as a nasal decongestant (in such products as Sudafed and in combination preparations such as Actifed), but it is not generally appreciated that it is equally effective a bronchodilator as is ephedrine. Pseudoephedrine has the distinct advantage of less pressor activity and is, therefore, safer for use in patients with hypertension or cardiovascular problems. The appropriate adult oral dose is 60 mg three or four times a day; children can be given the syrup in a dosage of 1 mg/kg four times a day. Pseudoephedrine is a popular mucosal constrictor, and it is useful for patients with nasal congestion and mild bronchospasm. A large number of proprietary preparations are available. Table 5–24 lists some of the simple products on the market.

Methoxyphenamine

The structure of methoxyphenamine (orthomethoxy-beta-phenylisopropyl methylamine hydrochloride) is somewhat similar to that of ephedrine, although it has a methoxy group in the benzene nucleus at position 2 (Table 5–12). It has beta-2 activity comparable to that of ephedrine, but it has less beta-1 activity and no alpha-adrenergic effects. Thus, methoxyphenamine is a potent bronchodilator,[77] with the advantage of no significant pressor or cardiovascular side effects; indeed, it may cause a slight fall in blood pressure. It is also alleged to have antihistamine action and it is less likely than ephedrine to cause insomnia (in fact, large doses cause drowsiness). Side effects include dry mouth, nausea and faintness.

There is controversy regarding the full

TABLE 5–25. COMPARISON OF THE "OLDER" ORAL SYMPATHOMIMETIC BRONCHODILATORS

	Ephedrine	Pseudoephedrine	Methoxyphenamine	Protokylol
BRAND NAMES	Various	Sudafed, etc.	Orthoxine	Ventaire
CLINICAL PROPERTIES				
Bronchodilator	+	+	+	+
Decongestant	+	++	±	±
Pressor agent	+	±	−	±
Cardiac stimulator	+	±	±	+
Central stimulant	+	±	±	+
Antiallergy agent	+	+	+	±
Antihistaminic	−	−	+	−
DOSE (adult) (3 or 4 times a day)	15–50 mg.	30–60 mg.	50–100 mg.	2–4 mg.

adrenergic effect of methoxyphenamine; it is possible that it has some ability to cause blockade of alpha and beta receptors. The evidence suggests that this agent should be a useful oral bronchodilator, but although it has been available for many years (for example, as Orthoxine), it is rarely employed. The drug is available in tablet and syrup forms; the adult dose is 50 to 100 mg four times a day; half this dosage is appropriate for children. The drug has not been used as an aerosol. Methoxyphenamine may be used as an alternative to ephedrine, although it is doubtful that this drug has much of a role in the current bronchodilator market (Table 5–25). Its main use may be for allergic patients with asthma who have hypertension; such patients should avoid ephedrine because of its pressor effects.

Protokylol

Protokylol was synthesized in 1954; it differs from most other bronchodilators in that it has a complex cyclic substituent added to the amino group of the catecholamine molecule. Chemically, protokylol is a derivative of protocatechuyl alcohol.

This drug has had a checkered history. It was made available in the United States years ago as Caytine, which was marketed in oral, parenteral and aerosol forms.[78] The product was not promoted vigorously, and it gradually fell into disuse. Recently, it was reissued in the form of a hydrochloride salt as a tablet, called Ventaire. It is possible, but unlikely, that the aerosol and parenteral preparations will be reissued in the future.

Protokylol has not been adequately studied, but evidence suggests that the oral preparation is similar to ephedrine, with an onset of action in 30 to 90 minutes, and an effect persisting up to four hours. It is equal to ephedrine in potency as a bronchodilator, and it has the same or more central nervous system side effects, according to the manufacturer's (Marion Laboratories) literature. However, it has little or no alpha-adrenergic activity, and it probably causes less beta-1 stimulation than does ephedrine, which suggests that it is apparently safer than ephedrine for use in hypertensive patients. In general, protokylol is similar to methoxyphenamine (Table 5–25), but it may be a better bronchodilator. The exact properties and values of both of these oral agents requires much better definition than is currently available, and, until such information

is obtained, these two drugs will remain relatively obscure.

Dosage and Recommendations. The appropriate dose of oral protokylol for adults is 2 mg three or four times a day; some patients may require half this dosage, and others may need twice as much. Protokylol has not been approved for children. Although Ventaire was, until recently, promoted quite vigorously, experience with this drug is inadequate, and it is difficult to recommend it except for trial use in a patient who has not benefited appropriately from other oral bronchodilators.

Metaproterenol

Metaproterenol is a derivative of isoproterenol; it has been available since 1961. In Europe the drug is called orciprenaline; it is marketed in the U.S. as Alupent and as Metaprel. These products are identical; they consist of a racemic mixture of two isomers of metaproterenol prepared as the sulfate. Metaproterenol is structurally similar to isoproterenol except that it is a resorcinol and not a catecholamine (Figure 5–3); that is, it has two hydroxy groups, which are at positions 3 and 5 (the meta-orientation) in the benzene nucleus rather than at 3 and 4 (Table 5–12). This difference renders metaproterenol immune from degradation by sulfatization and by COMT; it is excreted mainly as glucuronic acid conjugates. This bronchodilator is effective when given by mouth, and it is a long-acting drug with a persistence of effect lasting about five hours.[79] Overall, metaproterenol has been reported to be 10 to 40 times less active than isoproterenol as a beta-receptor stimulator.[1]

Although it is claimed that metaproterenol has no beta-1 effects when given by inhalation,[80] it is not correct to claim that it is a selective beta-2 stimulator, since, when it is given intravenously, metaproterenol produces as much an increase in heart rate as does isoproterenol.[81] Aerosolization of metaproterenol produces as rapid an onset of bronchodilation and reaches a peak as early as does an equivalent dose of isoproterenol;[82] the effect of metaproterenol persists for at least one hour longer.[80]

In spite of claims made for metaproterenol that attribute advantages to the drug, it has not been clearly demonstrated that most of these attributes are genuine. Thus, it is implied by some workers that metaproterenol offers advantages of minimal side effects, no tachyphylaxis and no paradoxic reactions.[82, 83] However, these claims have also been made for isoproterenol, when the drug is given by aerosol in the appropriate dosage. Yet, the much greater experience with this drug has demonstrated that, in fact, many patients do suffer side effects, and a few suffer from tachyphylaxis or paradoxic responses. More extensive studies of metaproterenol would probably reveal the potential for the same problems; indeed, many patients do develop tachycardia, with palpitations, nervousness and tremor after oral dosing with 20 mg;[79] apparent tachyphylaxis has also been noted. However, the oral syrup has been used successfully in children on a long-term basis, and has proved to be effective, without evidence of tachyphylaxis.[84] Thus, metaproterenol is a new bronchodilator that differs from isoproterenol by the dual virtues of being effective by the oral route and having a longer half-life (Table 5–13). Metaproterenol aerosol has been compared to isoetharine-phenylephrine (Bronkometer), and was found to cause bronchodilatation for about twice as long (four hours versus two hours).[85]

Dosages and Recommendations (Table 5–26)

ORAL. The oral dosage of metaproterenol that is recommended by the manufacturers for adults is 20 mg three times a day. However, many patients develop tremor and tachycardia with this dosage, and it is advisable to start at a dosage of 10 mg three times a day.[79] Until recently the marketed tablets were 20 mg in size, but now 10 mg preparations are available. Syrups are also marketed and are particularly useful when unusual dosages are required.

METERED AEROSOL. The metered aerosol powder form is used in similar fashion to other bronchodilators; in each patient the minimal required number of puffs should be established by individual trial. Each puff releases 650 mcg of metaproterenol as a micronized powder. Patients must be cautioned to try to limit the use of this aerosol to routine treatments about every six hours; if the response is inadequate, the patient may try 1 to 3 puffs every three to four hours, although 12 puffs a day should not be exceeded. No preparation of metaproterenol is available for IPPB usage; since the drug does not offer sufficient advantages, it is very unlikely that such a preparation will be marketed.

INTRAVENOUS. Intravenous metaproterenol has been found to be safe and effective in the treatment of asthma, but it is no more effective than isoproterenol, and it causes a similar degree of cardiovascular receptor effects[81]. Thus, it cannot be recommended for intravenous use.

One can certainly recommend the aerosol preparation of this drug, although other long-acting bronchodilators may be superior. The oral preparations provide a useful alternative to ephedrine, methoxyphenamine and protokylol, but no clear advantages over these drugs have been demonstrated. The oral syrup preparation has been of value in the long-term therapy of asthmatic children, and it could be considered one of the oral bronchodilators of choice in children over the age of six.[84] Thus, it is advisable for the practicing physician to keep metaproterenol in the bronchodilator armamentarium, since an individual patient may find this drug preferable to others.

In the final analysis, the relative cost of metaproterenol compared with other bronchodilators will determine the role of this drug in therapeutics. Most probably, this drug will have a limited life span in the very competitive bronchodilator market that is now opening up (Table 5–27), although, at present, it is one of the oral bronchodilators of choice, and it offers a useful metered aerosol alternative to patients who respond inadequately to the other available metered drugs.

TABLE 5–26. METAPROTERENOL

| AVAILABILITY | Brands | | Dosage | |
	ALUPENT	METAPREL	CHILDREN	ADULTS
Tablet	10,20 mg	10,20 mg	10–20 mg 3–4 times/day (usual daily dose is	10–20 mg 3–4 times/day
Syrup	10 mg/5 ml	10 mg/5 ml	1.3–2.6 mg/kg)	10–20 mg 3–4 times/day
Metered aerosol (powder)	0.65 mg/puff	0.65 mg/puff	1–3 puffs q3–6 h (maximum 12 puffs/day)	2–3 puffs q3–6 h (maximum 12 puffs/day)

TABLE 5–27. COMPARISON OF THE "NEWER" SYMPATHOMIMETIC BRONCHODILATORS SUITABLE FOR ORAL ADMINISTRATION

	Metaproterenol	Fenoterol	Terbutaline	Salbutamol
Other Names	Orciprenaline	Hydroxyphenylorciprenaline, Th 1165 a		Albuterol
Brand Names	Alupent*, Metaprel*	Berotec	Brethine*, Bricanyl*, Feevone	Proventil, Ventolin
Dosage in Adults				
Aerosol solution	0.65–2.0 mg q3–6 h	0.4 mg q8 h	0.25–1.5 mg q4–8 h	0.1–1 mg q6–8 h
Metered aerosol	2–3 puffs q3–6 h*		1–4 puffs q4–8 h	1–4 puffs q6–8 h
Oral	10–20 mg q6–8 h*	7.5 mg q8–12 h	2.5–5 mg q6–8 h	2–4 mg q.i.d.
Subcutaneous	Not advised		0.25–0.5 mg q4–6 h*	Not established
Intravenous	Not advised		Not established	0.1–0.4 mg
Persistence of Effect	3–5 hours	8 hours	4–7 hours	4–6 hours
Comments	Useful oral medium-acting drug; aerosol may offer some advantages; may be displaced by newer oral bronchodilators. However, currently is considered a drug of choice.	Long-acting drug suitable for oral and aerosol use; available in Europe, where it is considered to be one of the best selective bronchodilators; has not yet been introduced into the U.S	Valuable long-acting drug with variable beta-1 side effects; alternative to epinephrine for subcutaneous therapy; causes more side effects than salbutamol, but less tendency for a fall in PaO₂	Appears to be one of the best selective bronchodilators; has also been used for intravenous administration for status asthmaticus, circulatory support, and to inhibit premature labor

*Available in U.S. Salbutamol may not reach the market in the U.S.

Fenoterol
(Hydroxyphenylorciprenaline, Th 1165a)

This derivative of metaproterenol was discovered in 1964 and has been available in Europe since 1967, where it has been considered to be one of the best sympathomimetic bronchodilators.[4] The molecule has a large moiety inserted in the terminal amino group of the resorcinol chain; and this results in extreme beta-2 receptor selectivity (Table 5–12). Its similarity to metaproterenol ensures that it is resistant to COMT, and it can be given by mouth as well as by aerosol (Table 5–27). When given either orally or by aerosol it produces significant bronchodilatation for at least eight hours, with minimal cardiovascular or central nervous system side effects. The optimal oral dose for adults appears to be 7.5 mg two or three times a day;[86] the corresponding aerosol dose is about 400 mcg.[87] Fenoterol clearly is a considerable improvement when compared with its parent compound, metaproterenol;[88] it appears to be four times as active as a bronchodilator, and has more selective beta-2 receptor properties.[1, 88a, 88b]

Terbutaline

One of the most recently introduced (1969) of the European series of bronchodilator drugs is terbutaline.[89] It reached the American market relatively quickly (1974) and is marketed as Bricanyl and Brethine. In Australasia the drug is called Feevone.

Structure and Metabolism. The drug is the N-tertiary butyl analogue of metaproterenol (Table 5–12), and is made available as terbutaline sulfate. Since it is a resorcinol derivative (Figure 5–3) it is not affected by COMT or by sulfatization. Although incompletely absorbed,[90] it is effective when given orally, and it is relatively long-acting (Table 5–27). Thus, measurable bronchodilatation may persist for over seven hours following an oral dose of 5 mg of terbutaline.[71, 91, 92] The effect persists for at least four hours after a subcutaneous dose of 0.5 mg,[92] and lasts over five hours following an aerosol treatment.[91] Since the amino group of the ethanolamine chain is highly substituted, terbutaline would be expected to have potent beta-2 effects with little beta-1 and alpha activity. The drug is conjugated in the bowel wall and liver, but a large proportion is excreted unchanged.[90] After oral administration, about 30 per cent appears in the urine; after intravenous administration, over 90 per cent is excreted by the kidney.[7]

Actions. There is good evidence that terbutaline is one of the most selective beta-2 adrenergic stimulators,[93] but it does have cardiovascular side effects, which need to be considered in some detail. Since the drug is a potent beta-2 stimulator, not only does it cause bronchodilation, but it also results in peripheral vasodilation. If sufficient terbutaline is given, particularly by a systemic route, the resulting widespread vasodilation causes a fall in blood pressure. The reflex response to this hemodynamic change consists of an appreciable increase in heart rate;[94] thus, tachycardia may occur, even though this is not a direct result of stimulation of heart muscle beta-1 receptors. Since the body responds as a complex, holistic, interreacting unit rather than as a series of isolated muscles, a "beta-1" effect can be obtained reflexly, rather than as a primary receptor stimulus. Thus, in practice, terbutaline does have definite cardiovascular side effects when given in large enough doses.[71, 94]

Since beta-2 stimulants have an effect on neuromuscular receptors, the more potent bronchodilator quality of terbutaline is accompanied by a correspondingly marked tremor. Some patients also develop palpitations and other undesirable sympathomimetic side effects following larger doses of terbutaline, but the effect varies markedly in different subjects[91, 95]. The use of the aerosol preparation obviously reduces the incidence of all side effects; tremor does not occur after aerosol administration.[93] In view of the fact that animal studies clearly show that terbutaline is a far more selective beta-2 stimulator than is epinephrine, the clinical literature on these drugs contains various surprises, such as reports that compare subcutaneous injections of 0.5 mg or 1 mg of terbutaline with 0.25 mg or 0.5 mg of epinephrine: the terbutaline caused more tachycardia than did the epinephrine for the same degree of bronchodilatation.[92, 96, 96a] Studies such as this do little to clarify the issue of which drug is "better" or "more selective," but they do illustrate that the newer bronchodilators offer only limited advantages.

Terbutaline was first marketed as a subcutaneous preparation in the U.S., and it was hoped that it would offer a safer and more effective alternative to subcutaneous epinephrine for the treatment of bronchospasm. These hopes have not been fulfilled, and the subsequent marketing of the oral form similarly failed to revolutionize the treatment of bronchospasm. However, oral terbutaline in a 5 mg dose, when compared with 25 mg ephedrine, has the following advantages: earlier onset and longer duration of effect, greater bronchodilatation with less side effects and less likelihood of developing tachyphylaxis.[92a, 92b]

When compared with metaproterenol, terbutaline seems to have almost identical bronchodilator effects, although it is longer acting and is more potent, weight for weight, when given orally or by aerosol.[93] Oral terbutaline, in a dose of 5 mg, produces significantly greater protection against exercise-induced asthma than does 20 mg metaproterenol.[97] A single oral dose of 5 mg terbutaline produces significantly more bronchodilatation over a period of six hours than does a 20 mg dose of metaproterenol.[97] Both drugs, when given subcutaneously, can cause a slight fall in blood pressure, but metaproterenol causes more tachycardia. Thus, terbutaline can certainly be considered superior to metaproterenol.[1] An additional value of drugs such as terbutaline is that they increase tracheal mucociliary transport.[98]

Dosages and Recommendations. Terbutaline is made available in the U.S. as the sulfate for oral and subcutaneous administration (Table 5–28). Use of the drug in children under the age of 12 is probably safe, but dosage recommendations are not yet available.

ORAL. The usual oral dose of terbutaline for adults is one 5 mg tablet three or four times a day; tablets are scored, and half the 5 mg dose can readily be obtained and may be adequate in many subjects. Usually it is best to start on the lower dosage for the first two

TABLE 5–28. TERBUTALINE

Availability	Brands		Dosage	
	BRETHINE	BRICANYL	ADULTS	CHILDREN
Tablets	2.5 mg 5 mg	2.5 mg 5 mg	2.5–5 mg t.i.d.	0.75–4.5 mg t.i.d.
Elixir (3 mg/10 ml)*			2.5–5 mg t.i.d.	0.75–4.5 mg t.i.d.
Subcutaneous injection		1 mg/ml	0.25 mg; repeat if necessary in 15–30 mins; maximum: 0.5 mg q4 h	0.005–0.01 mg/kg q 4–6 h
Aerosol*				
Metered aerosol*		0.25 mg/puff	0.25–0.5 mg q4 h 1–2 inhalations q4 h (maximum: 8 inhalations/24 hr)	0.25–0.5 mg q4 h 1–2 inhalations q4–6 h (maximum: 8 inhalations/24 hr)

*Not available in U.S.

weeks of therapy. Young children should receive 1.25 to 2.5 mg three times a day. Both tablets and syrups are available; there is no significant bioavailability advantage of one form over the other.[99] The syrup has not been introduced in the U.S. as yet.

SUBCUTANEOUS. The subcutaneous dose is 0.25 mg, and can be repeated once or, with caution, twice, at half hourly intervals. However, most adult patients obtain adequate bronchodilatation with the smaller dose, whereas 0.5 mg causes a much greater incidence of side effects.[1, 92] In general, a dosage of 0.5 mg during a four hour period should not be exceeded. Although it is not advised that terbutaline be injected intramuscularly, this route has been safely used by investigators; in this regard, selective beta-2 drugs are safer than drugs such as epinephrine, which have vasoconstrictor properties.

AEROSOL. The aerosol is not yet available in the U.S., but, when approved, it should be administered in the same fashion as other aerosol bronchodilators: 1 to 4 puffs (each provided 250 mcg or 375 mcg terbutaline, depending on the metered product available) three to four times a day. The drug could also be given by various nebulizer devices or with IPPB, using a dosage of 0.25 to 0.5 ml (0.25 to 0.5 mg) of the solution, either diluted or undiluted. Although as much as 1.5 mg has been given by inhalation at one time without causing significant side effects,[91] it should not be necessary for a patient to take a total of more than eight inhalations (2 mg) a day. The problem of tremulousness does not occur after aerosol administration, whereas it can be a major difficulty with oral therapy.[99a] However, if oral therapy is initiated with minimal doses of terbutaline, adaptation to the tremorogenic effect may occur, and then the bronchodilator dose can be increased and tremor may not appear.[92b]

Terbutaline offers an important alternative for subcutaneous treatment, which may be preferable in patients who cannot tolerate epinephrine. Patients with hypertension or cardiac disease should be given terbutaline in preference to epinephrine. The oral drug may prove helpful to individual patients who do not respond appropriately to other bronchodilators, and it should be tried when a more specific beta-2 effect is desired.

Although it is unlikely that terbutaline aerosol will prove to be dramatically superior to the more established drugs for most patients with bronchospasm, there are undoubtedly many patients who will find this drug to be the best bronchodilator for their particular condition. Terbutaline may be considered one of the standard oral bronchodilators, but its overall value awaits the outcome of definitive comparison studies. The current evidence suggests that terbutaline will be most effective with least side effects when administered by air-compressor or IPPB nebulization, and it should become a useful alternative to other bronchodilators for this form of administration.

Salbutamol

Although salbutamol was introduced in 1968, and had been used in Europe before terbutaline, it has been very slow to enter the U.S. market, mainly because of technical problems in complying with FDA evaluation requirements. Salbutamol has probably been the topic of more scientific papers[100] than has terbutaline, and it is extraordinary to find that this excellent product has experienced such a delay in finding its way into American medicine. Unfortunately, there have been incredible problems that have prevented the entry of the drug into the U.S. market, and it now appears that it may never obtain FDA approval for its release. Recently, it has been accused of causing the development of mesovarian leiomyomas in rats; although this can hardly be relevant to the human, the FDA is unlikely to allow salbutamol to be used in either men or women patients.[100a]

Structure and Metabolism. Salbutamol is classified as a saligenin (Figure 5-3): the 3-hydroxy group in the catecholamine nucleus is replaced by a -CH_2OH group, that protects the molecule from sulfatization and from COMT (Table 5-12). Most of an administered oral dose of salbutamol is conjugated in the bowel and liver, but the metabolites formed have not been identified, and it is possible that a novel conjugate may be produced.[101] It is excreted in the urine partly unchanged and partly as a glucuronide; other metabolites are also identifiable. The side chain of salbutamol is the same as that found in terbutaline, since it also has an N-tertiary butyl substituent. Salbutamol is marketed under the trade name Ventolin in most countries; the drug is known as albuterol in the U.S., and it had been planned to market it with the trade name Proventil. (Table 5-27).

Actions. The molecular structure of salbutamol results in a selective beta-2 stimulator comparable to terbutaline (Table 5-13). The drug is, perhaps, the most potent and the safest of the sympathomimetic bronchodilators. It has been compared with most of the other commonly used agents,[102] and in general, oral doses of salbutamol that produce the same amount of bronchodilatation as do the other test drugs cause less cardiovascular side effects and more prolonged bronchodilatation. Salbutamol is a slightly more powerful bronchodilator than terbutaline when 5 mg oral doses of these drugs are compared.[103] However, in practice, the aerosol form does not differ appreciably from terbutaline.[104]

There is evidence to suggest that salbutamol is the safest of the bronchodilators for the intravenous therapy of bronchospasm.[68] It is a peripheral vasodilator, and the resulting fall in blood pressure can cause a reflex increase in heart rate, although this tends to be of minor degree. Moreover, intravenous administration does not appear to cause a significant fall in PaO_2, nor does it cause cardiac arrhythmias; in this regard, it offers safer and superior therapy than that obtained by using isoproterenol for intravenous treatment of severe asthma. The drug also appears to cause stimulation of the respiratory center, and thus may have an additional value in respiratory failure.[105] The added safety of salbutamol makes it a more suitable intravenous drug for providing circulatory support in patients who have undergone open-heart surgery.[23] Salbutamol, in common with other selective beta-2 stimulators, is safer for the treatment of asthma in any patient who is liable to develop cardiac irritability or myocardial ischemia.

Oral therapy with selective beta-2 drugs, including salbutamol, does have the distinct disadvantage of causing a significant incidence of fine finger tremor, which can make delicate hand work quite difficult. Moreover, there is much individual variation in patients, and appreciable numbers find that oral salbutamol causes less effective bronchodilation than does aerosol therapy. It is possible that the sublingual administration of the drug can result, at least in some patients, in more effective bronchodilation with a lower incidence of side effects.

Administration of salbutamol by aerosol produces an equally long lasting bronchodilatation as does oral therapy, but with much less side effects. The maximum response following aerosol therapy is delayed: thus, isoproterenol takes only about 15 minutes to produce maximal bronchodilatation, whereas the peak response after salbutamol may take up to one hour to develop.[106] It is of interest to find that a number of workers in Great Britain have reported the usefulness of IPPB in delivering an aerosol of salbutamol.[21, 67, 107] Most of these reports comment on the value of this form of therapy in asthmatics; certainly, on the basis of the published experience, salbutamol may be considered the best drug for IPPB treatments of bronchospastic conditions. In this regard, salbutamol is very similar to terbutaline, but may have the disadvantages of causing more "wasted" ventilation (by increasing the dead space/tidal volume ratio) and a tendency for a fall in PaO_2.[108] Thus, terbutaline may have less adverse effects on ventilation/perfusion relationships. Overall, terbutaline may cause a slightly greater incidence of side effects such as tremor and headache,[103] although aerosolized terbutaline produces negligible cardiovascular effects.[109]

It should be appreciated, however, that the various reports of side effects are always based on experiences with relatively few patients, and that the differences between drugs may not be significant in the general population of patients throughout the world. Indeed, metabolic studies by workers in England emphasize that most of an aerosolized drug may, in fact, be swallowed and then broken down or absorbed in the gastrointestinal tract,[110] casting further doubt on the validity of many reported trials comparing aerosolized agents. Each physician who prescribes bronchodilators should always be willing to compare different drugs on the individual patient, in order to determine whether any one agent is particularly suitable.

There are claims that salbutamol has some unusual clinical values. Intravenous administration of the drug has been reported to inhibit premature labor. The oral and inhalational preparations for this purpose have been more controversial,[24, 111, 112] and cannot be recommended. Salbutamol infusion can cause a fall in serum potassium, probably as a result of an intracellular migration of potassium, secondary to insulin release,[105] from stimulation of pancreatic beta-2 adrenoreceptors.[113] Salbutamol has also been reported to reduce the hyperkalemia associated with attacks of the rare disease familial periodic paralysis.[114] It is probable, though, that epinephrine and other sympathomimetic drugs would have similar effects to those that have been attributed to salbutamol; for example, intravenous metaproterenol has also been shown to effectively delay delivery in premature labor.

Dosages and Recommendations. Salbutamol, when it is available, must be considered one of the best bronchodilators; it is suitable for intravenous, oral and aerosol use.

ORAL. The appropriate oral dose for adults is probably 4 mg four times a day; if tremor develops with this dosage, 2 mg may prove to be effective without causing side effects. However, since salbutamol is comparable to terbutaline, the same dosage range may be considered suitable: 2.5 to 5 mg four times day. There is doubt about the comparative value of oral salbutamol as a member of the bronchodilator armamentarium.[4]

METERED AEROSOLS. Metered aerosols of salbutamol have become very popular in the U.K., and, in recent years, more salbutamol has been prescribed than isoproterenol. The metered product releases 100 mcg per puff; patients should take 1 to 4 puffs three to four times a day. When given by IPPB, a standard safe and effective dosage is 2 ml of the 0.5 per cent solution,[115] which provides 10 mg of the drug—only a fraction of which is actually deposited in the respiratory tract. The 0.5 per cent concentration appears to be optimal, and should be preferred to the 0.25 per cent or 1 per cent preparations.[115]

INTRAVENOUS. The suggested intravenous dose for the treatment of bronchospasm in adults is 100 mcg initially, followed by 300 mcg in 15 minutes if the response is inadequate; each injection should be given over the course of five minutes. The optimal dose for adults may be 300 mcg.[116] Salbutamol can also be given by intravenous infusion, using a rate of 4 mcg per minute, or by choosing a dosage of 0.05 to 0.2 mcg/kg per minute for one hour;[68] a total dosage of 0.2 mg given over a period of five minutes may be optimal.[116a] These forms of administration may become standard therapy for status asthmaticus,[117] since the intravenous drug is tolerated so well, although an increase in heart rate and some tremor may be produced. However, the same dose given by aerosol is more effective and has a longer-lasting effect when given to patients with less severe bronchospasm.[117a] There may be advantages in giving salbutamol intramuscularly; it is well-tolerated and effective in a dose of 10 mcg/kg.[117b]

In practice, there is little to choose between the long-acting bronchodilator aerosol drugs metaproterenol, terbutaline and salbutamol (Tables 5–13 and 5–27). For oral or systemic therapy, the experience with terbutaline is limited, whereas that with salbutamol is more extensive. At present, salbu-

TABLE 5–29. SYMPATHOMIMETIC BRONCHODILATORS
CURRENTLY UNDER INVESTIGATION*

Agent	Other Names	Chemical Relationship	Comments
CARBUTEROL	SKF 40383	Similar to salbutamol with urea substituent at C3 in benzene nucleus	Long lasting, highly selective beta-2 stimulator
CLENBUTEROL		Similar to salbutamol with substituents at C3, C4 and C5 in benzene nucleus	Similar to salbutamol, but more potent
HEXOPRENALINE	Ipradol, Etoscol	Contains two linked catecholamine moieties	Similar to metaproterenol, but superior
IBUTEROL		Di-isobutyric acid ester of terbutaline	More powerful than terbutaline
PIRBUTEROL	pyrbuterol, CP-24,314-1	Similar to salbutamol but has a pyridine ring instead of a benzene ring	Longer lasting than salbutamol, with fewer side effects
QUINTERENOL	quinprenaline	Quinolone derivative	Very long-acting; has beta-1 activity
RITODRINE	Premar, Pre-par, Yutopar	Related to fenoterol	
SALMEFAMOL	AH 3923	Similar to fenoterol	Long-acting, very potent, very low incidence of side effects
SOTERENOL		Sulfonanilide substituent at C3 in benzene nucleus of isoproterenol	Toxic to animals: drug now abandoned
TRIMETOQUINOL	Inolin, Tretoquinol	Isoquinoline, related to resorcinol, with cyclized side chain terminating in a tri-substituted ring	Long-acting

*The exact names and spellings of these drugs have varied in different reports in the literature.

tamol clearly appears to have advantages over metaproterenol, both orally and as an aerosol,[118] but it might not be better than terbutaline. Further clarification of the comparative effects of these drugs is still required.

OTHER SYMPATHOMIMETIC BRONCHODILATORS

Numerous drugs have been shown to have bronchodilator properties, and many of these would probably be suitable for clinical use.[2, 11] However, the expense and difficulty of bringing a new drug to the market suggest that very few additional drugs will become available unless they can be shown to have exceptional advantages. Thus, a selective beta-2 stimulator free of nervous and muscular stimulatory properties would be a welcome addition. At present, there is little to suggest that such an agent has been found.

Table 5–29 lists the main investigational bronchodilators reported to have valuable properties; some may prove to be of sufficient clinical value to merit their introduction into the competitive commercial market.[1, 4, 12] The most promising are salmefamol and soterenol; both have already received considerable attention in the recent literature.[1, 4, 12, 14, 119] Other useful agents are carbuterol,[120, 121, 122a] clenbuterol,[123] hexoprenaline,[87, 124] ibuterol,[125] pirbuterol,[126] quinterenol[127] and trimetoquinol.[1, 128] Less information is available on hoquizil,[129] isoprophenamine (clorprenaline)[12] and ritodrine (Premar).[12] Several derivatives of ephedrine may be of some value as bronchodilators and as "cough medicines;" these include dioxethedrin, etafedrine (Nethamine, Nehaphyl) and hydroxyephedrine.[130]

Unfortunately, the evaluation of new bronchodilator drugs is a difficult and expensive enterprise;[131] the successful agents that reach the commercial marketplace constitute a small fraction of all those that undergo consideration. It is unlikely that any new adrenergic agent will offer outstanding advantages that will make it the "wonder drug" that so many asthmatics crave. It is more realistic for physicians to obtain greater understanding of and capability with the numerous existing agents[130] than to place their faith on future developments in the pharmaceutic industry.[132, 133] Nevertheless, it can be expected that useful new bronchodilators will be marketed; the pharmacologically knowledgeable physician will welcome these extensions to the therapeutic smorgasbord for the additional flexbility in the treatment of bronchospasm that they offer.

REFERENCES

1. Alexander, M. R., Hendeles, L. and Guernsey, B.: The beta-2 agonist bronchodilators. Drug Intel. Clin. Pharm. 11:526–532, 1977.
1a. Avner, S. E.: β-Adrenergic bronchodilators. Pediatr. Clin. North Am. 22:129–139, 1975.
1b. Brandon, M. L.: Newer medications to aid treatment of asthma. Ann. Allergy 39:117–128, 1977.
2. Brittain, R. T., Jack, D. and Ritchie, A. C.: Recent β-adrenoreceptor stimulants. Adv. Drug Res. 5:197–253, 1970.
2a. Brittain, R. T., Dean, C. M. and Jack, D.: Sympathomimetic bronchodilator drugs. Pharmac. Ther. B 2:423–462, 1976.
2b. Jenne, J. W.: The clinical pharmacology of bronchodilators. Basics of RD (Published by American Thoracic Society) 6 #1, Sept., 1977.
3. Leifer, K. N., Wittig, H. J. and Rhoades, R. B.: Therapeutic advances in asthma. Cutis 15: 841–847, 1975.
4. Leifer, K. N. and Wittig, H. J.: The beta-2 sympathomimetic aerosols in the treatment of asthma. Ann. Allergy 35:69–80, 1975.
5. Paterson, J. W. and Shenfield, G. M.: Bronchodilators. Part I. B.T.T.A. Review 4:25–40, June, 1974.

6. Paterson, J. W. and Shenfield, G. M.: Bronchodilators. Part II. B.T.T.A. Review 4:61–74, Dec. 1974.
7. Rebuck, A. S.: Antiasthmatic Drugs I: Pathophysiological and clinical pharmacological aspects. Drugs 7:344–369, 1974.
8. Rebuck, A. S.: Antiasthmatic Drugs II: Therapeutic aspects. Drugs 7:370–390, 1974.
8a. Van Arsdel, P. P.: Drug therapy in the management of asthma. Ann. Intern. Med. 87:68–74, 1977.
9. van As, A.: Beta-adrenergic stimulant bronchodilators. In New Directions in Asthma. M. Stein (Ed.). Park Ridge, Ill., American College of Chest Physicians, 1975.
10. Van den Brink, F. G.: The pharmacology of bronchiolar muscle relaxation. Bull. Physiopath Respir. 8:475–486, 1972.
10a. Webb-Johnson, D. C. and Andrews, J. L.: Bronchodilator therapy. N. Engl. J. Med. 297: 476–482, 1977.
10b. Weinberger, M. and Hendeles, L.: Management of asthma. 2. Antiasthmatic drugs. Postgrad. Med. 61:95–103, May, 1977.
10c. Weinberger, M. and Hendeles, L.: The pharmacological basis of bronchodilator therapy. Rational Drug Therapy 11 #6, June, 1977.
11. Ziment, I.: The pharmacology of airway dilators. Respir. Therapy 4:51–56. May–June, 1974.

12. Jack, D.: Selectively acting β-adrenoreceptor stimulants in asthma. *In* Asthma: Physiology, Immunopharmacology, and Treatment. K. F. Austen and L. M. Lichtenstein (Eds.). New York, Academic Press, 1973.

13. Freedman, B. J.: Principles of comparative drug trials with special reference to bronchodilators. *In* Evaluation of Bronchodilator Drugs. D. M. Burley et al. (Eds.). Published by The Trust for Education and Research in Therapeutics, England, 1974, pp. 219–237.

14. Shenfield, G. M. and Paterson, J. W.: Clinical assessment of bronchodilator drugs delivered by aerosol. Thorax 28:124–128, 1973.

15. Wood, M.: Additives and combinations. Respir. Therapy 4:19–24, Sept.–Oct., 1974.

16. Orehek, J., Gayrard, P., Grimaud, C. and Charpin, J.: Patient error in use of bronchodilator metered aerosols. Br. Med. J. 1:76, Jan., 1976.

17. Bell, J. H., Brown, K. and Glasby, J.: Variation in delivery of isoprenaline from various pressurized inhalers. J. Pharm. Pharmac. 25 Suppl.:32p–36p, 1973.

18. Davies, D. S.: Pharmacokinetics of inhaled drugs. *In* Evaluation of Bronchodilator Drugs D. M., Burley et al., (Eds.). Published by The Trust for Education and Research in Therapeutics, England, 1974, pp. 151–165.

18a. Davies, R. J., D'Souza, M. F. and Simmonds, S. P.: Puffs per aerosol. Br. Med. J. 1:177, Jan., 1972.

19. Shore, S. C. and Weinberg, E. G.: Administration of bronchodilator to young children. Br. Med. J. 3:350, Aug., 1973.

20. Ziment, I.: Why are they saying bad things about IPPB? Respir. Care 18:677–689, 1973.

21. Choo-Kang, Y. F. J. and Grant, I. W. B.: Comparison of two methods of administering bronchodilator aerosol to asthmatic patients. Br. Med. J. 2:119–120, Apr., 1975.

21a. Reed, C. E.: Sites and mechanisms of airway obstruction in reversible obstructive airway disease. *In* Recent Advances In Asthma Therapy: Vanceril Inhaler. R. S. Farr, E. Middleton and S. L. Spector (Eds.). Miami, Symposia Specialists Medical Books (Schering Corporation), 1976, pp. 31–37.

22. Ahlquist, R. P.: Pharmacology of pressor agents on the systemic circulation. Semin. Drug Treat. 3:231–240, 1973.

23. Wyse, S. D., Gibson, D. G. and Branthwaite, M. A.: Haemodynamic effects of salbutamol in patients needing circulatory support after open-heart surgery. Br. Med. J. 3:502–503, Aug., 1974.

24. Hastwell, G. B.: Salbutamol aerosol in premature labour. Lancet 2:1212-1213, 1975.

25. Svedmyr, N. L. V., Larsson, S. A. and Thiringer, G. K.: Development of "resistance" in beta-adrenergic receptors of asthmatic patients. Chest 69:479–483, 1976.

26. Gazioglu, K., Kaltreider, N. L. and Hyde, R. W.: Effect of isoproterenol on gas exchange during air and oxygen breathing in patients with chronic pulmonary diseases. Am. Rev. Respir. Dis. 104:188–197, 1971.

27. Bergofsky, E. H.: The pharmacology of severe bronchial asthma. Am. J. Med. Sci. 267:225–227, 1974.

28. Brittain, R. T.: Pharmacology of recent beta-adrenoceptor stimulants. Proc. R. Soc. Med. 65:759–761, 1972.

29. Van Metre, T. E.: Adverse effects of inhalation of excessive amounts of nebulized isoproterenol in status asthmaticus. J. Allergy 43:101–113, 1969.

30. Keighley, J. F.: Refractory asthma and adrenergic aerosols. N.Y. State J. Med. 69:662–667, 1969.

30a. Trautlein, J., Allegra, J., Field, J. and Gillin, M.: Paradoxic bronchospasm after inhalation of isoproterenol. Chest 70:711–714, 1976.

31. Reisman, R. E.: Asthma induced by adrenergic aerosols. J. Allergy 46:162–177, 1970.

32. Conolly, M. E., Davies, D. S., Dollery, C. T. and George, C. F.: Resistance to β-adrenoceptor stimulants (a possible explanation for the rise in asthma deaths). Br. J. Pharmac. 43:389–402, 1971.

33. Benoy, C. J., El-Fellah, M. S., Schneider, R. and Wade, O. L.: Tolerance to sympathomimetic bronchodilators in guinea pig isolated lungs following chronic administration *in vivo*. Br. J. Pharmac. 55:547–554, 1975.

34. Inman, W. H. W.: Recognition of unwanted drug effects with special reference to pressurized bronchodilator aerosols. *In* Evaluation of Bronchodilator Drugs (D. M. Burley et al., Eds.). Published by The Trust for Education and Research in Therapeutics, England, 1974, pp. 191–206.

34a. Berk, J. L., Hagen, J. F., Koo, R. and Maly, G.: Pulmonary insufficiency produced by isoproterenol. Surg. Gynecol. Obstet. 143:725–726, 1976.

34b. Jenne, J. W. and Chick, T. W.: "Unresponsiveness" to isoproterenol. Chest 70: 691–693, 1976.

35. Davies, D. S.: Metabolism of isoprenaline and other bronchodilator drugs in man and dog. Bull. Physiopath. Respir. 8:679–682, 1972.

36. Symposium on isoproterenol therapy in asthma. Ann. Allergy 31:1–44, 1973.

37. Sherbell, S. and Lyons, H. A.: The effects of isoproterenol mistometer, with recommended use. J. Allergy Clin. Immunol. 52:321–327, 1973.

38. Aelony, Y., Laks, M. M. and Beall, G. N.: An electrocardiographic pattern of acute myocardial infarction associated with excessive use of aerosolized isoproterenol. Chest 68: 107–110, 1975.

39. Lockett, M. F.: Dangerous effects of isoprenaline in myocardial failure. Lancet 2:104–106, 1965.

40. Stolley, P. D.: Asthma mortality. Why the United States was spared an epidemic of deaths due to asthma. Am. Rev. Respir. Dis. 105:883–890, 1972.

41. Clark, D. G. and Tinston, D. J.: Cardiac effects of isoproterenol, hypoxia, hypercapnia and fluorocarbon propellants and their use in asthma inhalers. Ann. Allergy 30:536–541, 1972.

42. Paterson, J. W., Conolly, M. E., Davies, D. S. and Dollery, C. T.: Isoprenaline resistance and the use of pressurised aerosols in asthma. Lancet 2:426–429, 1968.

43. George, C. F., Blackwell, E. W. and Davies, D. S.: Metabolism of isoprenaline in the intestine. J. Pharm. Pharmac. 26:265–267, 1974.

44. Assael, R., Martt, J. M. and Okeson, G. C.: Frequency of isoproterenol hydrochloride-induced cardiac arrhythmia in 19 patients with

chronic obstructive pulmonary disease: a prospective study. Am. Rev. Respir. Dis. 111:743–747, 1975.

45. Shim, C., and Williams, M. H., Jr.: Cardiac response to repeated doses of isoproterenol aerosol. Ann. Int. Med. 83:208–211, 1975.

46. Downes, J. J., Wood, D. W., Harwood, I., Sheinkopf, H. N. and Raphaely, R. C.: Intravenous isoproterenol infusion in children with severe hypercapnia due to status asthmaticus. Crit. Care Med. 1:63–68, 1973.

47. Klaustermeyer, W. B., DiBernardo, R. L. and Hale, F. C.: Intravenous isoproterenol: rationale for bronchial asthma. J. Allergy Clin. Immunol. 55:325–333, 1975.

48. Williams, M. H., Jr. and Kane, C.: Dose response of patients with asthma to inhaled isoproterenol. Am. Rev. Respir. Dis. 111:321–324, 1975.

49. Light, R. W., Summer, W. R. and Luchsinger, P. C.: Response of patients with chronic obstructive lung disease to the regular administration of nebulized isoproterenol. Chest 67:634–639, 1975.

50. Segal, M. S. and Ishikawa, S.: Isoproterenol aerosols. Ann. Allergy 34:205–209, 1975.

51. Parry, W. H., Martorano, F. and Cotton, E. K.: Management of life-threatening asthma with intravenous isoproterenol infusions. Am. J. Dis. Child 130:39–42, 1976.

52. Harris, L. H.: Effects of isoprenaline plus phenylephrine by pressurized aerosol on blood gases, ventilation, and perfusion in chronic obstructive lung disease. Br. Med. J. 4:579–582, Dec., 1970.

53. Stone, D. J., Zaldivar, C. and Keltz, H.: The effects of very low doses of nebulized isoproterenol, nebulized saline, and intravenous isoproterenol on blood gases in patients with chronic bronchitis. Am. Rev. Respir. Dis. 101:511–517, 1970.

54. Cohen, A. A. and Hale, F. C.: Comparative effects of isoproterenol aerosols on airway resistance in obstructive pulmonary diseases. Am. J. Med. Sci. 249:309–315, 1965.

55. Cohen, B. M.: Ventilatory responses to aerosols of isoproterenol and isoproterenol-phenylephrine. Curr. Ther. Res. 4:601–609, 1962.

56. Freedman, B. J., Meisner, P. and Hill, G. B.: A comparison of the actions of different bronchodilators in asthma. Thorax 23:590–597, 1968.

57. Kallos, P. and Kallos-Deffner, L.: Comparison of the protective effect of isoproterenol with isoproterenol-phenylephrine aerosols in asthmatics. Int. Arch. Allergy 24:17–26, 1964.

58. Grant, J. L., Werfelman, N., Cook, M. R. and Metherall, W.: Comparison of isoproterenol and isoproterenol-phenylephrine aerosols. Chest 60:129–132, 1971.

59. Harris, L.: Comparison of the effect on blood gases, ventilation, and perfusion of isoproterenol-phenylephrine and salbutamol aerosols in chronic bronchitis with asthma. J. Allergy Clin. Immunol. 49:63–71, 1972.

59a. Singer, O. P. and Wilson, W. J.: Laryngotracheobronchitis: 2 years' experience with racemic epinephrine. Can. Med. Assoc. J. 115:132–134, 1976.

60. Gardner, H. G., Powell, K. R., Roden, V. J. and Cherry, J. D.: The evaluation of racemic

61. Berman, B. A.: Bronchial asthma. *In* Current Pediatric Therapy. B. Gellis and B. M. Kagan (Eds.). Philadelphia, W. B. Saunders Company, Vol. 6, 1973. pp. 701–707.

62. Cohen, B. M.: Studies with isoetharine. I. The ventilatory effects of aerosol and oral forms. J. Asthma Res. 4:209–218, 1967.

63. Lands, A. M.: Absorption profile of the bronchodilator drug isoetharine. Arch. Int. Pharmacodyn. Ther. 138:462–472, 1962.

64. Miller, J.: The profile of a beta receptor stimulant bronchodilator. Ann. Allergy 25:520–527, 1967.

64a. Spector, S. L., Hudson, L. and Petty, T. L.: Effect of Bronkosol and its components on cardiopulmonary parameters in asthmatic patients. J. Allergy Clin. Immunol. 59:371–376, 1977.

65. Blacow, N. W. (Ed.). Martindale: The Extra Pharmacopoeia. London, The Pharmaceutical Press, 26th ed., 1972, p. 18.

66. Linehan, W. and Griffin, J. P.: Oral preparations of isoetharine compared with orciprenaline and choline theophyllinate. Brit. J. Dis. Chest 65:44–51, 1971.

67. Cooke, N. J., Kerr, J. A., Willey, R. F., et al.: Response to rimiterol and salbutamol aerosols administered by intermittent positive-pressure ventilation. Br. Med. J. 2:250–252, May, 1974.

68. Marlin, G. E. and Turner, P.: Intravenous treatment with rimiterol and salbutamol in asthma. Br. Med. J. 2:715–719, June, 1975.

69. Bianco, S., Kamburoff, P. L. and Prime, F. J.: Comparison between the bronchodilator and cardiovascular effects of inhaling 0.5 mg. rimiterol ('Pulmadil') and 0.2 mg. salbutamol. Curr. Med. Res. Opin. 3:30–35, 1975.

70. Weinberger, M.: Use of ephedrine in bronchodilator therapy. Pediatr. Clin. North Am. 22:121–127, 1975.

70a. Pickup, M. E., May, C. S., Ssendagire, R. and Paterson, J. W.: The pharmacokinetics of ephedrine after oral dosage in asthmatics receiving acute and chronic treatment. Br. J. Clin. Pharmac. 3:123–134, 1976.

71. Tashkin, D. P., Meth, R., Simmons, D. H., and Lee, Y. E.: Double-blind comparison of acute bronchial and cardiovascular effects of oral terbutaline and ephedrine. Chest 68:155–161, 1975.

72. Lyons, H. A., Thomas, J. S., and Steen, S. N.: Theophylline and ephedrine in asthma. Curr. Ther. Res. 18:573–577, 1975.

73. Muittari, A. and Mattila, M. J.: Bronchodilator action of drug combinations in asthmatic patients: ephedrine, theophylline and tranquilizing drugs. Curr. Ther. Res. 13:374–385, 1971.

74. Weinberger, M., Bronsky, E., Bensch, G. W., et al.: Interaction of ephedrine and theophylline. Clin. Pharmacol. Ther. 17:585–592, 1975.

75. Bierman, C. W., Pierson, W. E. and Shapiro, G. G.: Exercise-induced asthma. Pharmacological assessment of single drugs and drug combinations. J.A.M.A. 234:295–298, 1975.

76. Weinberger, M. M. and Bronsky, E. A.: Evaluation of oral bronchodilator therapy in asthmatic children. J. Pediatr. 84:421–427, 1974.

77. Bresnick, E., Beakey, J. F., Levinson, L. and

Segal, M. S.: Evaluation of therapeutic substances employed for the relief of bronchospasm. V. Adrenergic agents. J. Clin. Invest. 28:1182–1189, 1949.

78. Wilson, R. H. L. and Wilson, N. L.: Evaluation of a new bronchodilator aerosol and its components in pulmonary emphysema. Clin. Pharmacol. Ther. 7:189–195, 1966.

79. Chervinsky, P. and Chervinsky, G.: Metaproterenol tablets: their duration of effect by comparison with ephedrine. Curr. Ther. Res. 17:507–518, 1975.

80. Chervinsky, P. and Belinkoff, S.: Comparison of metaproterenol and isoproterenol aerosols: spirometric evaluation after two months' therapy. Ann. Allergy 27:611–616, 1969.

81. McEvoy, J. D. S., Vall-Spinosa, A. and Paterson, J. W.: Assessment of orciprenaline and isoproterenol infusions in asthmatic patients. Am. Rev. Respir. Dis. 108:490–500, 1973.

82. Sobol, B. J. and Reed, A.: The rapidity of onset of bronchodilation: a comparison of Alupent and isoproterenol. Ann. Allergy 32:137–141, 1974.

83. Hurst, A.: Metaproterenol, a potent and safe bronchodilator. Ann. Allergy 31:460–466, 1973.

84. Emirgil, C., Dwyer, K. and Sobol, B. J.: A comparison of the duration of action and the cardiovascular effects of metaproterenol and an isoetharine-phenylephrine combination. Curr. Ther. Res. 19:371–378, 1976.

85. Brandon, M. L.: Long-term metaproterenol therapy in asthmatic children. J.A.M.A. 235:736–737, 1976.

86. Steen, S. N., Smith, R., Kuo, J., Ziment, I. and Beall, G. N.: Evaluation of fenoterol in patients with chronic obstructive airway disease. Am. Rev. Respir. Dis. 113 Suppl.:111, 1976.

87. Benjamin, C.: A comparative study of the bronchodilator effects of five β-adrenoceptor stimulant drugs in patients with reversible broncho-obstruction. Med. Proc. 18:35–40, 1972.

88. Beardshaw, J., MacLean, L. and Chan-Yeung, M.: Comparison of the bronchodilator and cardiac effects of hydroxyphenylorciprenaline and orciprenaline. Chest 65:507–511, 1974.

88a. Steen, S. N., Smith, R., Kuo, J., Ziment, I. and Beall, G.: Comparison of the bronchodilator effects of oral therapy with fenoterol hydrobromide and ephedrine. Chest 72:291–295, 1977.

88b. Steen, S. N., Smith, R., Kuo, J., Ziment, I. and Beall, G. N.: Comparison of the bronchodilator effects of aerosol fenoterol and isoproterenol. Chest 72:724–730, 1977.

89. Carlstrom, S. (Ed.): Studies on terbutaline, a new selective bronchodilating agent. Acta Med. Scand. Suppl. 512:1–48, 1970.

90. Davies, D. S., George, C. F., Blackwell, E., et al.: Metabolism of terbutaline in man and dog. Br. J. Clin. Pharmac. 1:129–136, 1974.

91. Glass, P. and Dulfano, M. J.: Evaluation of a new beta$_2$ adrenergic receptor stimulant, terbutaline, in bronchospasm. III. Aerosol administration. Curr. Ther. Res. 18:425–432, 1975.

92. Sackner, M. A., Greeneltch, N., Silva, G. and Wanner, A.: Bronchodilator effects of terbutaline and epinephrine in obstructive lung disease. Clin. Pharmacol. Therap 16:499–506, 1974.

92a. Wilson, A. F., Novey, H. S., Cloninger, P., Davis, J. and White, D.: Cardiopulmonary effects of long-term bronchodilator administration. J. Allergy Clin. Immunol. 58:204–212, 1976.

92b. Larsson, S., Svedmyr, N. and Thiringer, G.: Lack of bronchial beta adrenoceptor resistance in asthmatics during long-term treatment with terbutaline. J. Allergy Clin. Immunol. 59:93–100, 1977.

93. Brogden, R. N., Speight, T. M. and Avery, G. S.: Terbutaline: a preliminary report of its pharmacological properties and therapeutic efficacy in asthma. Drugs 6:324–332, 1973.

94. Sackner, M. A., Dougherty, R., Watson, H. and Wanner, A.: Hemodynamic effects of epinephrine and terbutaline in normal man. Chest 68:616–624, 1975.

95. Freedman, B. J.: Trial of new bronchodilator terbutaline in asthma. Br. Med. J. 1:633–636, Mar. 1971.

96. Amory, D. W., Burnham, S. C. and Cheney, F. W., Jr.: Comparison of the cardiopulmonary effects of subcutaneously administered epinephrine and terbutaline in patients with reversible airway obstruction. Chest 67:279–286, 1975.

96a. Smith, P. R., Heurich, A. E., Leffler, C. T., Henis, M. M. J. and Lyons, H. A.: A comparative study of subcutaneously administered terbutaline and epinephrine in the treatment of acute bronchial asthma. Chest 71:129–134, 1977.

97. Morse, J. L. C., Jones, N. L. and Anderson, G. D.: The effect of terbutaline in exercise-induced asthma. Am. Rev. Respir. Dis. 113: 89–92, 1976.

98. Wood, R. E., Wanner, A., Hirsch, J. and Farrell, P. M.: Tracheal mucociliary transport in patients with cystic fibrosis and its stimulation by terbutaline. Am. Rev. Respir. Dis. 111: 733–738, 1975.

99. Sitar, D. S., Piafsky, K. M. and Ogilvie, R. I.: The relative bioavailability of terbutaline (Bricanyl) elixir and tablet formulations. Curr. Ther. Res. 19:266–273, 1976.

99a. Trautlein, J., Allegra, J. and Gillin, M.: A long-term study of low-dose aerosolized terbutaline sulfate. J. Clin. Pharmacol. 16:361–366, 1976.

100. Symposium on salbutamol. Postgrad. Med. J. Suppl. 47:1–133, Mar., 1971.

100a. Poynter, D., Harris, D. M. and Jack, D.: Salbutamol: lack of evidence of tumor induction in man. Br. Med. J. 1:46–47, Jan., 1978.

101. Evans, M. E., Walker, S. R., Brittain, R. T. and Paterson, J. W.: The metabolism of salbutamol in man. Xenobiotica 3:113–120, 1973.

102. Owen, J. A.: A bronchodilator well-known in Europe. Hospital Formulary, pp. 386–388, Aug., 1975.

103. Legge, J. S., Gaddie, J. and Palmer, K. N. V.: Comparison of two oral selective β_2-adrenergic stimulant drugs in bronchial asthma. Br. Med. J. 1:637–639, Mar., 1971.

104. Choo-Kang, Y. F. J., MacDonald, H. L. and Horne, N. W.: A comparison of salbutamol

and terbutaline aerosols in bronchial asthma. Practitioner 211:801–804, 1973.

105. Leitch, A. G., Clancy, L. J., Costello, J. F. and Flenley, D. C.: Effect of intravenous infusion of salbutamol on ventilatory response to carbon dioxide and hypoxia and on heart rate and plasma potassium in normal men. Br. Med. J. 1:365–367, Feb., 1976.

106. Snider, G. L. and Laguarda, R.: Albuterol and isoproterenol aerosols. A controlled study of duration of effect in asthmatic patients. J.A.M.A. 221:682–685, 1972.

107. Shenfield, G. M., Evans, M. E., Walker, S. R. and Paterson, J. W.: The fate of nebulized salbutamol (albuterol) administered by intermittent positive pressure respiration to asthmatic patients. Am. Rev. Respir. Dis. 108:501–505, 1973.

108. Harris, L.: Comparison of cardiorespiratory effects of terbutaline and salbutamol aerosols in patients with reversible airways obstruction. Thorax 28:592–595, 1973.

109. Zsoter, T. T. and Epstein, S. W.: Effect of salbutamol on the peripheral circulation in man. Chest 64:465–471, 1973.

110. Walker, S. R., Evans, M. E., Richards, A. J. and Paterson, J. W.: The clinical pharmacology of oral and inhaled salbutamol. Clin. Pharmacol. Ther. 13:861–867, 1972.

111. Harris, D. M.: Salbutamol aerosol in premature labour. Lancet 1:37, 1976.

112. Hastwell, G. B.: Salbutamol aerosol in premature labour. Lancet 1:493, 1976.

113. Taylor, M. W., Gaddie, J., Murchison, L. E. and Palmer, K. N. V.: Metabolic effects of oral salbutamol. Br. Med. J. 1:22, Jan., 1976.

114. Wang, P. and Clausen, T.: Treatment of attacks in hyperkalaemic familial periodic paralysis by inhalation of salbutamol. Lancet 1:221–227, 1976.

115. Choo-Kang, Y. F. J., Parker, S. S. and Grant, I. W. B.: Response of asthmatics to isoprenaline and salbutamol aerosols administered by intermittent positive-pressure ventilation. Br. Med. J. 4:465–468, Nov., 1970.

116. Fitchett, D. H., McNicol, M. W. and Riordan, J. F.: Intravenous salbutamol in management of status asthmaticus. Br. Med. J. 1:53–55, Jan., 1975.

116a. Spiro, S. A., May, C. S., Johnson, A. J. and Paterson, J. W.: Intravenous injection of salbutamol in the management of asthma. Thorax 30:236, 1975.

117. Williams, S. J., Parrish, R. W. and Seaton, A.: Comparison of intravenous aminophylline and salbutamol in severe asthma. Br. Med. J. 4:685, Dec., 1975.

117a. Hetzel, M. R. and Clark, T. J. H.: Comparison of intravenous and aerosol salbutamol. Br. Med. J. 2:919, Oct., 1976.

117b. Semple, P. d'A. and Legge, J. S.: Salbutamol by various routes. Br. Med. J. 2:1449, Dec., 1976.

118. Choo-Kang, Y. F. J., Simpson, W. T. and Grant, I. W. B.: Controlled comparison of the bronchodilator effects of three β-adrenergic stimulant drugs administered by inhalation to patients with asthma. Br. Med. J. 2:287–289, May, 1969.

119. Lal, S., Dash, C. H. and Gribben, M. D.: An economical method of comparing inhaled bronchodilators in reversible diffuse airways obstruction. With special reference to a β-2 stimulant, salmefamol. Thorax 29:317–322, 1974.

120. Funahashi, A. and Hamilton, L. H.: A study of a new bronchodilator: carbuterol. Am. Rev. Respir. Dis. 113:398–400, 1976.

121. Saleeby, P. R. and Ziskind, M. M.: Clinical study on carbuterol (SKF 40383), a new selective bronchodilator agent aerosol: double-blind comparison with isoproterenol aerosol. Curr. Ther. Res. 17:225–233, 1975.

122. Rhoades, R. B., Leifer, K. N., Bloom, F. L. and Wittig, H. J.: Spirometric comparison of carbuterol and isoproterenol aerosol therapy in bronchial asthma. Am. Rev. Respir. Dis. 114:79–86, 1976.

122a. Cockcroft, D. W., Donevan, R. E. and Copland, G. M.: Carbuterol: a double-blind clinical trial comparing carbuterol and salbutamol. Curr. Ther. Res. 19:170–179, 1976.

123. Anderson, G. and Wilkins, E.: A trial of clenbuterol in bronchial asthma. Thorax 32:717–719, 1977.

124. Benjamin, C. and van As, A.: Clinical trial of intravenous hexoprenaline in asthma. S. Afr. Med. J. 46:599–603, 1972.

125. Arner, B. and Magnusson, P. O.: Comparison between ibuterol hydrochloride and terbutaline in asthma. Br. Med. J. 1:72–74, Jan., 1976.

126. Steen, S. N., Ziment, I. and Thomas, J. S.: Pyrbuterol: a new bronchodilator. Phase I-Single dose study. Curr. Ther. Res. 16:1077–1081, 1974.

127. Bleecker, E., McKinney, W., Lyons, H. and Steen, S. N.: Bronchodilator effects of quinterenol sulfate—a preliminary clinical study. Anesth. Analg. 48:7–9, 1969.

128. Buckner, C. K. and Abel, P.: Studies on the effects of enantiomers of soterenol, trimetoquinol and salbutamol on beta adrenergic receptors of isolated guinea-pig atria and trachea. J. Pharmacol. Exp. Ther. 189:616–625, 1974.

129. Scillitani, B., Thomas, J., Brewer, T. F., Lyons, H. and Steen, S. N.: Hoquizil—a new oral bronchodilator. Acta Anaesth. Scandinav. Suppl. 37:299–302, 1970.

130. Aviado, D. M. and Salem, H.: Sympathomimetic bronchodilator preparations available in the United States. Rev. Allergy 24:441–450, 1970.

131. McMahon, F. G. (Ed.): Evaluation of Gastrointestinal, Pulmonary, Anti-Inflammatory and Immunological Agents. Mount Kisco, N.Y. Futura Publishing Company, 1974, Chs. 8, 9.

132. Giles, R. E. and Herzig, D. J.: Pulmonary and antiallergy drugs. *In* Annual Reports in Medicinal Chemistry. R. V. Heinzelman (Ed.). New York, Academic Press, 1975. Vol. 10, Ch. 9.

133. Campbell, A. B. and Soyka, L. F.: Selective beta$_2$-receptor agonists for the treatment of asthma—therapeutic breakthrough or advertising ploy? J. Pediatr. 89:1020–1026, 1976.

6

PHOSPHODIESTERASE INHIBITORS

Drugs that inhibit the enzyme phosphodiesterase result in the persistence of cyclic 3',5'-AMP in the cells; thus, these drugs potentiate the process of bronchodilation, and they also interfere with the liberation of mediators that cause bronchospasm. Phosphodiesterase inhibitors are valuable both in the treatment and the prophylaxis of bronchospasm and are therefore employed in chronic maintenance therapy and in the acute management of status asthmaticus. Although clinical custom has favored utilizing these drugs as secondary agents to the sympathomimetics, their role is currently changing, and they should now be regarded as primary drugs.

At present, the only important phosphodiesterase inhibitors are the *methylxanthines,* all of which are related to *theophylline,* the prototype drug in this class. In the past few years, theophylline has become the subject of extraordinary pharmacologic interest, and it is now one of the few drugs for which detailed pharmacokinetic information has become common knowledge for practicing physicians. Many hospitals currently provide laboratory determinations of serum levels for this drug; very few other medications are accorded this degree of pharmacologic attention.

METHYLXANTHINES

The methylxanthines are 3-methylated xanthines (Figure 6–1). This class of alkaloids is widely spread throughout the plant world; however, most of the drugs in use today are produced synthetically. The important popular beverages, coffee, tea, cola and cocoa, owe their effects to the methylxanthine content of caffeine, theobromine and theophylline. Pure caffeine and theobromine are still occasionally used as clinical drugs, but less so than in previous years.

Theophylline, which is 1:3 dimethyl dioxypurine (dimethylxanthine), was introduced into medicine in 1900; *aminophylline,* its main salt, was made available 10 years later. Although the xanthines were known to be respiratory stimulants and to be of value in cardiac and pulmonary asthma since the beginning of this century, it was not until 1936 that intravenous aminophylline became established as a major treatment for asthma. At present, a considerable number of proprietary medications contain theophylline or aminophylline. There are a smaller number of marketed products that contain other methylxanthine derivatives. Aminophylline is of particular importance, since it is given by the intravenous route in the management of acute bronchospasm.

METABOLISM AND SERUM LEVELS OF THEOPHYLLINE

Oral theophylline is well absorbed from simple preparations in which it is compounded.[1] About 10 per cent is excreted unchanged in the urine; the remainder is inactivated, at a variable rate, by demethylation and oxidation by the liver microsomal system, and excreted mainly as mono- and di-methyluric acids. Complete demethyla-

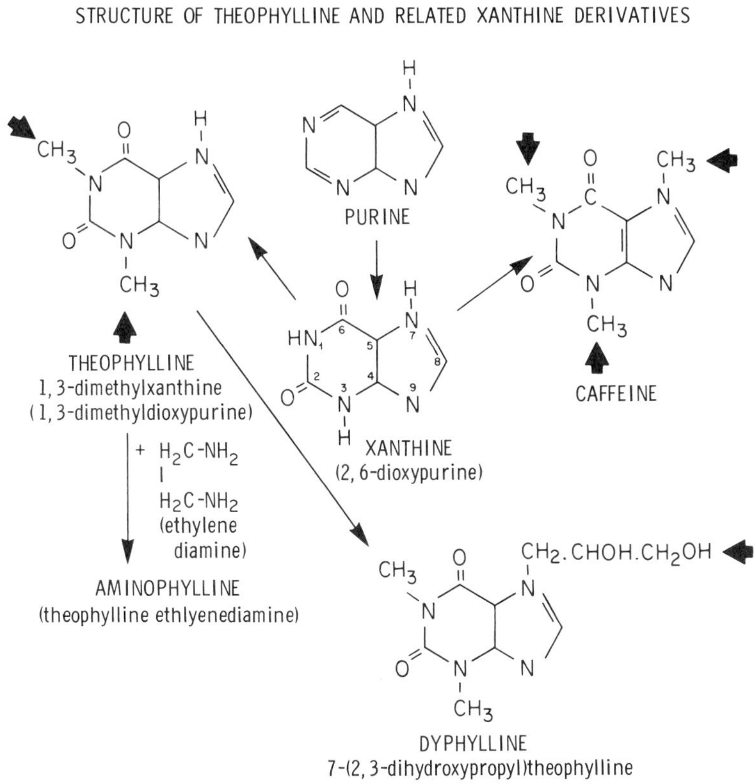

STRUCTURE OF THEOPHYLLINE AND RELATED XANTHINE DERIVATIVES

Figure 6–1. Structure of theophylline and related xanthine derivatives. The thick arrows point to significant groups that characterize each molecule. Xanthine is a purine derivative; caffeine and theophylline are derived from xanthine. Aminophylline is theophylline dissolved in the solvent ethylenediamine. Dyphylline is tne dihydroxypropyl derivative of theophylline.

tion of the xanthine metabolites does not occur. There is, therefore, no increase in excretion of uric acid following theophylline administration. Thus, gout would not be exacerbated, although certain laboratory methods for determining uric acid will give falsely elevated values if the patient has been taking methylxanthine drugs. Similarly, since xanthine oxidase is not involved in theophylline degradation, drugs used in the treatment of gout that inhibit this enzyme do not have any effect on theophylline pharmacokinetics.

The serum half-life of theophylline in normal adults is usually around 8 hours with a range of 3.0 to 9.5 hours; it rarely exceeds 10 hours.[1a] The half-life in children is shorter, ranging from 1.5 to 9.5 hours with a mean of about 3.6 hours.[2, 3] However, there is considerable variation between individuals, and with repeated doses in a given subject the half-life may increase somewhat,[4] although tachyphylaxis does not appear to occur even after continued use of the drug for years. If a patient is unable to metabolize and clear the drug normally (such as may occur for unknown reasons, although, more often, heart failure or hepatic insufficiency

is at fault), the serum half-life may be as long as 28 hours.[5] The marked variation in half-lives among individual patients cannot be predicted before initiating therapy, but physicians should be aware that patients do require some individual care in achieving the appropriate dosage. More recently, marked variations in theophylline kinetic parameters have been found in individual patients on repeated testing.[6, 7] However, more careful studies suggest that changes in clearance do not occur in healthy subjects, and even in growing children clearances may remain constant for many months.[7a, 7b]

Although a therapeutic effect may appear with theophylline serum levels at or above 5 mcg/ml,[4] many studies have revealed that optimal bronchodilation is achieved with levels over 10 mcg/ml.[2] A major problem in theophylline therapy is that toxicity begins to appear with serum levels slightly above the therapeutic range, which most investigators consider as 10 to 20 mcg/ml of serum.[8] The fact that there is a relatively narrow therapeutic range, which is very close to the toxic level, has led to a great interest in the pharmacokinetics of this drug. As a consequence, theophylline is now one of a

TABLE 6–1. THEOPHYLLINE PHARMACOKINETICS

| | Serum Half-Lives | | |
	Usual Range (Hours)	Mean (Hours)	Comments
ADULTS	3–9.5		Increases in presence of diseases that decrease clear-
nonsmokers		9	ance; decreases in cigarette smokers, and in patients
smokers		5.5	exposed to hydrocarbon fumes
CHILDREN	1.2–10	3.5	Marked variation at different ages

Therapeutic Response*	Peak Serum Level (mcg/ml or mg/l)
No effect	5
Suboptimal therapeutic level	5–10
Optimal therapeutic range	10–20
Anxiety appears	>15
Gastrointestinal toxicity appears	>15
Usual toxic level	20
Arrhythmias likely to occur	>30
Convulsions may occur	>40

*Patients who have not been previously exposed to theophylline may develop adverse effects independent of serum level during initial acute administration of drug.

handful of commonly used drugs for which determinations of serum levels are considered to provide useful information in clinical practice. Indeed, the torrent of papers that has expounded on the value of serum levels during the past few years has convinced many physicians that such determinations constitute a criterion of standard practice in patients receiving theophylline drugs. This concern about serum levels is appropriate in many cases, but it should be realized that the majority of patients can be adequately managed without resorting to the trouble and expense of obtaining checks on the theophylline level. The young adult with asthma who is otherwise healthy usually responds well to standard dosage; the guidance provided by serum level monitoring is not an essential requirement. Younger or older patients and those with abnormal theophylline metabolism do require more careful dosing; serum levels can be helpful in such cases.

In normal individuals, toxic symptoms appear as the serum level of theophylline approaches 20 mcg/ml, but some patients tolerate levels above 30 mcg/ml. Although it is desirable to give the methylxanthines in such a manner as to achieve the therapeutic range and avoid the toxic range, this objective is not practical in most patients, since it is obtained only by giving a constant rate venous infusion of the drug. However, the use of the reliable sustained-release products that are now available results in a more controlled serum level for patients on chronic oral therapy.

The correlation of adverse symptoms with serum levels is shown in Table 6–1; these side effects are not always manifested at the appropriate serum level, and some patients may go on to develop seizures without premonitory gastric, cerebral or cardiac symptoms if the serum level is allowed to rise too high.

MONITORING OF SERUM LEVELS

Recently, the monitoring of serum levels has become a more practical consideration, since rapid and relatively inexpensive techniques involving high-pressure liquid chromatography are becoming available.[9] Unlike the older Schack-Waxler method (which used ultraviolet spectrophotometry), the newer techniques can accurately measure theophylline levels in the presence of its metabolites, other xanthines (such as caffeine) or other drugs. A new radioimmunoassay method will allow determinations to be made rapidly, inexpensively and with greater practical ease.[9a] However, many workers are satisfied with high quality liquid chromatography assays, and this technique will probably be the standard for most hospitals during the next few years. Recently, a simplified semi-microspectrophotometric technique has been reported to be suitable for office use.[10] If assays can be made as inexpensively as simple pulmonary function tests, then monitoring of theophylline levels will become a standard practice. The ideal assay would be one that was rapid and easy to carry out, inexpensive yet accurate, requiring very small volumes of blood, and not affected by the presence of other drugs in the serum. Meanwhile, awareness of the potential pitfalls in conventional assay methods should be maintained.[10a, 10b]

If it is decided that serum theophylline levels need to be monitored in any individual, the following considerations should be kept in mind:

(a) The patient should not receive any non-therapeutic xanthine (tea, cola, chocolate) on the day of the determination, unless a high-pressure liquid chromatography method of measurement or immunoassay is used.

(b) For frequent determinations, *saliva* can be used instead of serum, since the saliva level parallels, and is about half (actually 55 per cent), the serum level.[5] However, in such cases, the drug should not be given by mouth unless it is protected from contact with the oral mucosa. Saliva is obtained by first having the patient thoroughly rinse out the mouth; the subject then chews on an inert material, such as a Parafilm ball.[5] A few ml of the saliva that results should be collected in a glass container. It may be advisable to determine the exact ratio of saliva/serum levels in individual patients by comparing simultaneous plasma and saliva levels on one or two occasions. Recently, it has been reported that the obtaining of saliva specimens from many patients results both in technical difficulties and unreliable assay results,[10c] and the technique is no longer recommended.

(c) Samples should be taken at appropriate intervals, so that levels can be determined for purposes of solving specific problems. If a patient complains of nausea, a theophylline level should be obtained on a serum sample taken within one to two hours of oral dosing; if the serum level is in the toxic range, dosage reduction can be made. In contrast, if a patient on a relatively large dosage of a theophylline preparation does not experience adequate control of bronchospasm, a serum level determination should be made prior to the administration of a maintenance dose; if the level is inadequate, the dosage can be increased, or the time between successive dosings may need to be shortened. In many situations, several serum or saliva determinations will be required to gain an insight into an individual's pharmacokinetic handling of theophylline.

For general evaluation, determination of the peak serum level can be utilized; sampling should be carried out about two hours after oral dosing. If a sustained-release preparation is taken every eight hours, blood for a serum level determination should be taken four hours after the last dose. It should be noted that for most patients on chronic therapy, a single peak level of theophylline is the only determination that the physician will require as a check on the appropriateness of the dosage schedule. Some further suggestions with regard to the use of determinations of serum levels of the theophylline are discussed later in this chapter.

FACTORS AFFECTING DOSAGES OF THEOPHYLLINE AND AMINOPHYLLINE

Pharmacokinetic studies by several different workers have been published that offer precise guidelines to theophylline dosages. However, such precision is neither appropriate nor possible in many patients, and an obsessive desire to comply with such guidelines is bound to result in frustration. Furthermore, new guidelines are published at frequent intervals, as a consequence of the high level of interest in elucidating what normal and abnormal factors govern the pharmacokinetics of theophylline and its derivatives.[10d, 10e] Although various nomograms have been published,[11, 11a] they rapidly become outdated. Until a full understanding of theophylline pharmacokinetics has been worked out, sound clinical judgment and experience will continue to provide the best guide to theophylline dosage.[3]

Jenne and co-workers[12] confirmed earlier work by Turner-Warwick[13] that showed that adults require a theophylline serum level of 10 to 20 mcg per ml for optimal bronchodilation. To achieve this, adult patients must first be given a loading dose of the drug, followed by maintenance dosages every six hours. For intravenous therapy, an initial loading dose (in the form of aminophylline) is required, but it has not been clearly established whether intermittent maintenance dosages are preferable to a continuous infusion that provides an identical total 24-hour dose.

If the recommended loading dose of aminophylline is administered rapidly by the intravenous route, a blood sample taken after the infusion is completed will usually reveal a theophylline level in excess of 20 mcg/ml, which is in the toxic range. Successive dosings lead to a gradual increase in the mean serum level, until a stable situation is attained. Intermittent therapy will always result in peaks and valleys, whereas a continuous infusion will result in a plateau. Many physicians feel that the peaks achieved in intermittent therapy, every four to six hours, result in more effective therapy, whereas the advocates of continuous infusion delivery feel that equally effective therapy is attained by the infusion, without the dangers of the toxic levels produced at each peak of intermittent dosing.

The best method of administering intravenous aminophylline is debatable, although, in practice, it may not be an important issue, since most patients generally do well with either approach. Furthermore, it is often impossible to ensure continuous intravenous infusion, unless an infusion pump is utilized and the patient is monitored carefully, since intravenous therapy is notoriously prone to difficulties and hazards that interfere with precise administration. Fortunately, intravenous therapy is rarely essential in resistant cases of status asthmaticus for more than one to two days, and it is usually possible to discontinue this form of treatment within the first 36 hours.

For the patient who does not require intravenous therapy, oral and rectal routes are available; of course, the alimentary orifices are less suited to continuous infusions. Thus, in practice, most patients who are given aminophylline, theophylline or related methylxanthines obtain these medications by intermittent dosing. Several slow-release formulations are available for oral

use, and provided their reliability is completely established, these preparations offer some advantages with regard to effectiveness and toxicity.[8, 14] Other preparations, such as rapidly dissolving tablets, may offer advantages, but further studies are required to determine the best forms of theophylline for oral administration.

Pharmacokinetic studies of theophylline and aminophylline have confirmed the need for a loading dose followed by an appropriate maintenance regimen. However, certain variables need to be taken into consideration (Table 6–2).

(a) Children can tolerate, and probably require, proportionally larger dosages than do adults, since they eliminate the drug at a rate as much as 60 per cent greater than that of adults.[5] It has now been shown that even young children and babies require proportionally larger doses than do older children and adults.[7b]

(b) Impaired liver activity results in a decreased ability of the body to handle the methylxanthines;[14a] symptoms of overdosage occur if standard dosage is maintained, since drug accumulation will result. Elderly and cirrhotic patients are at particular risk, and often require a reduction in dosage, or at least an avoidance of high-dose therapy.[14b]

(c) Prolonged administration of a methylxanthine may result in the induction of enzymes that alter the metabolism of these drugs. This, however, is an unusual problem, since most patients do not experience any decrease in the effectiveness of the theophyllines even after years of use. However, if the drug does seem to lose its therapeutic efficacy after a time, the dosage should be

TABLE 6–2. MODIFICATIONS NEEDED IN THEOPHYLLINE DOSAGES

Situations Requiring Increased Dosage	Situations Requiring Decreased Dosage
Children 2 months to 16 years	Premature neonates (theophylline treatment rarely justified)
Cigarette smokers, and patients exposed to hydrocarbon fumes	Elderly patients with borderline cardiac and hepatic function
Patients with suboptimal blood levels or blood levels below 10 mcg/ml	Cirrhosis, hepatic insufficiency
Patients with acidosis (possibly)	Heart failure, cor pulmonale, acute pulmonary edema, pneumonia
Patients who are known to have a high tolerance to theophylline, i.e. rapid metabolizers	Patients who manifest toxic symptoms on standard dosage
Patients on high protein diet	Patients who have received theophylline therapy in previous 24 hours
	Patients with alkalosis (possibly)
	Patients with fever and toxemia
	Patients taking a macrolide antibiotic (troleandomycin and erythromycins)

cautiously increased to see if a favorable response can be obtained.

(d) Specific factors or individual biologic variation may result in an individual patient responding in an inappropriate fashion to the recommended dosage. The influence of associated diseases or the medications used to treat them may be important.[15] Diseases such as heart failure, pneumonia[16] and acute pulmonary edema,[17] as well as hepatic insufficiency, have been reported to decrease theophylline clearance, and there can be no doubt that reports of other diseases with similar effects on xanthine kinetics will appear in the literature. Recently, it was reported than an acidotic patient, such as one with acute respiratory failure, requires a higher loading dose of theophylline to achieve a therapeutic level than does an alkalotic patient.[18] The effects of various drugs on theophylline kinetics will undoubtedly be a profitable area for future studies. At present, relatively little is known, other than the fact that some agents do interfere with the chronotropic actions of theophylline, for example, phenothiazine, reserpine, beta-blockers such as propranolol and ganglion-blockers such as hexamethonium and reserpine.[3] Recently, the macrolide antibiotics, troleandomycin and erythromycin salts, were reported to result in an increase in the serum levels achieved by theophylline.[18a, 18b]

(e) Oral administration of the methylxanthines can result in variable serum levels of theophylline, depending on factors such as the presence of food in the stomach. Better absorption is thought to occur if the drug is administered with fairly large volumes of water. Absorption is optimal when the drug is given before eating, and is less impaired when dosing is carried out after a high protein meal rather than after a high fat or high carbohydrate meal.[19] However, the presence of food in the stomach does not seem to significantly affect the absorption of the theophyllines. People who consistently eat high protein diets eliminate theophylline more rapidly and require slightly increased dosages.[19a]

(f) The preparation used probably does have some effect on the absorption of an oral form of methylxanthine.[19a] Although it has been suggested that phenobarbital-containing combination preparations interfere with theophylline absorption, this does not appear to be so.[20] An alcoholic elixir of theophylline is better, or at least more rapidly, absorbed than tablet forms; newer, microfine crystal tablet forms however, are claimed to be very well absorbed. In general, any oral liquid or simple tablet appears to be well absorbed, whereas some enteric-coated preparations and sustained-release products have less reliable absorption.[20a, 20b, 20c, 20d]

(g) Theophylline half-life may be significantly decreased in cigarette smokers,[8, 21] because inhaled polycyclic hydrocarbons apparently induce hepatic ribosomal enzymes that metabolize theophylline. Similarly, patients who live in a polluted atmosphere may metabolize theophylline more rapidly; as yet, experience in Los Angeles has not confirmed that this is of practical significance. Since patients who require theophylline for the treatment of chronic obstructive lung disease are, all too often, confirmed smokers, there may be a need to adjust the dosage should the patient quit smoking.

PHARMACOLOGIC EFFECTS
(Table 6-3)

There are primary, therapeutically desirable, effects and secondary, undesirable, side effects attributable to theophylline and its derivatives.

Primary Effects. Since the methylxanthines have beneficial effects on many organs in the body, theophylline and its derivatives are used in the treatment of several conditions besides bronchospasm. However, the most valuable effects are found to occur in the respiratory system, and these drugs are correctly regarded as being primarily bronchodilators. The following *therapeutic effects* are recognized:

RESPIRATORY EFFECTS. Theophylline is a powerful relaxer of bronchial muscles, and it can be used as a routine drug in chronic maintenance therapy or for the acute treatment of bronchospasm; it is a major therapy for status asthmaticus. Many physicians now regard theophylline or aminophylline as the agent of choice for the treatment of an exacerbation of asthma that is not responsive to the patient's conventional sympathomimetic drugs. Although subcutaneous epinephrine is often favored as the first agent to try in status asthmaticus, it may be appropriate to bypass this drug and give the patient intravenous aminophylline. Now that terbutaline and salbutamol have been shown to be

TABLE 6–3. PHARMACOLOGIC EFFECTS OF THEOPHYLLINE

Respiratory	Decreases bronchospasm Stimulates respiration and increases respiratory response to hypoxia Corrects Cheyne-Stokes breathing (aminophylline) May increase or decrease PaO_2 Alleviates cardiogenic pulmonary edema
Cardiac	Inotropic effect may increase cardiac output (reflex decrease may occur secondarily) May decrease cardiac output (after rapid intravenous administration of aminophylline) Chronotropic effect may result in tachycardia May decrease right atrial pressure in cor pulmonale
Vascular	Vasodilator of pulmonary vessels, causing a decrease in pulmonary hypertension Vasodilator of coronary vessels, causing an increase in coronary flow Vasoconstrictor of cerebral vessels
Blood Pressure	May increase or decrease (or may cause severe fall in) blood pressure
Involuntary Muscle	Causes relaxation (for example, of biliary duct, ureter)
Kidney	Increases renal plasma flow and glomerular filtration, may cause diuresis Can cause potassium diuresis, leading to hypokalemia
Nervous System	Stimulates
Stomach	Irritates (mainly related to serum level of theophylline)
Adrenal Gland	Releases catecholamines (which affect heart rate and blood pressure)

of value in this situation, these new drugs may be tried first by the subcutaneous or intravenous route; however, even if the response is relatively satisfactory, intravenous aminophylline will usually be required also.

Theophylline and other methylxanthines are also of value in maintenance and prophylactic therapy in patients with chronic bronchospasm. An investigational agent, *ICI 58,301,* which is a phosphodiesterase inhibitor, has been shown to have superior properties as a prophylactic, since it is more effective as a preventative of bronchoconstriction than as a bronchodilator.[22] However, the methylxanthines currently available seem to be equally effective in each role.

It has long been known that aminophylline, when given as an intravenous injection, can convert Cheyne-Stokes periodic breathing to a normal, regular pattern. There is evidence that it is the ethylenediamine component of aminophylline that regularizes and stimulates respiration in these patients by its action on the respiratory center; the theophylline component of aminophylline seems to potentiate the effect.[23] This appears to be the only therapeutic property of ethylenediamine; its other pharmacologic effects probably are mostly adverse. Theophylline administration to a patient with obstructed airways often increases depth of breathing and improves expectoration, but it

does not increase frequency of breathing and it is not a mucolytic. Aminophylline increases the ventilatory response to hypoxia, but not to hypercapnia.[23a]

CARDIAC EFFECTS. The xanthines have a direct stimulatory effect on the heart, resulting in an increase in cardiac output. The response of the heart rate is variable. Initially, there is usually an increase, but there is a secondary reflex slowing of the heart, apparently attributable to stimulation of the central vagal nuclei by xanthines. Recent studies have shown that the chronotropic effect of aminophylline has three components: a major direct effect on autonomic centers, a lesser effect due to local catecholamine release, and a peripheral vagolytic action.[24] In some patients, the cardiac output shows a secondary decrease after, perhaps, half an hour. Overrapid administration can cause complex and adverse cardiodynamic reactions, which are generally explained as constituting "overstimulation" of the heart. Measurable improvements can be found in patients with cardiac failure following an optimal dose of theophylline: these include increased coronary flow, increased cardiac work and output, and a decrease in right atrial pressure.

The initial response to theophylline is thus beneficial in heart failure, and the drug (conventionally given as intravenous aminophylline) is of value in the initial treatment of pulmonary edema. However, other appropriate therapy (oxygen, diuretics, digoxin) must also be provided, or else the secondary effects after the first hour may be detrimental. Excessive dosage of the methylxanthines produces effects comparable to those elicited by stimulation of beta-1 adrenergic receptors, although the phosphodiesterase inhibitors do not act on the adrenergic receptors. The response to excessive amounts of intravenous aminophylline or rectal theophylline is complex, since it involves the direct effect of the drug, not only on the heart, but also on the blood vessels, with further secondary reflex responses.

VASCULAR EFFECTS. In general, the xanthines act as vasodilators. The most significant vascular effect is pulmonary vasodilation, and theophylline appears to be one of the most powerful and effective drugs for the reduction of pulmonary hypertension. This action on the pulmonary vasculature can result in a fall in PaO_2 in bronchospastic patients, since the vasodilation may cause an increase in the shunt through the lungs. However, the decrease in bronchospasm and improved mucokinesis generally result in an improvement in gas exchange, with an increase in PaO_2 as a consequence.

The xanthines are thought to cause coronary vasodilation, as already pointed out, but the exact response to therapeutic dosing with intravenous aminophylline is controversial. The drug was once thought to be of value in the treatment of coronary artery disease, but currently this is not regarded as a valid use for the xanthines.

It is of interest that the xanthines appear to act in the opposite way on the blood vessels of the brain, and cause cerebral vasoconstriction. These drugs have been shown to be effective in the treatment of some cases of hypertensive headache, but a further claim that migraine can also be treated is not generally accepted. It is noteworthy that some habitual coffee drinkers develop a withdrawal syndrome accompanied by headaches when caffeine is withheld; thus, it appears that methylxanthines do affect cerebral vessels. However, headaches, which may be migrainous, are not uncommon side effects of theophylline therapy, particularly in children. Thus, it is difficult to support the old claim that this drug is effective in the treatment of headaches.

The overall peripheral vasodilation that follows the administration of large doses of the xanthines causes a decrease in venous return and can result in hypotension. However, the strong inotropic effect of the drug on the heart, and the central vasoconstrictor effect that follows secondarily, may combine to produce hypertension. Thus, the effect on blood pressure is variable, and depends on several factors, such as the dose of drug, the route and rate of administration, prior dosage with xanthines, the presence of other drugs in the body, and the state of the cardiovascular and autonomic nervous systems.

EFFECTS ON INVOLUNTARY MUSCLE. Besides producing relaxation of bronchial muscle, the xanthines can relax other involuntary muscles. Xanthines may be of value in the treatment of biliary colic and renal colic; however, these effects are of relatively little practical value.

RENAL EFFECTS. The xanthines improve blood flow to the kidney both directly (by vasodilating renal vessels) and indirectly (by increasing cardiac output); the result is an increase in the glomerular filtration rate. Moreover, these drugs appear to have a direct action on the renal tubules, resulting in decreased tubular reabsorption. Theophylline, therefore, acts as a diuretic; this property is fairly powerful, although it is short-lived. The drinking of coffee and tea also causes a slight methylxanthine-induced diuresis; caffeine and theobromine are sometimes used clinically as mild diuretics.

The diuretic effects of theophylline, coupled with its beneficial effects on bronchospasm and pulmonary hypertension, as well as its stimulation of the failing heart, account for the great value attributed to this drug in the management of the pulmonary edema that may be associated with congestive heart failure.

EFFECTS ON VOLUNTARY MUSCLE. The xanthines improve the functioning of skeletal muscle and decrease the sense of fatigue. This is one of the explanations for the benefits ascribed to tea and coffee. It is less certain that theophylline and its pharmacologic derivatives confer any significant muscular benefit when given for the usual clinical indications.

CENTRAL NERVOUS SYSTEM EFFECTS. The methylxanthines enjoy traditional and widespread popularity, partly accounted for by the central stimulating effects conferred by the various infusions of natural xanthine products that are consumed in such liberal quantities. Theophylline and the other derivatives that are employed clinically do have some stimulatory effect on the brain,

TABLE 6–4. ADVERSE EFFECTS OF THEOPHYLLINE THERAPY

Cardiovascular	Palpitations, tachycardia, arrhythmias Hypotension, vasomotor collapse, shock Hypertension, headache
Gastrointestinal	Anorexia, nausea, vomiting, thirst, abdominal distress, indigestion, abdominal pain, diarrhea Hematemesis, melena
Nervous System	Anxiety, irritability, agitation insomnia, tremulousness, mania Dizziness, faintness Twitching, seizures
Allergy*	Rashes, anaphylaxis
Blood Gases	Fall in PaO_2
Other	Diaphoresis Hematuria Hypokalemic alkalosis

*Allergic responses are probably caused by the ethylenediamine in aminophylline.

but this is of a much lower order than that found with caffeine. In general, the central nervous system stimulation caused by theophylline is not a significant primary effect of the drug, but can be manifested as a common, and sometimes serious, side effect.

GASTRIC EFFECTS. The stomach is the

TABLE 6–5. PRECAUTIONS REQUIRED WITH THEOPHYLLINE THERAPY

Relative Contraindications*	Absolute Contraindications†
Extremes of age	
Tachycardia Cardiac failure with hypoxemia Unstable blood pressure	Uncontrolled tachyarrhythmia Uncontrolled hypertension
Seizure history Severe anxiety	Uncontrolled seizures Agitated tremulousness
Active liver disease Peptic ulcer history Nausea Diarrhea	Hepatic failure Active peptic ulcer Vomiting Gastrointestinal bleeding
Hyperthyroidism	Thyroid storm
Glaucoma	
Hypersensitivity to ethylenediamine in aminophylline	Use by a physician who is unfamiliar with the drug
Failure of recent theophylline therapy	Inadequate supervision of patient's therapy

*Relative contraindications–theophyllines may be given, but great care must be taken.
†Absolute contraindications–theophyllines should be avoided unless the risk of withholding treatment is greater than the risk of the possibly severe side effects.

only organ whose stimulation by the methylxanthines results in entirely undesired side effects. The full explanation for the adverse actions of the drugs is not certain, but the xanthines do stimulate acid secretion, and they may cause reverse peristalsis, thereby resulting in gastric discomfort and nausea.

Undesired Side Effects. When the xanthines are given for the treatment of bronchospasm, certain undesirable side effects may occur[25] (Table 6–4). Although a predisposition to these toxic effects does not necessarily constitute a contraindication to xanthine therapy, the drugs should be used with great care when there is a special risk (Table 6–5). The appearance of side effects is related to the theophylline serum level (see Table 6–1).

The most common problems are anorexia, nausea and vomiting; these symptoms frequently appear when a patient is receiving maximal therapy in cases of severe bronchospasm, but they may also trouble the patient on lower-dose chronic theophylline therapy. In many patients diarrhea occurs, and rarely gastric bleeding results in hematemesis or melena. The exact mechanism involved in the adverse gastric effects is still unclear, but it appears that a serum level of around 15 mcg/ml or greater may induce nausea.[8] The effect could be a central one, caused by stimulation of the vomiting center in the medulla, or it may be a direct toxic effect on the gastric mucosa of the medication in the stomach or of the absorbed drug circulating in the blood stream. The problem appears to be greater if oral therapy is given, suggesting that a topical action on the gastric mucosa is concerned; indeed, actual stomach discomfort or abdominal pain may be experienced by some patients. Certain of the derivatives of theophylline appear to be less likely to cause gastric irritation when given orally, and this quality is the basis for much of the pharmaceutic competition in the marketing of various methylxanthine preparations. There are an increasing number of reports that demonstrate that nausea and vomiting might not occur as presenting features of toxicity, and that some patients experience more serious complications as a first indication that the theophylline level in the blood has reached a toxic level.[26]

The cardiovascular side effects are seen mainly with intravenous aminophylline; palpitations, tachycardia, and arrhythmias may occur, and are relatively common with serum levels in excess of 30 mcg/ml. Rapid injection of the drug, or administration of too large a dose, can result in serious or fatal consequences; however, the full explanation for this outcome is not established. Both hypotension and hypertension can be produced, and any disturbance in blood pressure may aggravate the cardiac status and result in a considerable decrease in cardiac output with consequent vasomotor collapse. It is possible that some of these serious reactions are due to hypersensitivity to the drug, although idiosyncratic reactions are very rare.[27] The various cardiodynamic responses are complex and difficult to explain, but the possibility of inducing potentially fatal reactions necessitates extreme caution when giving intravenous aminophylline or large doses of methylxanthine by other routes.

There are claims that an acute respiratory arrest may also be produced as a result of the toxic action of the drug on the respiratory center. Furthermore, the pulmonary vasodilation that the xanthines cause may be manifested as a right-to-left shunt with a fall in PaO_2; this can exacerbate the cardiorespiratory problems. These toxic effects of the xanthines are likely to be potentiated by concomitant sympathomimetic drug therapy.

The cerebral effects of the methylxanthines are similar to those of the sympathomimetic drugs. Thus, anxiety, irritability, restlessness, insomnia and tremulousness can occur, although these symptoms are less pronounced than they are with sympathomimetic therapy. Other nervous system side effects include dizziness, faintness, lightheadedness and, often, headache. A particular problem with intravenous aminophylline is the danger of drug-induced seizures, which can be fatal; this complication is usually dose-related, occurring mainly with high theophylline serum levels, over 40 mcg/ml.[15] Patients with liver disease and heart failure appear to be more susceptible to such severe reactions after standard doses.[28] Decreased clearance may occur in ill patients with cor pulmonale or pneumonia, or just with fever; in such high-risk groups even oral administration of theophylline, in a dose that would be appropriate for the individual when healthy, can cause a higher serum level, and result in a grand mal seizure.[29]

Children may have a relatively greater tolerance for xanthine therapy than adults, but reports of sudden death are alarmingly common in the pediatric literature. Rectal administration may be particularly dangerous in this respect if overzealous suppository therapy is used, especially in children under the age of six. Occasionally, adults and children show allergic responses, particularly to aminophylline; these are usually no more serious than skin rashes,[30] but anaphylactic reactions can occur.

Overdosage with aminophylline or theophylline can result in a toxic syndrome characterized by frequent vomiting, marked thirst, severe agitation and mania, cardiac arrhythmias, convulsions and shock; the end result may be death. Overdosages of theophylline drugs can be treated by resin hemoperfusion.[29a]

CONTRAINDICATIONS

The methylxanthines are difficult to use correctly and careful dosing is always required; and in certain cases the drugs should be avoided, if this is feasible (Table 6–5). A major contraindication to the use of these drugs is created when patient supervision is suboptimal; this warning applies particularly to the intravenous administration of aminophylline. The drugs are dangerous in patients with myocardial disease or cardiac arrhythmias and in subjects with unstable blood pressure. They should be given with great care to patients with hyperthyroidism, or with anxiety or a history of seizures, since these states can be exacerbated. Most theophylline preparations are poorly tolerated by patients with peptic ulcer disease, and they should not be given if the patient is nauseated or vomiting. Glaucoma is also said to be a contraindication.

Elderly patients and those with circulatory disease or poor hepatic function require careful monitoring to avoid overdosage. Similarly, additional care is needed when the drugs are given to children, particularly those who are under six years of age. Precautions should be taken to prevent toxicity; this may necessitate intensive cardiovascular monitoring and serial determinations of blood levels of the drug when potentially toxic amounts are being given. Theophylline may interact with certain drugs[3, 18a, 18b, 31] (Table 6–6), but the results are of relatively minor importance. In general, aminophylline should not be mixed with other drugs, since incompatibilities are fairly common.[32]

TABLE 6–6. THEOPHYLLINE : DRUG INTERACTIONS

Drug	Result
INTERFERENCES	
Lithium	Excretion increased by theophylline (especially if sodium bicarbonate is added)
Oral anticoagulants	Increased plasma prothrombin and Factor V observed in animals that are also given theophylline (not significant)
Phenobarbital, barbiturates	Reduce hepatic oxidative microsomal enzymes; may decrease theophylline catabolism
Polycyclic hydrocarbons	(From tobacco smoke or smog) induce microsomal catabolic enzymes, and thereby shorten serum half-life of theophylline
Beta-blockers	Theophylline antagonizes propranolol and vice versa
Phenothiazines, ganglion blockers, reserpine	Antagonize chronotropic effect of theophylline
Chlordiazepoxide	Theophyllines antagonize fatty acid mobilization that chlordiazepoxide causes.
POTENTIATIONS	
Sympathomimetic agents	Increased bronchodilation, and beta-1 and beta-2 side effects
Diuretics	Increased diuretic effect; can cause hypokalemia
Digitalis glycosides	Potentiate effects on heart; increased tendency to vomiting
Troleandomycin (TAO), erythromycins	Inhibit theophylline clearance
INCOMPATIBILITIES (in intravenous solutions)	(In general, avoid combining with other drugs)
ACTH	Precipitates when added to aminophylline
Calcium salts	Precipitate in aminophylline solution
Potassium penicillin	Slowly precipitates in aminophylline solution
Cephalothin, chloramphenicol, methicillin, erythromycin, tetracycline	May deteriorate in presence of aminophylline
Pressor amines (e.g. isoproterenol)	Deteriorate in presence of aminophylline
Acidic solutions	Precipitation may occur
Other incompatibilities	e.g. phenothiazines, phenytoin, hydroxyzine, meperidine

Note: Elixirs of theophylline that contain alcohol can cause severe reactions in patients taking disulfiram (Antabuse), metronidazole or chlorpropamide.

PHARMACOLOGY OF INDIVIDUAL METHYLXANTHINES

The important methylxanthines for the treatment of respiratory diseases are theophylline and aminophylline, and their related derivatives. They are utilized mostly for the treatment of bronchospasm.

THEOPHYLLINE
(Table 6–7)

Theophylline has a low solubility in water, requiring 120 parts of water to dissolve 1 part of theophylline; theophylline is 20-fold more soluble in the industrial solvent ethylenediamine, the product being aminophylline. It is also more soluble in ethyl alcohol, 1 part dissolving in 80 of alcohol. Numerous products are available, differing in factors such as solvents and pharmaceutic formulation, and there are many combination preparations. Various salts of theophylline are also used commercially; these are discussed in a later section.

There are three groups of medications in which theophylline is the active component: (1) elixirs, tablets and capsules of theophylline for oral use; (2) rectal preparations of theophylline; (3) combinations of theophylline and other drugs for oral use. The most important commercial products are listed in Table 6–8.[33-35]

Oral Preparations of Theophylline. Since theophylline has low solubility in water, the drug is usually given in solid form, or as alcoholic elixirs; however, nonalcoholic syrups and simple solutions are now marketed.

TABLETS AND CAPSULES. Tablets of anhydrous theophylline are favored by many physicians, and since there is adequate documentation of the acceptability and effectiveness of such tablets,[35a] which are relatively inexpensive, they should be regarded as the drugs of choice. A more soluble anhydrous product, originally available in Australia (as Neulin), has recently been introduced

TABLE 6–7. THE THEOPHYLLINES

ACTION	Inhibit phosphodiesterase
BENEFICIAL EFFECTS	Relieve bronchospasm, improve cardiac action, diuretic
THERAPEUTIC RANGE	10–20 mcg/ml serum
ADVERSE EFFECTS	Gastric irritation, cerebral overstimulation, myocardial irritation, change in blood pressure (with rapid intravenous administration of aminophylline)
TOXICITY EXACERBATED BY	Extremes of age, cardiac failure, hypoxia or hepatic insufficiency
SOLUBILITY	Low solubility in water, soluble in alcohol, soluble in ethylenediamine (as aminophylline), soluble in alkaline solutions
DOSAGE FORMS	Theophylline—tablets, elixirs, rectal solutions Aminophylline—tablets, intravenous solution, suppositories Other derivatives—mainly oral forms Combination products—oral forms
USUAL DOSE	Theophylline: adults 150–300 mg qid or 2.5–4.5 mg/kg q6h children 3–5 mg/kg q6h Aminophylline: loading dose (I.V.) 5–7 mg/kg maintenance 200–400 mg qid (adults) 3–6 mg/kg q6h (children)

as Theolair.[36] This preparation consists of tablets of microfine crystals that are apparently well tolerated by the stomach, and are rapidly absorbed to produce a relatively high blood level that persists for over six hours. A new micropulverized form of theophylline, Bronkodyl, is alleged to possess similar virtues. A number of sustained release preparations are available, such as Theograd (theophylline in an inert matrix,[37] not available in the U.S.), and Theo-Dur, which is alleged to result in a peak serum level after six to ten hours following administration and to produce a smooth plateau level in the therapeutic range with 12-hourly administration. Other long-acting preparations may be equally effective; recently, a number of them have been shown to offer consistent and complete absorption[35a] (Table 6–8).

TABLE 6–8. THEOPHYLLINE PREPARATIONS

Brand Name	Fluid Preparation (mg/15 ml) and Alcohol Content %	Capsules or Tablets (mg)	SR* Oral (mg)	Suppositories (mg)
Accurbron	150 (7.5%)			
Aerolate	160 (10%)		65, 130, 260	
Aqualin Supprettes				125,500
Bronkodyl	80 (20%)		100, 200	
Elixicon	300 (0%)			
Elixophyllin**	80 (20%)	100, 200	125, 250	
Lanophyllin	80 (20%)			
Liquophylline	80 (20%)			
Optiphyllin	80 (20%)			
Oralphyllin	80 (20%)			
Slo-Phyllin**	80 (0%)	100, 200	60, 125, 250	
Somophyllin**		100, 200, 250		
Synophylate LA Cenules			260	
Theo II	160 (10%)			
Theobid Duracaps			130, 260	
Theo-Dur**			100, 200, 300	
Theograd†			350	
Theolair**		125, 250		
Theolix	80 (20%)			
Theolixir	80 (20%)			
Theolline	80 (20%)			
Theon	150 (20%)	150		
Theophyl**	112.5 (5%)	100, 225	125, 250	
Theophylline (various products)	80 (20%)	100, 200		
Theospan	80 (1%)	200	260	

*SR = sustained release preparations. These should be administered q8–12h.
†Not available in United States.
**Bioavailability of these capsule or tablet preparations has been shown to be consistent and complete.
All these products require a prescription.

Among recently introduced formulations is a chewable tablet (Theophyl) that may be particularly suitable for children: the theophylline is microencapsulated and it therefore does not impart a taste. The sustained-release beads of Slo-Phyllin Gyrocaps can be removed and scattered on a spoonful of food and are thereby readily accepted and swallowed by children.[35a] Such alternatives to liquid preparations of theophylline offer useful practical advantages.

Various long-acting preparations are used to produce continuous therapeutic serum levels, with the advantage of smoother control of bronchospasm for selected patients, but appropriate dosage adjustments may be difficult to make, particularly in patients who have varying or unusual serum half-lives of theophylline.[37a, 37b] However, in most patients, including children, serum levels are predictable enough after an initial assessment of the response to several days of appropriate dosing has been made. In such cases, long-acting preparations of complete bioavailability result in excellent pharmacologic therapy and offer the conveniences of twice a day dosage, uninterrupted sleep and improved patient compliance.

SOLUTIONS. Various elixirs are marketed[35] in which theophylline is dissolved in 20 per cent alcohol (for example, as Elixophyllin, which is also formulated as a capsule of theophylline in polyethylene glycol) to produce hydroalcoholic solutions suitable for gastric absorption. Oral administration can result in blood levels that are comparable, within 15 to 30 minutes, to those obtained by giving an equivalent dose of aminophylline intravenously; peak levels are usually attained within an hour.[38] Elixirs probably do not provide more consistent absorption or more reliable serum levels than do other liquid preparations or solid formulations of good bioavailability.

Some patients object to the taste of these hydroalcoholic preparations; they are unsuitable if the patient has gastritis. Similarly, the elixirs may be undesirable for alcoholics, and they are contraindicated if the patient is taking disulfiram (Antabuse) or metronidazole (Flagyl), since alcohol reacts adversely with these drugs. A similar problem is seen in some patients on oral antidiabetic agents, such as chlorpropamide. If a patient is also taking a sedative or an antihistamine, the alcohol may potentiate the depressant effects of these drugs. Each ml of a 20 per cent theophylline elixir provides about one calorie, which may be significant to obese patients.[25] Several products have recently been introduced that have less alcohol: Theospan contains 1 per cent alcohol, while Slo-Phyllin and Elixicon are alcohol free. Such products are more suitable for children, who should not be given elixirs containing alcohol.

Rectal Preparations of Theophylline. Theophylline is available as suppositories, which are erratically, but often rapidly, absorbed; indeed, it is possible to produce dangerously high blood levels when the standard (that is, excessive) dose suppositories are given to small children. Theophylline is too insoluble to form an enema solution, but its derivative, theophylline monoethanolamine, provides a convenient and effective aqueous solution that is marketed as a unit for rectal administration.

Inhalational Preparations of Theophylline. The low solubility of theophylline is such that a suitable aqueous solution for intravenous or intramuscular administration cannot be produced. A saturated aqueous solution (Microphyllin), which contains 12.5 mg/ml, has been used in inhalation therapy, but it is still too dilute, and it is of poor effectiveness compared with sympathomimetic agents.[39, 40] The alcoholic solutions of theophylline, although of adequate concentration, are too irritating for inhalation.

Combination Products Containing Theophylline. Many oral antiasthmatic preparations contain theophylline in combination with ephedrine and, often, with an expectorant; usually, a tranquilizer is added to the mixture to counteract the central nervous system stimulation that theophylline and ephedrine cause. Several publications list the large numbers of these products[25, 33-35]; only the principles of their use need be considered here. These oral tablets, capsules, pulvules, elixirs and other preparations contain a surprising range of doses of theophylline or related agents; the content of theophylline or the equivalent amount of a related drug in the more popular products varies from about 15 mg to over 300 mg per unit dose! This extraordinarily wide diversity implies that some products are ineffective, whereas others are potentially toxic; although the rest may be acceptable, the various combinations are unlikely to contain optimal amounts of each component.

The rationale for combining theophylline and ephedrine was based on the concept that these drugs act synergistically as bronchodilators, and that by giving suboptimal dosages of each, the unwanted side effects caused by each drug would be decreased. Although synergism can occur, objective evidence on the benefits of various combination products is lacking.[41, 42] Indeed, it has been recently shown that theophylline alone serves to cause adequate bronchodilation, whereas the addition of ephedrine does not augment this effect but does cause potentially dangerous side effects, such as cerebral stimulation.[43]

Thus, it would be better to prescribe the appropriate dose of theophylline alone, without ephedrine, in which case a tranquilizer would not be required. It therefore seems that this form of combination therapy is an example of unsound pharmacology. In general, the use of combination preparations in clinical practice should be gradually abandoned, notwithstanding the fact that many patients seem to do well on them. It can be presumed that patients would do equally well, or better, using the correct oral dose of theophylline; in addition, one of the more modern oral sympathomimetic agents, such as metaproterenol or terbutaline, could be added if required. These comments should not be construed as advice to discontinue a combination product in a patient who appears to derive benefit from it, but, certainly, all physicians should strive for more rational therapy. Therefore, new patients should probably not be started on combination medications, unless treatment with theophylline or aminophylline alone has been evaluated and found to be unsuitable.

DERIVATIVES OF THEOPHYLLINE

Although there are a number of derivatives of theophylline, the most important is aminophylline. The prime objective of therapy with any derivative is to obtain a serum level of free theophylline in the therapeutic range. The only real advantages offered by the derivatives are those attributable to the improvements in bioavailability that they might offer. Prescribers should realize that the available derivatives provide less than 100 per cent free theophylline, with values ranging from 48 per cent to 85 per cent.

Aminophylline

The low solubility of theophylline in water militates against the drug's being given by intramuscular or intravenous injection. For obscure reasons, ethylenediamine was chosen to make a double salt with theophylline. The resulting compound is relatively soluble in water (one part in five parts water), and is suitable for intravenous use. This combination product was introduced into medicine as aminophylline in 1910.[44]

Aminophylline is used mainly as an intravenous drug for the management of acute bronchospasm. The drug is also used in tablet form for oral administration; it is also present in many combination oral preparations. Rectal preparations are available as solutions or suppositories. The major commercial products are listed in Table 6–9. Aminophylline contains 79 to 87 per cent theophylline,[49a] and although dosages should be related to this fact, it is clear from a perusal of standard textbooks that many authorities fail to give rational dosage recommendations. Unfortunately, individual variations in metabolic degradation make completely rational dosing difficult. Jenne advises that in the average adult, intravenous treatment can be started with a loading dose of 500 mg aminophylline followed by 300 mg four times a day.[8, 12] About 10 per cent of patients will develop nausea or vomiting on this regimen; this should be anticipated. Dosages should be increased or decreased by 100 mg a day to find the optimal dosage. Small patients and those with liver disease or chronic cardiac failure should be started on a maintenance dose of 200 mg four times a day.[8]

Whenever aminophylline is given *intravenously,* it should not be administered rapidly: at least 10 to 15 minutes should be taken in usual cases; if it is given more rapidly a physician should monitor the procedure, and the patient should be examined for evidence of acute cardiovascular or nervous system toxicity (Table 6–10). Patients may develop giddiness, weakness, diaphoresis and hypotension, and the injection may have to be discontinued. It has been suggested that the shock-like reaction that may follow rapid intravenous injection is a result of precipitation occurring when alkaline aminophylline is exposed to venous blood of lower pH.[34] Intravenous salbutamol (see Chapter 5) offers the important advantage of equivalent effectiveness whereas it can safely be given relatively rapidly over the course of one minute, without serious side effects.[45]

Oral administration of aminophylline tablets can be successfully employed, in spite of a lingering prejudice against this form of therapy. Most adult patients can tolerate the

TABLE 6–9. AMINOPHYLLINE PREPARATIONS

Major Brands	Injection (mg/10 ml) VIAL)	Tablets (mg)	SR* Oral (mg)	Liquids or Elixirs (mg/15ml)	Suppositories† (mg)	Enemas (mg)
Aminophylline**	250,500††	100,200			100,250,350,500	
Aminodur						
Dura-Tabs†			300			
Lixaminol				250 (in 20% alcohol)		
Mini-Lix				100 (in 20% alcohol)		
Rectalad				315		300/3 ml; 450/4.5 ml
Somophyllin				315 (no alcohol)		300/5 ml

*SR = sustained-release product.

**Trade names include Aminophyllin, Cardophyllin, Carena, Diophyllin, Genophyllin, Ionphyllin, Metaphyllin, Phyllindon, Teholamine, Theophyldine

†Bioavailability of these products is poor.

††More concentrated solutions are also available.

All these products require a prescription

Note: The anhydrous theophylline content of these aminophylline preparations is actually 79% although it is more customary to use the figure 85%.

500 mg tablet; if the drug is taken in a fasting state and is accompanied by water, absorption leading to a therapeutic level occurs reasonably rapidly, and peak blood levels are produced within one to two hours.[28] Enteric-coated preparations are not well absorbed, and these should not be used, but slow-release preparations can give acceptable results (for example Aminodur Dura-Tabs[8]). The latter produces peak levels about six hours after administration; the levels are lower than those obtained with an elixir, but they are within the therapeutic range. Whether the oral preparations of aminophylline are superior to those of theophylline has not been established; there is probably little practical difference. Different generic aminophylline preparations appear to have equivalent bioavailability and can be prescribed with confidence.[46] It is noteworthy that aminophylline is less expensive than theophylline when equivalent doses are given by oral or rectal administration.

Aminophylline *suppositories* are still popular, although there is inadequate evidence to support claims for their virtues. The suppositories are unreliably absorbed, and blood levels are lower than with oral administration of tablets of the same strength.[47] Moreover, patients often find them irritating, and many fail to retain suppositories. However, some patients seem to respond more favorably to rectal administration, and they attain an adequate therapeutic response with minimal gastric side effects.

Rectal solutions of aminophylline appear to be superior to suppositories.[48] Some of the marketed products are well accepted by patients, and they give a blood level that is equivalent, at one hour, to that resulting from the same dose given intravenously. Such enemas can be used once or twice a day for many years either prophylactically or therapeutically in the management of chronic asthma. Particular care is needed in children to avoid overdosage.

Both aminophylline and theophylline have been investigated as *inhalational* agents (see

TABLE 6–10. PRECAUTIONS TO BE TAKEN WITH INTRAVENOUS ADMINISTRATION OF AMINOPHYLLINE*

1. Give with particular care to small children and elderly patients, or those with major extra-pulmonary disease.
2. Use smaller doses if patient has had theophylline drug within 24 hours.
3. The loading dose should always be given under direct physician supervision.
4. In general, give the lower level of suggested dosages initially, and gradually increase to the upper level if necessary.
5. The drug should be administered slowly, and no more rapidly than 40 mg per minute.
6. The drug must be used with great care if patient has severe nausea, vomiting, a bleeding peptic ulcer, hyperexcitability, seizure disorder, cardiac arrhythmias, unstable blood pressure or known sensitivity to theophylline drugs.
7. Monitor patient's response, and discontinue administration if adverse effects occur (particularly cardiovascular or neurologic).
8. After initial loading dose is given, further administration can be given by intermittent dosing or by continuous infusion.
9. Reduce maintenance dose by as much as 33% if patient has congestive heart failure or is hypoxic, and by about 50% if patient has hepatic insufficiency.
10. In obese patients, calculate appropriate dosages on basis of lean body mass.

*For further details, see Table 6–15.

TABLE 6–11. THEOPHYLLINES IN INHALATION THERAPY

Preparation	Formulation	Comment
Aminophylline	Powder	Has been reported to be of some benefit; not used in recent years:
	Aqueous solution	Irritating and of little proven benefit
Theophylline (Microphyllin)	Saturated aqueous solution	Well-tolerated, but not very effective
Dyphylline	Aqueous solution	Rarely used, but its solubility and non-irritant properties suggest it would be well tolerated. Effectiveness remains unknown. (Present in Noradran Inhalant, see Table 6–19)
Theophylline sodium glycinate	Aqueous solution	Never used, but its solubility suggests it could be effective; however, its low percentage of free theophylline is a disadvantage

Table 6–11). In general, studies have shown that aerosol therapy can result in bronchodilation, but the theophyllines are not as effective as the sympathomimetic drugs. Aminophylline is a very alkaline drug (pH 10), and it is incompatible with acidic solutions; in fact, theophylline (which itself is slightly acidic) may be liberated from the compound in the acid environment of the stomach, which might account for the gastric irritation that is often caused. The theophyllines can also cause local irritation when given by the rectal route; similarly, aerosol administration can irritate the lungs. Moreover, in the lungs, aminophylline may release ethylenediamine, which has an ammoniacal quality, and this may cause further irritation of the airways. Micropowdered theophylline and aminophylline have been reported to be effective and well-tolerated when given by inhalation,[49] but this form of treatment has never gained acceptance. Solutions of aminophylline cannot be recommended, since they are bitter in taste, irritating to the mucous membranes and have been shown to be unsuccessful when given by inhalation to asthmatics.[50] Various solutions (alcoholic or aqueous) of theophylline may be more effective and less irritating, but there is little need to use theophylline and its derivatives in inhalation therapy, since better agents are available at present. However, if a reliable inhalational preparation were to become available, this would be a welcome therapeutic achievement.

Aminophylline is too irritating for intramuscular administration, as are solutions of theophylline in alcohol or water. The alkalinity of aqueous aminophylline is a major factor in its overall tissue irritant quality, and this has provided the rationale for the introduction of various salts of theophylline, which are neutral.

Oxtriphylline

The choline salt of theophylline (choline theophyllinate or theophylline cholinate) is more stable, more soluble and less irritating than aminophylline[44] Although it has been claimed that this derivative is better absorbed from the gastrointestinal tract, careful studies suggest that this does not appear to be so for the tablet formulation, and it is doubtful that the elixir preparation offers significant advantages, although it is absorbed more rapidly than the tablet.[5] Further proof will be required to convince the discriminating practitioner that oxtriphylline is better than other theophylline derivatives. The drug is made available as Choledyl.

The decreased gastric irritation claimed for oxtriphylline may simply be the result of giving the comparatively smaller dose of theophylline (64 per cent) contained in Choledyl tablets; if equivalent serum levels of theophylline are achieved, adverse gastric symptoms will be experienced by many patients. Oxtriphylline is relatively popular for oral use, but the drug is often prescribed in suboptimal dosage. The dose recommended by the manufacturers is 100 to 400 mg four times a day in adults, and 15 mg/kg a day in four divided doses in children; larger doses may be required for optimal effect. In adults, the standard dose should probably be 400 mg four times a day. A recent recommendation has been 600 mg loading dose followed by 400 mg every six hours, for a total of three doses a day.[51] Oxtriphylline is compared with other derivatives in Table 6–12.

TABLE 6–12. THEOPHYLLINE DERIVATIVES

Derivative	Main Proprietary Products	Tablets or Capsules (mg)	SR (mg)	Liquids (mg/15 ml) Alcohol Content %	Injections (mg/ml)	Suppositories (mg)	Enemas (mg/unit)	Average Theophylline (Per Cent)	Approx. Dose Yielding 10 mg/kg Free Theophylline	Approximate Comparative Adult Dose (mg)	Comments
Theophylline ethylenediamine (aminophylline)	See Table 6–9	+	+	+	+	+	+	85†	12 mg/kg	300	Standard alternative to theophylline; main product for intravenous use
Theophylline monoethanolamine	Fleet Monotheamin Generic products	100,200				500 250,500	250,500	75	14 mg/kg	325	Alleged to be particularly well tolerated and effective when given by rectum; very stable product
Dihydroxypropyl-theophylline (dyphylline, hyphylline, diprophylline)	Airet Circair Dilor Lutyllin Neothylline	200 200 200,400 200,400 200,400	400	100 (10%) 160 (20%) 100 (20%) 160 (18%)	250 250 250			70††	14 mg/kg	325	Nonirritating derivative; suitable for intramuscular use
Theophylline cholinate (oxtriphylline)	Choledyl Generic products	100,200 400		300 (20%)				64	16 mg/kg	350	Popular alternative for oral use
Theophylline sodium acetate	Theocin soluble							60	16 mg/kg	375	More soluble than theophylline; rarely used
Theophylline sodium glycinate	Asbron* Glynazan Panophylline Synophylate Theofort	324 330		330 (20%) 330 (20%) 320 (20%)	400	780		51	20 mg/kg	500	Very soluble in water; nonirritating; can be given intravenously; has been given by inhalation
Theophylline calcium salicylate	Phyllicin Quadrinal* Theokin* Verequad*							48	21 mg/kg	500	Popular oral agent, with no outstanding advantages

*Combination products, see Table 6–16.
†Correct figure is actually 79%.
††Dyphylline does not provide free theophylline, but is equivalent to 70% theophylline.

Dyphylline

Dyphylline (hyphylline) is the only derivative of theophylline used medically that is an actual chemical variation of the theophylline molecule rather than a simple salt. Dyphylline is dihydroxypropyl theophylline; in England it is known as *diprophylline* (Table 6–12). It is available as tablets, elixirs and as an intramuscular preparation, under such names as Dilor and Lufyllin. It is 40 times more soluble in water than is theophylline, and it results in a neutral solution (Table 6–13). It is stable in gastric acid and it appears to be relatively nonirritating to the stomach. The drug has only 70 per cent free theophylline activity equivalency.

Dyphylline is less irritating to all tissues than theophylline and its alkaline derivatives; because of this it is the only bronchodilating methylxanthine suitable for intramuscular use. This would suggest that claims that the drug causes minimal gastric irritation are correct. However, the claim that it is a very effective bronchodilator at well-tolerated doses[52] requires further clarification. Unfortunately, oral dyphylline produces a lower serum level than an equivalent dose of theophylline,[53] and the serum half-life of dyphylline is short (about two hours, compared with three to five hours for theophylline)[54]. Thus, the formerly recommended oral dosage of dyphylline of about 3 mg/kg three or four times a day was inadequate;[13] in fact, about 15 mg/kg four or more times a day is required, and this could result in side effects. The manufacturers used to recommend a 200 mg oral dosage for adults, but this was undoubtedly suboptimal, and a dose as high as 1,000 mg every four to six hours may be more appropriate;[54] such doses may still be adequately tolerated, but side effects may be expected.[55] When higher dose levels are used the advantages of this product over other forms of theophylline are likely to be lost.

Since dyphylline is very soluble and is relatively nonirritating, it may be expected that the aqueous solution would be effective and well accepted when given by the inhalational route. Although there is reason to believe that dyphylline would be the most suitable theophylline derivative for aerosolization, the drug has not yet been given by this route in any controlled trial; however, it is one of the constituents in the British proprietary aerosol bronchodilator, Noradran Inhalant (see Table 6–19). The drug does not appear to have been demonstrated to be suitable for intravenous use.

Further studies are required in order to determine if dyphylline is as valuable a bronchodilator as its properties suggest. However, its short serum half-life is a definite disadvantage,[55a] and pharmacokinetic studies may suggest a required dosage that would be no less toxic than the appropriate dosage of any other form of theophylline. Moreover, if larger doses are necessary for a full therapeutic effect, the cost relative to that of theophylline or aminophylline becomes a factor.

Other Theophylline Derivatives
(Table 6–12)

Theophylline sodium glycinate (theophylline sodium aminoacetate) is a buffered salt that is very soluble in water; it is better tolerated by the stomach than is theophylline. It also offers the advantage of versatility, in that it can be given orally, rectally and intravenously, and it has also been used as an aerosol, employing 2 ml of a 5 to 10 per cent solution every four hours. There is relatively little experience with this drug in comparison with the preceding agents, and it is therefore difficult to recommend it, although its properties suggest that it is worthy of further therapeutic consideration.

Theophylline sodium acetate is another buffered, less irritating product; it is available for oral use, but it has no special advantages.

Theophylline calcium salicylate is marketed in a number of proprietary tablets and elixirs, usually in combination with other drugs such as ephedrine and a mucokinetic agent. It is not clear what properties make this preparation commercially popular, but it is present in many combination products.

Theophylline monoethanoloamine (theophylline olamine) is particularly recommended for rectal use as an enema or as

TABLE 6–13. SOLUBILITY OF THEOPHYLLINE AND DERIVATIVES

1 gram of	dissolves in ____ ml water	to give a ____ solution
Theophylline	120	slightly acidic
Aminophylline	5	markedly alkaline
Dyphylline	3	neutral

suppositories, although it is also available for oral administration.

Proxyphylline, acepifylline, bamiphylline, bufylline, etamiphyllin and *etophylline* are derivatives used in the United Kingdom and Europe because they are less irritating than theophylline and aminophylline. Other theophylline derivatives are also known but are not used.[56] Related investigational agents include *quazodine* and *ICI 58,301*. The value of all these agents still needs to be determined.

RECOMMENDATIONS REGARDING ADMINISTRATION OF THEOPHYLLINE AND DERIVATIVES

The methylxanthines should be considered standard therapy in every patient with bronchospasm. They are usually essential in the management of acute bronchospasm and status asthmaticus, and they are of value in the chronic, daily treatment of most patients with moderate or severe chronic obstructive pulmonary disease. A loading dose is always required, since a single maintenance dose does not produce an adequate serum level.

ACUTE TREATMENT

In acute bronchospastic attacks that do not respond to the patient's usual therapy, *aminophylline* is generally required (see Table 6–14). A loading dose should be administered intravenously over the course of 10 to 30 minutes; particular care is required in young children and in old people, and in the presence of heart disease, cor pulmonale, hepatic impairment, and central nervous system excitation. The drug should be given cautiously and in reduced dosage if any theophylline-containing drugs have been given to the patient in recent days (Table 6–10).

The minimal loading dose should be in the region of 5 to 7 mg/kg in adults[57] and a similar loading dose can be given to children, including infants. The need for a loading

TABLE 6–14. DOSAGES OF AMINOPHYLLINE

Dosage	Amount	Comments
Adults		
LOADING DOSE	6 mg/kg (range 5–7 mg/kg), *average dose 400 mg*	Give dose over course of 10–30 minutes, with monitoring of response.
Decrease by 50%	(a) if patient has received a theophylline in previous 24 hours (b) if patient is in shock, heart failure or liver failure, or is hypoxic	Reduce dosage if there are uncertainties as to patient's liability to develop toxicity. Obtain a serum level if in doubt.
Increase by 50%	(a) if effect is suboptimal (b) in smokers who tolerate the drug	Increased dosage may be required if bronchospasm breakthrough occurs. Serum level must be checked when high dosage is used.
MAINTENANCE DOSE	0.5 mg/kg/hr or 1.15 gm/24 hr, *average dose 250 mg q6h*	Aminophylline can be given by continuous drip or by bolus every 6 hours.
Increase each dose by 50–100 mg	(a) if effect is suboptimal (b) in patients with increased clearance rate, e.g. in smokers	Increased dosages must be monitored for adverse reactions. Dosage changes should be made every 3 days until optimum is achieved: check serum level if in doubt.
Decrease each dose by 50–100 mg	(a) if toxic effects develop (b) in patients with poor cardiac or hepatic function	Decreased clearance can be deduced from clinical state or from serum levels. If slight nausea is only adverse problem, one or two doses can be skipped.
Children		
LOADING DOSE	6 mg/kg (given over 15–30 minutes)	If unimproved, give additional 3 mg/kg within 1–2 hours; check serum level.
MAINTENANCE DOSE	0.7–1.3 mg/kg/hr (depending on age)	Larger dosages are tolerated by younger children.
Dosage adjustments	Increase by 25% every 3 days	Usually, a suboptimal dosage is given initially, and increases are made using serum level for guidance (see Table 6–17).

dose in very small children has now been established, and this is unlikely to cause serious side effects; some physicians recommend a loading dose in children of 4 mg/kg given as a bolus over the course of five minutes.[5] Recent studies[58] have shown that theophylline clearance in neonates is substantially lower than it is in older children; therefore, a smaller dose requirement should be observed in neonates or premature infants who require aminophylline. The first loading dose should be given with careful monitoring, preferably by a physician, and, if undesirable findings appear, the full dose should not be administered. In acute asthma, it is advisable for the physician to administer the drug from a syringe, while reassuring and encouraging the patient; in this acute situation, the "bedside manner" potentiates the bronchodilating qualities of the aminophylline.

After giving a loading dose, subsequent therapy can be given intravenously by a continuous drip, but if this is not convenient, six hourly bolus administrations can be prescribed. In *adults*, the usual loading dose is 6 mg/kg (about 350–450 mg), and the subsequent maintenance dosage is governed by the clinical status of the patient. For the average adult who is not a smoker and is in otherwise good health, about 0.5 mg/kg is given every hour: this should produce a serum theophylline level of 10 to 20 mcg/ml. Cigarette smokers require larger doses, while patients with impaired clearance require smaller maintenance doses; women probably require up to 30 per cent larger doses than do men.[59] Maintenance doses are listed in Table 6–15 and are discussed later. In *children*, the dose formerly used was 12 to 15 mg/kg per day or 400 mg/meter[2] per day, by continuous drip or in three to four divided doses; however, more recently, Weinberger[35a] recommended giving the maximum adult dosage of about 1 mg/kg per hour, which is twice as great as the former recommendation. If several days of intravenous therapy are required, dosage changes may be needed on the basis of the clinical response or the appearance of side-effects, such as nausea, vomiting or cardiac or nervous system irritability. An additional problem with children is that the theophylline clearance rate may vary markedly during an acute illness.[58a] If higher dosages appear to be required, serum levels must be utilized for guidance.

An attempt can be made to evaluate the rate of clearance of theophylline from the blood by making determinations on serum or saliva specimens taken one hour, three hours and six hours after a dose of theophylline. However, the clearance rate may change after the first day or two of therapy. In most cases it is, therefore, more practical to do occasional checks on the serum level to make sure the correct therapeutic range of 10 to 20 mcg/ml is being maintained. Furthermore, if greater precision in dosing is considered to be necessary in a patient, the following equation can be used as a basis for determining the required infusion rate to produce a selected serum level:[59]

$$\text{plasma concentration} = \frac{\text{infusion rate}}{\text{clearance}}$$

Once a clearance rate has been established, subsequent changes that may be needed in the infusion rate can be established. The clearance rate can vary from 1.2 ml/kg per minute in a normal adult to as low as 0.35 ml/kg per minute in patients with problems such as liver disease.[59, 60] In similar fashion, the half-life (T/2) of theophylline can be determined in an individual patient, and the volume of distribution estimated, so as to employ a formula that has been provided for calculating a dosage regimen.[38] Hospitals that choose to utilize these concepts of theophylline kinetics as a guide to individual patient dosing will, of course, require the ready availability of a rapid, inexpensive and accurate method of assaying theophylline levels — as well as an individual who can use the information that is generated.

As an alternative to aminophylline, *theophylline sodium glycinate* can be given intravenously; this agent has only about 50 per cent theophylline, and, therefore, an appropriate initial loading dose for adults would be at least 10 mg/kg, followed by about 1.5 to 2.5 gm per 24 hours in divided doses. In some instances, effective emergency treatment can be given orally or rectally using an appropriate amount (for example, 300 to 500 mg) of a well-absorbed theophylline preparation, such as *elixir of theophylline, anhydrous theophylline tablets* (such as Theolair) or an enema of *theophylline monoethanolamine*. Aminophylline suppositories could also be used, but are not as effective or as well tolerated as the other alternatives in most patients. More recently, rectal solutions of aminophylline have been claimed to be effective when given in a unit of 300 to 450 mg of aminophylline.[14] Intramuscular *dyphylline* is another alternative: at least 500 mg (in 2 ml solution) should be given; this dose may need to be repeated several times. The disadvantage of dyphylline is the uncertainty as to the appropriate dose; the advantage is that the drug is suitable for intramuscular use.

Chronic Maintenance Therapy. When a patient is maintained on theophylline or one of its derivatives, it is important to give optimal dosages. It is very difficult to be sure that this is achieved by any fixed regimen; the dosage prescribed should be reviewed periodically and adjusted if necessary. The required amount in one group of adults varied from 400 to 3200 mg a day,[8] and even greater variation can be expected. Maintenance therapy can be given at dosage levels varying from low to high,[2] depending on the patient's response. Most patients will respond well to any standard tablet preparations, and they do not require elixirs or other specially formulated rapidly absorbed preparations. The aim of maintenance therapy is to achieve a satisfactory blood level for most of the time; appropriate doses at frequent enough intervals with any preparation will attain this objective. Thus, a manufacturer who boasts that a newly formulated product results in very rapid absorption should be considered to be appealing to a very limited market of patients who use oral theophyllines for acute treatment of an asthma attack rather than for chronic therapy. In general, any simple theophylline preparation can be used in maintenance therapy: the usual adult dosage is 2.5 to 4.5 mg/kg four times a day or 150 to 300 mg four times a day. Older children require about 2.5 to 3 mg/kg four times a day, while young children may need as much as 5 mg/kg four times a day. Current recommendations are summarized in Table 6–15.

Initially, patients should be started on a simple theophylline preparation or aminophylline tablets. Oral drugs should be given with water just before eating, for optimal absorption and minimal gastric irritation. If any simple preparation is not tolerated, then a less irritating derivative should be tried, using the appropriate dosage, although most alternatives (including the various theophylline salts and hydroalcoholic solutions) appear to be rarely needed for chronic oral use.[41] There is no adequate established basis on which to recommend one preparation rather than another, other than the comparative costs of the agents. Recently, sustained-action tablets have been promoted vigorously, and the market has become very competitive. There is some evidence to suggest that long-acting preparations provide superior control of bronchospasm,[35a] but their main advantage is the convenience of less frequent dosing.

In general, there is little indication for chronic administration by any route except the oral,[42] although occasional patients seem to have a better response to rectal administration.[3] In a few patients, it may be worth considering the use of the inhalation prepa-

TABLE 6–15. RECOMMENDED MAINTENANCE DOSAGES OF THEOPHYLLINE AND AMINOPHYLLINE*

	Theophylline			Aminophylline			
			SUGGESTED DAILY DOSE				SUGGESTED DAILY DOSE
	(mg/kg q6h)	(mg/kg/day)	(mg)	(mg/kg/hr)	(mg/kg q6h)	(mg/kg/day)	(mg)
CHILD†							
Age 2 months–9 yrs	6	24	–	1.3	7.5	30	–
Age 9–12 yrs	5	20	–	1.1	6.5	25	–
Age 12–16 yrs	4.5	18	900	1	6	23	1100
Age 16 and over	3	13	900	0.7	4	16	1100
ADULTS							
Average patient, smoker	4.5	18	1200	0.9	5.5	21	1500
Average patient, non-smoker	2.5	10	800	0.5	3	12	1000
Presence of heart failure, cor pulmonale or hypoxia	2.0	8	500	0.4	2.5	10	600
Presence of hepatic insufficiency	1.2	5	350	0.25	1.5	6	400
Presence of cardiac and hepatic insufficiency	0.5	2	150	0.1	0.6	2.5	200

*These recommendations are based on information provided by L. Hendeles, Pharm. D.

†To avoid toxicity, initiate maintenance theophylline therapy at a dosage of 16 mg/kg/day or 400 mg/day, whichever is less. Increase dose if tolerated in 25% increments at 3 day intervals to recommended dosages as tolerated.

In all cases, doses are based on lean body weight. Women may require up to 30% larger doses.

ration Microphyllin in conjunction with a sympathomimetic agent, since the mixture may have a synergistic effect. Certainly, theophylline is one agent that would be much safer if it could be given by inhalation, since side effects are so readily produced by oral administration when aiming for a blood level high enough to be effective. Although there are so many inhalational sympathomimetics available at present, there could still be some justification for utilizing a low-dose aerosol of a phosphodiesterase inhibitor, which may be an effective bronchodilator for patients who have developed tachyphylaxis to the sympathomimetic agents.

Combination Products in Maintenance Therapy. The concept of *synergistic combination therapy* has been extremely popular in the treatment of bronchospasm. Although there are numerous combination products of aminophylline or theophylline with ephedrine, the addition of ephedrine is usually undesirable, since it increases the side effects without making any marked contribution to the bronchodilator effect.[43] It is usual to add barbiturates to the mixture (as in Tedral and many other popular combination products), but there are many disadvantages to these agents, including the possibility of their inducing enzymes that may bring about the more rapid degradation of the active drugs used to treat bronchospasm.[61] Although it had been thought that added drugs could interfere with theophylline absorption, it has been shown that neither ephedrine nor phenobarbital affect the bioavailability of theophylline from combination preparations.[20] Hydroxyzine is more desirable as a tranquilizer than are barbiturates,[41] since not only is it free of enzyme-inducing activity, but it has been shown to have antihistaminic and bronchodilator properties that are of possible value in the treatment of asthma and bronchitis; the combination product Marax is popular, and may have some advantages in the mild asthmatic of nervous disposition.

Other drugs are often included in proprietary combination preparations for oral and rectal use.[25, 33-35] Some of these agents may be useful, although their benefit can be difficult to prove; thus, antacids are sometimes added, in the hope that they will counteract the irritant effect of the theophyllines on the stomach. Expectorant drugs are incorporated in many products, although these agents are generally present in subtherapeutic amounts; furthermore, they are liable to increase gastric irritation and nausea, since most of the oral expectorants are stimulants of the vagal afferents in the stomach. The more popular combination preparations are detailed in Table 6-16.

Dosage Adjustment in Maintenance Therapy. Most physicians attempt to find the appropriate amount of the theophyllines by increasing the dosage until the patient experiences nausea; at that point the dosage should be slightly decreased, and then maintained if it is well tolerated. This method does have problems; in particular, some patients may develop other, potentially more serious, toxic reactions before they experience nausea.[26, 28] When higher than average doses appear to be necessary, the serum level should be determined periodically and attempts should be made to keep the level below 20 mcg/ml.[43] If combination tablets are used, the appropriate theophylline dose will be difficult to attain, since excessive amounts of the other drugs in the preparation will be given. Thus, the best pharmacologic approach is to avoid combination products, and to manipulate the dosage of theophylline, or a derivative, using empiric guidelines and clinical judgment, supplemented by determinations of serum (or saliva) levels, if necessary.

CHILDREN. The maintenance dosage of theophylline for children under the age of 16 has been altered recently as a result of the careful work of Weinberger and others.[7b, 60a] Initially, the drug should be given in a dosage of 16 mg/kg/day or 400 mg/day, whichever is less, in 4 divided doses, or as sustained release preparations that can be given every 8 to 12 hours. If the response is suboptimal the dosage can be increased every three days until objective and subjective improvement occurs or until significant side effects occur; a serum level on the third day may be helpful. In general, the eventual dosage required is related to age, being proportionally greater in children less than 9; children over the age of 16 require the same dose as a healthy, but cigarette-smoking, adult (presumably, children who smoke may need increased dosages, or, more appropriately, forceful counselling). One serum check of the theophylline level may be advisable once the optimum dosage regimen has been achieved. Once the correct dosage is established in a child, serum levels should be checked every six months and changes in dosage instituted if necessary (see Table 6-17).

ADULTS. The dosage recommendations for adults have recently been revised as a

TABLE 6–16. COMBINATION PRODUCTS OF THEOPHYLLINE AND ITS DERIVATIVES *

Trade Name	Generic or Chemical Name	Tablets or Capsules (mg)	Contents Per 15 ml Elixir or Suspension (mg)	Percentage of Theophylline	Equivalent Amount of Theophylline Delivered
Amesec	Aminophylline	130		85	111 mg/capsule
	Ephedrine HCl	25			
	Amytal	25			
Amodrine†	Aminophylline	100		85	85 mg/tablet
	Racephedrine	25			
	Phenobarbital	8			
Asbron G	Theophylline sodium glycinate	300	300	50	153 mg/in-lay tablet
	Glyceryl guaiacolate	100	100		153 mg/15 ml elixir
Asma Lief†	Theophylline	130		100	130 mg/tablet
	Ephedrine	24			
	Phenobarbital	8			
Bronchobid	Theophylline	260		100	260 mg/timed action capsule
	Pseudoephedrine	50			
Broncomar	Theophylline	100	150	100	100 mg/tablet
	Pseudoephedrine	30	30		150 mg/15 ml elixir
	Glyceryl guaiacolate	100	150		
	Butabarbital		15		
Brondecon	Oxtriphylline	200	300	64	128 mg/tablet
	Glyceryl guaiacolate	100	150		192 mg/15 ml elixir
Bronitin†	Theophylline	130		100	130 mg/tablet
	Ephedrine	24			
	Guaifenesin	100			
	Methapyrilene	16			
Bronkaid†	Theophylline	100		100	100 mg/tablet
	Ephedrine	24			
	Guaifenesin	100			
	Mg trisilicate	74.5			
Bronkolixir	Theophylline		45	100	45 mg/15 ml elixir
	Ephedrine		36		
	Phenobarbital		12		
	Glyceryl guaiacolate		150		
Bronkotabs†	Theophylline	100		100	100 mg/tablet
	Ephedrine	24			
	Phenobarbital	8			
	Glyceryl guaiacolate	100			
Dibron	Theophylline	200		100	100 mg/capsule
	Phenylpropanolamine	25			
Dilor G	Dyphylline	200	300	70	140 mg/tablet
	Glyceryl guaiacolate	200	300		210 mg/15 ml liquid
Duovent	Theophylline	130		100	130 mg/tablet
	Ephedrine	24			
	Phenobarbital	8			
	Glyceryl guaiacolate	100			
Elixophyllin-KI	Theophylline		80	100	80 mg/15 ml elixir
	Potassium iodide		130		
Emfaseem	Dyphylline	200	100	70	140 mg/capsule
	Glyceryl guaiacolate	100	50		70 mg/15 ml liquid
Hylate	Theophylline	200	150	100	200 mg/tablet
	Glyceryl guaiacolate	100	100		150 mg/15 ml syrup
Isofil	Theophylline	200		100	200 mg/tablet
	Noscapine	30			
Isuprel Compound	Theophylline		45	100	45 mg/15 ml elixir
	Ephedrine		12		
	Isoproterenol		2.5		
	Phenobarbital		6		
	Potassium iodide		150		

| Trade Name | Generic or Chemical Name | Contents Per | | Percentage of Theophylline | Equivalent Amount of Theophylline Delivered |
		Tablets or Capsules (mg)	15 ml Elixir or Suspension (mg)		
Lufyllin EPG	Dyphylline	100	150	70	70 mg/tablet
	Ephedrine	16	24		105 mg/15 ml elixir
	Guaifenesin	200	300		
	Phenobarbital	16	24		
Marax	Theophylline	130	97.5	100	130.0 mg/tablet
	Ephedrine	25	18.75		97.5 mg/15 ml syrup
	Hydroxyzine	10	7.5		
Mudrane	Aminophylline	130		85	111 mg/tablet
	Ephedrine	16			
	Phenobarbital	21			
	Potassium iodide	195			
Neothylline-G	Dyphylline	100	300	70	70 mg/tablet
	Glyceryl guaiacolate	50	150		210 mg/15 ml elixir
Phedral†	Theophylline	129.6		100	129.6 mg/tablet
	Ephedrine	24.3			
	Phenobarbital	8.1			
Primatene M†	Theophylline	130		100	130 mg/tablet
	Ephedrine	24			
	Methapyrilene	16			
Primatene P†	Theophylline	130		100	130 mg/tablet
	Ephedrine	24			
	Phenobarbital	8			
Quadrinal	Theophylline calcium salicylate	130	195	48	62 mg/tablet
	Ephedrine	24	36		93 mg/15 ml
	Phenobarbital	24	36		suspension
	Potassium iodide	320	480		
Quibron	Theophylline	150	150	100	150 mg/capsule
	Glyceryl guaiacolate	90	90		150 mg/15 ml elixir
Quibron Plus	Theophylline	150	150	100	150 mg/tablet
	Guaifenesin	100	100		150 mg/15 ml elixir
	Butabarbital	20	20		
Slo-phyllin GG	Theophylline	150	150	100	150 mg/capsule
	Glyceryl guaiacolate	90	90		150 mg/15 ml syrup
Synophylate GG	Theophylline sodium glycinate	300	300	51	153 mg/tablet
	Glyceryl guaiacolate	100	100		153 mg/15 ml syrup
Tedral †	Theophylline	130	195	100	130 mg/tablet
	Ephedrine	24	36		195 mg/15 ml
	Phenobarbital	8	12		suspension
Tedral-SA	Theophylline	180		100	180 mg/sustained
	Ephedrine	48			action tablet
	Phenobarbital	25			
Thalfed†	Theophylline	120		100	120 mg/tablet
	Ephedrine	25			
	Phenobarbital	8			
Theokin	Theophylline calcium salicylate	448	448	48	215 mg/tablet
	Potassium iodide	450	450		215 mg/15 ml elixir
Verequad†	Theophylline calcium salicylate	130	195	48	62 mg/tablet
	Ephedrine	24	36		93 mg/15 ml
	Phenobarbital	8	12		suspension
	Glyceryl guaiacolate	100	150		

*These products are selected from those in Physicians' Desk Reference, 1978, and Handbook of Non-Prescription Drugs, 1977.

†These products are available without prescription.

Note: Guaifenesin is the new name for glyceryl guaiacolate; both names are now in use.

TABLE 6-17. GUIDELINES FOR USE OF SERUM LEVELS OF THEOPHYLLINE*

Peak Theophylline Level (mcg/ml)	Approximate Adjustment in Daily Dose Required		Comments
	INCREASE	DECREASE	
<5	100%		Discontinue drug if patient is asymptomatic; reinstitute appropriate dosage when necessary if symptoms return or are expected to recur.
5–7.5	50%		
8–10	20%		
11–13	10%		Increase dose only if patient is symptomatic.
14–20	–	–	If side effects occur, reduce dose by 10%.
21–25		10%	Reduce dosage even in absence of side effects.
26–30		25%	Omit one dose and reduce successive doses, then repeat serum level.
31–35		33%	
>35		50%	Omit two doses, decrease successive doses and repeat serum level.

NOTE: Serum levels should be taken 2 hours after most recent dose or 4 to 6 hours after a dose of sustained-release preparation. Serum levels will be meaningful if patient has been on dosage regimen for at least 48 hours without a missed dose.

*Based on information provided by L. Hendeles, Pharm. D.

result of the work of Weinberger and Hendeles and their colleagues, and lower dosages than were formerly advised are currently suggested (see Table 6–15). The average theophylline dosage for adults with normal extrapulmonary organs who are not cigarette smokers is 2.5 mg/kg every 6 hours: the daily dosage is in the region of 200 mg four times a day. Cigarette smokers may require doses that are at least 50 per cent larger; and 300 mg four times a day is usually appropriate. Smaller doses are effective in patients with cardiac failure or hypoxia, and even smaller doses in patients with hepatic insufficiency. Individuals with both liver and heart failure may require only 50 mg three times a day, and monitoring of serum levels is particularly important in these patients. Dosage adjustments of 50 to 100 mg can be made, on the basis of clinical response and side effects,

every few days when initiating therapy, but care should be taken to avoid excessive dosing. Few adults will require theophylline in dosages greater than 6 mg/kg four times a day. Young women cigarette smokers who live in a smoggy area and who eat charbroiled foods as part of a high-protein diet are most likely to need the highest dosages to maintain an appropriate serum level.

The standard therapeutic agents should be tablet preparations (regular or sustained-release), elixirs, or non-alcoholic solutions of aminophylline or theophylline, since these formulations are usually well tolerated. For a more rapid effect, oral solutions, rectal solutions or intravenous administration are required. If a patient develops adverse gastric reactions, one of the other oral derivatives could be tried. In rare cases, a rectal preparation could be considered for

TABLE 6-18. COMPARISON OF THEOPHYLLINE AND AMINOPHYLLINE PREPARATIONS

	Theophylline	Aminophylline
Use in acute situations	Hydroalcoholic elixirs and most simple oral preparations are well absorbed fairly rapidly, but response may be variable.	Intravenous aminophylline offers the most rapid and consistent effect.
Maintenance therapy with short-acting preparations	Most oral products are suitable, with no proven advantages over oral aminophylline preparations.	Oral preparations are effective, and are less expensive than theophylline preparations.
Use of long-acting preparations	Can provide adequate nocturnal or round-the-clock therapy, and tends to result in more consistent serum levels. Several products have consistently excellent bioavailability.	The long-acting aminophylline may lack reliable bioavailability.
Rectal preparations	Suppositories only are available, and they lack reliable bioavailability.	Suppositories and rectal solutions are available; only the solutions offer reliable bioavailability, but their expense precludes routine use.

TABLE 6–19. INHALATIONAL PRODUCTS CONTAINING PAPAVERINE THAT ARE MARKETED IN ENGLAND

Trade Name	Adrenaline (Epinephrine)	Isoprenaline (Isoproterenol)	Papaverine	Atropine Methonitrate	Pituitary Extract*	Hyoscine	Diprophylline (Dyphylline)
Compound Adrenaline and Atropine Spray	0.8%		0.8%	0.1%			
Asma-Vydrin	0.55%		0.88%	0.14%	0.75%		
Asthmosana	0.3%		0.88%	0.14%	0.4%	0.025%	
Brovon Inhalant	0.5%		0.88%	0.14%			
Neo-Rybarex	0.4%		0.15%	0.1%	0.4%		
Riddobron Inhalant	0.5%		0.88%	0.14%	0.4%		
Riddofan	1.5%		0.05%	0.14%			
Riddovydrin Inhalant	1%		0.88%	0.75%	+		
Rybarex	0.4%		0.08%	0.1%	0.2%		
Rybarvin	0.4%		0.08%	0.1%	0.2%		
Silbe Asthma Inhalant	1%		0.95%	0.125%	4%	0.05%	
Compound Isoprenaline Spray		1%	2.5%	0.2%			
Noradran Inhalant		1%	0.99%				5%

*Both anterior and posterior pituitary extract are used; there is no available information to suggest that these hormones have a bronchodilator effect. These combination products are presented for interest; they are not recommended.

maintenance therapy, although, in general, these formulations should be used only for emergency treatment. Most of the alternatives to oral tablets of aminophylline and theophylline are considerably more expensive. In all cases, the appropriate dose of a product should be calculated on the basis of the free theophylline content or equivalency. When long-acting preparations are used, adjustments in dosage have to be made particularly carefully.

Many patients develop some gastrointestinal symptoms when taking daily theophylline or aminophylline. Such effects can often be circumvented by having the patient take the medication when food is in the stomach; some individuals will find that antacids help the symptoms. If more serious problems appear, such as agitation or sleeplessness, the patient may need to reduce the frequency or dosage (for example, from every six hours to every eight hours), or to miss an occasional dose. Occasionally it is helpful to advise the patient to reduce the intake of other xanthines, such as chocolate, cola, tea and coffee. Persistent problems provide cause for changing to another preparation of theophylline, which might prove to be better tolerated.

Establishing the correct theophylline dosage and the most appropriate preparation for an individual patient can be a very time-consuming enterprise, and it is usually sufficiently acceptable to utilize a suboptimal but well-tolerated dosage. Nevertheless, it is becoming very clear that there is great variability in theophylline dosage requirements in different patients, and that both intravenous and oral therapy can lead to toxicity in subjects with decreased theo-phylline clearance. Unfortunately, the relatively minor complications of nausea and vomiting may not occur as the first indications of toxicity in some patients.[62] For these reasons, great care is needed when giving theophylline preparations to patients who may have diminished clearance, and suboptimal dosages should generally be accepted. It is an expensive counsel of perfection to advise that frequent checks of serum levels be obtained, but the trend of recommendations is in this direction. Certainly, when the patient appears to require large dosages, such as greater than 20 mg/kg/day or more than 1,200 mg/day in an average adult, a check of the serum level would be prudent.

The large number of competitive products has made the task of choosing an oral agent extremely confusing. In general, aminophylline appears to offer a number of advantages over the various theophylline formulations (Table 6–18), and until comparative studies for the various products are carried out using aminophylline as the basic standard, the initial choice of an oral preparation should be based primarily on relative costs. It is important to recognize that rapid absorption and prolonged effective serum levels are more often interesting pharmacologic parameters rather than significant therapeutic advantages of relevance to the clinical management of bronchospastic patients.

OTHER PHOSPHODIESTERASE INHIBITORS

Papaverine is the only other drug, commonly available, that has been shown to inhibit the enzyme phosphodiesterase. However, there are no good studies demonstrating the comparative effectiveness of this drug in the management of bronchospasm, and in clinical practice papaverine is used only as a vasodilator and as a nonspecific relaxant of smooth muscle. Even in these situations, the drug has not been shown to be unequivocally successful, and it is therefore rarely used. However, papaverine may be of value as a vasodilator in certain circumstances, and it has been given intravenously in the treatment of pulmonary and arterial embolism.

In the United Kingdom, papaverine enjoys a surprising popularity as a possible bronchodilator. It is incorporated in several proprietary aerosol mixtures, in widely varying dosages (Table 6-19); however, there is no proof that it confers any additional benefit to the sympathomimetic agents in the mixtures.

ICI 58,301 is one of a number of investigational agents that are phosphodiesterase inhibitors. This oral drug has been of value in the prophylaxis of bronchospasm, but it does not appear to be as successful for acute therapy.

REFERENCES

1. Weinberger, M.: Bronchodilator therapy. N. Engl. J. Med. 298:219–220, 1978.
1a. Levy, G.: Pharmacokinetic control of theophylline therapy, *In* Clinical Pharmacokinetics, a Symposium. American Pharmaceutical Association, Academy of Pharmaceutical Sciences. October, 1974, pp. 103–110.
2. Piafsky, K. M. and Ogilvie, R. I.: Dosage of theophylline in bronchial asthma. N. Engl. J. Med. 292:1218–1222, 1975.
3. Segal, M. S.: Methylxanthines, *In* Current Respiratory Care. K. F. MacDonnell and M. S. Segal (Eds.) Boston, Little, Brown and Company, 1977. Ch. 20.
4. Nicholson, D. P. and Chick, T. W.: A re-evaluation of parenteral aminophylline. Am. Rev. Respir. Dis. 108:241–247, 1973.
5. Ellis, E. F.: Asthma in childhood: Clinical pharmacology of theophylline in asthmatic children, *In* New Directions in Asthma. M. Stein (Ed.). Park Ridge, Illinois, American College of Chest Physicians, 1975, Ch. 19.
6. Resar, R., Walson, P., Perry, D. and Barbee, R.: Intra-patient variability of theophylline kinetics in adults with chronic obstructive pulmonary disease. Am. Rev. Respir. Dis. 115 #4 Pt. 2:155, 1977.
7. Walson, P. D., Strunk, R. C. and Taussig, L. M.: Intrapatient variability in theophylline kinetics, J. Pediatr. 91:321–324, 1977.
7a. Weinberger, M.: Variation in theophylline clearance rate. J. Allergy Clin. Immunol. 60:271–272, 1977.
7b. Wyatt, R., Weinberger, M. and Hendeles, L.: Oral theophylline dosage for the management of chronic asthma. J. Pediatr. 92:125–130, 1978.
8. Jenne, J. W.: Rationale for methylxanthines in asthma, *In* New Directions in Asthma. M. Stein (Ed.). Park Ridge, Illinois, American College of Chest Physicians, 1975, Ch. 24.
9. Weddle, O. H. and Mason, W. D.: Rapid determination of theophylline in human plasma by high-pressure liquid chromatography. J. Pharm. Sci. 65:865–868, 1976.
9a. Neese, A. L. and Soyka, L. F.: Development of a radioimmunoassay for theophylline: application to studies in premature infants. Clin. Pharmacol. Ther. 21:633–641, 1977.
10. Warren, S. L.: A simple office procedure for the monitoring of theophylline levels in asthma. Ann. Allergy 38:198–201, 1977.
10a. Banner, A. S., Berman, E., Sunderrajan, E. et al.: Drug interferences with the spectrophotometric assay of theophylline. N. Engl. J. Med. 297:170, 1977.
10b. Hendeles, L., Matheson, L. and Bighley, L.: Drugs interfering with theophylline. N. Engl. J. Med. 297:670, 1977.
10c. Hendeles, L., Burkey, S., Bighley, L. and Richardson, R.: Unpredictability of theophylline saliva measurements in chronic obstructive pulmonary disease. J. Allergy Clin. Immunol. 60:335–338, 1977.
10d. Kordash, T. R., Van Dellen, R. G. and McCall, J. T.: Theophylline concentrations in asthmatic patients after administration of aminophylline. J. A. M. A. 238:139–141, 1977.
10e. Chrzanowski, F. A., Niebergall, P. J., Mayock, R. L., Taubin, J. M. and Sugita, E. T.: Kinetics of intravenous theophylline. Clin. Pharmacol. Ther. 22:188–195, 1977.
11. Jusko, W. J., Koup, J. R., Vance, J. W., Schentag, J. J. and Kuritzky, P.: Intravenous theophylline therapy: nomogram guidelines. Ann. Intern. Med. 86:400–404, 1977.
11a. Koup, J. R., Schentag, J. J., Vance, J. W., Kuritzky P. M., Pyszczynski, D. R. and Jusko, W. J.: System for clinical pharmacokinetic monitoring of theophylline therapy. Am. J. Hosp. Pharm. 33:949–956, 1976.
12. Jenne, J. W., Wyze, E., Rood, F. S. and MacDonald, F. M.: Pharmacokinetics of theophylline. Application to adjustment of the clinical dose of aminophylline. Clin. Pharmacol. Ther. 13:349–360, 1972.
13. Turner-Warwick, M.: Study of theophylline plasma levels after oral administration of new theophylline compounds. Br. Med. J. 2:67–69, July 1957.
14. Segal, M. S.: Aminophylline: a clinical overview. Advances in Asthma and Allergy 2:17–35, Fall 1975. (Published by Fisons Corp.).
14a. Piafsky, K. M., Sitar, D. M., Rangno, R. E. and Ogilvie, R. I.: Theophylline disposition in patients with hepatic cirrhosis. N. Engl. J. Med. 296:1495–1497, 1977.
14b. Ogilvie, R. I., Sitar, D. S. and Rangno, R. E.: Theophylline in liver disease. N. Engl. J. Med. 297:1123–1124, 1977.

15. Jacobs, M. H. and Senior, R. M.: Theophylline toxicity due to impaired theophylline degradation. Am. Rev. Respir. Dis. 110:342–345, 1974.

16. Powell, J. R., Vozeh, S., Hopewell, P. C., Costello, J., Sheiner, L. and Riegelman, S.: Theophylline clearance (Cl) in acutely ill patients with asthma and chronic obstructive pulmonary disease (COPD) with and without congestive heart failure (CHF) and pneumonia. Am. Rev. Respir. Dis. 115 #4 Pt. 2:152, 1977.

17. Piafsky, K. M., Sitar, D. S., Rangno, R. E. and Ogilvie, R. I.: Theophylline kinetics in acute pulmonary edema. Clin. Pharmacol. Ther. 21:310–316, 1977.

18. Resar, R., Walson, P., Fritz, B. and Barbee, R.: Effect of arterial pH on intravenous theophylline loading in chronic obstructive pulmonary disease. Am. Rev. Respir. Dis. 115 #4 Pt. 2:155, 1977.

18a. Kozak, P. P., Cummins, L. H. and Gillman, S. A.: Administration of erythromycin to patients on theophylline. J. Allergy Clin. Immunol. 60:149–151, 1977.

18b. Weinberger, M.: Variation in theophylline clearance rate. J. Allergy Clin. Immunol. 60:271–272, 1977.

19. Welling, P. G., Lyons, L. L., Craig, W. A. and Trochta, G. A.: Influence of diet and fluid on bioavailability of theophylline. Clin. Pharmacol. Ther. 17:475–480, 1975.

19a. Fixley, M., Shen, D. D. and Azarnoff, D. L.: Theophylline bioavailability: a comparison of the oral absorption of a theophylline elixir and two combination theophylline tablets to intravenous aminophylline. Am. Rev. Respir. Dis. 115:955–962, 1977.

19b. Kappas, A., Anderson, K. E., Conney, A. H. et al.: Influence of dietary protein and carbohydrate on antipyrene and theophylline metabolism in man. Clin. Pharmacol. Ther. 20:643–653, 1976.

20. Welling, P. G., Domoradzki, J., Sims, J. A. and Reed, C. E.: Influence of formulation on bioavailability of theophylline. J. Clin. Pharmacol. 16:43–50, 1976.

20a. Hendeles, L., Weinberger, M. and Bighley, L.: Absorption characteristics of various oral theophylline dosage forms. Presented to the American Congress of Allergy and Immunology, New York, March, 1977.

20b. Hendeles, L., Weinberger, M. and Bighley, L.: Absolute bioavailability of oral theophylline. Am J. Hosp. Pharm. 34:525–527, 1977.

20c. Spangler, D. L., Kalof, D. D., Bloom, F. L. and Wittig, H. J.: Theophylline bioavailability following oral administration of six sustained-release preparations. Ann. Allergy 40:6–11, 1978.

20d. Katz, R. M., Rachelefsky, G. and Siegel, S.: The effectiveness of the short- and long-term use of crystallized theophylline in asthmatic children. J. Pediatr. 92:663–667, 1978.

21. Powell, J. R., Thiercelin, J. F., Vozeh, S., Sansom, L. and Riegelman, S.: The influence of cigarette smoking and sex on theophylline disposition. Am. Rev. Respir. Dis. 116:17–23, 1977.

22. Richards, A. J., Walker, S. R. and Paterson, J. W.: A new anti-asthmatic drug (ICI 58301): blood levels and spirometry. Brit. J. Dis. Chest 65:247–252, 1971.

23. Meyers, F. H., Jawetz, E. and Goldfien, A.: Review of Medical Pharmacology. Los Altos, Calif., Lange Medical Publications, 3rd ed., 1972, p. 117.

23a. Lakshminarayan, S., Sahn, S. E. and Weil, J. V.: Effect of aminophylline on ventilatory responses in normal man. Am. Rev. Respir. Dis. 117:33–38, 1978.

24. Urthaler, F. and James, T. N.: Both direct and neurally medicated components of the chronotropic actions of aminophylline. Chest 70:24–32, 1976.

25. Tong, T. G.: Aminophylline – a review of clinical use. Drug. Intel. Clin. Pharm. 7:156–167, 1973.

26. Hendeles, L., Carmichael, J., Bighley, L. and Richardson, R. H.: Nausea and vomiting as a clinical indicator of I.V. aminophylline toxicity. Clin. Res. 24:509A, 1976.

27. Simons, F. E. R., Pierson, W. E. and Bierman, C. W.: Current status of the use of theophyllines in children. Pediatrics 55:735–737, 1975.

28. Zwillich, C. W., Sutton, F. D., Neff, T. A., Cohn, W. M., Matthay, R. A. and Weinberger, M. M.: Theophylline-induced seizures in adults. Correlation with serum concentrations. Ann. Intern. Med. 82:784–787, 1975.

29. Matthay, R. A., Matthay, M. A. and Weinberger, M.: Grand mal seizure induced by oral theophylline. Thorax 31:470–471, 1976.

29a. Lawyer, C., Aitchison, J., Sutton, J. and Bennett, W.: Treatment of theophylline neurotoxicity with resin hemoperfusion. Ann. Intern. Med. 88:516–517, 1978.

30. Wong, D., Lopapa, A. E. and Haddad, Z. H.: Immediate hypersensitivity reaction to aminophylline. J. Allergy Clin. Immunol. 48:165–170, 1971.

31. Weinberger, M., Hudgel, D., Spector, S. and Chidsey, C.: Inhibition of theophylline clearance by troleandomycin. J. Allergy Clin. Immunol. 59:228–231, 1977.

32. VanDerLinde, L. P., Campbell, R. K. and Jackson, E.: Guidelines for the intravenous administration of drugs. Drug. Intel. Clin. Pharm. 11:30–55, 1977.

33. Berman, B. A. and Greenberg, B. L.: In defense of theophylline for asthma. Patient Care 8:107–119, 1974.

34. Salem, H. and Aviado, D. M.: Xanthine bronchodilator preparations available in the United States. Rev. Allergy 24:624–630, 1970.

35. Salem, H. and Jackson, R. H.: Oral theophylline preparations – a review of their clinical efficacy in the treatment of bronchial asthma. Ann. Allergy 32:189–199, 1974.

35a. Weinberger, M.: Theophylline for treatment of asthma. J. Pediatr. 92:1–7, 1978.

36. Cohen, A., Johnson, C. and Re, O.: A rapidly dissolving theophylline tablet. Curr. Ther. Res. 17:497–505, 1975.

37. Mitenko, P. A. and Ogilvie, R. I.: Bioavailability and efficacy of a sustained-release theophylline tablet. Clin. Pharmacol. Ther. 16:720–726, 1974.

37a. Jenne, J. W.: The clinical pharmacology of bronchodilator drugs. Basics of RD (Published by American Thoracic Society) 6 #1, Sept., 1977.

37b. Weinberger, M. and Hendeles, L.: The pharmacological basis of bronchodilator therapy. Rational Drug Therapy 11 #6, June, 1977.

38. Kern, J. W. and Lipman, A. G.: Rational theophylline therapy: a review of the literature with a guide to pharmacokinetics and dosage calculations. Drug Intel. Clin. Pharm. 11:144–153, 1977.

39. Ziment, I., Kuo, J. and Steen, S. N.: Microphyllin for bronchospasm. Proceedings of the Fourth Asian and Australasian Congress of Anaesthesiologists, Singapore, 1974, pp. 348–349.

40. Stewart, B. N. and Block, A. J.: A trial of aerosolized theophylline in relieving bronchospasm. Chest 69:718–721, 1976.

41. Muittari, A., and Mattila, M. J.: Bronchodilator action of drug combinations in asthmatic patients: ephedrine, theophylline and tranquilizing drugs. Curr. Ther. Res. 13:374–385, 1971.

42. Weinberger, M. and Riegelman, S.: Rational use of theophylline for bronchodilatation. N. Engl. J. Med. 291:151–153, 1974.

43. Weinberger, M., Bronsky, E., et al.: Interaction of ephedrine and theophylline. Clin. Pharmacol. Ther. 17:585–592, 1975.

44. Grover, F. W.: Oxtriphylline glyceryl guaiacolate elixir in pediatric asthma: with a theophylline review. Ann. Allergy 23:127–147, 1965.

44a. Floyd, R. A. and Bartlett, L. N.: Percent theophylline in aminophylline. Drug Intel. Clin. Pharm. 12:177, 1978.

45. Femi-Pearse, D., George, W. O., Ilechukwu, S. T., Elegbeleye, O. O. and Afonja, A. O.: Comparison of intravenous aminophylline and salbutamol in severe asthma. Br. Med. J. 1:491, Feb., 1977.

46. Loren, M., Miklich, D. R., Chai, H. and Barwise, G.: Aminophylline bioavailability and the across-time stability of plasma theophylline levels. J. Pediatr. 90:473–476, 1977.

47. Lillehei, J. P.: Aminophylline. Oral vs. rectal administration. JAMA 205:530–533, 1968.

48. Segal, M. S. and Weiss, E. B.: Rectal aminophylline (blood levels with concentrated solutions). Ann. Allergy 29:135–138, 1971.

49. Taplin, G. V., Gropper, A. L. and Scott, G.: Micropowdered aminophylline or theophylline inhalation therapy in chronic bronchial asthma. Ann. Allergy 7:513–539, 1949.

50. Segal, M. S., Levinson, L., Bresnick, E. and Beakey, J. F.: Evaluation of therapeutic substances employed for the relief of bronchospasm. VI. Aminophylline. J. Clin. Invest. 28:1190–1195, 1949.

51. Bulow, K. B., Larsson, H. and Leideman, T.: Plasma theophylline level and ventilatory function in chronic obstructive pulmonary disease during prolonged oral treatment with choline theophyllinate. Europ. J. Clin. Pharmacol. 8:119–123, 1975.

52. Levine, E. R.: An effective oral medication for long term bronchodilation. Ann. Allergy 23:403–413, 1965.

53. Isaksson, B. and Lindholm, B.: Blood plasma level of different theophylline derivatives following parenteral, oral and rectal administration. Acta Med. Scand. 171:33–38, 1962.

54. Simons, F. E. R., Simons, K. J. and Bierman, C. W.: The pharmacokinetics of dihydroxypropyl theophylline: a basis for rational therapy. J. Allergy Clin. Immunol. 56:347–355, 1975.

55. Hudson, L. D., Tyler, M. L. and Petty, T. L.: Oral aminophylline and dihydroxypropyl theophylline in reversible obstructive airway disease: a single-dose, double-blind, crossover comparison. Curr. Ther. Res. 15:367–372, 1973.

55a. Hendeles, L. and Weinberger, M.: Dyphylline: the "untheophylline" xanthine bronchodilator. Drug Intel. Clin. Pharm. 11:424, 1977.

56. St. John, M. A.: Pulmonary function studies for evaluation of oral theophylline compounds in the treatment of asthma. Clin. Med. 75:35–42, 1968.

57. Mitenko, P. A. and Ogilvie, R. I.: Rational intravenous doses of theophylline. N. Engl. J. Med. 289:600–603, 1973.

58. Arianda, J. V., Sitar, D. S., Parsons, W. D., Loughnan, P. M. and Neims, A. H.: Pharmacokinetic aspects of theophylline in premature newborns. N. Engl. J. Med. 295:413–416, 1976.

58a. Leung, P., Kalisker, A. and Bell, T. D.: Variation in theophylline clearance rate with time in chronic childhood asthma. J. Allergy. Clin. Immunol. 59:440–444, 1977.

59. Hendeles, L., Bighley, L., Richardson, H., Hepler, C. D. and Carmichael, J.: Frequent toxicity from IV aminophylline infusions in critically ill patients. Drug. Intel. Clin. Pharm. 11:12–18, 1977.

60. Petty, T. L.: Intravenous aminophylline dosage: use of serum theophylline measurement for guidance. J.A.M.A. 235:2110–2113, 1976.

61. Zaske, D. E., Miller, K. W., Strem, E. L., Austrian, S. and Johnson, P. B.: Oral aminophylline therapy: increased dosage requirements in children. J.A.M.A. 237:1453–1455, 1977.

62. Vozeh, S., Upton, R. A., Riegelman, S. et al: Bronchodilator therapy. N. Engl. J. Med. 298:220, 1978.

63. Jacobs, M. H., Senior, R. M. and Kessler, G.: Clinical experience with theophylline: relationships between dosage, serum concentrations, and toxicity. J.A.M.A. 235:1983–1986, 1976.

7

CORTICOSTEROIDS

INTRODUCTION

The adrenal corticosteroid hormones have an amazingly wide repertoire of therapeutic values; numerous synthetic derivatives are also used medically. The most important corticosteroids are classified into two groups, *glucocorticoids* and *mineralocorticoids*. The glucocorticoids affect the metabolism of glucose and have profound effects on the other basic metabolic processes; they also have an extraordinary range of antiinflammatory properties. The mineralocorticoids affect water and electrolyte balance, but do not have significant antiinflammatory effects. The natural glucocorticoids all have some mineralocorticoid activity. Thus, the natural adrenal corticosteroids have a variety of major effects, but the glucocorticoid or mineralocorticoid properties predominate in a given steroid hormone. The major mineralocorticoid is *aldosterone,* and the main glucocorticoid, which is produced by the adrenal cortex, is *hydrocortisone* (cortisol).

The natural glucocorticoids, and their synthetic derivatives, which have more powerful and specific antiinflammatory action (with correspondingly less mineralocorticoid properties), are of major importance in the treatment of many diseases. They are very effective in the management of asthma and various other lung diseases, and are a major weapon in the respiratory pharmacopeia. Several naturally occurring glucocorticoids have been identified and synthesized, and an ever-increasing number of synthetic glucocorticoids have been introduced into therapeutics. Hydrocortisone and cortisone, the two most important natural glucocorticoids, are still of value. Hydrocortisone is more potent than cortisone, while the new synthetic agents are much more potent than either of them. All the glucocorticoids have powerful effects on immunologic processes, and they are used extensively in the treatment of numerous noninfectious diseases that are characterized by pathologically inappropriate immune or inflammatory reactions.

Structure of the Glucocorticoids

The corticosteroids are derived from cholesterol; they consist of three and a half benzene rings. The antiinflammatory corticosteroids all contain a chain of two carbon atoms attached to the 17 position, and they are known as C-21 steroids; the OH group at 17 results in these steroids also being known as 17-hydroxycorticoids (Fig. 7–1). The steric configuration of the active antiinflammatory steroids always shows the following invariable features: an =O group at position 3, a double bond between positions 4 and 5, an OH group at position 11, and a =CO at position 20.[1] Cortisone, and the synthetic derivative prednisone, are 11-keto compounds, and lack glucocorticoid activity until converted in the body into the 11-β-hydroxyl compounds, hydrocortisone and prednisolone respectively. Additional drugs have been synthesized which have more powerful antiinflammatory effects and less action on electrolyte metabolism; thus, the addition of a fluorine atom at the 9α position increases all activity, whereas a methyl group at position 16 decreases sodium retaining potency. Although derivatives containing a fluorine atom are more potent, they are more likely to cause myopathy. Small modifications in molecular structure can have profound effects on the various properties of the corticosteroids. The pharmaceutical industry has introduced an extraordinary number of

STRUCTURAL FORMULAE OF SHORT-ACTING GLUCOCORTICOIDS

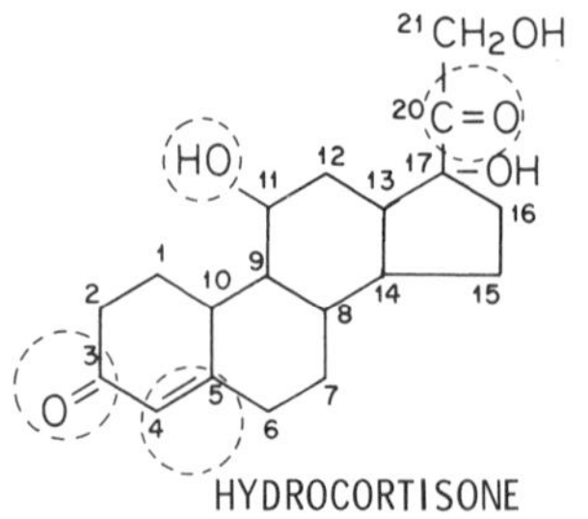

HYDROCORTISONE
Basic structure is C 21
glucocorticosteroid
(Groups essential for
antiinflammatory action
are circled)

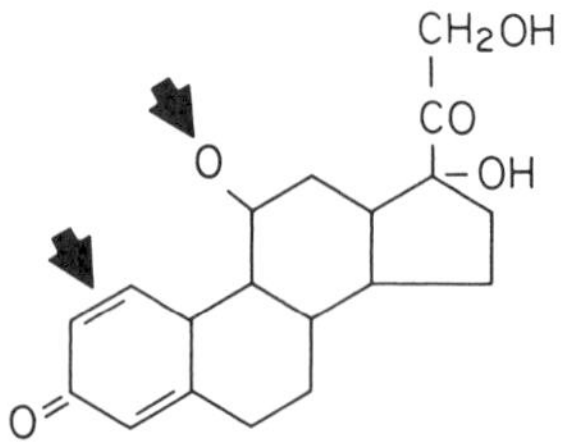

PREDNISONE
Differs from hydrocortisone
by double bond between C1
and C2, and C=O at C11 (arrowed)

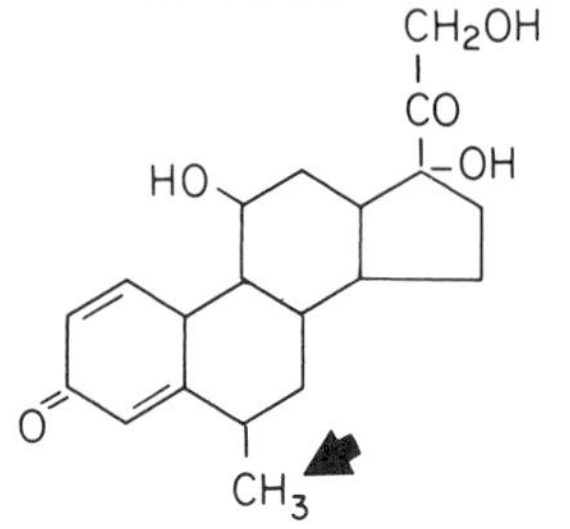

METHYLPREDNISOLONE
Differs from prednisolone
by CH$_3$-(methyl) group in
6 α position (arrowed)

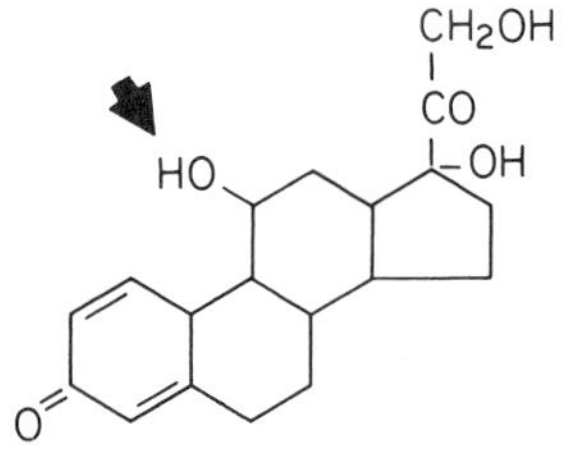

PREDNISOLONE
This is obtained from
prednisone by conversion
of C=O at 11 to 11 β
hydroxyl group (arrowed)

Figure 7–1.

glucocorticoids that are tailored for various specific therapeutic uses.[2] All the topical glucocorticoid preparations that are used in clinical therapy are 11-β-hydroxyl compounds.

Mechanism of Action of Glucocorticoids

The mode of action of the glucocorticoids in their curtailing of immunologic reactions is incompletely understood. Numerous studies have revealed a bewildering variety of complex effects, but it is not possible to fully explain the dramatic ability of steroid therapy to control disease processes, such as those involved in asthma.[3-5]

In general, physiologic concentrations of glucocorticoids contribute a "permissive" effect for many metabolic effects mediated by peptide hormone and catecholamines in which the steroids are not directly involved.[6] In the absence of normal amounts of glucocorticoids, various other hormones do not function appropriately, whereas administration of the steroid facilitates the hormonal effects. The cellular level of steroid action has been elucidated to a considerable degree (see Figure 7–2); through a sequence of complex events, the glucocorticoids bring about specific protein synthesis.[7, 8] The extraordinary complexity of these events is illustrated by the fact that the steroid hormones can produce specific RNA and protein synthesis in a tissue, while suppressing RNA and protein synthesis in other, or even the same, tissue.[6] The most basic glucocorticoid effect is the inhibition of amino acid incorporation into protein in peripheral tissues.[8a]

The glucocorticoids protect tissues from the inflammatory damage that characterizes many diseases by nonspecific interference in the pathologic processes at several points (Table 7–1). Thus, these hormones interfere with the migration of leucocytes into the damaged site in a tissue, and they help maintain the integrity of the affected blood vessels in the microcirculation. It is thought that a basic effect of corticosteroids is the alteration of the surface properties of the granulocytes, thereby reducing their adherence to vascular epithelium and their ability to phagocytose.[8b] By these various actions, the steroids decrease leakage from blood vessels; they also cause some vasoconstriction, and thus reduce a basic component in the inflammatory response. Corticosteroid

Corticosteroid
↓
Cytoplasmic Receptor
↓
Steroid-Receptor Active Complex
↓
Binding to Nuclear DNA
↓
Activation of Transcription Mechanism
↓
Production of New Messenger — RNA
↓
Stimulation of Ribosomal Synthesis
↓
Production of New Active Proteins (? e.g. adenylate cyclase)
↓
Action On Target-Cell Processes (e.g. bronchodilation)

Figure 7-2. Mechanism of action of glucocorticoids.

TABLE 7-1. GENERAL ANTIINFLAMMATORY EFFECTS OF GLUCOCORTICOIDS

Actions	Significance
Maintain microcirculation (vascoconstriction) by suppression of kinin activity	Prevents leakage of fluid from blood vessels, with formation of tissue edema
Inhibit migration of leucocytes and mast cells	Decreases exudation and migration of inflammatory cells (phagocytes, macrophages, etc.)
Reduce polymorph stickiness and margination in blood vessels	Impairs polymorph activity
Cause lymphopenia, monocytopenia and eosinopenia	Unknown significance
Maintain cell-membrane integrity	Protects cells from damage by noxious events, and prevents the intracellular sequestration of water that would swell and damage cells
Stabilize lysosomal membranes in mast cells, etc.	Prevents release of mediators which induce inflammatory reactions
Reduce tissue stores of histamine and other mediators	Decreases availability of mediators which cause inflammatory reaction
Potentiate catecholamine activity	Enhances sympathomimetic responsiveness
Enhance cardiac inotropy and improve circulatory function	Improves cardiopulmonary function in conditions of severe stress, such as shock

TABLE 7-2. IMMUNOLOGIC REACTIONS PRODUCING ASTHMA

	Type I	Type III
TYPE OF REACTION	"Anaphylactic reaction," atopic, immediate hypersensitivity	"Toxic-complex reaction," delayed hypersensitivity
IMMUNOLOGIC MECHANISM	Antigen + IgE (reagin); antigen + IgG (in nonatopic subjects)	Excess antigen + IgG and IgM + complement ⟶ precipitins
EFFECT ON IMMUNE CELLS	Release of histamine, etc. from mast cells	Release of lysosomal enzymes from leucocytes
SKIN TEST	Extravascular reaction, immediate wheal and flare (as in "Prausnitz-Kustner reaction")	Intravascular reaction ⟶ increased vascular permeability ⟶ extensive, poorly defined local edema ("Arthus reaction")
SYMPTOMS	Asthma; or rhinitis, urticaria or anaphylaxis (may be followed by Type III reaction)	Asthma with fever, malaise, leucocytosis; hypersensitivity reactions; extrinsic alveolitides (usually preceded by Type I reaction)
ONSET OF ASTHMA	Acute; maximal in 10–20 minutes	Gradual over 4–8 hours; maximal by 8 hours (some reactions start within 1 hour, maximal at 3 hours)
RESOLUTION	1–2 hours	1–3 or 4 days (some reactions resolve within 3 hours)
RELIEVED BY SYMPATHOMIMETICS	Yes; good response	Poor response
INHIBITION BY CROMOLYN	IgE-mediated: Yes IgG-mediated: No	Yes
INHIBITION BY GLUCOCORTICOIDS	No	Yes

therapy usually causes a decrease in the count of peripheral blood eosinophils, monocytes and lymphocytes, while increasing the polymorphonuclear leucocyte count.[8c]

There are several distinct ways in which glucocorticoids serve to counteract the abnormal processes that characterize asthma. Steroids are of value in both intrinsic and extrinsic (allergic) asthma, and these remarkable drugs are successful in both the prophylaxis and the treatment of various types of asthma. The clearest understanding of the bronchospastic mechanisms exists with regard to allergic asthma. Immunologists believe that there are two components to the allergic asthmatic response (Table 7-2), although these distinct phases are difficult to identify in clinical practice. The susceptible (atopic) patient who is exposed to a specific allergen may develop an early asthmatic response, which may subside spontaneously after one or two hours. Subsequently, a more sustained attack of asthma may develop, which becomes maximal within eight hours, and may persist for up to four days in the absence of appropriate treatment.[9]

There is evidence that the initial Type I reaction is mediated by the interaction of the antigen with a specific antibody (or immunoglobulin, Ig) in atopic subjects; this antigen, IgE, is also termed reagin. In some nonatopic patients, as well as in some subjects who have IgE antibodies, there is another "short-term homocytotropic antibody," STS-IgG, which may also react with antigen.[9] These antigen-antibody reactions occur on the surface of mast cells, and result in the release of histamine, SRS-A and other mediators of bronchospasm. This release phenomenon in reagin-mediated reactions can be inhibited by cromolyn; however, rather surprisingly, the release of mediators is not inhibited by glucocorticoids. Thus, steroids do not protect patients against this immediate bronchospastic reaction, nor do they provide effective therapy for the wheezing and dyspnea; isoproterenol and other sympathomimetics do, however, provide rapid relief.

In certain patients, the Type I reaction is followed a few hours later by a Type III delayed reaction, which occurs if there is a relative excess of the antigenic stimulus. This additional antigenic material combines with other antibodies, of the IgG and IgM classes, and, in the presence of serum complement, forms precipitins.[10] These in turn cause a release of leucocyte lysosomal enzymes, that induce a sustained inflammatory response, which can persist for several days: this response is similar to that occurring in the Arthus reaction, which can be induced by skin-testing the patient with the antigen. The susceptible patient who experiences a Type III reaction in the lung develops persistent bronchospasm with sputum production, and may also develop myalgias, malaise and fever. In some patients, the antigen may be responsible for a more severe reaction at the alveolar level, causing an allergic alveolitis (or hypersensitivity pneumonitis) such as occurs with farmer's lung. As yet, it is unclear what determines whether a patient develops predominant bronchospasm or alveolitis. However, both responses can be inhibited by corticosteroids; Type III asthma can also be prevented by cromolyn. The glucocorticoids are additionally successful both in the treatment of this delayed asthmatic response and in the management of allergic alveolitis, whereas, of course, cromolyn does not offer effective treatment (in contrast to prophylaxis); isoproterenol and other bronchodilators may not be successful either.[9] Clinically, status asthmaticus corresponds to the Type III reaction.

Therapeutic Effects of Glucocorticoids in Asthma

When one examines the factors involved in the asthmatic response, it is possible to identify several sites at which the glucocorticoids may intervene.[8, 11]

General Effects. A major contention is that the steroids, particularly when given in pharmacologic amounts, stabilize the membranes of all lysosomes, thereby preventing the release of their content of hydrolytic enzymes that would digest the cell and cause an inflammatory response in the tissue. However, although there is evidence to suggest that lysosomal stabilization may be involved in laboratory experiments,[12] there is much less certainty that the phenomenon occurs under either physiologic or pathologic conditions.[7, 8b, 8c, 13] Further confirmation is required before it can be accepted that this effect on lysosomes is a major component of the therapeutic outcome of pharmacologic administration of corticosteroids.[6]

Inhibition of DNA synthesis is an important basic consequence of glucocorticoid activity, but this does not explain the value of the steroids in the therapy of asthma. However, there is good evidence that the steroids inhibit the formation as well as the storage and release of histamine and other mediators that cause bronchospasm;[14] and this is probably one of the most important effects of steroid therapy. Other basic properties of the steroids, such as their ability to inhibit vasodilation (or to actually cause vasoconstriction[13]) and cellular migration, may play a role in reversing or preventing the asthmatic response. Certainly, steroid administration results in a decrease in circulating lymphocytes, eosinophils and in tissue mast cells;[8b] these characteristic effects are undoubtedly important factors in the control of asthma.

Specific Effects. More specific suggestions have been made to explain the value of steroid therapy in intrinsic as well as extrinsic asthma (Table 7–3). It has been suggested that the glucocorticoids have a direct relaxant effect on bronchial muscle, but no mechanism for this hypothetical action has been proposed;[14] in practice, the steroids cannot be regarded as direct bronchodilators. There is evidence that glucocorticoids potentiate the actions of beta-2 receptor stimulators, and restore responsiveness to standard sympathomimetic therapy.[15] These clinical findings have received a number of different explanations.[15-17] Thus, the glucocorticoids may cause increased production, availability, and activity of adenylate cyclase, the enzyme situated at the beta-2 receptor site.[16] The "permissive" effect of glucocorticoids is a general property that can be invoked to explain the lowering of the threshold of beta-2 receptors that have become, for various reasons, relatively unresponsive to sympathomimetic stimulation.[7] It has also been suggested that the corticoids can inhibit the enzyme COMT, which breaks down catecholamines.[8] There is but little evidence, however, to suggest that the glucocorticoids act directly to stimulate beta-2 receptors.[14] Another possible mechanism by which the glucocorticoids facilitate bronchorelaxation is by, somehow, increasing the availability of cyclic 3',5'-AMP, particularly

TABLE 7–3. SPECIFIC "BRONCHODILATOR" EFFECTS OF GLUCOCORTICOIDS

Effect	Significance
Restoration of "permissiveness" at beta-receptors	Improves effectiveness of sympathomimetic drugs
Inhibition of catechol O-methyl transferase (COMT)	Increases availability of catecholamines
Increase in adenylate cyclase production and activity	Provides additional receptor sites for sympathomimetic stimulation
Decrease in the responsiveness of cholinergic and alpha receptors (decrease ATPase and cyclic GMP activity)	Increases resistance to induction of bronchospasm
Stimulation of cyclic 3',5'-AMP production or activity	Enhances basic bronchospasmolytic process
Inhibition of phosphodiesterase production or activity	Increases cyclic 3',5-AMP availability
May interfere with action of prostaglandin synthetase	Decreases availability of $PGF_2\alpha$ (a bronchoconstrictor)

in response to sympathomimetic drug stimulation.[17] Although the corticoids do not appear to increase the level of c-AMP directly, they may serve to inhibit the production or the activity of phosphodiesterase, which breaks down c-AMP.[6] Another suggestion is that the glucocorticoids interfere with the bronchoconstrictive mechanisms activated by cholinergic and alpha-adrenergic receptor stimulation.[8] Thus, steroids may cause a reduction in ATP-ase activity, which is involved in the alpha-adrenergic response, and they may also decrease the production of the bronchoconstrictive prostaglandin, $PGF_{2\alpha}$.

It is of interest that glucocorticoids do not appear to significantly interfere with the production of antibodies by the body's immune system,[7] nor do they prevent antibody reacting with antigen,[13] and they do not interfere with the metabolism of complement.[11] Thus corticosteroids do not prevent the initial events in the Type I and Type III reactions involved in antigen-induced asthma.[9] Their main role in this form of asthma is to prevent the release of lysosomal enzymes. In contrast, cromolyn acts at an earlier stage to prevent the release of mediators from mast cells. Thus, the glucocorticoids are mainly of value in the prophylaxis of Type III allergic asthma, some forms of intrinsic asthma, and in the treatment of status asthmaticus.

A further suggestion that has been made with regard to the value of administered steroids in the treatment of asthma is related to the fact that some patients do not show the usual immunologic responses (such as a decreased eosinophil count) to steroid therapy. Thus, there may be an abnormality in cortisol metabolism in some patients, whereby the normal permissive effect of endogenous corticoids is lost. These patients may require relatively large doses of steroids to restore the permissive effect at beta-2 receptor sites.[18]

Additional Effects. Glucocorticoids may offer important contributions at additional points in the complex interreactions that occur in asthma. Thus, these drugs have a euphoriant action, which increases the patient's sense of well being; this could counterbalance the anxiety and depression that may contribute to an asthmatic patient's liability to attacks of bronchospasm. The steroids are of value in the management of hay fever, allergic rhinitis, conjunctivitis and atopic eczema; these other diseases may interact, in a cyclic fashion, in an atopic patient's susceptibility to asthma, and the interruption of these other problems may be of indirect benefit to the asthmatic component in the overall disease process.

One further important benefit of corticosteroid therapy in asthma is related to the mucokinetic effect. Thus, as Hirsch[19] points out, glucocorticoid therapy decreases mucus volume and appears to alter its composition favorably; it also results in improved ciliary clearance, and, by relieving bronchospasm, helps alleviate the overall problem of mucus stasis. To quote Hirsch: "Were it not for the side effects of this drug, it would be a virtually perfect treatment for asthma."

Thus, there are many ways in which corticosteroid therapy may be of value in the therapeutic management of asthma. Furthermore, these remarkable hormones are useful in a number of other pulmonary diseases, although, in general, the benefits are less dramatic than those obtained in asthma. Although there are serious gaps in our understanding of the disease mechanisms and of steroid actions, there is adequate clinical experience to help direct us in the oral, systemic and topical use of these powerful agents in the treatment of asthma and other disorders of the respiratory tract.

Topical Steroids

For topical therapy, only 11-β-hydroxyl glucocorticoids are of value.[13] The 11-keto compounds, hydrocortisone and prednisone, must be converted (mainly by the liver) to the active hormones, and therefore these two agents are relatively ineffective unless given systemically. They are relatively unsuitable for topical dermatologic therapy, and would not be expected to be successful if given by inhalation. Glucocorticoids that are suitable for topical application are rendered water-soluble by the addition of phosphate or succinate groups to the molecule. These salts are hydrophilic compounds, which are highly polar, and they penetrate poorly when applied to the skin. On the other hand, fatty acid esters of the steroids (such as acetate preparations) are able to penetrate into the deeper layers of the skin; they are only slowly absorbed and, therefore, they exert a powerful topical effect. Certain substituents may profoundly increase the antiinflammatory properties of many of the glucocorticoids: the acetonide of triamcinolone and the dipropionate of beclomethasone constitute extremely powerful topical agents that are very effective in the treatment of skin disease.

These latter agents have more recently been shown to be very effective when applied topically to the respiratory mucosa; moreover, they are poorly absorbed into the blood stream, and therefore have little systemic effect. The advantages of these properties have been clearly demonstrated in the therapeutic administration of such steroids in the inhalational treatment of asthma. It is possible that these preparations may also prove to be of value in other pulmonary diseases that respond to steroid therapy, although clinical evidence is not available as yet for diseases such as sarcoidosis and alveolitis.

Adverse Effects of Glucocorticoids

The glucocorticoids have numerous potent effects on the body, with the "glucose" effect being a relatively minor consideration (see Table 7–4). Most of the side effects that accompany therapeutic administration of the drugs begin to appear only after a few days or weeks. The development of these hormonal consequences of steroid therapy can be minimized by using the smallest possible dose, or even by trying to manage the disease by administering the drug on alternate days. This latter regimen is often very successful in the management of childhood asthma, and may be equally successful in many adults. More recently, the introduction of powerful aerosol preparations has provided a remarkable improvement in the benefit:toxicity therapeutic ratio.[20]

In the Boston Collaborative Drug Surveillance Program of about 1800 patients who received prednisone, the most frequently used corticosteroid, about 16 per cent developed adverse effects.[21] Two-thirds of these reactions appeared during acute courses, and higher dose therapy caused more problems, particularly psychiatric reactions.

The common adverse effects can be grouped as follows:

Cushingoid Effects.[7, 22, 23] Prolonged use of relatively high doses of glucocorticoids results in a condition similar to Cushing's syndrome, which is found in patients with overactivity of the adrenal cortex. The patients gain weight in a characteristic and unsightly fashion, resulting in swelling ("mooning") of the face, central obesity with a "buffalo hump" over the back of the neck, and stretch marks (striae) over the limbs and trunk; the limbs remain relatively slender. Fat pads may also develop in the mediastinum, resulting in a widened cardiac border in the chest x-ray. The skin texture changes: acne and hirsutism often appear; a thin, fragile skin (susceptible to bruising and ecchymoses), associated with poor healing ability, is also a frequent consequence.

Other Cushing's syndrome complications may appear. Problems such as weakness associated with muscle atrophy and suppression of growth in children are manifestations of a general interference with metabolism, which may be correlated with factors such as an increase in calcium excretion, which usually occurs with steroid

TABLE 7–4. COMPLICATIONS THAT MAY BE ASSOCIATED WITH GLUCOCORTICOID THERAPY

Site	Unpleasant Effects	Dangerous Effects
Skin	Acne, hirsutism, striae, flushing, facial erythema, increased perspiration	Loss of subcutaneous tissue, poor wound healing
Vascular	Petechiae, bruising	Thromboemboli, vasculitis, periarteritis nodosa
Appearance	Fat deposition (facial mooning, buffalo hump, truncal obesity, etc.)	Stunting of growth in children
Central nervous system	Insomnia, restlessness, agitation	Altered personality, psychosis (euphoria, mania, depression, confusion), pseudotumor cerebri
Cardiovascular	Edema (due to sodium retention), nocturia	Hypertension, heart failure, arrhythmias
Metabolic	Electrolyte disturbance, calcium loss, alkalosis, negative nitrogen balance, hyperlipidemia	Diabetogenic effect, hyperosmolar non-ketotic coma
Musculoskeletal	Weakness (due to myopathy, hypokalemia and wasting), osteoporosis	Vertebral and other fractures, aseptic bone necrosis of femoral and humeral heads
Endocrine	Menstrual disorders, menopausal symptoms, impotence	Hypothalamic-pituitary-adrenal axis suppression
Gastrointestinal	Nausea, vomiting, fatty liver, increased appetite, esophagitis	Increased risk of peptic ulceration (in rheumatoid arthritis), large bowel perforation, pancreatitis
Ocular	Exophthalmos, posterior subcapsular cataract, sixth-nerve palsies (diplopia)	Papilledema, increased risk of fungal and viral keratitis
Immunologic	Suppression of skin responses to antigenic tests, depression of immunologic responses	Impaired response to infections, susceptibility to dissemination of vaccinations, opportunistic infections
Fetus		Risk of teratogenicity in first trimester, possible adrenal insufficiency in newborn infant

TABLE 7–4A. GLUCOCORTICOID WITHDRAWAL SYNDROME

Emotional "letdown," depression

Malaise, headache, fatigue, lethargy, weakness

Orthostatic hypotension, dizziness and fainting

Anorexia, nausea

Hypoglycemia

Weight loss

Conjunctivitis, rhinitis

Pseudorheumatism (arthralgias, myalgias, stiffness)

Desquamation of skin

Exacerbation of primary disease

Exacerbation of secondary disease, e.g. dermatitis, conjunctivitis, rhinitis

Withdrawal symptoms may be alleviated by antihistamine therapy.

therapy. Fluid retention with edema and even heart failure and hypertension are seen, particularly with those agents with marked mineralocorticoid activity. Psychiatric complications are common, and include euphoria, depression and other psychoses; these problems are more directly related to the dose of the drug than are the other acute complications.[21] Serious damage may occur in particular organs, and the following problems may develop with iatrogenic cushingism, although they do not appear to occur in spontaneous Cushing's syndrome:[24] osteoporosis, which may be accompanied by spontaneous fractures and a tendency for aseptic necrosis of the femoral and humeral heads; ophthalmic complications including posterior subcapsular cataracts, glaucoma and exophthalmos; pancreatitis; benign intracranial hypertension. One of the most common and potentially serious complications of chronic corticosteroid administration is osteoporosis and the secondary problems related to the weakness of the affected bones. The condition arises as a dose-related phenomenon, particularly in post-menopausal women. Although most accounts of steroid therapy dutifully list the commonly accepted complications, there is doubt about the frequency of occurrence of some of these alleged side effects. In particular, evidence has gradually accumulated to show that the association of peptic ulceration with steroid therapy is, in fact, mythical,[25] although it is common to see this listed as a frequent and serious complication.

Endocrine function may be severely disturbed in both iatrogenic and spontaneous Cushing's syndrome, since the corticosteroids suppress pituitary activity. The most common endocrine complication is a tendency toward overt diabetes, in addition to the metabolic hyperglycemia caused by the direct glucocorticoid effect. Menstrual irregularities are relatively frequent, and some virilism may occur in women; men may develop impotence. These effects are due to complex consequences of the negative biofeedback action of steroids on the hypothalamic-pituitary-adrenal axis. Following a prolonged course of steroid therapy, it takes six to nine months or more for the axis to recover its normal function. A depressive effect on the axis can be detected after as little as five days on a moderate dose of prednisone.[24]

Impairment of Immunologic Status. The ability of glucocorticoids to suppress immunologic activity is both a therapeutic advantage and a special hazard. Patients on steroids are more susceptible to the usual infections, and are at risk of developing unusual infectious diseases (such as nosocomial or opportunistic infections in hospitals), and severe complications (such as dissemination of viral or fungal infections, or severe reactions to immunization procedures). Steroid therapy may completely suppress Type IV lymphocyte-mediated hypersensitivity reactions, thereby causing prior positive skin tests to mycobacterial and fungal antigens to become negative. During the course of therapy, underlying quiescent infection with granulomatous infectious diseases, such as tuberculosis, may flare up in an insidious fashion.

Steroid Dependency. A dubious benefit of glucocorticoid therapy is that not only do patients obtain symptomatic and pathologic improvement of the disease being treated, but they also experience a steroid-induced sense of well being and euphoria, often associated with a disappearance of minor aches and pains. Thus, when the physician attempts to reduce the dose of the drug, not only may the original disease undergo a recrudescence, but the patient may lose the sense of physical and mental well being and may develop withdrawal symptoms such as anorexia, nausea, lethargy, headache, fever, weight loss and hypotension; many patients experience myalgias, stiffness and joint pains ("pseudorheumatism"). This withdrawal syndrome (Table 7–4A) may appear after a very brief course of steroids, and has even occurred after a single moderately large dose of prednisolone.[24] For these reasons, once a course of steroids is embarked upon, it often becomes difficult to wean the patient from the drugs—and a state akin to addiction appears. The steroid withdrawal syndrome has not been fully explained.[24]

The problem of dependency has a further dimension. The patient's own adrenals lose their normal capability of responding to a stressful situation by increasing corticosteroid output. Therefore, if the steroid-dependent patient is faced with the stress of intercurrent illness, trauma or an operation, the administered dose will have to be increased to compensate for the iatrogenic adrenal gland suppression. This need for additional drug coverage in times of stress can persist for several months after a prolonged course of steroid therapy has been discontinued. If steroid therapy is discontinued in a dependent patient, serious adrenal insufficiency may develop. This condition mimics Addison's disease, secondary to pathologic destruction of the adrenal gland. The patient becomes weak and debilitated, with low blood pressure and marked susceptibility to stress. An intercurrent illness may precipitate an addisonian crisis, in which the steroid deficient patient may go into a potentially fatal shock-like state.

It is possible that periodic administration of the pituitary hormone, adrenocorticotropic hormone (ACTH), may stimulate the adrenal glands and prevent the development of disuse atrophy of these glands. However, ACTH therapy will exacerbate the suppression of the pituitary gland, which is a major iatrogenic problem in the steroid-dependent patient, and current thinking generally opposes the use of ACTH.

Pregnant women who require glucocorticoid therapy should not be deprived of these drugs, but it must be recognized that the safety of such therapy has not been completely demonstrated. It is advisable to try to avoid steroids during the first trimester, although there is no proof that teratogenic problems are likely. If steroids are given to a pregnant woman, the new-born child should be watched for several months for any evidence of hypoadrenalism.

PHARMACOLOGY OF GLUCOCORTICOSTEROIDS

The adrenal glands produce, under basal conditions, 15 to 30 mg of corticosteroids a day, of which 10 to 25 mg is hydrocortisone (cortisol). Normal diurnal secretion increases during sleep; in the average person there is maximal output between 4 A.M. and 8 A.M. The secretion of steroids by the adrenal glands is controlled by ACTH, which is released by the anterior lobe of the pituitary gland; there is a constant biofeedback mechanism whereby ACTH release is diminished by the rising level of cortisol in the blood. Severe stress stimulates the pituitary axis and results in increased ACTH secretion. The normal diurnal decrease in cortisol secretion during sleep cannot be correlated with the common experience that asthma attacks often develop during the night; nocturnal steroid therapy is not advocated for this problem.[26]

In addition to glucocorticoids, the adrenal gland also secretes mineralocorticoids and other steroid hormones that affect sexual function. The so-called glucocorticoids do have a minor degree of mineralocorticoid activity, and can produce some retention of sodium, which may, in susceptible patients, result in the development of edema and hypertension. However, edema does not usually appear when cortisol or synthetic glucocorticoids are given therapeutically, since these (with the exception of cortisone) tend to increase free water clearance.[27]

The synthetic glucocorticoids offer greater antiinflammatory potency with diminished mineralocorticoid activity. A major advance has been the synthesis of agents that offer potent local effectiveness with minimal systemic absorption, suitable for selective topical therapy. However, the synthetic preparations not only have many of the same therapeutic effects of the natural glucocorticoids, but they also have the same propensity to cause most of the adverse effects that characterize Cushing's syndrome when they are given in large enough dosage.

The natural glucocorticoids can be given orally, intravenously and topically. When given by inhalation therapy they are well absorbed by the respiratory mucosa and, therefore, systemic effects can follow topical administration. This makes the natural steroids, hydrocortisone and cortisone, unsuitable for aerosol therapy.

The biologic potency of different steroid preparations correlates to some extent with the plasma half-life of each agent. However, the half-lives vary from half an hour (cortisone) to over five hours (dexamethasone),[8a] whereas the biologic effect lasts as long as two and a half days. The plasma half-life is determined mainly by the rate of metabolic degradation of the steroid, which occurs mainly in the liver, whereas the biologic effect is related to the intracellular activity of the hormone in various target tissues. The most significant target organ is the pituitary gland; reports on biologic half-lives are usually based on the duration of suppression of hypothalamic-pituitary activity (for example, endogenous ACTH secretion).[3] It is of interest that the half-lives of prednisolone, methylprednisolone, dexamethasone and triamcinolone are markedly affected by the dose employed and by other less well-defined factors.[3] The increased half-lives of synthetic steroids can be correlated with differences in plasma protein binding, tissue binding and metabolism by liver enzymes.[1]

Certain drugs have a marked effect on glucocorticoid metabolism (Table 7–5). Barbiturates induce liver microsomal hydrolysing enzymes that potentiate prednisolone and dexamethasone metabolism;[28] thus, steroid dosages may have to be increased when these other drugs are administered concurrently. This can be a problem, since many oral combination products used in bronchodilator therapy contain phenobarbital. Another commonly used drug, phenytoin (diphenylhydantoin, Dilantin), used in the management of seizures, has a similar potentiating effect on the hepatic metabolism of glucocorticoids;[29] phenytoin also increases the rate of biliary and renal excretion of dexamethasone.[30] Barbiturates and phenytoin are often used together in the management of epilepsy; thus, the epileptic asthmat-ic patient can present a difficult therapeutic challenge. Other tranquillizers (such as diazepam, nitrazepam and hydroxyzine) may have an effect on steroid metabolism, since they have been shown to decrease plasma cortisol titers. High dose salicylate therapy may also potentiate glucocorticoid activity by displacing the steroids from albumin binding sites.[31]

In contrast, certain drugs potentiate steroid activity; the macrolide antibiotics (such as erythromycin) have a particularly marked effect.[32] There is evidence that parabens, which are used as preservatives in pharmaceutic solutions of various drugs, including steroid preparations, may have a bronchodilator effect, thereby serving to potentiate the glucocorticoid products marketed in such solutions.[33] Both propyl and methyl paraben can inhibit phosphodiesterase; this has been suggested as a mechanism by which these agents could potentiate corticosteroids.

The natural corticosteroids are transported in the plasma by albumin and also by a specific alpha globulin known as *transcortin* or *corticosteroid binding globulin* (CBG). Exogenous steroids, such as prednisone, may displace endogenous cortisol from the CBG binding sites, and thereby increase the availability of the hormone to the tissues; by this means, small doses of prednisone may have a surprisingly marked effect on disease processes. Although about 80 per cent of the circulating cortisol is bound to CBG, most exogenous steroids, such as dexamethasone, are not so bound, and rapidly diffuse into the

TABLE 7–5. FACTORS INFLUENCING GLUCOCORTICOID EFFECTIVENESS

Factor	Potentiates Effect	Decreases Effect	Mechanism
Phenytoin		+	
Barbiturates		+	Induce microsomal enzymes that
Other tranquillizers (?)		+	increase steroid catabolism
Ephedrine		+ (dexamethasone)	
Erythromycin	+		Decreases steroid catabolism (?)
Parabens	+ (increase anti-asthma effect)		Inhibit phosphodiesterase
Low serum albumin	+		Decreases binding of steroid; leaves more steroid available
High dose salicylate	+		Binds with albumin, and may displace steroid
Liver disease		+ (prednisone)	Prednisone must be converted by the liver to the active derivative prednisolone

tissues;[3, 6] thus, small doses are more effective than equal doses of cortisol. In patients with hypoalbuminemia, less hydrocortisone is bound to serum albumin; therefore, a relatively high proportion is available to the tissues. For this reason, patients with a low serum albumin more readily develop toxic side effects from prednisone therapy.

USE OF GLUCOCORTICOIDS

The corticosteroids are powerful and valuable therapeutic drugs, with potent, dangerous, and sometimes long-lasting side effects.[34] They should be administered only when simpler and less dangerous forms of therapy have failed; courses should be designed to last as short a time as possible. The minimal effective dosage should be used, and once the disease state is under control an attempt should then be made to wean the patient from the drug. Fortunately, many side effects are reversible if the dosage can be substantially reduced, or steroid therapy discontinued. Impaired renal function does not increase the incidence of steroid toxicity, but in hepatic insufficiency the half-life of prednisolone is increased and administration of the standard dosages of prednisone or prednisolone to cirrhotics results in an increased frequency of side effects. Thus, multiple problems may occur in liver disease: conversion of prednisone to

prednisolone is impaired, the decreased serum albumin (a common consequence of cirrhosis) results in decreased binding of hydrocortisone and prednisolone, and there is a decreased rate of metabolic breakdown of glucocorticoids.

If long term therapy is required, it is important to follow certain rules (see Table 7–6):

(1) Minimal dosages should be established, and a marked increase in the dose should be made promptly to cover an exacerbation or intercurrent stress situation.

(2) Frequent attempts should be made to wean the patient from steroids, using various alternative drugs, such as cromolyn in allergic asthmatics. If steroid therapy has been given more than 10 to 14 days, the drug must be tapered, and not withdrawn abruptly. The process of weaning always needs to be carried out carefully and patiently; it may require weeks or months in some patients.

(3) In allergic patients, an ongoing effort should be made to eliminate the allergen or to control the hypersensitive state. Thus, hyposensitization therapy may be useful in the few situations in which a clear-cut allergy cannot be controlled by other means.

(4) Total control of a disease should not necessarily be aimed for with steroid therapy; careful judgment is always needed to balance an acceptable persistence of symptoms against the development of tolerable

TABLE 7–6. HOW TO MINIMIZE SIDE EFFECTS AND COMPLICATIONS OF GLUCOCORTICOID THERAPY

Follow These Rules	
Use minimal dose*	Never rely on steroids alone to control disease
Increase dose to cover stress	Do not withdraw steroids rapidly
Continually attempt to wean patient off steroids	Do not allow patient to increase dosage irresponsibly
Administer daily single dose of steroid at breakfast	Caution patient not to take the dose of steroid at bedtime
Try to use alternate day dosage regimen	Caution patient not to use a haphazard dosage regimen
Use aerosol therapy for asthma	Do not use steroids in combination preparations
Control weight gain by dietary regulation	Do not permit liberal use of salt in patient's diet
Give antacids and dietary advice if patient is susceptible to peptic ulcer	There is no need for routine antacid therapy in average patient
Try to use most suitable and least expensive steroid preparation	Do not use steroids with marked mineralocorticoid effect, particularly if patient has heart, kidney or liver disease, or has hypertension, obesity or edema
Carry out routine medical check-ups	Do not allow patients to go for long periods without medical supervision
Be alert to the development of masked infections	Do not vaccinate against smallpox, and defer other immunizations; consider use of isoniazid in patients with positive PPD.

*Side effects are minimal if the daily dose of steroid is less than 25 mg hydrocortisone or 6 mg prednisone (or the equivalent amount of another agent).

complications that can also be accepted. Certainly the asthmatic patient should not rely on steroids alone to control bronchospasm; the physician should ensure that a complete regimen of other bronchodilator drugs is maintained.

(5) Single oral morning doses should be given in most situations requiring chronic administration, so as to minimize the suppression of the pituitary diurnal rhythm, thereby resulting in minimal disturbance of the hypothalamic-pituitary-adrenal (HPA) axis. However, this approach does not reduce the risk of producing cushingism.

(6) Alternate day therapy should be tried when feasible, particularly in growing children with relatively stable disease.

(7) Topical preparations should be used when possible, such as suitable aerosol steroids for the treatment of asthma and, perhaps, other hypersensitivity respiratory tract disorders.

(8) Different steroid preparations exist; the appropriate preparation should be used when a clear advantage can be discerned. In particular, preparations with a pronounced mineralocorticoid effect may need to be avoided, since these drugs result in sodium retention; thus, they can cause electrolyte and fluid balance problems and can increase underlying hypertension.

(9) Dietary control is needed if a patient develops indigestion or is susceptible to weight problems. Although there is no definite proof that steroid therapy results in a serious ulcerogenic hazard, most physicians tend to give routine antacid therapy. This is clearly not a necessity in the average patient. Patients should be advised to take their steroids after meals if peptic symptoms occur. All patients should receive advice regarding diet in order to forestall the gain in weight that usually occcurs with steroid therapy as a result of appetite stimulation.

(10) The patient should be kept under ongoing observation to ensure early detection and control of complications. Diseases such as diabetes usually require additional efforts to control them when the patient is on steroid therapy.

(11) Since steroid therapy causes a decrease in circulating eosinophils, periodic eosinophil counts can be used as an objective means of monitoring the adequacy of therapy. In acute asthma, a marked fall in the eosinophil count should occur within eight hours of initiating steroid therapy; if this does not happen, an increase in the dosage of the drug should be considered.

(12) Patients who have a positive PPD skin test when chronic steroid therapy is instituted may be at increased risk of developing overt tuberculosis. However, this risk may have been exaggerated, and recent work shows that asthmatics do not appear to be at significant risk unless they have had active tuberculosis previously or unless the chest x-ray shows evidence of tuberculous activity.[34a, 34b] Patients at particular risk of reactivation can be given a daily prophylactic dose of isoniazid (INH) while on steroid therapy. It should be noted that individuals over the age of 35, and those who are alcoholics or who have liver disease, are at greater risk of developing INH-induced hepatitis, and this risk of prophylactic therapy has to be taken into consideration in each individual patient.

(13) Patients with chronic liver disease associated with hypoalbuminemia may require smaller amounts of maintenance steroid dosage than usual. Hypoalbuminemia in the absence of hepatic insufficiency does not require this adjustment in dosage. It is probably advisable to use prednisolone rather than prednisone in patients who have hepatic insufficiency, and lower dosages than usual may be appropriate.

(14) Patients who require barbiturate or diphenylhydantoin therapy may require increased amounts of glucocorticoid for maintenance therapy.

(15) The primary physician must be aware of the possiblities for the development of insidious and serious complications of steroid therapy that affect organs for which the physician has inadequate special knowledge, such as the eye. It is, therefore, important to refer a patient for consultation to a specialist as soon as suspicious symptoms or findings appear on routine follow-up. This consideration further emphasizes the complexity of management entailed in chronic steroid therapy and provides an additional reason for avoiding this form of therapy if possible.

(16) Once a patient has completed a prolonged course of steroid therapy, the physician must remain aware of the necessity for careful evaluation of any illness that the patient develops during the following year, since a state of steroid dependency may be resurrected as a result of stress. Stressful events such as major surgery require coverage by steroid therapy to forestall the steroid withdrawal syndrome that is a consequence of persisting HPA axis depression. Any patient who has received the

TABLE 7–7. CONTRAINDICATIONS TO STEROID THERAPY*

Major Contraindications	Other Contraindications
In children	Responsiveness to less dangerous drugs
Uncontrolled peptic ulcer disease	Unreliability of patient
Generalized osteoporosis	Inadequate supervision
Psychosis	Adverse response to prior steroid trial
Severe diabetes mellitus	Obesity
Susceptibility to infections	Chronic infections
Glaucoma, cataract	

*Glucocorticoids should be avoided, if possible, in patients with these contraindications. If steroid is deemed necessary, minimal dosage, alternate-day therapy or aerosol administration should be preferred to routine daily oral therapy.

equivalent of 20 to 30 mg of prednisone a day for more than a week, or lesser doses for more than a month, may require steroid coverage for stressful events during the year after the steroid course has terminated. In selected cases, it is advisable to perform various tests that evaluate pituitary function to determine whether the HPA axis has recovered; if the tests reveal impairment, additional glucocorticoid coverage will be indicated at the time of an intercurrent illness or surgical event.

Although there are few absolute contraindications to glucocorticoid therapy, the potential risk in certain patients must be taken into account (Table 7–7). There is a major risk of stunting growth in children, and long-term steroid therapy should be avoided if possible. Patients with underlying problems such as active peptic ulceration, osteoporosis or psychosis may suffer deterioration in these states when given steroids. Diabetes is more difficult to manage when the patient is on glucocorticoids; subjects troubled by recurrent infections or those with glaucoma or cataracts may suffer exacerbations of these problems. Corticosteroid therapy should be avoided in such cases if adequate control of this dangerous form of treatment cannot be provided, or if less potent drugs can be utilized instead.

GLUCOCORTICOID AGENTS

The important glucocorticoids in therapeutics are already numerous, and additional derivatives continue to be marketed. However, hydrocortisone is still one of the most valuable agents, and all other glucocorticoids should be compared with this prototype drug.

HYDROCORTISONE

Hydrocortisone (cortisol) is the major steroid produced by the adrenal gland (Table 7–8). Normal adult adrenals release 10 to 25 mg of this hormone a day, mainly in the early morning hours. The plasma half-life for elimination is 80 to 115 minutes, although, of course, the physiologic effect persists for about 24 to 36 hours.[24] The normal plasma level varies with a diurnal rhythm between 5 and 30 mcg/100 ml.[3, 35] During stressful circumstances, the amount released may increase tenfold, but the plasma level rarely exceeds 60 mcg/100 ml. In replacement therapy, 25 to 37.5 mg a day is usually required; doses in excess of 75 mg a day may cause electrolyte disturbances.[2] The appropriate dose for suppressive therapy varies with the disease entity; recommended daily dosages vary from about 40 mg to over 4000 mg a day. Patients who have been on steroid therapy seem to have an increased rate of metabolic degradation of hydrocortisone in the liver, and the plasma half-life decreases.[35]

Hydrocortisone (in its basic form as cortisol) is only slightly soluble; more suitable therapeutic products with greater solubility are prepared by forming esters at the 21-hydroxyl position of the molecule (see Fig. 7–7 and Table 7–9). The most soluble forms are *hydrocortisone sodium phosphate* and *hydrocortisone sodium succinate*. These derivatives are favored for parenteral therapy; they have a rapid onset of action and a short duration of action, and are therefore useful for emergency treatment of acute conditions, such as status asthmaticus, and for replacement therapy in acute adrenal insufficiency (for example, in addisonian crisis). Some derivatives are particularly useful for oral use; these include *hydrocortisone cypionate,* which is not very soluble, but is administered as a suspension that is more palatable and is

TABLE 7–8. HYDROCORTISONE (CORTISOL)

Main steroid hormone produced by adrenal cortex
Normal daily production is 10–25 mg
Normal plasma level varies between 5 and 30 mcg/100 ml
Dosage required for replacement therapy in adrenal insufficiency: 25–37.5 mg a day
Dosages for maintenance suppressive therapy usually vary between 40 mg and about 100 mg a day; sometimes larger doses are advocated
Dosage for status asthmaticus: 4 mg/kg, then 1 mg/kg q1h. Average daily dose for adults is less than 2 gm (but up to 4 gm may be needed)

TABLE 7–9. HYDROCORTISONE

Derivative	Brand Name	Tablets (mg)			Oral Suspensions	Injections
		5	10	20		
Hydrocortisone	USP products	+	+	+		25 mg/ml, 50 mg/ml (I.M.)
	Cortef	+	+	+		25 mg/ml (I.M.)
	Hydrocortone		+	+		
Hydrocortisone cypionate	Cortef Fluid				10 mg/5 ml	
Hydrocortisone sodium phosphate	USP products					50 mg/ml (I.M., S.C., I.V.)
	Hydrocortone Phosphate					50 mg/ml (I.M., S.C., I.V.)
Hydrocortisone sodium succinate	Solu-Cortef					100 mg, 250 mg, 500 mg and 1000 mg vials (I.V., I.M.)

I.M. = intramuscular; S.C. = subcutaneous; I.V. = intravenous

Note: *Hydrocortisone acetate* and *Hydrocortisone butylacetate* are available as intramuscular, intraarticular and ophthalmic preparations for local therapy.

more slowly absorbed than hydrocortisone.

Hydrocortisone has been given by inhalation in the treatment of asthma in the form of *hydrocortisone acetate*, which is less soluble than hydrocortisone, and is poorly absorbed; these qualities make it suitable for topical therapy, and the preparation is mostly used for dermatologic application and for intra-articular injection. Nebulization of a powder preparation of 15 mg of the acetate three times a day has been found to be of value in controlling chronic asthma.[36, 37] However, much of the nebulized aerosol is deposited in the oropharynx, and is then swallowed and absorbed; some absorption will also occur through the respiratory mucosa. It has been found that systemic side effects can be produced following prolonged use of the aerosol form when the drug is given in sufficient quantity to control asthma.[20] Since hydrocortisone and its esters do not offer proven advantages when given by nebulization, this form of administration is rarely used, and cannot be recommended.

CORTISONE

Although cortisone was the first natural adrenocorticosteroid to be used therapeutically, it is relatively rarely used at present. Cortisone develops glucocorticoid activity only after it is metabolized: the keto group at carbon atom 11 is converted in the body to an alcohol group, as occurs in hydrocortisone (Table 7–10). This conversion occurs fairly rapidly and therefore cortisone has a shorter half-life in the plasma than does hydrocortisone, 30 minutes ver-

sus about 90 minutes (see Table 7–10). The conversion occurs mainly in the liver, but can occur in other tissues. Cortisone has 25 per cent less glucocorticoid potency than does hydrocortisone and has pronounced mineralocorticoid properties. Its main therapeutic value is in replacement therapy for patients with adrenal insufficiency, in which the combination of glucocorticoid and mineralocorticoid properties is required.

Cortisone is insoluble in water, and for use in therapeutics the *acetate ester* has been prepared by substitution at the 21 carbon atom. Cortisone acetate is not only more soluble, but also has greater stability and prolonged activity. The drug has been used orally and systemically in the treatment of pulmonary diseases,[14] but it offers no therapeutic advantages, and causes more severe side effects than do the newer steroids. Aerosolized cortisone does not appear to have been used in the treatment of asthma. Since cortisone must first be converted to hydrocortisone, and this change occurs mainly in the liver, there is no rationale for giving cortisone by the inhalational route.

At present, there are few therapeutic situations when cortisone is the preferred drug, apart from some cases of Addison's disease or acute adrenal insufficiency. If an asthmatic patient has been on long-term corticosteroid therapy that is stopped because of improvement, a new stressful situation (such as a sudden severe asthma attack) may provoke an acute addisonian crisis; in these circumstances, the combined gluco-

TABLE 7–10.   THE ANTIINFLAMMATORY GLUCOCORTICOIDS

Drug	Relative Gluco-corticoid Potency	Equivalent Oral Dose (mg)	Relative Mineralo-corticoid Potency	Serum Half Life (minutes)	Physiologic* Half Life (days)	Important Substituents in Steroid Molecule
SHORT-ACTING						
Cortisone	0.8	25	0.8	30	$<\frac{1}{2}$	$C_{11}{=}O$
Hydrocortisone (Cortisol)	1	20	1	80–115	$<\frac{1}{2}$	$C_{11}{-}OH$
INTERMEDIATE-ACTING						
Prednisone	3.5	5	0.8	60	$\frac{1}{2}$–$1\frac{1}{2}$	$C_{11}{=}O;\ C_1{=}C_2$
Prednisolone	4	5	0.8	115–252	$\frac{1}{2}$–$1\frac{1}{2}$	$C_{11}{-}OH;\ C_1{=}C_2$
Methylprednisolone	5	4	0–0.5	78– 188+	$\frac{1}{2}$–$1\frac{1}{2}$	$C_{11}{-}OH;\ C_1{=}C_2;\ C_6{-}CH_3$
Triamcinolone	5	4	0	200+	$\frac{1}{2}$–2	$C_{11}{-}OH;\ C_1{=}C_2;\ C_9{-}F;\ C_{16\alpha}{-}OH$
LONG-ACTING						
Dexamethasone	25–40	0.75	0	110–300+	$1\frac{1}{2}$–2+	$C_{11}{-}OH;\ C_1{=}C_2;\ C_{9\alpha}{=}F;\ C_{16\alpha}{=}CH_3$
Betamethasone	25–30	0.60	0	300+	$1\frac{1}{2}$–2+	$C_{11}{-}OH;\ C_1{=}C_2;\ C_{9\alpha}{=}F;\ C_{16\beta}{=}CH_3$
Beclomethasone			0	?	$1\frac{1}{2}$–2+	$C_{11}{-}OH;\ C_1{=}C_2;\ C_{9\alpha}{=}Cl;\ C_{16\beta}{=}CH_3$

*The physiologic half-life is an indication of the persistence of the biologic effect of the glucocorticoid on the tissues.

corticoid and mineralocorticoid properties of cortisone make this drug particularly suitable for the initial treatment of the patient.

PREDNISOLONE

Prednisolone is a synthetic derivative that differs from hydrocortisone in having a double bond between carbon atoms 1 and 2 (see Fig. 7–1). This alteration does not affect the mineralocorticoid properties, but enhances glucocorticoid potency fourfold. For these reasons, prednisolone is preferable to hydrocortisone for routine management of inflammatory hypersensitivity diseases on a long-term basis, although it is not suitable for replacement therapy in adrenal insufficiency. The half-life of prednisolone is reported to be longer than that of cortisol, in that it ranges from 115 to 252 minutes;[24] the longer half-life may occur in patients who have been on steroid therapy for some time.

Prednisolone is mostly given by the oral route, but it can be applied topically. The highly soluble esters are used in systemic therapy; these include *prednisolone sodium phosphate* and *prednisolone sodium succinate* (Tables 7–11 and 7–12). *Prednisolone sodium acetate* and *prednisolone tebutate* are less soluble, but are suitable for intramuscular and intraarticular injection therapy. The sodium phosphate and acetate esters are also suitable for topical administration. Intravenous prednisolone can be given, but it takes longer to achieve its peak effect than does hydrocortisone;[39] therefore, the latter drug is preferable. Indeed the intravenous preparation of prednisolone is not generally available.

Inhalation therapy with prednisolone can be of benefit in asthma,[38] but it is not recommended, since an effective dosage free of adverse complications cannot readily be achieved.

TABLE 7–11   PREDNISOLONE DERIVATIVES

Drug	Solubility	Use
Prednisolone acetate	Low	Ophthalmic, I.M., intra-articular, soft tissues
Prednisolone butylacetate	Low	Intraarticular, soft tissues
Prednisolone sodium phosphate	High	Ophthalmic, I.V., I.M.
Prednisolone sodium succinate	High	I.V., I.M.
Prednisolone tebutate	Low	Intraarticular, soft tissues

TABLE 7–12. REPRESENTATIVE PREDNISOLONE PREPARATIONS*

Brand Names	Tablets (mg)			Injections (mg/ml)					Route
	1	2.5	5	20	25	40	50	100	
PREDNISOLONE									Oral
Delta-Cortef			+						
Fernisolone-P			+						
Prednis			+						
Predoxine			+						
Ropredlone	+		+						
Sterane			+						
USP preparations	+	+	+						
PREDNISOLONE ACETATE									I.M. only
Durapred								+	
Fernisolone					+				
Meticortelone					+				
Predcor					+	+			
Ropredlone					+	+	+		
Savacort					+	+	+		
Sterane					+				
USP preparations					+		+	+	
PREDNISOLONE NA PHOSPHATE									I.M. or I.V.
Hydeltrasol				+					
PSP				+					
Savacort				+		+			
Sodasone				+					
PREDNISOLONE NA SUCCINATE									I.M. or I.V.
Meticortelone							+		

*Additional brand name preparations are marketed. Combinations of prednisolone acetate and prednisolone sodium phosphate (2:1) are available for I.M. injection.

PREDNISONE

The most popular oral glucocorticoid is prednisone (Table 7–13). This synthetic derivative has a structure similar to that of cortisone, but prednisone has a double bond between carbon atoms 1 and 2 (Fig. 7–1). Thus, the relationship of prednisone to cortisone is comparable to the relationship between prednisolone and hydrocortisone. Prednisone is very similar to prednisolone; however, prednisone must be metabolized to prednisolone before it becomes biologically active. Normally, this conversion occurs very rapidly in the liver;

TABLE 7–13. PREDNISONE

Standard oral glucocorticoid
Available only in tablet form*
Well absorbed when given by mouth
Inexpensive and reliable preparations available
Usual dosage range: 5–80 mg/day (adults and children)
Exceptional (unproven value) doses range up to 250 mg/day
Converted to prednisolone by liver
Reduced dosage advisable in hepatic insufficiency with hypoalbuminemia

*Pediatric suspension can be prepared by pharmacists.

prednisone, therefore, has a shorter plasma half-life (60 minutes) than prednisolone, and it is slower in onset of action.[24] Prednisone effectiveness may be markedly decreased in patients with hepatic disease, and, in such circumstances, prednisolone is a more suitable drug. It is of interest that hepatic conversion of prednisone to prednisolone occurs with much greater efficiency than does the conversion of cortisone to cortisol.[40]

Prednisone is usually given by oral administration, and it is less suited for administration by any other route. It is not made available as salts or esters, and is currently available only as tablets. Although the drug has probably been given by aerosol, there are no reports to support this practice.[41] On the other hand, there is little to suggest that any other steroid preparation is better than oral prednisone for the acute or chronic management of most respiratory diseases that require glucocorticoid suppressive therapy, and prednisone (or perhaps even better, prednisolone) is recommended for routine oral therapy unless large doses are needed, when a drug with less mineralocorticoid activity is preferable.[31] About 70 different companies make prednisone tablets, and some are inferior. Meticorten is consis-

TABLE 7–14. PREDNISONE PREPARATIONS

Brand Name	Tablets (mg) 1	2.5	5	10	20	50
Delta-Dome			+			
Deltasone		+	+	+	+	+
Fernisone			+			
Keysone			+			
Lisacort			+			
Maso-Pred			+			
Meticorten	+		+			
Orasone	+		+	+	+	
Paracort			+			
Pred-5			+			
Prednicen-M			+			
Prednisone		+	+	+	+	
Ropred	+	+	+		+	
Servisone			+			
SK-Prednisone			+			
Sterapred			+			
USP preparations	+	+	+	+	+	

tently reliable and is relatively inexpensive;[42] Deltasone and Orasone have also been documented to provide reliable bioavailability (see Table 7–14).

Meprednisone is similar to prednisone, but has a methyl substituent in the 16β position. It is alleged to cause less salt and water retention. However, there appears to be relatively little experience in the use of this agent, which is rarely employed in clinical practice.

METHYLPREDNISOLONE

The addition of a CH_3-group to carbon atom 6 of prednisolone results in the synthetic product methylprednisolone (Fig. 7–1 and Table 7–10). This derivative offers greater glucocorticoid potency than prednisone. Different authorities list methylprednisolone as having from 0 to 50 per cent of the mineralocorticoid effect of prednisone, and the evidence suggests that it has very little effect on electrolyte balance. The half-life of this derivative varies according to the dose given, and investigators have reported it to range between 78 and 188 minutes.[24] The drug has an effect that lasts up to 36 hours. For routine therapy in nonacute situations, methylprednisolone offers no pharmacologic advantages; moreover, the oral preparation is comparatively expensive. The *21-succinate ester* is very soluble and is claimed to be particularly suitable for intravenous administration in emergencies because of its rapid onset of action. Since this parenteral product is comparable in price to hydrocortisone, and causes less electrolyte disturbance, it may be more suitable than hydrocortisone for high dose intravenous therapy. The *acetate ester* also has a rapid onset, and it has a longer duration of effect; it is mainly used as an intramuscular depot preparation for treatment of musculoskeletal problems, but 80 mg injections every two weeks have been reported to successfully control severe hay fever.[31] No insoluble topical derivative has been prepared, such as could be of value in topical aerosol therapy; therefore, methylprednisolone cannot be recommended for inhalation. Available products are listed in Table 7–15.

Methylprednisolone sodium succinate has acquired the reputation of possessing special properties suited to the emergency management of serious diseases, such as status asthmaticus, aspiration pneumonia, and adult respiratory distress syndrome. However, there is, in fact, little convincing evidence to support the specific use of this agent in these clinical situations; indeed, further proof is needed before methylprednisolone can be recommended as the steroid of choice in any disease. It may be a useful agent for initial intravenous treat-

TABLE 7–15. METHYLPREDNISOLONE PREPARATIONS

Derivative	Brand Name	Tablets or Capsules (mg) 2*	4*	16	Injections I.M.† (mg/ml) 20	40	80	I.V. or I.M. (mg/vial) 40	125	500	1000
Methylprednisolone	Medrol	+	+	+							
Methylprednisolone acetate	Depo-Medrol				+	+	+				
	D-Med					+	+				
	Medralone					+	+				
	Pre-Dep					+	+				
Methylprednisolone sodium succinate	A-Methapred							+	+	+	+
	Solu-Medrol							+	+	+	+

I.M. = intramuscular; I.V. = intravenous
*Sustained release capsules, as well as rapidly absorbed tablets, are available (as Medules).
†The intramuscular product is probably suitable only for local tissue effect.

ment of extremely ill patients who require a glucocorticoid with relatively little mineralocorticoid activity. A major difficulty with this drug is that clear dosage guidelines have not yet been established. Some of the proponents of intravenous methylprednisolone have suggested that the sodium succinate component of this preparation of the drug has a specific value in that it "stabilizes" the molecule. Wilson[43] has proposed that methylprednisolone sodium succinate has substantially different properties from other available steroid preparations which endow the drug with enhanced effectiveness in the prevention and treatment of pulmonary cellular damage. In spite of similar claims from other workers, there is no adequate proof that the drug offers a unique advantage in the therapy of lung disease in the human. Furthermore, there is still insufficient evidence on which to base the often made claim that huge "pharmacologic" doses of intravenous methylprednisolone (or, indeed, other glucocorticoids) are required in the treatment of various emergencies, such as status asthmaticus and the many types of the adult respiratory distress syndrome.[23, 44]

TRIAMCINOLONE

Triamcinolone contains a fluorine atom at carbon atom 9, and a hydroxyl group at 16; it is a fluorinated, hydroxylated derivative of prednisolone (Figure 7–3). These substitutions result in a glucocorticoid that is both more selective (because of the hydroxyl group) and more potent (because of the fluorine atom). The drug is a potent antiinflammatory steroid with little mineralocorticoid effect and is very similar to methylprednisolone. Triamcinolone is said to result in less weight gain than other steroid preparations; indeed, it tends to cause a sodium and water diuresis, and it may cause some anorexia, whereas most other glucocorticoids stimulate the appetite.[27] Thus, a patient may actually lose weight when taking this drug. On the other hand, triamcinolone has a catabolic effect on muscle, and may cause myopathy and weakness with chronic administration. It is also said that triamcinolone can cause mental depression.[2] The action of triamcinolone persists for about 48 hours after a single dose, and it is therefore classified as intermediate-acting (Table 7–10). For this reason it is unsuited for alternate-day therapy.

The acetonide esters of the fluorinated steroids demonstrate a remarkably enhanced topical activity.[45] Thus, *triamcinolone acetonide* is a poorly soluble, highly potent, moderately long-acting, antiinflammatory drug that is particularly suited for intraarticular, intralesional and dermatologic topical therapy. Triamcinolone, as tablets, and *triamcinolone diacetate* (as a syrup or suspension) are suitable for oral therapy; the acetonide and diacetate can be given by the intramuscular route. The poorly soluble *triamcinolone hexacetonide* is suited only for intraarticular and intralesional administration.

Since triamcinolone acetonide is so potent when given topically, and since it is not readily absorbed, the drug is found to be relatively free of systemic side effects when used in therapeutic amounts in dermatologic therapy. Favorable experiences with this derivative in the topical treatment of skin diseases prompted trials of aerosols of the drug in the treatment of steroid-dependent asthmatics.[46–49] Investigators used fine suspensions of triamcinolone acetonide which were made available in metered dispensers, each activation of which apparently delivered 50–150 mcg of powdered aerosol of particle size 1 to 5μ; it is claimed that approximately half of the dose was delivered into the patient's respiratory tract.[48] The results appeared to be very impressive. Most patients were able to reduce oral steroid therapy, since the aerosol effectively controlled the asthma. Those patients who were cushingoid on oral therapy lost these adverse complications while maintained on the aerosol over the course of many months. The appropriate amount is 0.15 to 2.0 mg in four divided doses; doses up to 3.6 mg per day by aerosol have been given for two weeks without any adverse effect on endogenous corticosteroid levels.[49] The average dosage required to control asthma in adults in one investigation was found to be 4 puffs four times a day, that is, about 0.8 mg of triamcinolone acetonide.[48] The main problem with the aerosol is that some patients develop hoarseness and weakness of the voice,[47] but this does not appear to have been a major complication, and it could possibly be prevented by gargling after each treatment. Vocal changes do not appear to have arisen with the use of other aerosolized steroids, and it is possible that the weakness of the voice is caused by laryngeal muscle myopathy, which could be comparable to the skel-

STRUCTURAL FORMULAE OF LONGER-ACTING GLUCOCORTICOIDS

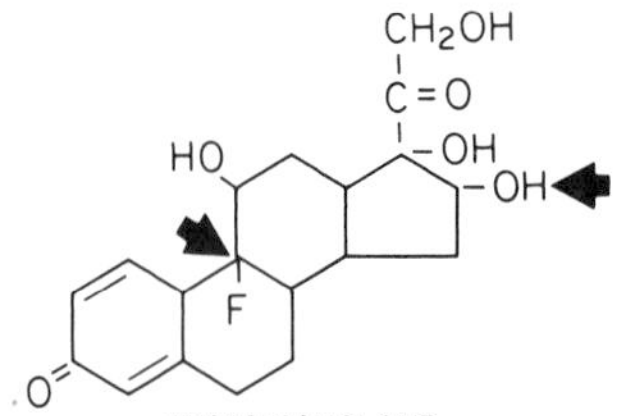

TRIAMCINOLONE
(9 α-fluoro, 16β-hydroxy, prednisolone)

Related to prednisolone; additional groups are an F (fluorine) at 9α, and an -OH (hydroxyl) at 16β

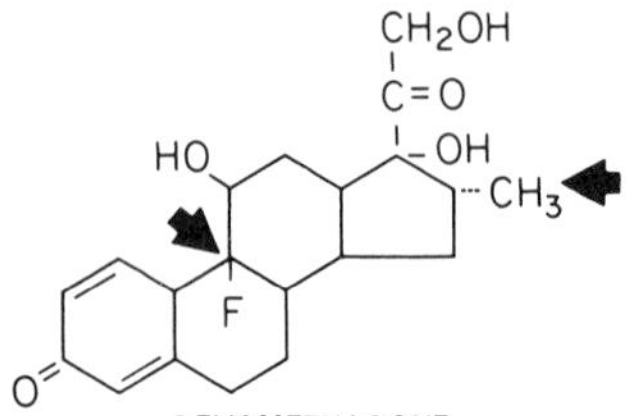

DEXAMETHASONE
(9 α-fluoro, 16 α-methyl, prednisolone)

Related to prednisolone; additional groups are an F (fluorine) at 9α, and a CH_3 (methyl) at 16β

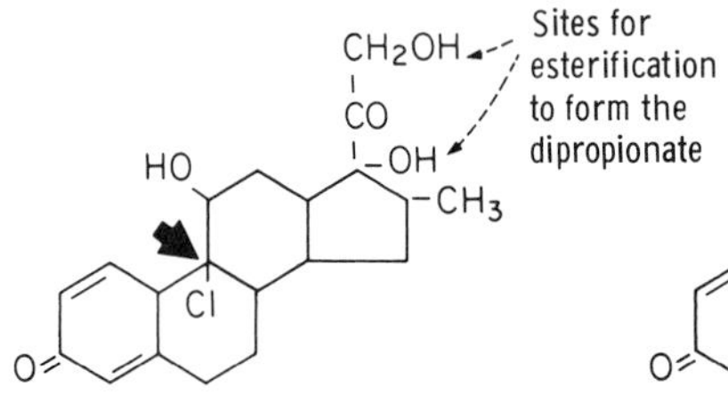

BECLOMETHASONE
(9α-chloro, 16β-methyl, prednisolone)

Differs from betamethasone in that there is a Cl (chlorine) atom at 9 rather than an F (fluorine) atom

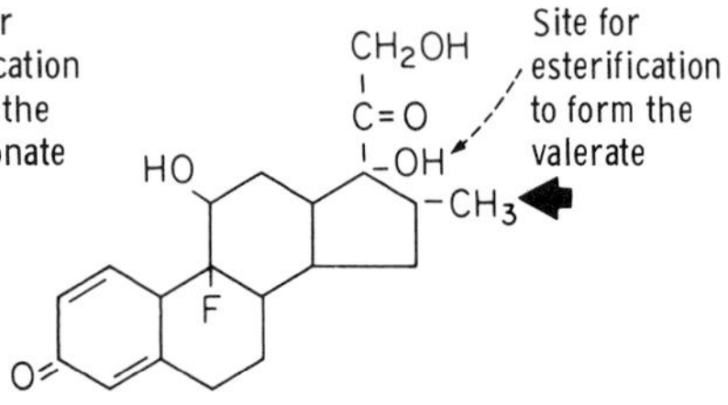

BETAMETHASONE
(9 α-fluoro, 16β-methyl, prednisolone)

Differs from dexamethasone in that the methyl group at 16 is in the β configuration rather than α

Figure 7–3.

etal muscle myopathy arising in patients receiving systemic triamcinolone. However, this is entirely speculative. Oropharyngeal candidiasis occurs in up to 50 per cent of patients, but the problem is usually a transient one and does not necessitate discontinuance of the triamcinolone aerosol; furthermore, sore throat and hoarseness are not correlated with the development of candidiasis.[49a]

Triamcinolone acetonide is currently available as an aqueous suspension for injection into joints and soft tissue (Table 7–16), but this product is not approved for use as a respiratory inhalational drug. Since it is not a true solution, there may be some

TABLE 7–16. TRIAMCINOLONE PREPARATIONS

Derivative	Brand Name	Tablets (mg) 1	2	4	8	16	Syrup or Suspension	Injectable (I.M. or I.V.)	Topical
Triamcinolone	Aristocort	+	+	+	+	+			
	Kenacort	+	+	+	+				
	Rocinolone			+					
	SK-Triamcinolone		+	+	+				
	Triamcinolone*		+	+	+				
Triamcinolone acetonide†	Kenalog							10 mg/ml, 40 mg/ml (I.M.)	0.025–0.5%
Triamcinolone hexacetonide	Aristospan							5 mg/ml, 20 mg/ml	
Triamcinolone diacetate	Amcort							40 mg/ml	
	Aristocort						2 mg/5 ml		
	Aristocort Forte							40 mg/ml (I.M.)	
	Cenocort Forte							40 mg/ml (I.M.)	
	Kenacort						4 mg/5 ml		
	Triamcinolone*							40 mg/ml (I.M.)	
	Triam-Forte							40 mg/ml	

*The generic product is much less expensive than most brand name products.

†Triamcinolone acetonide has been given by inhalation in the management of asthma, but this is not an approved use. A marketed product (Kenalog) contains sodium chloride, 0.9% benzyl alcohol, 0.75% sodium carboxymethylcellulose, 0.04% polysorbate 80, and NaOH or HCl: however, this formulation is not recommended for nebulization. An approved aerosol form is expected to be marketed.

difficulty in nebulizing this product, and it cannot be recommended unless controlled studies first show it to be effective as an aerosol. If this product (or a more suitable derivative) were to be approved, it could probably be given by IPPB, using a solution of 40 mg/ml; 0.25 ml would then need to be diluted to 10 ml with saline. If 1 ml of this diluted solution (containing about 1 mg of the triamcinolone acetonide) is given by IPPB, about 10 per cent (100 mcg) might be expected to deposit in the lungs. Initially, one treatment a day could be given, while the oral steroid dosage is gradually reduced. If the aerosol does not control symptoms, the same dose could be given more often, up to four times a day. If this is still inadequate, the dose per treatment should slowly be increased up to 5 mg, by making appropriate dilutions. The alternative, and probably easier method, would be for the patient to be given a metered preparation providing 50 mcg (0.05 mg) per puff; the dosage would be up to 10 puffs four times a day.

Clearly, aerosolization of triamcinolone offers considerable promise, since it is possible to maintain asthmatic patients on this drug using only one-tenth the dose required for oral therapy.[48] It is to be hoped that this rational and highly desirable application of aerosol pharmacology will become standard treatment for respiratory patients who require long-term corticosteroid administration. Further work will be needed both to establish which of many potential aerosol preparations is most suitable, and to determine how many treatments a day constitute optimal therapy. However, triamcinolone may not be able to compete against other aerosols that have pre-empted its appearance on the market.

DEXAMETHASONE

The addition of a fluorine atom in the α-position at the 9-carbon atom and a methyl group in the α-position at the 16-carbon atom of prednisolone results in dexamethasone. It differs from triamcinolone only in that it has a 16α methyl group rather than a 16α hydroxyl group (Fig. 7–3). Dexamethasone has very potent antiinflammatory properties, with virtually no mineralocorticoid activity. It is one of the more effective glucocorticoid preparations available, and it has a long-acting effect on tissues, with detectable activity persisting

for longer than 48 hours. The half-life in the plasma ranges between 110 and 210 minutes, similar to the half-life of prednisolone (Table 7–10), thus illustrating that the length of the half-life cannot be correlated with the potency of the drug. Dexamethasone is said to cause relatively more stimulation of appetite, thus leading to greater weight gain than is usual with other steroid preparations.[50] It should be noted that recent studies have shown that dexamethasone may be more potent than is generally believed, since the actions of the glucocorticoids are governed by complex factors that make it difficult to evaluate their actions and their effects with accuracy.[50a]

Dexamethasone, itself, is used orally and topically, but, since it is relatively insoluble in water, it is not suitable for parenteral administration (Table 7–17). *Dexamethasone sodium phosphate* is soluble, and can be given by injection into joints and soft tissues as well as intravenously; it is also suitable for oral and topical administration. The potent topical effect of this preparation has resulted in the drug being utilized as a nasal aerosol spray for the treatment of allergic and inflammatory forms of rhinitis. Dexamethasone sodium phosphate has also been marketed as a metered aerosol for the inhalational treatment of asthma. Several studies have shown that this form of therapy is effective[14] but, as could be predicted from the known solubility of the preparation, systemic absorption occurs.[51, 52] Thus, when the aerosol is given in amounts sufficient to control chronic asthma, glucocorticoid side effects and adrenocortical suppression can develop, and the results appear to be no better than those obtained with oral therapy.[41, 51, 52] For these reasons, dexamethasone sodium phosphate aerosol should not be used for the treatment of asthma, and the metered product on the market should be withdrawn now that more effective and less dangerous corticosteroids are becoming available. Although dexamethasone sodium phosphate has also been given successfully by IPPB[53] (0.25 mg in 1 ml of saline), this practice also cannot be condoned.

European workers have claimed that the insoluble ester *dexamethasone isonicotinate,* which precipitates as relatively poorly absorbed microcrystals, is effective and safe when given by metered aerosol;[54] however, there is evidence that aerosol therapy with this derivative results in HPA axis depression.[55] The overall value of dexa-

TABLE 7–17. REPRESENTATIVE DEXAMETHASONE PREPARATIONS

Derivative	Brand Name	Tablets (mg)					Elixir	Injectable I.M. or I.V.	Inhaler
		0.25	0.5	0.75	1.5	4			
Dexamethasone	Decadron	+	+	+	+	+	0.5 mg/5 ml		
	Deronil			+					
	Dexameth			+					
	Dexamethasone*	+	+	+	+				
	Dexone		+	+	+	+			
	Gammacorten			+					
	Hexadrol		+	+	+	+	0.5 mg/5 ml		
Dexamethasone sodium phosphate	Decadron Phosphate							4 mg/ml (I.M., I.V.)	
	Dexasone							4 mg/ml (I.M., I.V.)	
	Decadron Respihaler†								18 mg/12.6 gm
	Decadron Turbinaire†								18 mg/12.6 gm
	Hexadrol phosphate							4 mg/ml (I.M., I.V.)	
	USP products*							4 mg/ml (I.M., I.V.)	
Dexamethasone acetate	Decadron-LA							8 mg/ml (I.M.)	

*The generic product is much less expensive than most brand name products.
†Inhalation products contain the equivalent of 15 mg dexamethasone base in metered cartridges which weigh 12.6 gm. Each actuation delivers approximately 100 mcg dexamethasone sodium phosphate (84 mcg dexamethasone base). Decadron inhalational products are as follows:
  Respihaler—for asthma. This product is no longer recommended.
  Turbinaire—for nasal use. Dose is 1–2 sprays 2 to 3 times a day.

methasone in asthma is questionable, since there is evidence that it has less potentiating action on the bronchodilator effectiveness of isoproterenol than either hydrocortisone or methylprednisolone.[16, 55a] The fact that dexamethasone is considerably less expensive than other intravenous glucocorticoids may influence physicians to prefer to use this preparation for massive pharmacologic therapy in conditions in which it has been shown to be at least as effective as hydrocortisone or methylprednisolone. It is of interest that ephedrine (but not theophylline) may cause an acceleration in the rate at which dexamethasone is metabolized.[55b]

Paramethasone is a derivative closely related to dexamethasone; the only difference is that the fluorine atom is attached to the 6-carbon atom. It is less potent than dexamethasone, but is otherwise comparable; however, it may be more likely to cause an increase in appetite. This preparation is made available only for oral use; it cannot be recommended.

BECLOMETHASONE

Beclomethasone is one of the newer glucocorticoids that has proved to be very successful as a topical dermatologic agent. The drug is structurally related to prednisolone, and differs in that it contains a chlorine atom at the 9-carbon atom, and a methyl group in the position at the 16-carbon atom. It has a long-acting effect of over 48 hours, as does dexamethasone (Table 7–10). The substitution of dipropionate in the side chain attached to the 17-carbon atom results in *beclomethasone dipropionate*, which is a relatively insoluble, potent, topical glucocorticoid that has been used as an inhalational preparation[20] (see Figure 7–3). It has been marketed for several years in England and elsewhere as a metered aerosol inhaler under the name of Becotide. This steroid drug had not been used, in any form, in the U.S., until it was introduced in 1976 as the metered aerosol preparation Vanceril.[55c]

This preparation has been the source of tremendous interest during the past few years; careful studies since the drug was introduced in England in 1968 have shown that the aerosolization of beclomethasone dipropionate may control chronic asthma without causing side effects or depressing the hypothalamic-pituitary-adrenal axis. The drug is far more suitable than prior inhalational agents such as dexamethasone, since beclomethasone dipropionate has 500 times as much topical antiinflammatory action as hydrocortisone or dexamethasone. Beclomethasone is much less active when given orally, being only about 30 times as effective as oral hydrocortisone, while the dipropionate is less active than dexamethasone when given orally. Since much of an aerosol drug is deposited in the oropharynx and swallowed, the lack of activity of the ingested beclomethasone is an important advantage; apparently, the swallowed beclomethasone dipropionate is absorbed in the gastrointestinal tract, and it is rapidly inactivated by the liver.[56] The lung can also absorb and inactivate the dipropionate; irrespective of the route of absorption, most of the drug and its metabolites are excreted in the feces. Very large doses of inhaled beclomethasone dipropionate can result in sufficient systemic absorption to cause adrenal suppression, but about 4 mg a day is required to produce this undesirable result.[57] In the usual aerosol dose of 400 mcg a day, the endocrinometabolic effects are minimal,[57a] and may amount to a slight disturbance of the glucose tolerance test in patients who had been dependent on oral glucocorticoid therapy.[57b] However, such patients have been effectively treated for many months without significant complications, other than slight candidiasis, or symptoms of pseudorheumatism, or an exacerbation of atopic eczema or associated nasal or sinus allergy; these problems may trouble many patients, but, in general, they tend to diminish with the passage of time.[57a-e]

Numerous recent investigations using aerosolized beclomethasone have demonstrated that the drug can be extremely beneficial in the management of asthma of adults and children.[57b-66a] Moreover, the topical therapy seems to reduce cough and sputum production more effectively than does oral prednisone.[59] Beclomethasone metered aerosol offers several important advantages: (1) A dosage of 50 to 200 mcg four times a day usually controls steroid-dependent asthma. (2) Evidence of hypothalamic-pituitary-adrenal axis depression does not occur with dosages under 1600 mcg a day.[61] (3) Since most patients do well with one or two puffs, each releasing 50 mcg of a microcrystalline suspension, significant systemic side effects are not produced, as the total daily dosage required is generally only 200 to 400 mcg. (4) Most patients who require oral steroids to control asthma can reduce the dosage by 50 per cent or more after starting on aerosolized beclomethasone, and cushingoid side effects and adrenal suppression gradually diminish as the substitution is made.[57e] Some patients improve markedly and have fewer problems with their asthma with beclomethasone than they experience with oral steroid therapy. A daily dosage of 300 to 400 mcg of aerosolized beclomethasone is claimed to be as effective as 7.5 mg of prednisone,[63] which is an oral dose associated with negligible complications. Studies have shown that beclomethasone in a dosage of 100 mcg four times a day provides safe and effective therapy for children with chronic asthma,[66a] but some evidence of adrenal suppression may be produced.[66b] The safety of long-term beclomethasone therapy in children needs further clarification.

Clearly, beclomethasone dipropionate aerosol therapy offers a major advance in the treatment of asthma. The main problem with this drug appears to be the liability of patients to develop oral candidiasis, but the incidence of this complication on the usual daily dosage of 400 mcg has been acceptable to most investigators. Thus, a recent study of 400 patients revealed a 4.5 per cent prevalence of oral thrush;[65] another study suggests that this complication is dose related.[65a] Even if more serious consequences appear following its long term use (such as topical changes in the respiratory tract) it is unlikely that the aerosol could be as harmful as the oral steroid therapy that it is designed to replace. It is regrettable that it takes so long for such a valuable drug, which has proved itself

TABLE 7–18. INHALATIONAL STEROIDS

Drug Preparation	Typical Total Daily Dose For An Adult	Comment
Hydrocortisone sodium succinate	Variable	No longer advocated
Dexamethasone sodium phosphate	400–2,000 mcg	No longer advocated
Dexamethasone isonicotinate	up to 1875 mcg	Investigational
Triamcinolone acetonide	800 mcg	Investigational
Beclomethasone dipropionate (Becotide,* Vanceril)	300–600 mcg	Appears to be best agent
Betamethasone valerate (Bextasol)	600–800 mcg	Similar to beclomethasone
Flunisolide	1000–2,000 mcg	Investigational

*Proprietary name in Great Britain; the drug is marketed as Beclovent in Canada.

throughout the world, to be introduced onto the market in the United States.[63] However, it is important to not expect the aerosol to be uniformly successful, since an appreciable proportion of asthmatic patients will undoubtedly find the drug to be of less value than conventional oral therapy. At present, this drug appears to be the best inhalational steroid (Table 7–18).

BETAMETHASONE

Betamethasone is 9α-fluoro-16β-methyl-prednisolone (Figure 7–3); it has the same structure as dexamethasone, and differs only in that, in the latter, the 16-methyl group is α-oriented. This minor difference results in betamethasone having very similar properties to dexamethasone, but with slightly more potent glucocorticoid activity. Thus, betamethasone is one of the most active of the antiinflammatory corticosteroids (see Table 7–10).

Betamethasone, like dexamethasone, is a long-acting drug with an effect persisting for over 48 hours. It is insoluble in water, but is effective when given by mouth, and it can be given by injection into joints and soft tissues; it is also used as a topical skin preparation. *Betamethasone acetate* is an insoluble derivative for repository injection therapy of joints and soft tissues. *Betamethasone disodium phosphate* is a soluble derivative also used in injection therapy; it is more rapid in its onset of action. These various derivatives have been relatively popular in the U.S. for the treatment of rheumatologic, dermatologic and other diseases; this contrasts with beclomethasone, which had not been marketed in the U.S. until the aerosol form was introduced recently (see Tables 7–18 and 7–19).

Betamethasone valerate is an insoluble ester that is a valuable dermatologic preparation (Valisone®). This derivative has 360

times the topical activity of hydrocortisone, although the base betamethasone possesses only 30 times the systemic activity of hydrocortisone. Since the valerate is poorly absorbed, it provides extremely potent topical therapy without systemic side effects. Betamethasone valerate has about three-quarters of the topical potency of beclomethasone dipropionate, and it also has been found to be of great value in the aerosol treatment of chronic asthma.[67] The aerosol drug is more effective than the oral preparation; daily treatment with 1 mg a day of the oral drug was of negligible clinical value in asthmatic children.[67] The oral drug, however, is of value for intermittent maintenance treatment of asthma in some patients, and offers the advantage that dosing is required only every three or four days.[8a]

Betamethasone valerate is available in England and elsewhere as Bextasol inhaler, a metered product that delivers 100 mcg of the micronized suspension per puff (twice the amount delivered by the Becotide inhaler, which delivers 50 mcg of beclomethasone dipropionate per puff). The drug appears to be comparable in action and in incidence of side effects to beclomethasone dipropionate, and it can be used in similar fashion[68]. The recommended dosage for betamethasone valerate in both adults and children is two inhalations four times a day, which results in 800 mcg per day; individual patient adjustments are always required. If the daily dose is restricted to 200 mcg a day, candidiasis is unlikely to appear. The main difference between betamethasone and beclomethasone aerosol is that the larger amount of the former drug released by each activation of the metered inhaler allows the patient to take fewer puffs than are required when the beclomethasone inhaler is used. However, it appears that twice as much betamethasone is required (800 mcg a day, compared with 400 mcg a day of beclomethasone).[69] The larger dosage of betamethasone

TABLE 7–19. BETAMETHASONE

Derivative	Brand Name	Tablets	Syrup	Injection I.M.	Topical
Betamethasone	Celestone	0.6 mg	0.6 mg/5 ml		
Betamethasone acetate	} Celestone Soluspan			{ 3 mg per ml	
Betamethasone sodium phosphate				{ 3 mg per ml	
Betamethasone sodium phosphate	Celestone Phosphate			4 mg per ml	
Betamethasone valerate	Valisone*				+

*Valisone is available as a topical agent for dermatologic use in U.S. Betamethasone valerate is marketed as Bextasol in England; this is a metered cartridge for inhalational use. Each activation delivers 100 mcg of the micronized suspension.

has not led to a greater incidence of side-effects, but it leads one to consider that beclomethasone is the more suitable preparation for general use in asthmatics.

RECOMMENDATIONS FOR STEROID ADMINISTRATION IN ASTHMA

Appropriate use of glucocorticoids in respiratory disease presents a rather difficult therapeutic problem, since the literature does not provide adequate guidelines.[70] Thus, there are dilemmas presented in making choices of a steroid preparation, route of administration, initial dosage, maintenance dosage and the method of dosing. Empirical regimens are usually employed, and it is fortunate that the wide latitude that results nevertheless produces a successful outcome in most situations. In this section, an attempt will be made to present the best documented approach to the problem of steroid dosage, with particular emphasis on the treatment of asthma.

Many products are available,[71] and each has particular advantages and disadvantages (Table 7–20). Hydrocortisone, as its sodium succinate salt, is the standard product for parenteral therapy and prednisone or prednisolone are the standard oral preparations. The physician who chooses to prescribe another product should recognize that most brand name derivatives are more expensive than prednisone,[42] and they can be justified only if specific circumstances warrant their use. Furthermore, preparations for intravenous use are many times more expensive than oral agents, and therefore parenteral therapy should be used only if oral administration is precluded.

Acute Administration

There is evidence that acute respiratory problems, such as most cases of status asthmaticus, respond to a plasma cortisol level of 100 to 150 mcg/100 ml.[35, 72] This level cannot be attained by maximal endogenous adrenal secretion, and therefore exogenous steroid administration is mandatory. Studies have shown that patients admitted to hospital with severe acute asthma usually have plasma cortisol levels in the normal range of 30 to 60 mcg/100 ml. Even patients who have been on low-dose steroid maintenance usually have normal plasma levels. Severe asthma, with acidemia, results in the highest levels, which still tend to be within the normal range.[73]

Hydrocortisone has been considered by most workers to be the drug of choice for intravenous administration in status asthmaticus, and there is little evidence to

TABLE 7–20. GLUCOCORTICOIDS USED IN THE TREATMENT OF ASTHMA

Drug	Advantages	Disadvantages
Hydrocortisone (Cortisol)	Intravenous therapy effective in status asthmaticus	May cause electrolyte disturbance
Cortisone	No advantages (converted to hydrocortisone by liver)	Marked mineralocorticoid effect
Prednisolone	Fairly rapid acting when given by mouth	Slightly more expensive than prednisone
Prednisone	Standard oral preparation; nonexpensive, effective	Not as effective in patients with liver disease
Methylprednisolone	Rapid acting; minimal mineralocorticoid side effects; unproven advantages in severe disease	Relatively expensive
Triamcinolone*	Potent; minimal mineralocorticoid side effects; not likely to produce weight gain; Acetonide used as aerosol	May cause myopathy and mental depression
Dexamethasone	Potent; minimal mineralocorticoid side effects; suitable for topical therapy	May markedly stimulate appetite; value in asthma has been controversial
Beclomethasone*	Potent; minimal mineralocorticoid side effects; dipropionate used as aerosol: not very active by oral route	Aerosol may cause hoarseness and oral candidiasis
Betamethasone*	Similar to, but more potent than, dexamethasone; valerate used as aerosol; less potent than beclomethasone dipropionate	Aerosol may cause hoarseness and oral candidiasis; may cause greater adrenal suppression than beclomethasone

*Suitable for inhalational administration in asthma.

suggest that other intravenous preparations are either inferior or superior. Methylprednisolone may be advantageous, since it is comparable in cost, and it is less likely to cause electrolyte abnormalities; however, this preparation does not offer any other proven pharmacologic advantage in status asthmaticus. Collins et al[73] suggest that hydrocortisone be used, with a loading dose of 4 mg/kg given as a bolus by intravenous injection; an adequate plasma level can then be maintained if an infusion is delivered at the rate of 1 mg per kg per hour. Alternatively, bolus injections of 4 mg/kg of hydrocortisone could be given every three hours, to provide a plasma cortisol level of 100 to 150 mcg/100 ml. This latter technique results in a larger total daily dose; the outcome does not appear to be any better.[73] Thus, continuous infusion is preferable, since fluid and electrolyte disturbances are less likely to occur, and adequate therapy is provided.[74, 75] When such an infusion is given to the average adult patient, a loading dose of about 300 mg of hydrocortisone is given, followed by a total 24 hour dosage of about 1500 to 2000 mg. Usually, potassium supplements are required: about 15 mEq should be given each eight hours, and serum electrolytes should be checked once or even twice a day while the hydrocortisone infusion is maintained.

Some patients may require larger doses of steroids to control status asthmaticus, particularly if the subject has recently been on steroid therapy: in these patients the rate of metabolic clearance of hydrocortisone is apparently increased.[35] Asthmatics who demonstrate such tolerance to steroids may have to be treated with two or more times the standard dosage[76] (Table 7-21). Thus, 3 to 4 gm hydrocortisone might be needed in the first 24 hours, although Collins et al report that their studies have never revealed the need for such large doses.[73, 76a] Many physicians believe that the larger dosage should always be given to patients who have recently been on steroid therapy, or to subjects taking barbiturates or phenytoin;[35, 75] obviously, such doses are also advisable for those patients who have previously demonstrated a need for higher-dose steroid therapy. In most cases, it is possible to control severe asthma within one to three days, and then the steroid dosage should rapidly be decreased; in those patients whose asthma clears completely, steroid therapy can be abruptly discontinued, and treatment with routine bronchodilators is continued. No serious side effects are likely to develop in such a short time, and no steroid dependency occurs.

It is important to recognize that the therapeutic effect of hydrocortisone (or any other steroid) may not appear for several hours. Indeed, one study suggested that a single dose of hydrocortisone in acute asthma may not have any significant effect on pulmonary function.[77] Most patients with asthmatic attacks who do not respond rapidly to sympathomimetic or xanthine therapy should be started on a steroid within one or two hours. A response may be noted after four to eight hours, and, in general, relatively high-dose steroid therapy should be administered for one to three days until the attack has substantially subsided.

Prednisone or *prednisolone* can be given intravenously or orally, usually by the latter route since intravenous preparations are not generally available. There is good evidence that both of these agents are well absorbed from the gastrointestinal tract during acute asthma, provided that the patient is not vomiting. Intravenous therapy

TABLE 7-21. STEROID THERAPY IN STATUS ASTHMATICUS*

Drug	Route	Initial Dose	Subsequent Dosage	For Inadequate Response†	Comment
Prednisolone	oral	40–60 mg	20 mg q4–6h	Use I.V. drug	For mild asthma attack
Prednisone	oral	40–60 mg	20 mg q4–6h	Use I.V. drug	
Betamethasone	oral	6–10 mg	1.2 mg q.d.	Use I.V. drug	
Dexamethasone	oral	7.5–12.5 mg	1.5 mg q.d.	Use I.V. drug	Dubious value
Methylprednisolone	oral/I.V.	0.8 mg/kg	5 mg/kg/24 hr e.g. 300 mg/24 hr	0.9–1.2 gm/24 hr	For severe asthma attack
Hydrocortisone	I.V.	4 mg/kg	1 mg/kg q1hr e.g. 1500 mg/24 hr	4.5–6 gm/24 hr	

*One of the above drugs should be used for first 1–3 days. Subsequently, oral prednisone can be used as in Table 7-23, or another drug can be given in equivalent daily dosage.

†Response may be inadequate for several reasons, including prior steroid therapy, phenytoin/barbiturate therapy, and intrinsic resistance. Such patients may require up to three times the standard dose.

with prednisolone has been shown to produce subjective and objective improvement in asthma beginning within one hour, with a peak effect at eight hours.[78] Prednisolone, when given orally in a single dose of 40 mg, results in improvement within two to three hours, with a peak effect at nine to twelve hours.[39] Thus, although there is a slight advantage to giving this drug by the intravenous route, it is not unreasonable to use the oral route if the patient can take the drug by mouth. Since intravenously administered hydrocortisone produces a beneficial effect within one hour with a peak effect at five hours, it does have a definite therapeutic advantage over oral prednisolone. Nevertheless, administering a steroid by the intravenous route in acute asthma is a matter of convention rather than a universal necessity. In all cases of status asthmaticus, bronchodilators should be utilized while awaiting the onset of the steroid effect.

Clearly, many patients with an acute asthma attack can be treated effectively with oral steroids, and they do not necessarily require the more conventional intravenous regimen. Patients on chronic maintenance therapy with oral steroids often discover that an exacerbation can be treated by doubling or tripling the normal daily oral dose for one to three days. Physicians worry about this use of a steroid as a "bronchodilator," but such a concern is not necessarily valid, provided the increased oral course is taken appropriately, used infrequently, and only when indicated for a severe exacerbation of asthma. Prednisolone is perhaps preferable to prednisone, since the former agent has a more rapid onset of action; furthermore, in patients with liver disease, prednisolone is more effective.

Many patients who are susceptible to frequent exacerbations of asthma must take prednisone or prednisolone for maintenance therapy; it is reasonable for their physicians to instruct them to double or triple the usual daily dose to about 40 to 60 mg when a severe exacerbation or an attack of asthma develops. A single dose of oral prednisone (40 mg) or intravenous hydrocortisone (200 mg) may completely abort an attack if given early enough, but, more often, two to three days of steroid therapy are required.[70] Some general guidelines regarding the use of prednisone are reviewed in Table 7–22.

TABLE 7–22. GENERAL RULES FOR STEROID THERAPY

1. Start suppressive therapy with high doses
   e.g. Hydrocortisone 100–500 mg q6h
   Prednisone 30–80 mg/day
   Daily dosage can be given in 1 or 2 divided doses.

2. Discontinue abruptly within 5 day; otherwise wean over next 1–10 weeks
   e.g. Prednisone 60 mg/d:
   reduce by 10–15 mg/day each week to 30 mg/day
   then, by 5 mg/day each week to 10 mg/day
   then, by 1 mg/day each week

3. With "long-term" therapy (more than 2 wks):
   try to avoid more than 10 mg prednisone/day in average adult
   try to avoid more than 6 mg prednisone/day in postmenopausal women
   try to avoid more than 5 mg prednisone/day in children

4. The use of 20 mg prednisone per day results in 50% adrenal suppression within 5 days. Use alternate-day regimen if patient requires more than 7.5 mg/day.

5. If patient has been on daily steroids for more than 2 years, alternate day regimen may need to be started with 3 to 4 times the usual daily dose.

For intensive short-term therapy, other long-acting steroid preparations could be used instead of hydrocortisone, prednisone or prednisolone (Table 7–21). Thus, a single dose of *betamethasone* (or perhaps *dexamethasone*) may completely alleviate an asthma attack, but the appropriate dosages and routes of administration have not yet been established; therefore, firm advice regarding the use of these alternative preparations for the treatment of status asthmaticus cannot be provided. Mild asthmatics who do not require daily steroids, and who experience exacerbations not more often than every month or two, could be advised to treat themselves with 40 mg of prednisone and 1.2 mg of betamethasone (or perhaps, as an alternative, 1.5 mg of dexamethasone), thus providing a brief but sufficiently prolonged emergency course of steroid therapy at the first sign of an impending attack. Alternatively, 7 to 10 mg of betamethasone could be taken, and, if necessary, a similar dose could be repeated the next day; if improvement occurs but some bronchospasm persists, 1.2 to 6 mg a day could be used for one or two more days, while the physician evaluates the situation and determines the need for a maintenance course of steroids.

High-dose steroid therapy can usually be given for about 48 hours, as described, without any important side effects. Electrolyte disturbances and fluid retention may become manifest in patients who are given larger doses of hydrocortisone, prednisone or prednisolone, but these problems are unlikely to be serious unless the patient has heart failure, hypertension or renal disease. In these patients, an agent such as *methylprednisolone,* which has little mineralocorticoid effect, is more suitable; the dosage should be equivalent to that recommended earlier for hydrocortisone.

In many patients in whom the bronchospastic crisis is well controlled by the initial steroid therapy, the drug can be withdrawn abruptly after two days, without any tapering or weaning schedule, although it is usually advisable to continue with a course of oral steroid therapy if the patient was ill enough to require hospitalization. The following problems should be watched for during intensive steroid therapy:[3] precipitation of ketoacidosis in a susceptible diabetic patient; superficial ulceration of the gastric mucosa with the possibility of bleeding; burning and itching at mucocutaneous junctions; impaired sleep; and, rarely, multifocal ventricular contractions.

Although the use of steroid therapy as described usually proves adequate, some patients require more vigorous treatment. When the asthmatic attack does not respond to standard dosages of steroids, much higher doses may be tried. Steroid resistance is most likely to occur in patients who have been on relatively large-dose steroids prior to the exacerbation.[35] Once the acute problem has resolved, the dosage of prednisone or prednisolone may need to be maintained at levels as high as 120 mg a day for some time in these patients.[3]

Maintenance Therapy

In most patients with glucocorticoid-responsive respiratory disease, high dosage therapy can be rapidly reduced after the first two or three days. A short-term course for less than two weeks rarely results in troublesome side effects. A vigorous effort should be made to wean all patients from steroids within this time period, since hypothalamic-pituitary-adrenal axis depression is likely to appear, and persist for several months, if therapy is continued for more than a few weeks. Successful weaning can be accomplished in asthmatics only if maximal routine bronchodilator therapy is used concomitantly to control bronchospasm; it is an error to rely on large doses of glucocorticoids alone to control symptoms. Many patients feel so much better on steroids that they may be reluctant to reduce the dosage. The physician has to insist on the extreme importance of reaching a low maintenance dosage, or, better still, discontinuing steroids completely, if this is at all possible.

Once an acute attack of asthma is controlled by oral or intravenous steroid therapy, the patient will frequently require oral therapy for a while longer. Prednisone or prednisolone are usually chosen, and either can be given as a single dose of 40 to 60 mg administered early in the day. If the patient progresses favorably, careful dosage reduction can be made at a rate of about 25 per cent every two days,[70] or alternatively, the dose is decreased by 5 to 10 mg a day. In some cases, it is not possible to continue this rate of reduction without causing an exacerbation of symptoms; it may then be necessary to reduce the dose by as little as 0.5 to 1 mg a day or even 1 mg a week. Rarely, an even slower reduction regimen will be required, particularly when an allergic patient is exposed to an unfavorable environment, such as a pollen season lasting several months. Similar weaning problems are encountered in patients who have developed iatrogenic cushingism as a result of long-term high dosage therapy, and it may not be possible to reduce the dosage by more than 1 mg of prednisone a month in some of these subjects. Table 7–23 provides a typical maintenance and weaning plan. Once a level equivalent to 7.5 mg of prednisone a day is reached, there is much less concern about further tapering, since this dosage is unlikely to result in severe physiologic consequences or to produce the clinical manifestations of Cushing's syndrome; this dosage of prednisone (or the equivalent dose of any other glucocorticoid) may be tolerated for years.[79]

In general, there is no need to use any agent other than the familiar prednisone or prednisolone. Growing children should never be put on maintenance therapy with a long-acting steroid, such as dexamethasone, since there is an increased susceptibility to retardation of growth with such agents. Some patients may require more specific glucocorticoids with less mineralocorticoid activity if they develop problems

TABLE 7–23. MAINTENANCE THERAPY WITH PREDNISONE FOR ADULT ASTHMATICS

Example†

Start oral therapy on 2nd or 3rd day of asthma attack

15 mg   qid

Reduce rapidly
i.e., discontinue drug
by 3rd to 5th day

Reduce slowly
i.e., 25% every 2–3 days
or 5–10 mg every day

20 mg every morning

Reduce
0.5–1 mg every day

Occasionally, slower
dosage reduction is
required

Often, more rapid
dosage reduction
can be made

10 mg every morning

Improvement

Mild exacerbation ⟶
double dose; stop
weaning schedule for
about 1 week

No improvement

7.5 mg every day

Reduction
in oral
dosage
with
addition
of aerosol
may be
possible

Poor control ⟶

May be maintained
indefinitely
or
may be discontin-
ued

Alternate-day
regimen should
be initiated*

Continue to
try to wean

*In many patients, the dose on alternate (even) days can be successively reduced without the need for a compensatory dosage increase on the adjacent (odd) day. In some patients, the dose on one day of each pair can be doubled, while the adjacent day's dose is abruptly reduced to zero. Modifications of this alternate day weaning program may be successful if carried out with careful supervision (see Table 7–29).

Day	Oral Dosage (mg)
1	(I.V. therapy)
2	15, 15, 15, 15 or 60
3	15, 15, 15, 15 or 60
4	15, 15, 15 or 45
5	15, 15, 15 or 45
6	15, 5, 15 or 35
7	15, 5, 15 or 35
8	15, 5, 5 or 25
9	15, 5, 5 or 25
10	20
11	19
12	18
13	17
14	16
15	15
16	14
17	13
18	12
19	11
20	10
22	20
30	19
31	18
32	17
33	30
34	10
35	30
36	7.5
37	30
38	5
39	30
40	2.5
41	30
42	—
43	30
44	—
45	25
46	—
47	22.5
48	—
49	20
50	—
	Continue weaning

†This example depicts the management that may be required by a very steroid-dependent adult asthmatic. The majority of patients, however, can be weaned much more quickly.

TABLE 7–24. PRECAUTIONS FOR PATIENTS ON GLUCOCORTICOID THERAPY

By Patient

Patient must understand drug, and should carry a card showing the dose of steroid being taken.

Patient should increase drug in stress, or if exacerbation of disease occurs or serious intercurrent illness develops.

Diet should include protein supplements with calorie restriction, and a low sodium and high potassium content.

Antacids should be taken for peptic symptoms, or known peptic disease, three or four times a day.

Special care must be taken of skin, with immediate treatment of injuries or infections.

Activity must be maintained, or physiotherapy instituted.

By Physician

Check patient regularly and ensure that drug is being used correctly.

Carry out periodic checks for weight gain, edema, hypertension, electrolyte disturbances, diabetic problems, change in chest x-ray, cataracts, glaucoma, myopathy, occult bleeding from bowel, mental changes, etc.

In patients predisposed to osteomalacia, increase calcium intake to the equivalent of one quart of milk a day, or Os-Cal tablets, one four times a day.

Consider use of anabolic hormones in older patients, especially postmenopausal women, if physical state deteriorates.

Monitor for occult or unusual infections, and for development of active tuberculosis.

Consider giving INH to patients with positive PPD skin test and radiologic evidence of inactive tuberculosis.

Try to wean patient from steroids or onto a safer regimen if possible. Avoid the use of long-acting preparations in growing children, since these agents are very likely to cause inhibition of growth.

related to electrolyte disturbance; however, equipotent therapy with such agents is much more expensive.[42]

Patients and physicians should continuously observe various precautions when prolonged steroid therapy is employed (Table 7–24). Breakdown of healed tuberculosis is a particular risk in many patients; prophylactic isoniazid (INH) may be advisable, particularly in younger subjects, if the PPD skin test is positive and the chest x-ray shows evidence of old tuberculosis.[34a] Diabetes may be unmasked if latent, or worsened if overt, and other complications may be precipitated in such patients, for example hypertension, urinary and other infections, glaucoma, and cataracts. In elderly patients, a catabolic state can be produced, and osteoporosis is a risk, especially in postmenopausal women. Various forms of therapy have been suggested for osteoporosis,[79a] including 50,000 units of vitamin D once a week and 1 gm of calcium lactate a day; hormones have also been advised, including conjugated estrogens (Premarin) 0.625 to 1.250 mg daily for 25 days a month in postmenopausal women. Fluoride administration has been suggested, but this agent is even more controversial than the other anabolic agents—which are, as yet, not generally recommended by all experts. Nevertheless, their use should be considered in patients who require relatively large doses of steroids and who develop problems attributable to osteoporosis. All patients on chronic glucocorticoid treatment should carry a warning card or bracelet inscribed with relevant information about the steroid

TABLE 7–25. PATIENT INFORMATION CARD*

Mr.
Mrs.
Ms. _____
is being treated for
_____
(disease)
with
_____
(glucocorticoid) ,
_____
(dose) . In a stress situation, dosage should be increased as follows:

1. *Mild stress* (e.g., slight injury, non-febrile illness): double the daily dose.

2. *Moderate stress* (e.g., influenza-like illness, minor surgery): triple the daily dose. Give equivalent dose of dexamethasone parenterally if oral intake is unreliable.

3. *Severe stress* (e.g., high fever, multiple trauma): increase dose to 100 mg hydrocortisone three or four times a day, or give equivalent dose of another preparation.

4. *Unexplained coma:* Give 4 mg dexamethasone intramuscularly, and seek medical help.

PHYSICIAN'S NAME

_____, M.D.

ADDRESS

_____

EMERGENCY PHONE NUMBER

_____

This card could be given to any patient on chronic glucocorticoid therapy; a bracelet or necklace with similar information could be used. The patient or relatives could be given a prepackaged syringe containing 4 mg dexamethasone for use in emergency (e.g., if patient is vomiting or is comatose). Patients on aerosol steroid therapy require some modification of this guide.

*The design of this card is based on that recommended by Streeton.[27]

therapy, such as that illustrated in Table 7–25.

If a patient relapses on maintenance therapy, it is important to increase the dose of the steroid sufficiently to suppress the exacerbation. It may be advisable to double or triple the dosage for a few days, and then taper down rapidly to the maintenance level during the following week.[80] Fortunately, relatively few patients require a chronic maintenance dose of more than 15 mg of prednisone a day, particularly if adequate routine treatment with other drugs and modalities is utilized.

Alternate Day Steroid Therapy

If a patient cannot be tapered down to an acceptable daily maintenance dose of a glucocorticoid without flare-up of the respiratory problem, the continuing risk of severe side effects makes it essential to consider a different approach. In recent years it has been found that many patients do well enough if the steroid is administered every other day; the undesired consequences are markedly reduced by this regimen.[79a, 81] On the day when no steroid dose is given, the patient can usually manage by taking larger doses of the routine bronchodilator drugs being used; in some cases, the patient may need to plan for less strenuous and demanding activities on the days when the low dose of steroid is taken.

There is convincing evidence that an adequate dose of a short-acting steroid given every 48 hours, as a single early morning dose, causes only minimal hypothalamic-pituitary-adrenal (HPA) axis feedback disturbance, and therefore results in only minimal adrenal gland suppression.[24] The underlying explanation is that normal endogenous cortisol secretion is maximal in the early morning, and lowest in the evening; thus feedback depression is greatest during the day, but the axis is enabled to become activated again during the night, thereby stimulating adrenal secretion during sleep. Thus, the early morning administration of a steroid mimics the natural secretory tide, and causes minimal endocrine feedback disturbance. If a sufficient dosage of the steroid is given, the beneficial therapeutic effect will persist for 48 hours, while the HPA axis will have time enough to recover completely. When an alternate-day regimen is established, there is only about one fourth the risk of endocrine disturbance for a given dose than there would be if that dose was given on a daily basis.[82] The proven advantages of an alternate-day regimen include less risk of cushingoid side effects, and a decreased susceptibility to infectious complications.[8b]

In practice, only prednisone, prednisolone or methylprednisolone have short enough half-lives to be successful in alternate day therapy. Other steroid preparations have a longer half-life, which results in more interference with the HPA axis. The endocrine side effects of the longer-acting agents could be avoided by giving these agents every three or four days,[3] but the respiratory disease is not adequately controlled on the days without therapy. Thus, longer-acting preparations have not been so successful when used on other than a daily basis.

When a patient is stabilized on a daily steroid regimen that employs a relatively large dose, a change to alternate day therapy should be attempted by using a plan such as that outlined in Table 7–23; other regimens have been published.[79a] Conversion to an alternate-day regimen is more easily accomplished if the patient has not been on daily therapy for more than a few weeks; in contrast, a history of daily therapy for months or years is a signal for greater care when changing to an alternate-day regimen. There is probably no advantage to alternate day therapy unless the dosage of prednisone on the "low-dose day" is kept below 7.5 mg;[70] it is, of course, best if this alternate-day dosage is reduced to zero. However, if a patient has been on chronic maintenance therapy with a daily glucocorticoid regimen, it may be helpful to carry out tests that evaluate HPA axis function before switching to an alternate-day regimen. If the tests reveal HPA insufficiency, it may be advisable to give a small dose of a short-acting glucocorticoid (for example, 10 mg hydrocortisone) on the afternoon of the second day to forestall the development of steroid deficiency problems during the latter part of that day.[24] Unfortunately, it is not possible at present to recommend any method of introducing alternate-day therapy that is absolutely trouble-free and safe.

If a patient on an alternate-day steroid regimen develops an exacerbation of the disease, each alternate-day's dose will need to be increased, and usually the drug will also need to be given on the steroid-free day. In such cases, the alternate-day regimen may have to be abandoned until the disease is stabilized again. Successful introduction of an alternate day regimen often requires that the patient accept an initial worsening of symptoms on the off-day. This should be managed by increasing the administration of routine bronchodilator drugs on that day. If the patient is adequately motivated, the transition to an alternate-day regimen can usually be made with reasonable comfort within a period of less than a month.

Aerosol Therapy

The recent advent of the newer topical glucocorticoids for aerosolization in asthma has created a considerable interest in this form of therapy[83] (Table 7–18). Although steroids have been used for many years in nebulization therapy, older agents such as cortisol, prednisone and dexamethasone have not proved to be of great value when their soluble derivatives are given by aerosolization. However, numerous recent reports on beclomethasone, betamethasone and triamcinolone clearly demonstrate that the introduction of the topical ester preparations of these agents has been extremely successful. Undoubtedly, steroid administration is destined to become a major consideration in the inhalational treatment of asthma. The possibility of topical steroid therapy for other respiratory diseases needs to be explored also. Although it is recognized that only a small proportion of an aerosolized dose is deposited in the lungs, studies reveal that appropriate metered doses produce good results with few side effects;[62] the fate of the uninspired portion of the steroid dose is relatively uncertain.

Any asthmatic patient who is dependent on maintenance oral therapy should be considered a candidate for an aerosol preparation. Very obstructed asthmatics may find it difficult to inhale the steroid aerosol, and some may find the particles cause irritation. Thus, a patient must be in a relatively good condition before the aerosol can be introduced into the management regimen; similarly, it may be necessary to suspend aerosol use if an exacerbation of the asthma develops. Since the transfer to aerosol therapy is particularly advantageous in children, persistent efforts should be made to achieve the substitution in young patients. However, overrapid transfer leaves patients vulnerable to steroid withdrawal; death can occur in such cases.[83a]

Great care is required when transferring any patient to an aerosol regimen, and the physician may need to supervise the procedure very closely. Usually, the aerosol preparation will be introduced, using three or four treatments a day, while the daily dosage of the oral drug is gradually tapered: one or two weeks are often required if the patient is on lower-dose oral therapy, but a month or more may be needed to effect a transfer from higher-dose therapy. If the daily dose of prednisone does not exceed 20 mg (or another oral drug is given in an equivalent dosage), it may be possible to completely wean the patient from the oral preparation. In the case of patients who are maintained on more than 20 mg of prednisone a day, complete transfer may not be possible, but sufficient reduction of oral dosage can usually be made to permit some recovery of the HPA axis and resolution of cushingoid features.[84] During the attempt to transfer from oral therapy, some withdrawal symptoms may occur, for example, lassitude, headaches, malaise, rhinitis, muscular and articular aching and emotional changes[34, 62] (Table 7–4A) lasting a week or more. The aerosol drug, when given in the maximal recommended dosage, will not result in a significant serum level, and thus will not contribute to systemic effects. The steroid-dependent patient is offered an enormous therapeutic advantage if an appropriate transfer to aerosol administration can be made. In Table 7–26 the various approaches to steroid therapy are outlined, utilizing the daily requirements of prednisone as a basis for introducing an alternate-day regimen or starting the patient on an aerosol steroid.

When metered products of topical steroids are available, they should probably be used as recommended by the manufacturers. Thus, metered beclomethasone dipropionate should be administered as two inhalations, each of 50 mcg, three or four times a day initially; about half as much suffices in children under the age of twelve. All complications are minimized by using dosages of not more than 200 mcg a day; thus, candidiasis of the oropharynx or larynx does not appear when such a dosage is employed.[67] Probably, the majority of suitably selected adult patients will not require more than 400 mcg a day.[61] It has not been established whether the best dosage regimen would be one or two aerosol treatments a day rather than three or four, but it is advisable for patients to try to reduce the inhalations to as few as possible. It would be expected that adequate

TABLE 7–26. DOSAGE REGIMENS OF PREDNISONE IN ASTHMA IN ADULTS

	Total Daily Dosage Required to Control Asthma		
	< 7.5 mg	7.5–20 mg	> 20 mg
Occurrence of HPA axis suppression	No	Yes	Yes
Occurrence of cushingoid effects	No	Usually	Yes
Conversion to alternate-day regimen†	Should be tried, although not essential	Should be tried	Should be tried, but may not succeed
Aerosol therapy† for asthma: Probability of success	High	Medium	Low
Recommendation	Not necessary	Determined effort should be made to switch to aerosol	Compromise of aerosol with reduced oral dosage should be attempted

†Alternate day or aerosol regimen must be aimed for in steroid-dependent children to avoid growth suppression.

control with minimal risk of systemic effects would result if the greater proportion of the daily dose is taken in the early morning.

Patients who find aerosol steroid therapy to be successful should be cautioned to not discard their routine bronchodilators: it is a serious error to rely on the steroid as the sole drug, since these preparations may be potentially more dangerous in the long run than most sympathomimetic-xanthine maintenance regimens. Thus, the steroid-dependent patient should be taught to utilize and adjust other bronchodilator therapy as indicated by variations in symptoms, and to remain on the lowest possible dosage of the aerosol steroid. If a moderate exacerbation of asthmatic symptoms should develop, the patient may try to increase the daily intake of beclomethasone to as many as 32 inhalations (1600 mcg) a day, but it is advisable to resort to oral prednisone (a dose of 10 to 15 mg or more) when faced with an evolving asthma attack. It is rare for an adult to require more than 20 inhalations (1 mg) a day, and children under 12 should not be allowed more than 10 inhalations (500 mcg) a day. Aerosol therapy with a steroid is unlikely to be effective in status asthmaticus, and the patient will generally require oral or parenteral short-acting glucocorticoids in this circumstance.

Betamethasone valerate can be used in similar fashion to beclomethasone, but the metered preparation delivers 100 mcg per activation: the recommended two inhalations three or four times a day therefore result in twice the total daily dose recommended for beclomethasone. There is no pharmacologic information to suggest that either of these two new topical steroids offers important advantages over the other, but consideration of dosages suggests that beclomethasone should be preferred.

In the United States, triamcinolone acetonide has been used for aerosol therapy, employing an investigational metered preparation that is not generally available.[85] Although a suspension of the drug is available on the market, it is formulated for use as intraarticular injection therapy, and it is not clear that this preparation is suitable for aerosol therapy. Moreover, beclomethasone and betamethasone might render triamcinolone superfluous. However, if triamcinolone does prove appropriate, it could be given in doses up to 2.4 mg a day,[48] although less than half as much should be regarded as a more appropriate dosage (about 0.8 mg a day[86]). This preparation could perhaps be given by IPPB, but further studies are required to determine the suitability of the preparation for nebulization, the appropriate amount to put in the nebulizer, and the number of treatments to be given each day. Results so far suggest that a patient who requires oral prednisone will be controlled by a daily aerosol dose of triamcinolone which is equivalent to less than 10 per cent of the necessary dose of prednisone.[48]

The complications of aerosol steroid therapy are annoying rather than serious;[20, 67, 87] also, aerosols have both advantages and disadvantages over oral therapy (Tables 7–27 and 7–28). The main problems have been oropharyngeal candidiasis; hoarseness and weakness of the voice occurs particularly with triamcinolone, whereas candidiasis appears to be a less frequent complication with this agent. These difficulties could possibly be avoided by using optimal inhala-

TABLE 7–27. COMPARISON OF ORAL AND AEROSOL STEROIDS FOR ASTHMA

	Oral	Aerosol
Advantage of Aerosol Preparations		
of cushingism with optimal dose	Yes	No
of suppression of HPA axis	Yes	No
Creation of steroid-dependency state	Marked risk	Less risk
Localization of therapeutic action	No	Yes
Advantages of Oral Preparations		
Ease of administration	Very simple	Relatively complex
Difficulty in administering to patients	Rarely	Young children, weak, uncooperative, etc.
Cost	Cheap	Relatively expensive
Well-established dosage schedules	Yes	No
Risks of therapy	Well established	Full risks not known yet
Chance for improper use (e.g., as "bronchodilator")	Moderate	High
Optimal preparations	Prednisone, prednisolone	Not established yet
Suitable for status asthmaticus	Often	Never
Risk of airway superinfection	Increased	May be relatively greater (candidiasis, etc.)
Local airway effects	None	Hoarseness, etc.

tional techniques to limit the deposition of the drug in the pharynx and larynx. Perhaps gargling with water after using the drug would remove excessive amounts from the oropharynx and prevent local complications; the use of an alcoholic solution (such as Cepacol) may be more effective, since these aerosol steroids are more soluble in alcohol than in water. If candidiasis does appear, it is likely to be manifested as a sensation of irritation or discomfort in the throat, with pain on swallowing; the patient may also notice hoarseness. White plaques (thrush) may be visible in the pharynx, and throat culture should grow out the fungus. Candidiasis can usually be managed by withdrawing the aerosol for a few days (and using oral steroids), but an antifungal drug, such as lozenges of nystatin, will readily cure the condition. Another possible problem is that inhaled steroids appear to predispose some patients to pulmonary infections,[58] including tuberculosis;[58a] these drugs should be used with special care in bronchiectasis, and in other cases in which the patient experiences frequent bouts of pneumonia or purulent bronchitis.

Other steroids will undoubtedly be developed for inhalational administration. Currently, *flunisolide* (Table 7–18) is being investigated, and preliminary studies reveal that the drug is of value when given intranasally in allergic rhinitis as well as when inhaled into the lungs in the management of asthma.[88] Future developments in the inhalational use of steroids promise to be interesting.

The more severely obstructed patients are less likely to do well on aerolized steroids; individuals who are unable to cooperate in taking inhalation therapy are usually precluded from this method of administration. It is difficult to forecast which asthmatic patients will do well on aerolized glucocorticoids, and it is therefore worth attempting the transfer in most patients who are maintained on oral steroids. Children in general seem to obtain better results than do adults; bronchitics with thick secretions obtain

TABLE 7–28. SPECIAL PRECAUTIONS WITH AEROSOL STEROID THERAPY

1. The aerosol steroid must be introduced gradually.
2. The aerosol must not be used as a bronchodilator, on an "as needed" basis.
3. Strict observance of the dosage schedule must be demanded by the physician.
4. When the aerosol is introduced and oral steroid therapy is discontinued, the patient and physician must remain aware of the possibility of adrenal insufficiency for the next year or so.
5. Patients who have depended on oral steroid therapy will need to restart systemic therapy if there is an exacerbation of the asthma, an intercurrent illness, or any other stress (see Table 7–25).
6. Any patient on aerosol steroids who is discovered to be very ill or in coma should immediately be given a systemic glucocorticoid in large dosage (Table 7–25).
7. Large doses of aerosol steroid can cause systemic effects and hypothalamic-pituitary-adrenal suppression.
8. The early morning serum hydrocortisone level should be checked to determine if it is near normal in cases of doubt.
9. Pharyngeal irritation and infection must be watched for, and treated immediately.

TABLE 7–29. DAILY MAINTENANCE STEROID THERAPY FOR ASTHMA

Day	Week	Scheme For Gradual Weaning From Prednisone (mg/day)				Scheme For Alternate Day Prednisone Therapy (mg/day)	Scheme For Introduction Of Aerosol	
							Oral Prednisone (mg/day)	Aerosol Beclomethasone*
1	1	I.V. Therapy				60	20	2 puffs qid
2						60		
3		15	15	15	15	80		
4		15	15	15	15	40		
5		15		15	15	90		
6		15		15	15	30		
7		20		15		90		
8	2	20		15		20	17.5	2–4 puffs qid
9		20		7.5		90		
10		20		7.5		10		
11		20				90		
12		19				5		
13		18				90		
14		17				5		
15	3	16				90	15	2–4 puffs qid
16		15				5		
17		14				85		
18		13				5		
19		12				85		
20		11				5		
21		10				85		
22	4	10				5	12.5	
23		9				80		
24		9				5		
25		8				80		
26		8				5		
27		7				80		
28		7				5		
29	5	7				75	10	
30		7				5		
31		7				75		
32		6				5		
33		6				75		
34		6				5		
35		6				70		
36	6	6				5	7.5 or stop	
37		5				70		
38		5				5		
39		5				70		
40		5				5		
41		stop				65		
42		—				5		
43	7	—				65	5 or stop	
44		For mild exacerbation				5		
45		start 60				65		
46		30				5		
47		15				60		Continue,
48		stop				—		or reduce to,
49		—				60		e.g., 1 puff tid
50	8	—				etc.	stop	

*Alternatively, cromolyn sodium aerosol therapy could be instituted.

poorer results. In all cases, patients should continue to use routine bronchodilators; if necessary, a small dose of oral steroids should be continued, and if an exacerbation of the asthma occurs the oral dosage must be increased.[58] Optimal results with aerosolized steroids are obtained if the patient precedes the dose with an aerosolized sympathomimetic bronchodilator: this will help open up the airways and thereby allow better distribution of the steroid, and will help prevent reactive bronchospasm.

In Table 7–29, suggested schemes are outlined for maintenance therapy in asthmatics. In general, a patient who requires intravenous therapy for status asthmaticus can be converted to an oral regimen within three days. Many patients can be weaned completely within five days, but others may require more gradual reduction in dosage to prevent exacerbations. Thus, it may take over a month or longer before steroids can be discontinued. If a mild exacerbation of the asthma occurs, the reinstitution of oral prednisone with rapid weaning may suffice. If a patient requires large dose therapy, such as 60 mg prednisone a day, then an attempt should be made to introduce alternate-day treatment; it may take a month or longer to achieve this if the patient is steroid dependent. Any patient who requires the equivalent of 7.5 to 20 mg or more of prednisone a day should be put on an aerosol, as shown, and an attempt should be made to discontinue the oral drug while relying on not more than 4 puffs four times a day of the aerosol preparation.

Whenever a patient has been maintained on oral glucocorticoid therapy prior to the introduction of aerosol therapy, the possibility of adrenal-hypophyseal insufficiency must be kept in mind. Although weaning symptoms of minor degree may be acceptable, more severe manifestations justify the reintroduction of oral steroids, at least temporarily, so that a more cautious weaning may be attempted. Any exacerbation of asthma, or the occurrence of any severe stress (illness, accident, and so forth), necessitates the reintroduction of adequate oral or parenteral therapy to cover the incident. The dangers of relying on the aerosol alone at such times must be impressed on the patient.

Corticosteroid Resistance in Asthma

Some patients with asthma do not respond adequately to the usual dose of a glucocorticoid. If an asthmatic requires more than 15 mg of prednisone, or its equivalent, daily, for at least two months, corticosteroid resistance can be considered to exist.[88a] This condition is mostly seen in adults with intrinsic asthma, and they are susceptible to frequent relapses, which often necessitate hospital management. Such cases of brittle asthma may necessitate very large doses of steroid, and then it may be weeks or months before a dosage reduction to a relatively safe level can be achieved in the individual patient. Models have been postulated to account for the phenomenon of steroid resistance, and factors such as an unidentified circulatory antiglucocorticoid have been invoked.[88a] Other possibilities include the loss or unavailability of cell receptor sites for glucocorticoids, increased protein-binding of steroids in the plasma, and enhanced steroid clearance or inactivation; none of these explanations has received experimental backing as yet. However, the abnormality probably exists at the beta-2 receptor sites, which are less sensitive to both sympathomimetic drugs and glucocorticoids.

A number of other factors may be involved in steroid-resistance.[88a] These patients may suffer from enhanced alpha receptor activity or increased cholinergic stimulation. Drugs such as phenobarbital and phenytoin, which induce the microsomal enzymes involved in steroid catabolism, can result in a diminished steroid effect; this action may be more potent for the synthetic glucocorticoids, whose actions may be particularly diminished in steroid-resistant patients. Ephedrine can also increase the clearance of some steroids, for example, dexamethasone.[55b] For these reasons, agents containing phenobarbital and ephedrine should be avoided in asthmatic patients who are steroid-resistant.

The problem of steroid resistance is more serious in women and children, who are more likely to suffer severe side effects from high-dose therapy than are adult males. These patients may fail to respond at all to aerosolized steroids, and the most their physicians can hope for is to achieve a reasonable alternate-day oral steroid program. Such individuals may need high-dose therapy for status asthmaticus (for example, the equivalent of 4 to 6 mg/kg hydrocortisone every four hours) following which oral treatment may be required with dosing every six to eight hours. As the patient stabilizes and improves, prednisone (or another oral preparation) can be given every 12 hours, although the total daily dose may need to remain high. If the patient remains very wheezy, twice daily therapy should be continued, with careful attempts to reduce the evening dose; eventually, a single daily administration in the morning may suffice. At that point, the patient will usually require a dose in excess of 60 mg of prednisone a day, and further efforts to introduce an alternate-day regimen should be attempted cautiously. At first, the dose on one day (say, the even day) should be increased, while, the next day, the dose should be dropped: the total dose given on a pair of days should be twice that of the stable daily dose achieved. Thus, if a daily dose of 60 mg had been reached, the even day's dose should be increased to 70 mg while the odd day's dose should be dropped to 50 mg; that is, 120 mg is given over the course of two successive days. The following even day, the dose can be increased to 80 mg, with a reduction to 40 mg the following day. In this fashion, it may be possible to reduce the dose of prednisone on odd days to 5 to 10 mg within two weeks, at which point an attempt should be made to reduce the large even-day dosage.[79a]

In all cases, the approach should be individualistic, and many months may be needed to achieve a satisfactory reduction in glucocorticoid dosage. In successful cases, complete cessation of steroid therapy may be the eventual outcome; in others, variable daily or alternate-day doses may still be required. In some patients, small doses, for example 10 mg prednisone, may be required every second day initially and the weaning process may lead to an extension of the days between doses, so that the 10 mg is given every third day, then every fourth day, and then stopped. Patients usually appreciate the efforts of physicians to arrive at a successful and physiologically acceptable maintenance regimen, even if the dosage schedule may appear to be somewhat bizarre. However, the "addiction" potential of glucocorticoids and the psychologic stresses affecting the patient with steroid-resistant asthma require a continuing and imaginative effort to establish the optimal low-dose regimen for the particular individual.

Poststeroid Therapy Vulnerability

Any patient who receives a course of steroids for life-threatening asthma is at risk of demonstrating acute steroid dependency during the following twelve months or so. The problem may arise in patients on a reduced maintenance dose of glucocorticoids as well as in those who have been completely weaned from steroids, and adrenal insufficiency may be precipitated by any severe stress, including intercurrent illness or accident, emergency or elective surgery, unusual physical or emotional strain, or an exacerbation of the underlying asthma. If the susceptibility of such patients to develop acute adrenal insufficiency is not recognized, especially when the stressful event is severe enough to necessitate hospitalization, the incidence of severe morbidity or mortality will be relatively high. Ideally, the patient or family will have been aware of the risk, and the physicians involved will be informed about the patient's steroid history; if the patient carries a warning card, such as that illustrated in Table 7–25, the chance of overlooking the latent steroid dependency will be lessened.

When an asthmatic patient thought to be steroid-dependent is scheduled for elective surgery, it is advisable to undertake a basic study of the HPA axis (for example, by performing a short-ACTH stimulation test). If the patient's adrenals demonstrate normal function, then the risk of a stress reaction is small; if the result is abnormal or equivocal, it is advisable to provide steroid coverage for the surgical procedure. For this purpose, cortisone is of value,[88b] since it has mineralocorticoid potency in addition to glucocorticoid properties; this is the only situation in which this adrenal steroid is of therapeutic value in the management of asthma: when it serves to provide temporary hormonal replacement for a depleted adrenal gland. On the night before surgery, cortisone acetate 100 mg can be given orally; a further 100 mg can be given intravenously, prior to the operation, and an additional 100 mg can be similarly administered in the recovery room. If the patient undergoes a lengthy procedure, 100 mg of hydrocortisone can be given intravenously during the operation. There is no need to administer ACTH as part of the management of the patient, although some physicians do recommend this. Following recovery from the procedure, daily oral prednisone (or, if necessary, an intravenous steroid, such as methylprednisolone) should be given in a weaning course appropriate to the patient's respiratory status and rate of recovery from the stress of surgery. Other regimens to cover surgery have been recommended[50, 88c, 88d] with larger or more frequent doses of cortisone if the stress is more severe: common sense is required, and the emphasis should be to give more steroid than is required if there is any doubt.

When an asthmatic patient who has been steroid dependent is exposed to other forms of stress, judgement will be needed to arrive at a suitable regimen of steroid coverage. In acute situations, 100 mg of cortisone can be given intramuscularly or intravenously, and 50 mg may be given every six or eight hours subsequently. If the stress is considered to be less severe, it may be more appropriate to give 100 mg of cortisone intramuscularly every day for a few days, particularly if there is evidence of adrenal unresponsiveness. An intravenous glucocorticoid could be used instead of or in addition to cortisone, or an oral glucocorticoid could be used also. In less stressful circumstances, such as occur when the patient's asthma undergoes periodic exacerbation, it may be adequate to simply double or triple the patient's current steroid dosage, or to arbitrarily select a high glucocorticoid dosage regimen. There are no absolute guidelines to offer for all eventualities, but the principle of providing coverage for stress with large-dose glucocorticoid therapy, with an adjuvant mineralocorticoid component (cortisone) if necessary, should be clearly recognized, and acted upon.

GLUCOCORTICOID THERAPY IN OTHER PULMONARY DISEASES

Corticosteroids have long been advocated for the treatment of many immunologic and inflammatory noninfectious pulmonary diseases in addition to asthma. The glucocorticoid ability to antagonize the inflammatory process has been invoked as a basis for the use of these powerful drugs, although the exact means by which they bring about their therapeutic effect is not always demonstrable. Similarly, the steroids are used in the management of some diseases, besides asthma, in which bronchospasm is involved, such as bronchitis.

Unfortunately, the benefits of glucocorticoid therapy in most of these assorted respiratory diseases is not so readily proved as are the results of steroid therapy in asthma.[89] Various dosage regimens are suggested, including massive "pharmacologic" doses. In general, such doses are recommended for potentially fatal infections, and in such cases numerous other modalities of therapy are employed simultaneously. It is, therefore, very difficult to isolate the contribution of the steroid, and at present it is fair to state that massive dose therapy is of relatively unproven value.

Some of the respiratory diseases that are commonly treated with glucocorticoids are discussed in the following section; various disease categories and examples are listed in Table 7–30. Undoubtedly, other pulmonary diseases have been treated by glucocorticoids, but the ones in the list are those that are more likely to be considered suitable for steroid therapy. The appropriate dosages of various preparations for each category of disease have not been established; Table 7–31 presents currently available data, but it must be realized that these broad guidelines are not categoric.

Chronic Obstructive Pulmonary Disease

Many patients with bronchitis-emphysema appear to have an asthmatic component, in that they have a chronic wheeze that under-

TABLE 7–30. RESPIRATORY DISEASES TREATED BY CORTICOSTEROIDS

Disease Categories	Examples
Asthma	Intrinsic and extrinsic
Allergic alveolitis	Farmer's lung, fungal hypersensitivity, bird fancier's lung
Pulmonary infiltrates with eosinophilia	Parasitic diseases, eosinophilic pneumonias
Other immunologic diseases	Drug hypersensitivity, Goodpasture's disease
Collagen vascular disease	Periarteritis nodosa, systemic lupus
Respiratory distress syndrome of newborn	Prophylactic treatment (of mother)
Adult respiratory distress syndrome	Shock lung, capillary leak syndromes, fat embolism
Pneumonias	Overwhelming tuberculosis or viral pneumonia
Inhalational injury	Aspiration pneumonia, drowning, chemical or fume injury, smoke or hot air inhalation
Tracheitis	Post extubation laryngotracheitis
Interstitial diseases of uncertain origin	Sarcoidosis
Malignancies	Carcinoma lymphomatosa, superior vena caval syndrome, adjuvant in chemotherapy
Hay fever	Allergic rhinitis, perennial rhinitis, conjunctivitis

TABLE 7-31. INITIAL DAILY DOSES OF STEROIDS IN VARIOUS DISEASES*

	Hydrocortisone (mg)	Prednisone and Prednisolone (mg)	Triamcinolone and Methylprednisolone (mg)	Dexamethasone (mg)	Betamethasone (mg)
Chronic asthma	80–240	20–60	16–48	3–9	2.4–7.2
COPD	100–200	25–50	20–40	3.8–7.5	4.8–7.2
Sarcoidosis	160–240	40–60	32–68	6–9	4.8–7.2
Allergic alveolitis	200–240	50–60	40–48	7.5–9	4.8–7.2
Fulminant TB	240–480	60–120	48–96	9–18	4.8–7.2
Status asthmaticus	300–2000+	75–250+	60–200+	11–35	9–30
"Shock lung"†	2000+		2000+	120+	

*These doses are based, in part, on manufacturers' recommendations, as summarized by Facts and Comparisons, Inc. The suggested ranges can be taken as guidelines, and are probably reasonable enough, both for adults and children. Each patient should receive an individualized dosage, which should be adjusted as necessary.

†The massive doses suggested by some investigators for use in "shock lung" strain one's credulity. These figures are provided for interest, and they are not to be regarded as established recommendations.

goes periodic exacerbations. In some cases, specific etiologic factors (for example, emotions, allergens, inhalational irritants), lead to an increase in wheezing; in some cases eosinophilia may also develop. When such patients fail to improve adequately on bronchodilators and routine respiratory therapy, it is often worth trying a course of steroids; in these cases, prednisone in low dosage (such as 5 mg a day) may be useful.[90] Some patients experience marked relief, with a decrease in wheezing, improved exercise tolerance, improved mucokinesis, less annoying coughing, and an increased sense of well-being. Careful clinical judgement is needed to decide whether maintenance steroid therapy should be utilized in a patient with predominant bronchitis, since secondary complications (such as superinfection, gastritis and steroid dependency) may occur. The risk of causing pulmonary superinfection suggests that aerosol glucocorticoids should not be used in wheezy patients who have purulent bronchitis. Whenever a patient is in the terminal phase of chronic obstructive pulmonary disease, the nonspecific benefits as well as the specific effects of steroid therapy may improve the quality of the last few months of that individual's life, and in such cases the prescribing of prednisone or another glucocorticoid may be worthwhile.

Bronchiolitis

The role of corticosteroid therapy in bronchiolitis has not been defined. Although steroids may not be of marked value in children, they may be beneficial in adults with this condition,[91] particularly if wheezing is present or if there is progressive hypoxemia. Since bronchiolitis in adults is difficult to diagnose, and may be mistaken for asthma, it is probable that many cases are being treated with steroids without physicians realizing that the "asthma" is, in reality, bronchiolitis.

Pulmonary Infections

Steroid therapy may be of value in overwhelming *tuberculosis* with hypoxemia, and such treatment should certainly be tried in a patient who presents with far-advanced tuberculosis, with severe toxemia and respiratory failure. There would seem to be no disadvantage to steroid therapy in such a situation, provided adequate antituberculosis chemotherapy is also administered.

The value of glucocorticoid therapy in severe *viral infections,* such as influenza pneumonia, has not been convincingly displayed. In a patient who is at risk of dying, there is a clear temptation to try large doses of steroids, but those who have resorted to this approach have found it difficult to determine whether the treatment was beneficial. Most workers seem to feel that although corticosteroids are generally contraindicated in viral infections of the respiratory tract, they are justified in severe viral pneumonia presenting as an acute respiratory distress syndrome.[92]

It must be recognized that glucocorticoid therapy is contraindicated in most pulmonary infections. In fact, routine steroid therapy may predispose patients to unusual, opportunistic infections. As a curious example, a recent report documented the development, in an asthmatic patient on steroid therapy, of an overwhelming pulmonary infestation with a nematode worm, *Strongyloides stercoralis*.[93]

Adult Respiratory Distress Syndrome

Various insults can result in the syndrome of pulmonary infiltrates associated with respiratory failure, which is known by names such as shock lung and adult respiratory distress syndrome. Viral pneumonia is one cause of this syndrome; other causes include severe trauma, fluid imbalance, sepsis, fat embolism and injury by noxious inhaled fumes or chemicals.

Many workers consider that corticosteroid therapy is of value in the treatment of this potentially lethal disease, but the issue remains controversial. Methylprednisolone in massive dosage (for example, up to 30 mg/kg every six hours) has gained a mixed reputation as being the steroid of choice in this condition.[94a] However, at the present time, it is not possible to recommend this particular agent or any other steroid as being of proven value. Furthermore, the popular but unfounded concept that massive, pharmacologic doses of specific agents may be beneficial can only suggest, at the present state of knowledge, that the usual beneficiary is the drug manufacturer rather than the patient. When a patient is dying from the adult respiratory distress syndrome, it is understandable for the physician to turn to corticosteroids in desperation. Large or massive doses of hydrocortisone (for example, 15 to 30 mg/kg a day) or dexamethasone (for example, 0.4 mg/kg every six hours) have been advocated as alternatives to the seemingly overvalued methylprednisolone. However, there are very few controlled investigations on which to base these recommendations for such extraordinarily huge amounts of these very expensive drugs.

Aspiration Pneumonia

The severe pulmonary injury that results from massive inhalation of vomited acid gastric contents presents a particular therapeutic dilemma. Many reports attest to the value of systemic corticosteroid therapy instituted promptly following the aspiration.[95, 96] However, it is not certain which preparation (if any) is best, what dosage should be used, how long a course of therapy should last, or, indeed, whether steroid therapy should be initiated if more than an hour or so elapses without treatment after the occurrence. Experimental studies using animals have produced variable results,[97] whereas clinical studies report more favorably for steroids.[98, 99] If steroids are of value, it is more likely that these benefits occur when the aspirate consists of gastric acid with a pH of less than about 2.5[97] One recent study suggested that corticosteroid therapy following gastric aspiration may have a harmful effect,[99a] but this has not been the experience of other workers.

Overall, steroid therapy appears to be favored but administration must be initiated within a few minutes, or at most an hour, of the event, or not at all. Although methylprednisolone is favored by some workers, and dexamethasone by others, it is doubtful that the agent used is a critical factor. Hydrocortisone could be regarded as suitable in most cases; the initial intravenous dose should be 200 to 500 mg; subsequently, 100 to 250 mg can be given every six hours for about three days (or the equivalent amount of prednisone can be given by mouth), following which the drug can be discontinued if the patient is responding satisfactorily. Methylprednisolone is a reasonable, and less expensive, alternative to hydrocortisone, when used in equivalent dosage. Although intrabronchial instillation of steroids was advocated by some workers in the past, there is no current data to support this approach, and therefore topical therapy is not advocated. However, the use of aerosolized steroids should probably be reconsidered, although careful studies will be required to evaluate this form of therapy.

Steroid therapy is advised for the treatment of a number of conditions that are similar to aspiration pneumonia, such as, drowning, smoke inhalation, respiratory tract burns from hot fumes, chemical injury and other inhalational injuries with noxious fumes or irritants. However, the value of steroids in these conditions (particularly in drowning) is still not completely settled.[100]

Oxygen Toxicity

There is some evidence that corticosteroids may have a beneficial effect on a patient's susceptibility to oxygen toxicity. However, the evidence at present is fragmentary and inconclusive, and therefore steroids should be used with caution in patients who are exposed to very high inspired oxygen concentrations, since some experimental animals fare worse when exposed to oxygen and steroids together.[101]

Respiratory Distress Syndrome of Neonates

Premature infants are susceptible to the development of a severe lung disease that was formerly called hyaline membrane disease. The condition is a consequence of the inability of the immature lung to manufacture surfactant. It has been found that this problem can be prevented by giving steroid therapy to the mother for 48 to 72 hours preceding a premature delivery, or by giving, for instance, one dose of a long-acting preparation (such as 12 mg betamethasone) to a woman who goes into premature labor.[102] There is evidence that the steroids cause enzyme induction in the surfactant-producing system of the fetal lung. At present, this use of steroids is still controversial,[102a, 102b] and recommendations have not been adequately developed. However, some workers suggest that treatment of the expectant mother with dexamethasone 12 mg per day for up to seven days may be advisable as a means of preventing neonatal respiratory distress.[103]

Sarcoidosis

This disease of unknown etiology has a predilection for the lungs and can cause extensive pulmonary destruction. Patients who are symptomatic, and have compromising, progressive pulmonary disease, may benefit from corticosteroid therapy.[104] The results are variable, but the available experience provides justification for a trial of therapy in a deteriorating patient;[70] however, glucocorticoid therapy does not help in most cases of sarcoidosis, and steroid drugs should not be used routinely.[105] Although the appropriate dosage is debatable, initial therapy with prednisone, 60 mg a day, is usually recommended. If a beneficial response occurs, the dosage should be gradually reduced; if the patient cannot be weaned from steroids without further deterioration, an effort should be made to stabilize the disease on an alternate-day regimen.[106] Although there is no information to support the use of inhalational steroids in pulmonary sarcoidosis, this form of therapy probably deserves consideration. Systemic steroid therapy may be of particular value in sarcoidosis complicated by progressive hypercalcemia,[107] since glucocorticoids appear to impair the absorption of calcium from the bowel by counteracting the effect of vitamin D.

Allergic Alveolitis
(Hypersensitivity Pneumonitis)

Various forms of allergic response to inhaled allergens occur, producing severe pulmonary changes such as those of farmer's lung. Fungi, in particular, may cause allergic alveolitis, and some patients also experience an asthmatic reaction; the immunologic response constitutes a Type III reaction.[9] In such cases, oral or intravenous glucocorticoids provide effective treatment.[70] Aerosol therapy with beclomethasone[107a] or triamcinolone[107b] has been used for allergic aspergillosis. In the absence of bronchospasm, the development of an allergic alveolitis accompanied by eosinophilia would constitute a strong indication for steroid therapy.[108] It should be noted that contaminated air conditioners[109] and home humidifiers,[110] which are colonized by certain fungi, can cause hypersensitivity pneumonitis; this can present a complex problem in the bronchospastic patient who is, theoretically, being protected or treated by air conditioning or humidification!

Steroids may also be of value in a variety of *interstitial diseases*,[70] ranging from pneumoconiosis with progressive fibrosis to conditions thought to be autoimmune in origin, such as Goodpasture's syndrome.[111] Similarly, steroids are indicated in collagen-vascular disorders affecting the lung, for example systemic lupus erythematosus, periarteritis nodosa. In all these conditions, it is possible that inhalational steroids, in addition to systemic administration, may be of benefit.

Malignant Disease

Corticosteroid therapy has a limited role in the management of malignant diseases affecting the lungs.[70] The glucocorticoids can be used as adjuvants to chemotherapy, and they may be of more specific value in carcinoma with lymphatic spread and in the management of the superior vena cava syndrome. The euphoria that glucocorticoids can cause provides additional justification for the use of one of these drugs in patients with symptomatic malignant disease.

Steroids may also be of value in the treatment of postradiation pneumonitis,[70] if initiated at an early stage of the disorder.

Laryngotracheitis

Various inflammatory conditions of the larynx and trachea are treated with steroids, although the value of these agents is not clearly established. Thus, the drugs are used in acute laryngitis or tracheitis (particularly following the removal of an endotracheal tube that has been in place for several days) and in the treatment of croup. Systemic therapy is of doubtful benefit, although it is possible that inhalational steroids may provide topical antiinflammatory effects that could be of value. More information is required before clear recommendations can be offered. Nevertheless, a short course of a glucocorticoid may be appropriate, and harmless, as an adjuvant in the management of patients with these clinical problems. Perhaps the advent of the new inhalational steroids will spur an interest in their use for the management of tracheitis or croup.

A more clear indication for steroids would be the development of an allergic edema of the epiglottis, pharynx or larynx causing obstruction of the upper airway. Emergency management of such conditions demands more rapidly-acting drugs (such as epinephrine) or procedures (such as tracheostomy), but steroids are indicated in subacute, chronic or recurrent cases.

Hay Fever

Various forms of allergic rhinitis, popularly called hay fever, respond well to glucocorticoid therapy. In recent years, depot injections of intramuscular methylprednisolone have been given every two weeks by workers who claim that this technique suppresses the allergy; however, there seem to be few advantages associated with this form of therapy.[31]

For many years, topical therapy has been used effectively in the prophylaxis and treatment of hay fever, and dexamethasone has been made available as a commerically marketed metered aerosol for intranasal administration. More recently, beclomethasone dipropionate has been shown to be effective,[112a] and it has been successful in nonallergic, perennial rhinitis.[112b] Other topical glucocorticoids are also providing promising results, and cromolyn is known to be successful in the treatment of allergic rhinitis. For further discussion see Chapters 8 and 9.

Intranasal topical therapy, although successful and relatively free of systemic side effects, can result in adverse local complications. Thus, nasal irritation and dryness are not uncommon complaints, and nasal septum perforation may follow as a rare consequence.[113]

Other Diseases

Most noninfectious pulmonary diseases have probably been treated with steroids, with greater or lesser degrees of success. Very few of these disorders can clearly be shown to have profited by administration of these "wonder drugs," and it is difficult to offer useful advice. However, it is of interest that manufacturers' literature claim that, in addition to the diseases discussed above, steroids are indicated for the treatment of berylliosis (a very rare hypersensitivity reaction to the metal beryllium) and Löffler's syndrome (a form of allergic pneumonia seen in the tropics).

CORTICOTROPIN (ACTH)

Corticotropin, also known as *adrenocorticotrophin* or *adrenocorticotropic hormone,* is more commonly and simply referred to as ACTH. The anterior lobe of the pituitary gland (adenohypophysis) produces ACTH, and releases it from storage when stimulated by another hormone, *corticotropin releasing factor* (CRF). The latter is produced in the hypothalamus in response to stress or stimulation by a variety of inputs; the CRF travels down the portal system in the pituitary stalk to the anterior lobe of the pituitary, where it results in secretion of ACTH into the systemic blood stream.

ACTH is a polypeptide, and it does not have a steroid structure; it does not, therefore, have the usual corticosteroid effects on isolated tissues, although it has been shown to have a direct relaxing effect on human bronchial smooth muscle strip preparations in vitro, probably by directly potentiating the adenylate cyclase-cyclic AMP system.[114] When used in therapeutics, ACTH serves to stimulate the intact functioning adrenal glands to secrete hydrocortisone and other corticosteroids. Thereby ACTH can bring about, indirectly, various glucocorticoid effects. Under normal physiologic circumstances, the release of ACTH by the pituitary controls adrenal activity, and in turn the released corticosteroids exert a negative feedback effect on the pituitary to decrease ACTH release. There is a natural diurnal circadian rhythm of adrenal-pituitary interplay, which is characterized by maximal corticosteroid release in the early morning in the normal individual. This biologic rhythm was discussed earlier in this chapter, when it was pointed out that glucocorticoid therapy should be given in the early part of the day to avoid disturbing the natural feedback relationship between the hypothalamus, pituitary and adrenal glands.

Although ACTH is able to cause a glucocorticoid-like effect, this hormone does differ from the adrenal steroids in many important aspects (Table 7–32). It is thought that ACTH may have some individual steroid-like properties that are not mediated through the adrenal gland; for example, in high doses it may cause adipokinesis (hypoglycemia, insulin resistance and ketosis). Since ACTH stimulates the adrenal gland, it results in mineralocorticoid hormone and androgenic hormone secretion, and therefore it has more profound secondary effects than those of hydrocortisone and other glucocorticoids. However, the maximal endogenous glucocorticoid production evoked by ACTH is small compared with the large doses of exogenous steroid that are administered therapeutically; therefore, ACTH has less potent antiinflammatory effects. However, ACTH causes fewer cushingoid side effects, and fewer general disturbances of body function. These advantages may be particularly important in children, since ACTH probably does not interfere with growth as much as does exogenous glucocorticoid therapy. Chronic administration of ACTH causes less pituitary suppression, and will not cause adrenal atrophy (indeed, adrenal gland growth may result); these are important advantages when compared with the serious pituitary and adrenal suppression that accompany chronic glucocorticoid therapy.

The main disadvantages of using ACTH as an alternative to glucocorticoid therapy are the following:

TABLE 7–32. COMPARISON OF GLUCOCORTICOIDS AND ACTH

Properties	Glucocorticoids	ACTH
PHYSIOLOGIC		
Requires functioning adrenal gland	No	Yes
Effect on adrenal glands	Atrophy	Stimulation
Effect on glucocorticoid secretion	Decreases	Increases
Effect on aldosterone secretion	Not altered	Increases
Effect on adrenal androgen secretion	Decreases	Increases
HPA axis suppression	Definite	Probable
CLINICAL		
Antiinflammatory effect	Considerable	Variable
Mineralocorticoid activity	Depends on preparation	Considerable
Androgenic effects in women	Slight	Marked
Pigmentation (chronic administration)	No	Yes
Diabetogenic effect	Yes	Yes
Causes cushingism	Yes (dose dependent)	May not (variable)
Catabolic action	Marked	Minimal
Impairment of growth in children	Yes	No
Value in asthma	Considerable	Debatable
Useful in stress situations	Yes	No
Suitable for severe disease	Yes (high dosage)	Not usually
THERAPEUTIC		
Routes of administration	Oral, parenteral, topical	Parenteral only
Therapeutic preparations	Many; well established	Few; not all established
Dosage schedules	Many established	Controversial
Persistence of pharmacologic effect	Depends on derivative	Six hours
Variable dose response	No	Yes
Reliable therapeutic effect	Generally predictable	Unpredictable
Acquired resistance to effects occur	No	Yes (due to antibodies)
Causes allergic reaction	Very rare	Occasional
Development of withdrawal syndrome	Common	Infrequent
Necessity for weaning	Yes	No

(1) The drug cannot be given by mouth and must be administered by parenteral injection at least three times a week in chronic therapy. Thus, it is not as suitable as oral steroid administration for domiciliary treatment.

(2) ACTH can cause troublesome androgenic effects in women, such as acne and hirsutism, and its mineralocorticoid effects can result in fluid and electrolyte problems. Since the first thirteen amino acids in the molecule of ACTH are identical in sequence to those of melanocyte-stimulating hormone (MSH, a pituitary hormone), chronic administration of ACTH can cause some generalized hyperpigmentation of the skin.

(3) Repeated courses of ACTH may result in the induction of antibodies. As a consequence, the therapeutic response may diminish, and, more important, patients may develop allergic reactions.

(4) The drug is not suitable for the management of serious exacerbations of disease states that respond to large doses of glucocorticoid therapy, because its action is unpredictable, and the maximal potency of its effect is limited. Similarly, ACTH is unlikely to be helpful in patients who develop an exacerbation of disease while on chronic glucocorticoid therapy.

(5) Preparations and therapy schedules have been poorly established.

In spite of these disadvantages, the drug has gained a definite but limited popularity.[79a, 115] Many physicians feel that ACTH has advantages over glucocorticoids in the treatment of a number of diseases including myasthenia gravis, multiple sclerosis, rheumatoid arthritis, Bell's palsy and ulcerative colitis. The androgenic effect of ACTH may be advantageous in diseases accompanied by severe muscle wasting; in contrast, glucocorticoid therapy generally exacerbates this problem. However, there is little reason to advocate the preferential use of ACTH over glucocorticoids in the management of most steroid-responsive lung diseases.

Numerous articles have suggested that ACTH may be of use in chronic asthma, particularly during childhood;[115] in the United Kingdom, the drug is already popular in the treatment of childhood asthma and certain other respiratory diseases.[116] ACTH has also been reported to be effective in status asthmaticus. Thus, Collins et al[73] used 1 mg of the British synthetic preparation, tetracosactrin depot (which is equivalent to cosyntropin), at 24 hour intervals in asthmatics who had not received corticosteroids previously; the patients improved, almost as rapidly as another group who were treated with hydrocortisone. Long-acting tetracosactrin in a dose of 1 mg can result in a sustained plasma cortisol level as high as 90 mcg per 100 ml, and the British workers concluded that tetracosactrin or ACTH provides satisfactory treatment in acute asthma, particularly for patients who have not previously received corticosteroids. However, there is relatively little literature to suggest that ACTH is as suitable as the established glucocorticoids in status asthmaticus or in the routine management of asthma in adults. There is, perhaps, more support for the use of ACTH in childhood asthma, but this is still controversial. A further use, of very limited value, would be the intermittent administration of ACTH to provide protection for an atopic patient during a brief pollen season.[117]

In the United States, the main use for ACTH is in diagnostic tests, where the effect of the hormone on adrenal secretion can be used to evaluate the function of the gland. This may be of particular value when a patient has been on long-term maintenance therapy with a glucocorticoid, in which case the function of the HPA axis is usually impaired. If the patient is admitted to the hospital, or if a major change in steroid therapy is contemplated, tests to evaluate adrenal function can provide useful information. Various established tests for the assessment of both pituitary and adrenal responsiveness are available, for example ACTH stimulation test, metapyrone tests, dexamethasone suppression test.[88c, 118]

One of the simplest of these tests of the adrenal cortex is the ACTH stimulation test.[119] Either 25 units of ACTH or 0.25 mg of cosyntropin is given intravenously early in the morning: the normal adult adrenal should secrete hydrocortisone in sufficient amount to achieve a plasma level of more than 17 mcg per 100 ml within half an hour. If a patient is on glucocorticoid therapy, a rise of more than 7 mcg per 100 ml above the basal level indicates that adequate adrenal function is present. The test is simple to carry out, since it necessitates only one intravenous injection and two venous blood samples for serum cortisol determination. Variations on this diagnostic test exist, including a longer test in which ACTH is given daily for two to four days and the plasma cortisol response is measured each day.

Some workers consider that if impaired adrenal responsiveness is found, function can be improved by giving a course of ACTH injections. When adrenal function is markedly impaired, the patient is unlikely to do well on a rapid weaning schedule, or if a switch from oral therapy to an aerosol steroid is attempted, and a slow changeover is advisable; ACTH administration may facilitate the process. However, it is still not clear that ACTH has value in any such case of suspected or proven adrenal suppression caused by glucocorticoid therapy.

Another controversial use of ACTH has been to provide "booster" doses periodically (for example, once a month) to patients on long-term glucocorticoid therapy, or in the management of asthmatics who have been weaned from glucocorticoids. These controversial uses for ACTH have gained a select following both in the U.S.[120, 121] and, more recently, in the U.K.[122, 123] The ACTH is thought to stimulate the adrenal glands, which may atrophy during the course of prolonged steroid therapy.[121] However, there is little proof that this objective is attained, and there is good evidence that booster doses of ACTH lead to further suppression of the hypothalamic-pituitary-adrenal axis.[27, 50, 124]

Further work is now needed to answer the following questions:

(1) Should ACTH be used in the acute management of asthma as an alternative to or in preference to glucocorticoids? Although this form of therapy has its advocates, few physicians have been persuaded that ACTH offers advantages.

(2) Should ACTH be used for chronic maintenance therapy in any asthmatic? This form of therapy has been utilized, particularly by pediatricians.

(3) Should periodic "booster" injections of ACTH be given to patients on glucocorticoids to decrease adrenal suppression?

(4) Should ACTH be part of the regimen in treating status asthmaticus in patients who are steroid-dependent? The evidence in support of such an approach is extremely tenuous.

(5) Should ACTH be employed when converting a patient from oral steroid maintenance treatment to an aerosol preparation? Some experts favor this approach, but it is not yet possible to provide definitive guidelines.

The following considerations regarding ACTH therapy may be worth further evaluation:

(1) When an ACTH stimulation test of a patient on long-term steroid therapy demonstrates significant adrenal suppression, 0.5 mg of a depot preparation of ACTH can be given twice a week for several weeks. Whether this will actually restore adrenal function is not certain, but this form of treatment has been reported on favorably by some authorities.

(2) When an attempt is made to withdraw from large dose steroid therapy in a stable asthmatic with iatrogenic cushingism, injections of 60 units of ACTH given intramuscularly every day for several days may be of value.

(3) Some patients can be transferred more easily from oral steroids to an aerosol preparation if a course of ACTH is given during the transition period:[123] 40 units a day, by intramuscular injection, for one week may be suitable.

(4) There are some asthmatic patients whose exacerbations do not respond adequately to glucocorticoids. Occasionally, such patients will respond to ACTH, and a daily dose of 5 to 90 units may be tried by intramuscular or intravenous injection. Probably the larger dose should be selected.

(5) If a patient in status asthmaticus has not received steroid therapy previously, treatment with ACTH may prove successful. The drug is given in a dose of 100 units of a depot preparation intramuscularly, followed by 100 units each day for three to five days until recovery. Such a form of treatment might be deemed advisable in patients who present contraindications to glucocorticoid therapy, such as psychosis, severe diabetes, infection or peptic ulceration. Whether ACTH would be significantly safer in such conditions, however, has not been established.

Although ACTH may be considered to have various possible roles in the treatment of asthma, there is little support for the use of the drug in any of these roles in the United States. Most of the recommendations for the therapeutic use of different preparations of ACTH have been suggested by British workers, and it is evident that further studies will be required before ACTH can be generally accepted as a useful drug in the management of asthma. The current indications for and disadvantages of ACTH are summarized in Table 7–33.

TABLE 7–33. ACTH

Production	Polypeptide hormone, produced by anterior lobe of pituitary gland; synthetic subunit preparation available (cortrosyn)
Action	Stimulates adrenal gland to secrete glucocorticoids, mineralocorticoids and sex hormones
Indications	Management of certain chronic inflammatory diseases (including asthma), especially in children Management of acute asthma (controversial) To stimulate adrenal gland that has been suppressed by glucocorticoid therapy (i.e. "booster therapy") As a test of adrenal gland responsiveness
Therapeutic Disadvantages	Requires administration by injection May cause allergic reactions May be ineffective form of therapy if adrenal gland is unresponsive, e.g. after prolonged steroid therapy Therapeutic value compared with glucocorticoids is disputed

TABLE 7–34. PREPARATIONS OF ACTH

Corticotropin Injection

	Solution units/ml			Powder units/vial		S.C.	I.M.	I.V.
	20	40	80	25	40			
ACTH or Corticotropin	+	+	+	+	+	+	+	
Acthar				+	+	+	+	+

Corticotropin Repository Injection

	units/ml		S.C.	I.M.	I.V.
	40	80			
ACTH Gel or Corticotropin Gel	+	+	+	+	+
H.P. Acthar Gel	+	+	+	+	+
Cortigel	+	+	+	+	+
Cortrophin Gel	+	+	+	+	
Cortrophin-Zinc	+			+	

Synthetic (α^{1-24} ACTH)
Cortrosyn (cosyntropin), I.M., I.V.   25 u (25 mcg)/ml
Synacthen (tetracosactrin)*
Synacthen-Zinc (repository tetracosactrin)*

*Available in U.K., but not in U.S.

If ACTH is tried a preparation suitable for administration by the intramuscular route once a day should be used; more frequent therapy or a very long-acting repository preparation would each be more harmful. Some children seem to do well enough with injections two or three times a week, although the inconvenience renders this form of treatment unsuitable for most pediatric asthmatics.

Preparations of ACTH
(Table 7–34)

Most commercial preparations of ACTH are biologic derivatives of animal pituitary glands, but synthetic derivatives are also marketed. These are made available in a number of formulations.

Short-acting Preparations. These consist of aqueous solutions, or lyophilized powders that can be dissolved in saline for injection. These products can be given subcutaneously, intramuscularly or intravenously.

Long-acting Preparations. The rate of absorption of intramuscular ACTH is delayed by preparing the drug as a repository product. This is achieved either by incorporating ACTH in gelatin, or by combining it with zinc hydroxide. A detectable effect persists for two to three days or longer.

Synthetic Preparations. In the U.S., a synthetic analogue is available that consists of the amino acids 1 to 24 of the ACTH molecule, α^{1-24} ACTH. This part of the molecule lacks antigenicity, and the preparation is unlikely to cause sensitivity reactions; it has the additional advantages of uniform potency by weight and rapid onset of action. The preparation available in the U.S. is rarely used other than in diagnostic tests to evaluate HPA function: it is known as *cosyntropin*. In the U.K., the preparation is known as *tetracosactrin*, and it is used therapeutically as well as diagnostically; however, its action is generally considered to be too short for the drug to be suitable for the treatment of asthma. Tetracosactrin has been complexed with zinc phosphate to form a long-acting preparation more suited for therapeutic administration. A further derivative of ACTH is the α^{1-18} peptide, which is suitable for administration by inhalation as a snuff; its therapeutic value has yet to be determined.

Administration of ACTH

The usual therapeutic dose of ACTH is 40 units a day, and it can be given by injection in four divided doses. Some authorities advocate giving as much as 80 units a day, but larger doses cannot achieve additional stimulation of the adrenal glands, since maximal glucocorticoid output is achieved with less than 80 units. In chronic maintenance therapy, various regimens are utilized, and dosages vary from one injection a day, to three injections a week, to one injection a month. For infrequent therapy regimens both the short-acting and long-acting preparations have been advocated.

The dose of cosyntropin that is suitable for adults is 0.25 mg (equivalent to 25 units of ACTH) for diagnostic tests, and larger doses (for example, 1 mg) for therapeutic purposes. The available preparations can be given intramuscularly or intravenously.

These preparations of ACTH can be given to children; the usual dose ranges from two-thirds to the full adult dosage. In general, preparations can be given subcutaneously, intramuscularly or intravenously in adults and children, but the repository forms for sustained action are administered only by the intramuscular route.

REFERENCES

1. Dluhy, K. G., Lauler, D. P., and Thorn, G. W.: Pharmacology and chemistry of adrenal glucocorticoids. Med. Clin. N. Amer. 57:1155–1165, 1973.
2. Liddle, G. W.: Clinical pharmacology of the anti-inflammatory steroids. Clin. Pharmacol. Ther. 2:615–635, 1961.
3. Melby, J. C.: Systemic corticosteroid therapy: pharmacology and endocrinologic considerations. Ann. Intern. Med. 81:505–512, 1974.
4. O'Malley, B. W.: Mechanisms of action of steroid hormones. N. Engl. J. Med. 284:370–377, 1971.
5. Zurier, R. B., and Weissman, G.: Anti-immunologic and anti-inflammatory effects of steroid therapy. Med. Clin. N. Amer. 57:1295–1307, 1973.
6. Thompson, E. B., and Lippman, M. E.: Mechanisms of action of glucocorticoids. Metabolism 23:159–202, 1974.
7. Baxter, J. D., and Forsham, P. H.: Tissue effects of glucocorticoids. Am. J. Med. 53:573–589, 1972.
8. Middleton, E.: Mechanism of action of corticosteroids. *In* New Directions in Asthma. M. Stein, (Ed.). Park Ridge, Ill., American College of Chest Physicians, 1975.

8a. Melby, J. C.: Clinical pharmacology of systemic corticosteroids. Ann. Rev. Pharmacol. Toxicol. 15:511–527, 1977.

8b. Fauci, A. S., Dale, D. C., and Balow, J. E.: Glucocorticosteroid therapy: mechanisms of action and clinical considerations. Ann. Intern. Med. 84:304–315, 1976.

8c. Claman, H. N.: Mechanism of action of steroids in reversible obstructive airway disease. In Recent Advances in Asthma Therapy: Vanceril Inhaler. R. S. Farr, E. Middleton and S. L. Spector (Eds.). Miami, Symposia Specialists Medical Books (for Schering Corporation), 1976. pp. 109–113.

9. Pepys, J., and Hutchcroft, B. J.: Bronchial provocation tests in etiologic diagnosis and analysis of asthma. Am. Rev. Respir. Dis. 112:829–859, 1975.

10. Turner-Warwick, M.: Provoking factors in asthma. Brit. J. Dis. Chest 65:1–20, 1971.

11. Claman, H. N.: How corticosteroids work. J. Allergy Clin. Immunol. 55:145–151, 1975.

12. Weissman, G.: Effects of corticosteroids on the stability and fusion of biomembranes. In Asthma: Physiology, Immunopharmacology, and Treatment. K. F. Austen and L. M. Lichtenstein (Eds.). New York, Academic Press, 1973. Ch. 14.

13. Haynes, R. C., Jr.: Hormonal drugs. Clin. Pharmacol. Ther. 16:945–953, 1974.

14. Aviado, D. M., and Carrillo, L. R.: Antiasthmatic action of corticosteroids: a review of the literature on their mechanism of action. J. Clin. Pharmacol. 10:3–11, 1970.

15. Ellul-Micallef, R., and Fenech, F. F.: Effect of intravenous prednisolone in asthmatics with diminished adrenergic responsiveness. Lancet 2:1269–1270, 1975.

16. Geddes, B. A., Jones, T. R., Dvorsky, R. J., and Lefcoe, N. M.: Interaction of glucocorticoids and bronchodilators on isolated guinea pig tracheal and human bronchial smooth muscle. Am. Rev. Respir. Dis. 110:420–427, 1974.

17. Logsdon, P. J., Middleton, E., Jr., and Caffey, R. G.: Stimulation of leukocyte adenyl cyclase by hydrocortisone and isoproterenol in asthmatic and nonasthmatic subjects. J. Allergy Clin. Immunol. 50:45–56, 1972.

18. McCombs, R. P.: Diseases due to immunologic reactions in the lungs. N. Engl. J. Med. 286:1245–1252, 1972.

19. Hirsch, S. R.: The role of mucus in asthma. In New Directions in Asthma. M. Stein (Ed.). Park Ridge, Ill., American College of Chest Physicians, 1975. Ch. 22.

20. Williams, M. H., Jr.: Corticosteroid aerosols for the treatment of asthma. JAMA 231:406–407, 1975.

21. Jick, H.: What to expect from prednisone. Drug Therapy 5:85–90, Aug., 1975.

22. Clifford, G. O., et al: Do's and don'ts for using steroids. Patient Care 8:74–101, Oct., 1974.

23. Streeten, D. H. P.: Corticosteroid therapy. II. Complications and therapeutic indications. J.A.M.A. 232:1046–1049, 1975.

24. Axelrod, L.: Glucocorticoid therapy. Medicine 55:39–65, 1976.

25. Conn, H. O., and Blitzer, B. L.: Nonassociation of adrenocorticosteroid therapy and peptic ulcer. N. Engl. J. Med. 294:473–479, 1976.

26. Soutar, C. A., Costello, J., Ijaduola, O., and Turner-Warwick, M.: Nocturnal and morning asthma. Relationship to plasma corticosteroid and response to cortisol infusion. Thorax 30:436–440, 1975.

27. Streeten, D. H. P.: Corticosteroid therapy. I. Pharmacological properties and principles of corticosteroid use. J.A.M.A. 232:944–947, 1975.

28. Brooks, S. M., Werk, E. E., Ackerman, S. J., et al.: Adverse effects of phenobarbital on corticosteroid metabolism in patients with bronchial asthma. N. Engl. J. Med. 286:1125–1128, 1972.

29. Choi, Y., Thrasher, K., Werk, E. E., et al.: Effect of diphenylhydantoin on cortisol kinetics in humans. J. Pharmacol. Exp. Ther. 176:27–34, 1971.

30. Haque, N., Thrasher, K., Werk, E. E., et al.: Studies on dexamethasone metabolism in man: effect of diphenylhydantoin. J. Clin. Endocrinol. Metab. 34:44–50, 1972.

31. Myles, A. B., and Daly, R. J.: Corticosteroid and ACTH Therapy. Baltimore, The Williams and Wilkins Company, 1974.

32. Itkin, I. H., and Menzel, M. L.: The use of macrolide antibiotic substances in the treatment of asthma. J. Allergy 45:146–162, 1970.

33. Geddes, B. A., and Lefcoe, N. M.: Respiratory smooth muscle relaxing effect of commercial steroid preparations. Am. Rev. Respir. Dis. 107:395–399, 1973.

34. David, D. S., Grieco, M. H., and Cushman, P., Jr.: Adrenal glucocorticoids after twenty years. A review of their clinically relevant consequences. J. Chronic Dis. 22:637–711, 1970.

34a. Editorial: Tuberculosis in corticosteroid-treated asthmatics. Br. Med. J. 3:266–267, July, 1976.

34b. Schatz, M., Patterson, R., Kloner, R., and Falk, J.: The prevalence of tuberculosis and positive tuberculin skin tests in a steroid-treated asthmatic population. Ann. Intern. Med. 84:261–265, 1976.

35. Dwyer, J. M.: Corticosteroids in asthma. Drugs 6:81–83, 1973.

36. Brockbank, W., Brebner, H., and Pengelly, C. D. R.: Chronic asthma treated with aerosol hydrocortisone. Lancet 2:807, 1956.

37. Helm, W. H., and Heyworth, F.: Inhalation of hydrocortisone acetate for bronchial asthma. Br. Med. J. 2:768–769, Sept., 1958.

38. Franklin, W., Lowell, F. C., Michelson, A. L., and Schiller, I. W.: Aerosolized steroids in bronchial asthma. J. Allergy 29:214–221, 1958.

39. Ellul-Micallef, R., Borthwick, R. C., and McHardy, G. J. R.: The time-course of response to prednisolone in chronic bronchial asthma. Clin. Sci. Mol. Med. 47:105–117, 1974.

40. Jenkins, J. S., and Sampson, P. A.: Conversion of cortisone to cortisol and prednisone to prednisolone. Br. Med. J. 2:205–207, Apr., 1967.

41. Bickerman, H. A., and Itkin, S. E.: Aerosol steroid therapy and chronic bronchial asthma. J.A.M.A. 184:533–538, 1963.

42. Oral corticosteroids. Med. Lett. 17 (24):99–100, 1975.

43. Wilson, J. W.: Treatment or prevention of pulmo-

nary cellular damage with pharmacologic doses of corticosteroid. Surg. Gynecol. Obstet. 134:675–681, 1972.

44. Petty, T. L.: A chest physician's perspective on asthma. Heart and Lung 1:611–620, 1972.

45. Maibach, H. I., and Stoughton, R. B.: Topical corticosteroids. Med. Clin. N. Amer. 57:1253–1264, 1973.

46. Falliers, C.: Corticosteroid aerosols in asthma. Lancet 1:606–607, 1973.

47. Williams, M. H., Jr., Kane, C., and Shim, C. S.: Treatment of asthma with triamcinolone acetonide delivered by aerosol. Am. Rev. Respir. Dis. 109:538–543, 1974.

48. Falliers, C. J.: Triamcinolone acetonide aerosols for asthma. I. Effective replacement of systemic corticosteroid therapy. J. Allergy Clin. Immunol. 57:1–11, 1976.

49. Kingston, R. S., Steen, S. N., and Thomas, J. S.: Triamcinolone acetonide aerosol in chronic bronchospastic disease. IRCS-Respiratory System 3:36, 1975.

49a. Pingleton, W. W., Bone, R. C., Kerby, G. R., and Ruth, W. E.: Oropharyngeal candidiasis in patients treated with triamcinolone acetonide aerosol. J. Allergy Clin. Immunol. 60:254–258, 1977.

50. Hess, E. V., and Goldman, J. A.: Corticosteroids and corticotropin in therapy of rheumatoid arthritis. In Arthritis and Allied Conditions. J. L. Hollander and D. J. McCarthy (Eds.). Philadelphia, Lea and Febiger, 8th ed., 1972. Ch. 31.

50a. Meikle, A. W. and Tyler, F. H.: Potency and duration of action of glucocorticoids: effects of hydrocortisone, prednisone and dexamethasone on human pituitary-adrenal function. Am. J. Med. 63:200–207, 1977.

51. Novey, H. S., and Beall, G.: Aerosolized steroids and induced Cushing's syndrome. Arch. Intern. Med. 115:602–605, 1965.

52. Siegel, S. C., Heimlich, E. M., Richards, W., and Kelley, V. C.: Adrenal function in allergy. IV. Effect of dexamethasone aerosols in asthmatic children. Pediatrics 33:245–250, 1964.

53. Rumble, L., Jr.: The use of nebulized steroids. J. Med. Assoc. Ga. 53:314–318, 1964.

54. Scotti, P., and Aresini, G.: Functional evaluation of a corticosteroid molecule activity, dexamethasone-isonicotinate, by aerosol dosage in obstructive lung disease. Respiration 32:227–236, 1975.

55. Sparkes, C. G.: Plasma cortisol levels in normal subjects after inhaled corticosteroids. Postgrad. Med. J. 50 (Suppl. 4):9–11, 1974.

55a. Dvorsky-Gebauer, R. J.: Potentiation of bronchodilators by glucocorticoids. Lancet 1:306–307, 1976.

55b. Brooks, S. M., Sholiton, L. J., Werk, E. E., and Allenau, P.: The effects of ephedrine and theophylline on dexamethasone metabolism in bronchial asthma. J. Clin. Pharmacol. 17:308–318, 1977.

55c. Farr, R. S., Middleton, E., and Spector, S. L. (Eds): Recent Advances in Asthma Therapy: Vanceril Inhaler. Miami, Symposia Specialists Medical Books (for Schering Corporation), 1976.

56. Martin, L. E., Tanner, R. J. N., Clark, T. J. H., and Cochrane, G. M.: Absorption and me-

tabolism of orally administered beclomethasone dipropionate. Clin. Pharmacol. Ther. 15:267–275, 1973.

57. Choo-Kang, Y. F., Cooper, E. J., Tribe, A. E., and Grant, I. W. B.: Beclomethasone dipropionate by inhalation in the treatment of airways obstruction. Br. J. Dis. Chest 66:101, 1972.

57a. Spitzer, S. A., Kaufman, H., Koplovitz, A., Topilsky, M., and Blum, J.: Beclomethasone diproprionate and chronic asthma. Chest 70:38–42, 1976.

57b. Yernault, J.-C., Leclercq, R., Schandevyl, W., Vivasoro, E., DeCoster, A., and Copinschi, G.: The endocrinometabolic effects of beclomethasone dipropionate in asthmatic patients. Chest 71:698–702, 1977.

57c. Ericksson, N. E., Lindgren, S., and Lindholm, N.: A double-blind comparison of beclomethasone dipropionate aerosol and prednisolone in asthmatic patients. Postgrad. Med. J. 51 (Suppl. 4): 67–70, 1975.

57d. Davies, G., Thomas, P., Broder, I., Mintz, S., Silverman, F., Leznoff, A., and Trotman, C.: Steroid-dependent asthma treated with inhaled beclomethasone dipropionate. Ann. Intern. Med. 86:549–553, 1977.

57e. Kass, I., Nair, S. V., and Patil, K. D.: Beclomethasone dipropionate aerosol in the treatment of steroid-dependent asthmatic patients. Chest 72:703–707, 1977.

57f. Williams, M. H.: Steroid aerosols in asthma. Ann. Intern. Med. 86:650, 1977.

58. Hodson, M. E., Batten, J. C., Clarke, S. W., and Gregg, I.: Beclomethasone dipropionate aerosol in asthma. Am. Rev. Respir. Dis. 110:403–408, 1974.

58a. Horton, D. J., and Spector, S. L.: Clinical pulmonary tuberculosis in an asthmatic patient using a steroid aerosol. Chest 71:540–542, 1977.

59. Boe, J., and Thulesius, O.: Treatment of steroid-dependent asthma with beclomethasone dipropionate administered by aerosol. Curr. Ther. Res. 17:460–466, 1975.

60. Cayton, R. M., et al.: Double-blind trial comparing two dosage schedules of beclomethasone dipropionate aerosol in the treatment of chronic bronchial asthma. Lancet 2:303–307, 1974.

61. Gaddie, J., Petrie, G. R., Reid, I. W., et al.: Aerosol beclomethasone dipropionate: a dose-response study in chronic bronchial asthma. Lancet 2:280–281, 1973.

62. Wilcox, J. B., and Avery, G. S.: Beclomethasone dipropionate corticosteroid inhaler: a preliminary report of its pharmacological properties and therapeutic efficacy in asthma. Drugs 6:84–93, 1973.

63. Editorial: Beclomethasone dipropionate aerosol in asthma. Lancet 2:1239–1240, 1972.

63a. Editorial: Topical steroids in asthma. Lancet 2:695, 1977.

64. Franklin, W., and Lowell, F. C.: Unapproved drugs in the practice of medicine. Beclomethasone—a case in point. N. Engl. J. Med. 292:1075–1077, 1975.

64a. Francis, R.S.: Long-term beclomethasone dipropionate aerosol therapy in juvenile asthma. Thorax 31:309–314, 1976.

65. Willey, R. F., Milne, L. J. R., Crompton, G. K.,

and Grant, I. W. B.: Beclomethasone dipropionate aerosol and oropharyngeal candidiasis. Brit. J. Dis. Chest 70:32–38, 1976.

65a. Toogood, J. H., Lefcoe, N. M., Haines, D. S. M., Jennings, B., Errington, N., Baksh, L., and Chuang, L.: A graded dose assessment of the efficacy of beclomethasone dipropionate aerosol for severe chronic asthma. J. Allergy Clin. Immunol. 59:298–308, 1977.

66. Lal, S., Harris, D. M., Bhalla, K. K., et al.: Comparison of beclomethasone dipropionate aerosol and prednisolone in reversible airways obstruction. Br. Med. J. 3:314–317, Aug., 1972.

66a. Klein, R., Waldman, D., Kershnar, H., Berger, W., Coulson, A., Katz, R. M., Rachelefsky, G. S., and Siegel, S. C.: Treatment of chronic childhood asthma with beclomethasone dipropionate aerosol: I. A double-blind crossover trial in nonsteroid-dependent patients. Pediatrics 60:7–13, 1977.

66b. Wyatt, R., Waschek, J., Weinberger, M., and Sherman, B.: Adrenal suppression from alternate-day prednisone and inhaled beclomethasone. J. Allergy Clin. Immunol. 61:151, 1978.

67. McAllen, M. K., Kochanowski, S. J., and Shaw, K. M.: Steroid aerosols in asthma: an assessment of betamethasone valerate and a 12-month study of patients on maintenance treatment. Br. Med. J. 1:171–175, Feb., 1974.

67a. Frears, J., Maizels, J., and Friedman, M.: Betamethasone valerate compared by the oral and inhaled routes in childhood asthma. J. Allergy Clin. Immunol. 57:391–395, 1976.

68. Dash, C. H.: Some observations on the use of corticosteroid aerosols in asthma. Postgrad. Med. J. 50(Suppl. 4):25–32, 1974.

69. Riordan, J. F., Sillett, R. W., Dash, C. H., and McNicol, M. W.: A comparison of betamethasone valerate, beclomethasone dipropionate and placebo by inhalation for the treatment of chronic asthma. Postgrad. Med. J. 50(Suppl. 4):61–64, 1974.

70. Kettel, L. J., and Morse, J. O.: Corticosteroids in the treatment of pulmonary disease. In Steroid Therapy. D. L. Azarnoff (Ed.). Philadelphia, W. B. Saunders Company, 1975. Ch. 20.

71. Salem, H., and Aviado, D. M.: Antiasthmatic preparations containing corticosteroids available in the United States. Rev. Allergy 24:819–822, 1970.

72. Collins, J. V., Harris, P. W. R., Clark, T. J. H., and Townsend, J.: Intravenous corticosteroids in treatment of acute bronchial asthma. Lancet 2:1047–1049, 1970.

73. Collins, J. V., Clark, T. J. H., Brown, D., and Townsend, J.: The use of corticosteroids in the treatment of acute asthma. Q. J. Med. 44:259–273, 1975.

74. Editorial: Corticosteroids in acute severe asthma. Lancet 2:166–167, 1975.

75. Editorial: Management of acute asthma. Br. Med. J. 4:65–66, Oct., 1975.

76. Rebuck, A. S., and Read, J.: Assessment and management of severe asthma. Am. J. Med. 51:788–798, 1971.

76a. Britton, M. G., Collins, J. V., Brown, D., Fairhurst, N. P. A., and Lambert, R. G.: High-dose corticosteroids in severe acute asthma. Br. Med. J. 2:73–74, Jul., 1976.

77. McFadden, E. R., Jr., Kiser, R., deGroot, W. J., et al.: A controlled study of the effects of single doses of hydrocortisone on the resolution of acute attacks of asthma. Am. J. Med. 60:52–59, 1976.

78. Ellul-Micallef, R., and Fenech, F. F.: Intravenous prednisolone in chronic bronchial asthma. Thorax 30:312–315, 1975.

79. Tuft, L., Marks, A. D., and Channick, B. J.: Long-term corticosteroid therapy in chronic intractable asthmatic patients. Ann. Allergy 29:287–293, 1971.

79a. Thorn, G. W., and Lauler, D. P.: Treatment schedules with steroids. In Bronchial Asthma: Mechanisms and Therapeutics. E. B. Weiss and M. S. Segal (Eds). Boston, Little, Brown and Company, 1976. Ch. 53.

80. Blumstein, C. G.: Drug treatment in bronchial asthma. Semin. Drug. Treat. 2:385–401, 1973.

81. Portner, M. M., Thayer, K. H., Harter, J. G., et al.: Successful initiation of alternate-day prednisone in chronic steroid-dependent asthmatic patients. J. Allergy Clin. Immunol. 49:16–26, 1972.

82. Lauler, D. P.: Alternate day therapy. In Steroid Therapy — a Clinical Update for the 1970's. G. W. Thorn (Ed.). MEDCOM Inc. (for the Upjohn Company), 1971, p. 46.

83. Turner-Warwick, M.: Corticosteroid aerosols: the future? Postgrad. Med. J. 50(Suppl. 4):80–84, 1974.

83a. Editorial: Deaths from asthma in children on aerosol corticosteroids. Br. Med. J. 1:1117, Apr., 1977.

84. Camerson, S. J., Cooper, E. J., Crompton, G. K., et al.: Substitution of beclomethasone aerosol for oral prednisolone in the treatment of chronic asthma. Br. Med. J. 4:205–207, Oct., 1973.

85. Kriz, R. J., Chmelik, F., doPico, G., and Reed, C. E.: A short-term double-blind trial of aerosol triamcinolone acetonide in steroid-dependent patients with severe asthma. Chest 69:455–460, 1976.

86. Williams, M. H., Jr.: Treatment of asthma with triamcinolone acetonide aerosol. Chest 68:765–768, 1975.

87. Milne, L. J. R., and Crompton, G. K.: Beclomethasone dipropionate and oropharyngeal candidiasis. Br. Med. J. 3:797–798, Sept., 1974.

88. Kammermeyer, J. K., Rajtora, D. W., Anuras, J., and Richerson, H. B.: Clinical evaluation of intranasal topical flunisolide therapy in allergic rhinitis. J. Allergy ꞏClin. Immunol. 59: 287–293, 1977.

88a. Brooks, S. M., and Werk, E. E.: Corticosteroid resistance in bronchial asthma: In Bronchial Asthma: Mechanisms and Therapeutics. E. B. Weiss and M. S. Segal (Eds.). Boston, Little, Brown and Company, 1976. Ch. 54.

88b. Stein, M., and Abdel-Rassoul, M. I.: Preoperative and postoperative considerations in patients with bronchial asthma. *In* Bronchial Asthma: Mechanisms and Therapeutics. E. B. Weiss and M. S. Segal (Eds). Boston, Little, Brown and Company, 1976. Ch. 66.

88c. Bass, B. F.: Steroids. Clin. Anesth. 10:249–267, 1973.

88d. Byyny, R. L.: Withdrawal from glucocorticoid therapy. N. Engl. J. Med. 295:30–32, 1976.

89. Cronin, M. P.: Steroids in respiratory therapy. Resp. Therapy 5:33–36, May–Jun., 1975.

90. Evans, J. A., Morrison, I. M., and Saunders, K. B.: A controlled trial of prednisone, in low dosage, in patients with chronic airways obstruction. Thorax 29:401–406, 1974.

91. Petty, L.: Intensive and Rehabilitative Care. Philadelphia, Lea and Febiger. 2nd ed., 1974. pp. 180–188.

92. Ferstenfeld, J. E., Schlueter, D. P., Rytel, M. W. and Molloy, R. P.: Recognition and treatment of adult respiratory distress syndrome secondary to viral interstitial pneumonia. Am. J. Med. 58:709–718, 1975.

93. Higenbottam, T. W., and Heard, B. E.: Opportunistic pulmonary strongyloidiasis complicating asthma treated with steroids. Thorax 31:226–233, 1976.

94. Jones, R. L., and King, E. G.: The effects of methylprednisolone on oxygenation in experimental hypoxemic respiratory failure. J. Trauma 15:297–303, 1975.

94a. Sladen, A.: Methylprednisolone: pharmacologic doses in shock lung syndrome. J. Thorac. Cardiovasc. Surg. 71:800–806, 1976.

95. James, P. M., and Myers, R. T.: Experience with steroids, albumin, and diuretics in progressive pulmonary insufficiency. S. Med. J. 65:945–948, 1972.

96. Toung, T. J. K., Bordos, D., Benson, D. W., Carter, D., Zuidema, G., Permutt, S., and Cameron, J. L.: Aspiration pneumonia: experimental evaluation of albumin and steroid therapy. Ann. Surg. 183:179–184, 1976.

97. Downs, J. B., Chapman, R. L., Modell, J. H., and Hood, C. I.: An evaluation of steroid therapy in aspiration pneumonitis. Anesthesiology 40:129–135, 1974.

98. Dines, D. E., Titus, J. L., and Sessler, A. D.: Aspiration pneumonitis. Mayo Clin. Proc. 45:347–360, 1970.

99. Ribaudo, C. A., and Grace, W. J.: Pulmonary aspiration. Am. J. Med. 50:510–520, 1971.

99a. Wolfe, J. E., Bone, R. C. and Ruth, W. E.: Effects of corticosteroids in the treatment of patients with gastric aspiration. Am. J. Med. 63:719–722, 1977.

100. Calderwood, H. W., Modell, J. H., and Ruiz, B. C.: The ineffectiveness of steroid therapy for treatment of fresh-water near-drowning. Anesthesiology 43:642–650, 1975.

101. Sahebjami, H., Gacad, G., and Massaro, D.: Influence of corticosteroid on recovery from oxygen toxicity. Am. Rev. Respir. Dis. 110: 566–571, 1974.

102. Editorial: Corticosteroids and the fetus. Lancet 1:74, 1976.

102a. Gluck, L.: Administration of corticosteroids to induce maturation of fetal lung. Am. J. Dis. Child. 130:976–978, 1976.

102b. Ballard, R. A., and Ballard, P. L.: Use of prenatal glucocorticoid therapy to prevent respiratory distress syndrome. Am. J. Dis. Child. 130: 982–987, 1976.

103. Caspi, E., and Schreyer, P.: Prevention of respiratory-distress syndrome by antepartum dexamethasone. Lancet 1:973, 1976.

104. Israel, H. L., Fouts, D. W., and Beggs, R. A.: A controlled trial of prednisone treatment of sarcoidosis. Am. Rev. Respir. Dis. 107:609–614, 1973.

105. Young, R. L., Harkleroad, L. E., Lordon, R. E. and Weg, J. G.: Pulmonary sarcoidosis: a prospective evaluation of glucocorticoid therapy. Ann. Intern. Med. 73:207–212, 1970.

106. Block, A. J., and Light, R. W.: Alternate day steroid in diffuse pulmonary sarcoidosis. Chest 63:495–500, 1973.

107. Mitchell, D. N., and Scadding, J. G.: Sarcoidosis. Am. Rev. Respir. Dis. 110:774–802, 1974.

107a. Hilton, A. M., and Chatterjee, S. S.: Bronchopulmonary aspergillosis—treatment with beclomethasone dipropionate. Postgrad. Med. 51 (Suppl. 4): 98–103, 1975.

107b. Pingleton, W. W., Hiller, F. C., Bone, R. C., Kerby, G. R. and Ruth, W. E.: Treatment of allergic aspergillosis with triamcinolone acetonide aerosol. Chest 71:782–784, 1977.

108. Slavin, R. G.: Immunologically mediated lung diseases. Postgrad Med. 59:137–141, Apr., 1976.

109. Banaszak, E. F., Thiede, W. H. and Fink, J. N.: Hypersensitivity pneumonitis due to contamination of an air conditioner. N. Engl. J. Med. 283:271–283, 1970.

110. Tourville, D. R., Weiss, W. I., Wertlake, P. T., and Leudemann, G. M.: Hypersensitivity pneumonitis due to contamination of home humidifier. J. Allergy Clin. Immunol. 49:245–251, 1971.

111. Editorial: Goodpasture's syndrome. Lancet 2: 916–917, 1970.

112. Morrison Smith, J., Clegg, R. T., Cook, N. and Butler, A. G.: Intranasal beclomethasone dipropionate in allergic rhinitis. Br. Med. J. 1:255, May, 1975.

112a. Mygind, N., Harsen, I., Pedersen, C. B., Prytz, S., and Sorensen, H.: Intranasal beclomethasone dipropionate aerosol in allergic nasal diseases. Postgrad. Med. J. 51 (Suppl. 4): 107–110, 1975.

112b. Tarlo, S. M., Cockcroft, D. W., Dolovich, J. and Hargreave, F. E.: Beclomethasone dipropionate aerosol in perennial rhinitis. J. Allergy Clin. Immunol. 59:232–236, 1977.

113. Miller, F. F.: Occurrence of nasal septal perforation with use of intranasal dexamethasone aerosol. Ann. Allergy 34:107–109, 1975.

114. Svedmyr, N., Andersson, R., Bergh, N. P., and Malmberg, R.: Relaxing effect of ACTH on human bronchial muscle *in vitro*. Scand. J. Respir. Dis. 51:171–176, 1970.

115. Siegel, S. C.: Corticosteroids and ACTH in the management of the atopic child. Pediatr. Clin. North Am. 16:287–304, 1969.

116. Editorial: Treatment of asthmatic children with steroids. Br. Med. J. 1:413–414, Feb., 1975.

117. Clark, T. J. H.: Corticosteroids. *In* Asthma. T. J.

H. Clark and S. Godfrey (Eds.). Philadelphia, W. B. Saunders Company, 1977. Ch. 15.

118. Melby, J. C.: Pituitary-adrenal function: considerations in asthma. *In* Bronchial Asthma: Mechanisms and Therapeutics. E. B. Weiss and M. S. Segal (Eds.). Boston, Little, Brown and Company, 1976. Ch. 52.

119. Kehlet, H., Blichert-Toft, M., Lindholm, J., and Rasmussen, P.: Short ACTH test in assessing hypothalamic-pituitary-adrenocortical function. Br. Med. J. 1:249–251, Jan., 1976.

120. Thorn, G. W.: Clinical considerations in the use of corticosteroids. N. Engl. J. Med. 274:775–781, 1966.

121. Harter, J. G.: Corticosteroids: their physiologic use in allergic disease. N.Y. State J. Med. 66:827–834, 1966.

122. Lowry, R. C., Mackay, J. S., Sheridan, B., and Weaver, J. A.: Intermittent-corticotrophin treatment: ventilatory tests in asthmatic subjects. Br. Med. J. 4:455–456, Nov., 1969.

123. Hugh-Jones, P., Pearson, R. S. B. and Booth, M.: Tetracosactrin for the management of asthmatic patients after long-term corticosteroids. Thorax 30:426–429, 1975.

124. Editorial: Steroid therapy and the adrenals. Lancet 2:537–538, 1975.

CHAPTER

8

CROMOLYN SODIUM

INTRODUCTION

For many centuries, the seeds of the Mediterranean plant *Ammi visnaga* have been used in medicine. An extract known as *khellin* or *visamin* has been recognized to possess smooth-muscle–relaxing properties; this drug has a long history of moderate success as a means of treating diseases such as biliary and renal colic, urethral spasm and bronchospasm. Khellin has only a mild bronchodilator action and causes too many side effects, such as nausea, to be of much value in clinical medicine. However, as often occurs in the history of pharmacotherapy, this ancient remedy was the basis for the development of an important modern drug.[1]

In the 1960's, a research team at Fisons, an English pharmaceutical company, began investigating the potential value of khellin and related agents. Khellin is the aglycone of a glycoside; it is also classified as a furanochrome. The chromone (benzopyrone) ring, which is the basic component of khellin, can be attached to another chromone ring, by an alkylene dioxy chain, to form a bischromone.

The Fisons team focussed its efforts on a series of chromone-2-carboxylic acids following the fortuitous discovery that one of these agents, when inhaled, inhibited the antigen-induced asthma of one of the researchers.[2] Eventually, one of a number of bischromones that were investigated was found to be most active as an inhibitor of allergic asthma. This agent was called *disodium cromoglycate* in England, and it was subsequently introduced into the United States under the name *cromolyn sodium*.

The drug was initially marketed in England in 1968; it was named Intal, because of its ability to interfere with allergy. The drug entered the U.S. in 1973, and is marketed as Aarane as well as Intal. Cromolyn is known as Lomudal or Inostral in many countries; it is also marketed in the United Kingdom as a nasal drug under the names Lomusol and Rynacrom.

CROMOLYN SODIUM
(Table 8–1)

Cromolyn sodium is a complex chemical with bilateral molecular symmetry, having the formula $C_{23}H_{14}Na_2O_{11}$; it is not related structurally to any other group of respiratory drugs (Figure 8–1).

Cromolyn is a white, odorless powder that leaves a slightly bitter aftertaste. Although it is hygroscopic, it is poorly soluble in water, and it is insoluble in organic solvents. The drug is not effective when given orally, and it cannot be given by any route except topical administration. Recently, a soluble preparation was introduced in the United Kingdom, but, in general, the drug must be administered as a powder by inhalation. Since the required dose is relatively large, a special turbo-inhaler was developed that enables the drug to be taken conveniently by the inhalational route.

Mode of Action

Cromolyn has a specific antiallergic effect quite different from that of any bronchodilator, although it is mainly of value as an

271

TABLE 8–1. CROMOLYN SODIUM

Chemical Structure	Bischromone structure, unrelated to any other antiasthma class of drug
Mechanism of Action	Blocks release of asthmagenic mediators from mast cell granules; may block bronchial muscle α-receptors
Effect	Prophylactic for many types of asthma; reduces dependency on glucocorticoid therapy (steroid-sparing effect)
Administration	Topical, as a powder or aqueous solution
Absorption	Less than 10% of a dose is absorbed through the lungs
Metabolism	Excreted unchanged by liver and kidneys
Side Effects	Irritation of throat; bronchospasm; skin rashes; hypersensitivity reactions (very rare)
Usual Dosage	Inhalation of contents of 1 capsule four to six times a day; dose can be reduced to 1–2 capsules a day or use as needed (e.g. before exercise) in many cases
Persistence of Effect	Major effect lasts two hours, lesser effect persists up to six hours. Some "carry-over" effect may last for several days

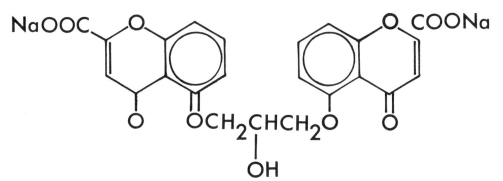

Figure 8–1. Cromolyn sodium. This drug is the disodium salt of the diabasic acid, 1,3-bis (2-carboxychromon-5-yloxy)-2-hydroxypropane. It is unrelated to any other available bronchodilator or antiasthmatic drug.

TABLE 8–2. COMPARISON OF CROMOLYN WITH GLUCOCORTICOID DRUGS

	Glucocorticoid	Cromolyn
Prevents release of mediators from mast cells	No	Yes
Potentiates cyclic 3′,5′-AMP mechanism	Yes	No
Prophylactic for Type I reactions	No	Yes
Prophylactic for Type III reactions	Yes	Yes
Interferes with Type IV reactions	Yes	No
Prevents allergic asthma	No	Yes
Prevents exercise-induced asthma	Variable	Yes
Prevents other forms of asthma	Usually	Variable
Effective in status asthmaticus	Yes	No
Success rate in all forms of asthma	90–100%	About 50%
Effective in hay fever	Yes	Yes
Effective in other diseases	Numerous	Very few
Age group achieving greatest benefit	All ages	Children (up to 70%)
Preparations available	Numerous	Only topical
Serious side effects	Numerous	Very few

"antiasthmatic."[2a] The drug has some of the same effects as glucocorticoids, in that it serves as a prophylactic antiasthma agent; however, it completely lacks any of the other glucocorticoid properties, including the adverse effects (Table 8–2). Cromolyn has no direct effect on smooth muscle, or on β-adrenergic receptors; it has no direct antagonistic activity against histamine or other mediators involved in the bronchospastic reaction.[2b] It is particularly effective in preventing Type I hypersensitivity reactions, and is somewhat less effective in inhibiting Type III reactions.[3] Cromolyn does have the ability to prevent the bronchoconstriction that can be induced by alpha-adrenergic agonists.[2a]

In vitro studies have demonstrated that cromolyn acts on the surface of the mast cells to stabilize the cell membrane and to protect it from the effects of antigen-antibody reactions that would otherwise release the mediators of bronchospasm. It is thought that cromolyn is able to prevent the calcium ion influx into mast cells that appears to trigger degranulation of cells that have been the site of antigen-antibody interaction.[4] Mast cell degranulation occurs as a consequence of cytoplasmic microfilament contraction; this phenomenon is dependent on the influx of calcium that follows the hypothesized opening of the "calcium gates" in the membrane by the antigen-antibody reaction. The protective effect of cromolyn on mast cell degranulation is not exhibited by any other antiasthma drugs, including the glucocorticoids. The probable site of action of cromolyn is illustrated in Figure 4–3.

Thus, it is believed that the main effect of cromolyn is at the level of the lung mast cells in order to prevent degranulation and the release of asthmagenic mediators. The drug may have similar effects on mast cells elsewhere (for example, the nasal mucosa), but cromolyn does not affect blood basophils or lymphocytes, and it does not interfere with hypersensitivity (Type IV reaction) skin tests. There is evidence that cromolyn inhibits cyclic 3′, 5′-AMP phosphodiesterase from several tissues, but this action is weak, and it is certainly not of significance in bronchial muscle;[5] moreover, it is arguable whether such an action occurs at all.[5a]

Cromolyn does not protect the asthmatic lung against the bronchospasm-inducing effects of inhaled histamine and similar provocative agents. However, the drug is of prophylactic value in preventing asthmatic symptoms in patients who are pretreated before exposure to an inhalational antigenic challenge.[6] The drug has been demonstrated to allow allergen and antibody combination to take place, but both the immediate and delayed mediator-induced bronchospastic reactions are prevented. In this respect, cromolyn has a more profound effect than prophylactic doses of glucocorticoids, which prevent the delayed (Type III) response rather than the immediate (Type I) response (see Table 7–2).

A further effect of cromolyn, that is not so well understood, is the ability of the drug to protect susceptible individuals from asthmatic attacks provoked by exercise[8, 8a] or hyperventilation.[9] It is possible that this property is related to its participation in the alteration of local prostaglandin release and action on small airways.[10] The drug sometimes benefits patients with intrinsic (non-allergic) asthma, but it appears that a relatively small proportion of patients with intrinsic disease respond to cromolyn.[11]

Use of Cromolyn in Asthma

Although there has been waxing and waning of enthusiasm for the use of cromolyn, the drug is clearly of major value in the prophylactic management of asthma (Table 8–3).[12] The drug is particularly effective in younger patients with extrinsic asthma, when there is known hypersensitivity to an allergen.[13–15] The prophylactic effect is manifested against both inhaled and ingested allergens of all types;[7] it is probable that the drug is more successful in allergic conditions characterized by the development of eosinophilia in the blood or the appearance of eosinophils in the mucosal secretions. The use of cromolyn has been of greatest benefit in patients who have been dependent on dangerous levels of maintenance glucocorticoid drugs, since the dosage of steroids can be reduced or discontinued in individuals who derive the full benefit of cromolyn therapy. This steroid-sparing effect of cromolyn has been reported particularly in children with severe intractable asthma.[16, 17]

Cromolyn therapy is not effective in all patients, even when there is a strong history of allergy or when the asthma has required corticosteroid therapy for control of the disease.[18] Controlled studies have shown that the drug is more effective in subjects under 17 years of age, particularly if the asthma first appeared before the age of 4.[13] The effect is less marked in patients with evidence of bronchial infection, or in those patients who have suffered more severe physiologic damage as indicated by pulmonary function evidence of chronic hyperinflation.[19] A success rate of over 80 per cent can be expected in patients with chronic perennial asthma who have an allergic history.[20] Studies of general populations of adult patients with asthma, however, suggest that only about 20 per cent show a dramatic improvement, while a further 30 per cent show a less striking benefit.[18] Certainly, the numerous reports indicate a variability in the success rate of cromolyn in different groups of patients, but perhaps 50 per cent of severe asthmatics may be expected to show some improvement with cromolyn therapy.[3] The best results may occur in those patients with labile asthma, who are difficult to control with bronchodilator drugs, and therefore require frequent courses of steroid therapy. The least success can be expected in older patients with intrinsic asthma of recent onset. However, some patients with intrinsic, nonallergic asthma do appear to benefit from cromolyn therapy, and since it cannot be predicted which asthmatic patients will respond, generous indications for a trial of the drug should be adopted. Cromolyn appears to retain its effectiveness in most patients for at least several years,[20] and tachyphylaxis has not been a problem.

Cromolyn may be of considerable value (though perhaps not as valuable as sympathomimetic bronchodilators and theophyllines) when given prophylactically to those asthmatic patients who develop bronchospasm mainly after exercise.[8, 8a, 21] The explanation for this success is uncertain, but it is of interest that another antimediator drug, diethylcarbamazine, may also be of value in the prophylaxis of exercise-induced asthma.[22, 23] (See Chapter 4.) This

TABLE 8–3. INDICATIONS IN ASTHMA FOR TRIAL OF CROMOLYN THERAPY

Youth	Children between 5 and 17
Allergy	Extrinsic asthma, with allergic history
Eosinophilia	Suggests patients may respond to therapy with cromolyn
Steroid-dependency	Marked or moderate steroid-sparing achieved with cromolyn
Intractability	Young people with chronic, intractable asthma
Long history	Asthma that started in early childhood
Exercise	Effort-dependent or post exercise asthma
Hay Fever	Asthma associated with hay fever
Occupation	Asthma caused by occupational exposure
Aspirin hypersensitivity	Asthma caused by aspirin in patients with nasal polyps
Other	May be given a trial in any type of asthma when disease is inadequately controlled by other drugs, or when there are contraindications to the use of routine bronchodilator therapy (e.g. cardiovascular or neurologic hyperirritability)

interesting property of cromolyn is being utilized in investigations into the mechanism of the curious form of asthma that is seen characteristically in children after they have carried out a period of exercise. An additional value of cromolyn is that it can prevent the asthma that is produced by aspirin in some patients with nasal polyps.[23a]

Use of Cromolyn in Other Diseases
(Table 8–4)

A few "allergic" conditions in addition to extrinsic asthma have been shown to respond to cromolyn therapy. The drug can inhibit certain delayed (Type III) reactions in the lung that characterize *allergic alveolitis* syndromes.[11] Thus, cromolyn inhalation may protect susceptible patients from the reactions implicated in aspergillosis and bird-fancier's lung. However, further studies of the value of the drug in preventing diseases such as farmer's lung are still required.

An important value of cromolyn has been clearly demonstrated in the prophylaxis of *allergic rhinitis* and other conditions that can be classified as *hay fever*.[24, 25] Nasal therapy with cromolyn may prove beneficial for many of these patients.[25a] Suitable preparations have already been marketed in Great Britain: Rynacrom is a 2 per cent solution used as a spray or as drops, while Lomusol has more recently been marketed as a metered nasal aerosol. This form of therapy is useful for children who suffer from constant nasal irritation with repetitive "colds;" these young patients are frequently noted to repeatedly rub or twitch their noses, this being a clue to the possible presence of nasal allergy. The drug may also be effective when used topically to control various types of allergic, seasonal or vernal *conjunctivitis*.

Other uses for cromolyn, or similar mast-cell stabilizing drugs, may be discovered in the future. However, present experience suggests that cromolyn has most success as an antiasthma drug, and it is not likely to prove to be of such outstanding value in other allergic diseases. It will be interesting to see if the protective benefit of cromolyn for lungs exposed to irritants which cause nonimmunologic damage (such as the alveolitis or pneumonia that results from damage secondary to various inhaled gases, chemicals, dusts, vapors and fumes) will be of practical value. Several studies have shown that cromolyn is protective against asthma induced by a variety of chemical fumes and inhalants.[7]

It is possible that cromolyn, or similar agents, may prove to be of benefit in other diseases. As an example, it has been shown that oral administration of the drug has protected infants from *gastrointestinal protein intolerance*, which causes diarrhea, vomiting and other symptoms in patients who are predisposed to this allergic syndrome.[26] More recently, studies have shown that the drug, when given orally or as an enema, can be of value in a significant proportion of patients with *ulcerative colitis*[27, 27a] or *proctitis*.[28] A recent report suggests that an ointment containing 10 per cent cromolyn is of value in the treatment of *atopic eczema* in children.[28a]

Problems with Cromolyn Use

One important factor in cromolyn therapeutics is that the drug may be able to protect the lung against only one type of asthmagenic stimulus at a time. A patient who is clearly allergic to two different allergens can be protected against one of these by prior inhalation of cromolyn; a subsequent challenge with the second allergen, during the period of protection against the initial allergen, may invoke bronchospasm unless a further inhalation of cromolyn is first administered.[4] Thus, a patient who is susceptible to multiple, varying asthmagenic stimuli may not derive adequate protection from cromolyn.

Another problem with cromolyn is that several weeks of therapy may be needed before an asthmatic patient starts to experience significant benefit. For this reason, some short-term trials have not found cromolyn to be as valuable as have longer-term trials. In the case of an individual patient who might be expected to benefit from the drug, a trial of therapy should be maintained for at least a month before conclusions on effectiveness can be drawn.

TABLE 8–4. DISEASE CONDITIONS HELPED BY PROPHYLACTIC CROMOLYN

Asthma—extrinsic (many cases)
         intrinsic (some cases)
Post-exercise bronchospasm
Allergic alveolitis
Hay fever, allergic rhinitis
Vernal conjunctivitis
Gastrointestinal protein intolerance
Ulcerative colitis
Ulcerative proctitis
Atopic eczema

Certain patients find it difficult to take the deep inhalations of the powder that are required for administration of the drug. This problem occurs particularly with children under the age of five, and in patients who are unable to understand or cooperate for any reason. Very dyspneic patients, who are unable to take deep, slow breaths, may also find it difficult to obtain adequate inhalational treatment; thus, cromolyn may not be of practical value to many patients with severe, perennial, extrinsic asthma unless the bronchospasm is first well controlled by appropriate use of bronchodilators or glucocorticoids.

Many asthmatics find that inhalation of cromolyn powder causes airway irritation, resulting in an immediate worsening of the bronchospasm, which is not only disturbing to the patient, but also prevents adequate deposition of the powder in the distal airways. For this reason, a bronchodilator should be given to such patients preceding the administration of cromolyn inhalation. A preparation is available in the United Kingdom that incorporates isoprenaline (isoproterenol) in the capsule with the cromolyn (Intal Compound).[11]

Side Effects of Cromolyn

Present evidence suggests that cromolyn is one of the most benign drugs available; it is certainly much less hazardous and has fewer annoying side effects than any other major drug used in the management of asthma. However, there are some fears that as experience with this new drug accumulates, latent toxic effects will gradually become manifest. The most significant side effects are listed in Table 8-5.

TABLE 8-5. SIDE EFFECTS OF CROMOLYN

Mechanical	Idiosyncratic*
Dry throat and mouth	Rashes (maculopapular,
Irritation of throat	urticarial)
Irritation of airways	Eosinophilic pneumonia
Coughing	Pulmonary granulomatosis
Reactive bronchospasm	Anaphylaxis
Exacerbation of status	Fever
asthmaticus	Angioedema
	Polymyositis
	Myocardiopathy

*With the exception of rashes, hypersensitivity reactions are extremely rare.

Note: Safety in pregnancy has not been established, and safety in long-term use has not yet been proved.

The main side effect is the irritation of the airways and possible bronchospasm that may be caused by the inhaled powder. Many asthmatics have very reactive airways, and the powder has a greater capacity to induce spasm in such cases than do the various other aerosol solutions used in the treatment of asthma. A minority of patients may not be willing to tolerate cromolyn because of these bronchospastic reactions; in the majority of cases, there is no significant reaction, or the spasm is minor and short-lasting. Patients who do suffer annoying bronchospasm should be advised to inhale a sympathomimetic bronchodilator, prophylactically, before taking cromolyn. Acceptance of the drug is usually enhanced if the physician encourages the patient to persist in using it for several weeks, so as to allow a fair evaluation.

Some patients, who do not necessarily develop bronchospasm after cromolyn administration, complain of pharyngeal and tracheobronchial irritation with symptoms of discomfort. In a small percentage of patients, the powder may cause annoying coughing paroxysms.[1] Such symptoms usually do not persist with repeated treatments, but occasional patients will refuse to accept cromolyn therapy because of these adverse effects. Other less specific symptoms, such as faintness, are unlikely to present serious problems; such complaints are often made by some patients even after placebo use.[12]

A small minority of patients appear to develop a hypersensitivity to cromolyn, manifested by the development of urticaria and maculopapular *rashes*.[1] The skin lesions rapidly disappear if cromolyn therapy is discontinued, and may or may not recur if the drug is reinstituted.[20] The development of *eosinophilic pneumonia* has been reported in two patients; one of these patients developed *pulmonary granulomatosis*.[29]

More disturbing has been the recent report of severe hypersensitivity responses in a group of six patients.[29] These reactions ranged from potentially fatal anaphylaxis to angioedema, polymyositis, myocardiopathy, and fever as well as pulmonary infiltrates and skin rashes. Analysis of the adverse immunologic reactions reveals that the syndromes may appear acutely or subacutely, usually after several months of continuous cromolyn therapy. These reactions are heterogeneous, and include humoral and cellular immunologic responses, with the relatively unusual finding of lymphocyte sensitization in some of the patients.[29]

TABLE 8–6. ADVANTAGES AND DISADVANTAGES OF CROMOLYN

Advantages	Disadvantages
1. May be dramatically effective as a prophylactic in some cases of asthma (particularly chronic allergic asthma in children).	1. Can be given only by topical administration.
2. Prevents exercise-induced asthma.	2. Solution for nebulization has not been established as yet.
3. May prevent some forms of occupational asthma.	3. Powder form irritates when given by inhalation.
4. Useful in other allergic diseases (especially hay fever).	4. Young, uncoordinated or very obstructed patients find it difficult to use Spinhaler.
5. Absence of glucocorticoid side effects.	5. Success rate in asthma is very variable and unpredictable.
6. Major side effects are rare.	6. Cromolyn is not a bronchodilator and is contraindicated in acute bronchospasm; it does not potentiate other bronchodilators.
7. Steroid-sparing effect in asthma.	7. Patients who had been on steroids may need to be restarted on steroids if an asthmatic exacerbation or intercurrent stress occurs.
8. No evidence of tachyphylaxis.	8. Several weeks of use may be required to evaluate effectiveness in any patient.
9. Use of aqueous solution forms of cromolyn will extend its acceptability (e.g., preparation can be given by nebulizer).	9. Long-term potential for toxicity is unknown.
10. The drug is safer than sympathomimetics, theophyllines or steroids for use in patients whose compliance is questionable.	10. Both the drug and the dispensing Spinhaler are relatively expensive.
	11. Efficacy is limited by difficulties in patients' compliance, and their acceptance of the drug and the inhalational technique required.

Note: Inhalational steroids may prove to be more satisfactory than cromolyn in many patients.

Fortunately, the incidence of side effects is rare; and though the impression has developed that cromolyn is safe in the vast majority of patients,[13] one must expect, as with all generally acceptable drugs, frequent minor and occasional serious problems. One fear had been that cromolyn might cause renal lesions, since a proliferative arterial lesion, mainly affecting the kidney, appeared in some monkeys tested with cromolyn. However, no evidence of a similar lesion has appeared in human subjects exposed to the drug, and the possibility of such an adverse reaction has been discounted. Several other toxic effects have been described in individual animal species (for example, hypotensive response in dogs following intravenous cromolyn), but none have been shown to occur in humans.[1]

Although serious side effects are rare, there are still enough problems associated with cromolyn use to force the conclusion that this drug is far from an ideal preventative of asthma. Unfortunately, the disadvantages of the drug more than counterbalance the undoubted advantages (Table 8–6).

Administration of Cromolyn

At present, cromolyn is made available world wide as a powder for inhalation or insufflation. Although the powder has only limited solubility and the solution is relatively viscous, it has nevertheless been given by aerosolization using an air-compressor nebulizer.[30] Very recently, Fisons in England released a nebulizer solution containing 20 mg cromolyn in a 2 ml aqueous solution.[31] This is particularly suitable for the treatment of infants and for very obstructed asthmatics who are unable to use the turbo-inhaler mechanism.

Cromolyn sodium is marketed as a micronized particle preparation for inhalation. More than 50 per cent of these particles are between 2 and 6 μ in size. These micronized particles are too fine to flow well in an airstream, and for that reason cromolyn is combined with lactose powder. The lactose contains a high percentage of particles between 30 and 60 μ in size; these coarse particles markedly improve the flow properties of the blend. Thus, lactose acts as an excipient, that is, an inert additive used to improve qualities of a preparation to permit more effective delivery to the tissues.

Cromolyn is available commercially packaged in gelatin capsules that contain 20 mg of the drug and an equal amount of lactose; the marketed products Aarane and Intal are identical. The powder blend is administered by means of a special turbo-inhaler (Spinhaler); the capsule is inserted in this device and two perforations are made by a simple mechanism. The patient inhales through the mouthpiece, and a plastic propeller-like rotor is thereby activated and causes the pierced capsule to undergo turbulent vibratory rotation. The powder is thus "fluidized," and is sucked out into the airstream, to enter the respiratory tract in the form of a finely particulate aerosol. The micronized particles of cromolyn reach the more peripheral airways, whereas the larger lactose particles are deposited mainly in the oropharynx and the trachea. These particles of lactose probably account for much of the irritation that many patients experience when they inhale Aarane or Intal.

The patient must be instructed to take several maximal inhalations in order to obtain as much of the powder from the capsule as possible. For initiation of cromolyn therapy, it is important that a respiratory therapist or some other competent individual instruct the patient and the family to follow the administering details enclosed in the package of the commercial product. The patient should demonstrate his or her technique initially and at a follow-up visit; dummy demonstration models are available for patients to practice on in a clinic or physician's office.

It should be realized that less than 10 per cent of the cromolyn (less than 2 mg) is actually retained in the respiratory tract. Much of the drug is swallowed, but little (less than 1 per cent) absorption occurs from the gastrointestinal tract. The drug deposited in the lung is absorbed into the blood stream, and is completely excreted in the bile and the urine within four hours. Since hepatic and renal clearance is required for elimination of cromolyn, reduced dosage may be advisable in patients with liver and kidney insufficiency. Unfortunately, cromolyn does not appear to be effective when given by any other route; indeed, it is hazardous to give a solution of the drug intravenously. At present in the U.S., the drug is not approved for administration except by means of a Spinhaler, but it is probable that solutions suitable for other forms of nebulization (for example, by using IPPB) will become available.

TABLE 8–7. RECOMMENDATIONS FOR USE OF CROMOLYN IN ASTHMA

Patient Selection
Patients dependent on more than 10 mg a day of prednisone
Younger patients with completely reversible bronchospasm who are poorly controlled by routine bronchodilators
Patients who suffer periodic, predictable bronchospasm when exposed to allergens or industrial irritants
Patients who develop post-exercise asthma.

Technique of Use of Capsules
Patient or family member must be taught how to use and maintain Spinhaler. In most patients, preliminary prophylactic use of an aerosol bronchodilator is advisable.
Patient must use correct technique, with several vital capacity inhalations, to breathe contents of capsule.
Throat should be rinsed or a candy sucked if pharyngeal irritation is produced.

Introduction of Cromolyn Therapy
PATIENT ON GLUCOCORTICOID THERAPY
Steroid-dependent patient should commence with cromolyn capsule inhalations 4–6 times a day, depending on severity of disease.
Four weeks of therapy are advisable to allow full benefits of cromolyn to appear, using 4–6 capsules a day.
If benefit appears, steroid reduction should be started, decreasing the dose by 10% a week.
If patient does well, cromolyn dosage may be reduced to one or two capsules a day.
Exacerbation of asthma or development of a stress situation will require the reinstitution of steroid therapy; cromolyn therapy may need to be abandoned temporarily.

PATIENT NOT REQUIRING GLUCOCORTICOID THERAPY
Occasional use of cromolyn as needed may be better than daily therapy (e.g., 1 capsule prior to exercise or prior to exposure to an occupational asthmagenic stimulus).

General
Routine bronchodilator therapy should be maintained.
Aerosol glucocorticoid therapy may prove to be more suitable for individual patients.
Cromolyn solublized in aqueous solution may be suitable for nebulization with air-compressor or by IPPB for very young, disabled or very obstructed patient.

Dosage and Recommendations
(Table 8–7)

The current recommendation is that adults and children should be started on a dosage regimen of one capsule of one of the available cromolyn preparations inhaled four times a day at spaced intervals. In more unstable cases, it may be advisable to initiate the drug with five to six administrations a day until an improvement appears, at which time the frequency can be reduced.[31] Correct technique must be utilized; if the inhaled drug causes bronchial irritation or wheezing, this can be treated by a routine bronchodilator. Subsequent administrations of cromolyn should be preceded by a prophylactic puff of a sympathomimetic aerosol. If oropharyngeal irritation occurs, this may be relieved by a drink of water, by sucking a candy or by gargling.

A definite impression of the prophylactic success of cromolyn is usually noted within a few days, but in some patients it may take up to one month before the effect becomes apparent.[12] In patients for whom cromolyn is most definitely indicated (for example, children who are steroid-dependent), encouragement to persist with the drug will be required if an early benefit is not noted. However, there are patients who never develop an adequate response, and there are many who develop a lasting antipathy to the drug. It is virtually impossible to persuade some patients to continue taking cromolyn for a full month's trial if an initial benefit does not occur, and it is rarely worth persisting with an unsuccessful trial for longer than a month.

If a response to cromolyn is noted, a patient on corticosteroid maintenance therapy should be gradually weaned, usually by decreasing the glucocorticoid dosage by about 10 per cent a week.[31] It is sometimes possible to entirely withdraw the steroid, but in other cases only a reduction in dosage can be attained. Nevertheless, it is a great benefit to reduce prednisone therapy to a daily dose of less than 10 mg; the steroid-sparing effect of cromolyn can help achieve this reduction. Some patients find that after the first few weeks they can safely reduce the daily dosage of cromolyn also, and such patients are able to retain control of the asthma with only one or two capsules a day. If sufficient improvement occurs, it may be possible to discontinue cromolyn therapy; the drug can be reinstituted later if the disease relapses.

It is a serious error to try to wean an asthmatic patient from other routine bronchodilator drugs when the patient is stabilized on cromolyn. In most patients, aerosol, or oral, sympathomimetics and theophylline derivatives provide safe and reliable bronchodilator therapy, which is of prophylactic value also. Moreover, these established agents are usually less expensive than cromolyn and their dosages can be increased if necessary to help treat an exacerbation of bronchospasm. Cromolyn is expensive, it is not a bronchodilator, and its long-term potential for toxicity remains unknown; therefore, it cannot be regarded as a primary drug in the management of asthma.

An important caution for patients who use maintenance cromolyn therapy is to realize that cromolyn is neither a bronchodilator nor a corticosteroid. Asthmatic patients who have used steroid therapy in the past will often need to restart steroids when they develop an intercurrent illness or stress while on cromolyn therapy. In some cases, increasing the cromolyn can be helpful when bronchospasm becomes exacerbated, but routine bronchodilators or steroids are often needed in such circumstances. If cromolyn therapy is stopped for any reason, steroids will often have to be reinstituted.

Cromolyn is available in Europe for the treatment of nasal allergies. A special dispenser of the powder is marketed, and the patient insufflates the powder into the nose. Although this preparation (Rynacrom) is not available in the U.S., it is possible that the Spinhaler could be used by an adept patient to treat the nasal mucosa. At present, no definite recommendations can be offered; in the future, an aqueous solution (comparable to the British product Lomusol) might be marketed.

Thus, cromolyn is a fascinating drug that can be remarkably successful in the prophylactic management of asthma (see summary in Table 8–7). It should be tried on all asthmatics who are poorly controlled by other modalities, especially by those who have difficulty tolerating other drugs. The drug can also be recommended for prophylactic use, as required, in patients who develop bronchospasm after exercising: one capsule used before the exercise may provide very effective protection.[10] Indeed, cromolyn appears to be as effective as theophylline, but neither drug is as effective as salbutamol when given in appropriate dosage to prevent exercise-induced asthma.[32] Cromolyn should be tried particularly in children who are steroid dependent in an attempt to reduce the dosage requirements of the steroid. However, the advent of the safer inhalational steroids may decrease the indications for cromolyn. Moreover, the expense and other problems associated with cromolyn militate against recommending the drug for all patients on steroids. Thus, if a patient is able to control asthma on less than 10 mg of prednisone a day without any side effects, there is little justification for introducing cromolyn therapy (cf. Tables 7–26, 7–29).

As greater experience evolves, it is probable that the familiar cromolyn products and the turbo-dispenser will rapidly become obsolete. Newer drugs that can inhibit mediator-induced bronchospasm will undoubtedly appear; at present, at least two oral agents, *AH 7725* and *doxantrazole,* have shown promise in preliminary investigations.[33, 33a, 34] Other drugs with similar actions include *bufrolin* (ICI 74,917) and *M & B 22,948.* All these agents appear to exert their antiallergic effects by blocking the antigen-induced transport of calcium.[34]

Undoubtedly, cromolyn is certain to be compared with the newer inhalational steroids, which may be as safe, as effective and as well tolerated as the various preparations of cromolyn. The future of cromolyn is thus obscure, although it is likely to be displaced either by inhalational steroids or by an innovative oral drug (such as AH 7725) that similarly inhibits mast-cell degranulation, or by a combination of these two alternatives. At present, however, cromolyn continues to receive favorable long-term reports,[35] and it must be regarded as a major therapeutic advance in the management of many asthmatic patients, regardless of whether the disease appears to be intrinsic or extrinsic.

REFERENCES

1. Intal (Cromolyn Sodium-Fisons), A Monograph. Bedford, Mass. Fisons Corporation, 1973.
2. Boorer, D.: The men who created Intal. Nurs. Times 67:890–891, 1971.
2a. Cox, J. C. G.: Disodium cromoglycate (cromolyn sodium) in bronchial asthma. *In* Bronchial Asthma: Mechanisms and Therapeutics, E. B. Weiss and M. S. Segal (Eds.). Boston, Little, Brown and Company, 1976. Ch. 56.
2b. Ryo, U. Y., Kang, B. and Townley, R. G.: Cromolyn therapy in patients with bronchial asthma. J.A.M.A. 236:927–931, 1976
3. Editorial. Disodium cromoglycate. Lancet 2:1299, 1972.
4. Townley, R. G.: Pharmacologic blocks to mediator release: clinical applications. Advances in Asthma and Allergy 2:7–16, Fall, 1975. (Published by Fisons Corporation, Bedford, Mass.).
5. Assem, E. S. K.: Inhibition of the release of mediators of immediate-type allergy *in vivo* and *in vitro.* Proc. R. Soc. Med. 66:1191–1198, 1973.
5a. Vardey, C. J. and Skidmore, I. F.: Mechanism of action of antiallergic drugs. Br. Med. J. 2:396, Aug., 1976.
6. Cox, J. S. G., Beach, J. E., Blair, A. M. J. N., et al: Disodium cromoglycate (Intal). Adv. Drug Res. 5:115–196, 1970.
7. Pepys, J.: Disodium cromoglycate in clinical and experimental asthma. *In* Asthma – Physiology, Immunopharmacology, and Treatment. K. F. Austen and L. M. Lichtenstein (Eds.). New York, Academic Press, 1973. Ch. 18.
8. Poppius, H., Muittari, A., Kreus, K. E., et al: Exercise asthma and disodium cromoglycate. Br. Med. J. 4:337–339, Nov., 1970.
8a. Chan-Yeung, M.: The effect of Sch 1000 and disodium cromoglycate on exercise-induced asthma. Chest 71:320–323, 1977.
9. Clarke, P. S.: Effect of disodium cromoglycate on exacerbations of asthma produced by hyperventilation. Br. Med. J. 1:317–319, Feb., 1971.
10. Rebuck, A. S.: Antiasthmatic drugs I: Pathophysiological and clinical pharmacological aspects. Drugs 7:344–369, 1974.
11. Anonymous: Disodium cromoglycate in allergic respiratory disease. Br. Med. J. 2:159–161, Apr., 1972.
12. Dykes, M. H. M.: Evaluation of an antiasthmatic agent cromolyn sodium (Aarane, Intal). J.A.M.A. 227:1061–1062, 1974.
13. Bernstein, I. L., Siegel, S. C., Brandon, M. L., et al: A controlled study of cromolyn sodium sponsored by the drug committee of the American Academy of Allergy. J. Allergy Clin. Immunol. 50:235–245, 1972.
14. Bruderman, I.: Cromolyn therapy. *In* New Directions In Asthma. M. Stein (Ed.). Park Ridge, Ill., American College of Physicians, 1975. Ch. 27.
15. Molk, L.: Blocking of induced asthma by cromolyn sodium. Ann. Allergy 30:321–325, 1972.
16. Chai, H., Molk, L., Falliers, C. J. and Miklich, D.: Steroid-sparing effects of disodium cromoglycate (DSC) in children with severe chronic asthma. Excerpta Medica Int. Cong. Series 232, pp. 385–391, Proc. VII Int. Cong. Allerg., Florence, Oct. 12–17, 1970.
17. Read, J. and Rebuck, A. S.: Steroid-sparing effect of disodium cromoglycate ("Intal") in chronic asthma. Med. J. Aust. 1:566–569, 1969.
18. Hyde, J. S.: Cromolyn prophylaxis for chronic asthma. Ann. Intern. Med. 78:966, 1973.
19. Burgher, L. W., Elliott, R. M. and Kass, I.: A perspective on the role of cromolyn sodium as an antiasthmatic agent. Chest 60:210–213, 1971.
20. Crisp, J., Ostrander, C., Giannini, A. et al: Cromolyn sodium therapy for chronic perennial asthma. (A double-blind study of 40 children). J.A.M.A. 229:787–789, 1974.

21. Patel, K. R., Kerr, J. W., MacDonald, E. B. and MacKenzie, A. M.: The effect of thymoxamine and cromolyn sodium on postexercise bronchoconstriction in asthma. J. Allergy Clin. Immunol. 57:285–292, 1976.

22. Orange, R. P. and Austen, K. F.: Guest Editorial—Prospects in asthma therapy: disodium cromoglycate and diethylcarbamazine. N. Engl. J. Med. 279:1055–1056, 1968.

23. Sly, R. M. and Matzen, K.: Effect of diethylcarbamazine pamoate upon exercise-induced obstruction in asthmatic children. Ann. Allergy 33:138–144, 1974.

23a. Gwin, E., Kerby, G. R. and Ruth, W. E.: Cromolyn sodium in the treatment of asthma associated with aspirin hypersensitivity and nasal polyps. Chest 72:148–154, 1977.

24. Capel, L. H. and McKelvie, P.: Disodium cromoglycate in hay fever. Lancet 1:575, 1971.

25. Glazer, I. and Leventon, G.: Topical treatment of hay fever with disodium cromoglycate (DSCG) solution. Int. Arch. Allergy Appl. Immunol. 49:125–128, 1975.

25a. Handelman, N. I., Friday, G. A., Schwartz, H. J. et al: Cromolyn sodium nasal solution in the prophylactic treatment of pollen-induced seasonal allergic rhinitis. J. Allergy Clin. Immunol. 59:237–242, 1977.

26. Frier, S., and Berger, H.: Disodium cromoglycate in gastrointestinal protein intolerance. Lancet 1:913–915, 1973.

27. Mani, V., Lloyd, G., Green, F. H. Y. et al: Treatment of ulcerative colitis with oral disodium cromoglycate. Lancet 1:439–441, 1976.

27a. Cella, G. D., Garibaldi, L. R. and Durand, P.: Ulcerative colitis and disodium cromoglycate. Lancet 1:1129, 1976.

28. Editorial: New treatment for ulcerative colitis? Br. Med. J. 1:2, Jan., 1976.

28a. Haider, S. A.: Treatment of atopic eczema in children: clinical trial of 10% sodium cromoglycate ointment. Br. Med. J. 1:1570–1572, 1977.

29. Sheffer, A. L., Rocklin, R. E. and Goetzl, E. J.: Immunologic components of hypersensitivity reaction to cromolyn sodium. N. Engl. J. Med. 293:1220–1224, 1975.

30. Williams, H. E. and Phelan, P. D.: Administration of disodium cromoglycate to young children. Br. Med. J. 2:488, May, 1973.

31. Advertisement. Thorax 31: pages v-vi, Apr., 1976.

32. Godfrey, S. and Konig, P.: Inhibition of exercise-induced asthma by different pharmacological pathways. Thorax 31:137–143, 1976.

33. Assem, E. S. K., Evans, J. A. and McAllen, M.: Inhibition of experimental asthma in man by a new drug (AH 7725) active when given by mouth. Br. Med. J. 2:93–95, Apr., 1974.

33a. Batchelor, J. F., Follenfant, M. J., Garland, L. G. et al: Doxantrazole, an antiallergic agent orally effective in man. Lancet 1:1169–1170, 1975.

34. Foreman, J. C. and Garland, L. G.: Cromoglycate and other antiallergic drugs: a possible mechanism of action. Br. Med. J. 1:820–821, Apr., 1976.

35. Grant, I. W. B., Turner-Warwick, M., Fox, W. et al: Sodium cromoglycate in chronic asthma. Br. Med. J. 1:361–364, Feb., 1976.

CHAPTER
9
MEDICATIONS FOR COUGHS AND COLDS

COUGHS

THE COUGH MECHANISM

The cough is a reflex respiratory maneuver, which, unlike the sneeze, can be considerably modified or controlled by voluntary effort. The airways and lung parenchyma are richly supplied by a variety of receptors, whose stimulation results in reflex modifying effects on respiration; some of these receptors play a major role in the cough mechanism. At present, there is still much confusion as to the specific receptors involved in the cough. The competing experiments and theories in the literature demonstrate the complexity of the cough mechanism, but fail to provide a clear explanation of the components involved.

Respiration is controlled by reflexes arising from the nose, larynx, trachea, lung epithelium and alveoli as well as from extrapulmonary receptors; it is probable that sufficient stimulation of any of the receptors involved can affect the cough mechanism. Three types of pulmonary vagal sensory reflexes involving three different pulmonary receptors can be identified:[1] (1) the slowly-adapting stretch receptors, which are involved in the Hering-Breuer inflation reflex and which mediate bronchodilation; (2) the rapidly adapting irritant receptors, which

control bronchoconstriction and expiratory constriction of the larynx, and which mediate hyperpnea; and (3) the Type-J receptors, whose stimulation results in rapid, shallow breathing and severe expiratory constriction of the larynx. There is agreement that the irritant receptors, whose supplying nerve fibers ramify in the airway epithelium, are of major importance in the cough reflex,[2] but there is no uniformity in concept on whether there is more than one type of irritant receptor.

Salem and Aviado[3] have postulated that there are two types of irritant receptors: *mechanoreceptors,* which are located mainly in the larynx, the lower trachea and the carina; and *chemoreceptors,* which are more abundant in the bronchioles and pulmonary parenchyma. Mechanical stimuli (such as coarse particles, foreign bodies, and instrumentation) or chemical stimuli (such as inhalations of irritating aerosols of citric acid or ammonia, or of bronchoconstrictor agents, including histamine and acetylcholine) can produce a cough; these stimuli can also cause bronchospasm. Salem and Aviado suggest that the prime event is bronchoconstriction (either by direct irritation or through a pulmonary reflex or by means of released humoral agents such as SRS-A), and that the contracting muscle fibers secondarily stimulate cough receptors in the

282

airways. This theory has not been proved, and since epithelial irritant receptors can still respond when bronchoconstriction is blocked by drugs such as isoproterenol,[2] there is good reason to doubt that the bronchoconstrictor theory is applicable in all cases of induced cough. Nevertheless, whatever the actual mechanism, stimulation of airway receptors constitutes the peripheral event in the pathogenesis of most forms of cough (Table 9–1).

The afferent nerve fibers that supply the cough receptors eventually enter into one of three major nerve trunks: the vagus nerve, the recurrent laryngeal nerve and the glossopharyngeal nerve. These nerves supply the cough center in the hindbrain. This center is probably located in the dorsolateral area of the medulla and in the descending vestibular and solitary tracts and their nuclei;[3] scattered areas in the medullary and pontine dorsolateral reticular formation also appear to subserve the brain's cough controlling center.[4, 5] The cough center consists of a coordinating neuronal network in close conjunction with the respiratory center and the

vomiting center;[5] it can be postulated that a "mucokinetic" center is also located in the same area of the hindbrain. Violent coughing interferes with normal respiration and can result in both vomiting and increased expectoration, presumably because the respective centers are secondarily activated by the discharge from the cough center.

The production of a cough involves a finely coordinated series of events that is based on the subservience of the respiratory center to the drive imposed by the cough center (see Table 9–1). Usually, the act is initiated by an inspiration that interrupts the regular respiratory rhythm. Next, the muscles of the thorax and abdomen rapidly contract, and compress the diaphragm against the lungs: the intrathoracic pressure usually increases to between 50 and 100 mm Hg, but can rise as high as 300 mm Hg.[3] During this phase, the larynx is kept closed and the gas in the trachea and airways is compressed. The high intrathoracic pressure narrows the pliable trachea to as little as 16 per cent of its normal cross-sectional area;[6] compression of the more peripheral airways

TABLE 9–1. COUGH MECHANISM

Components	Location	Comments
IRRITANT RECEPTORS		
Chemoreceptors	Mainly in bronchioles and pulmonary parenchyma	Stimulated by chemicals such as ammonia and citric acid, and by asthmagenic mediators such as histamine
Mechanoreceptors	Mainly in upper airways, trachea and carina	Stimulated by inert dusts and foreign bodies, and by sudden severe mechanical changes in their condition
AFFERENT NERVES		
Vagal (Xth nerve)	From superior laryngeal nerves and vagal roots	Afferents terminate at nuclei in medulla
Glossopharyngeal (IXth nerve)	From pharynx and carotid body	Afferents terminate at nuclei in medulla
CENTRAL CONNECTIONS		
Cough center	Dorsolateral region of medulla oblongata; pontine components exist	Interconnects with respiratory and vomiting centers and with cerebrum
Respiratory centers	Throughout the reticular formation of the medulla and pons	Rich afferent connections; control autonomic and somatic efferents
Associated connections	Cerebral centers	Involved in voluntary and psychogenic coughing
PERIPHERAL NERVES		
Phrenic nerve (C3–5)	Supplies diaphragm	Mainly involved in inspiratory phase of coughing
Recurrent branch of vagus (Xth)	Supplies glottic muscles	Glottic valve required for effective cough
T1–11 (intercostal) nerves	Supply intercostal muscles	Contract strongly during coughing
T6–L1 nerves	Supply abdominal muscles	Contract strongly during coughing

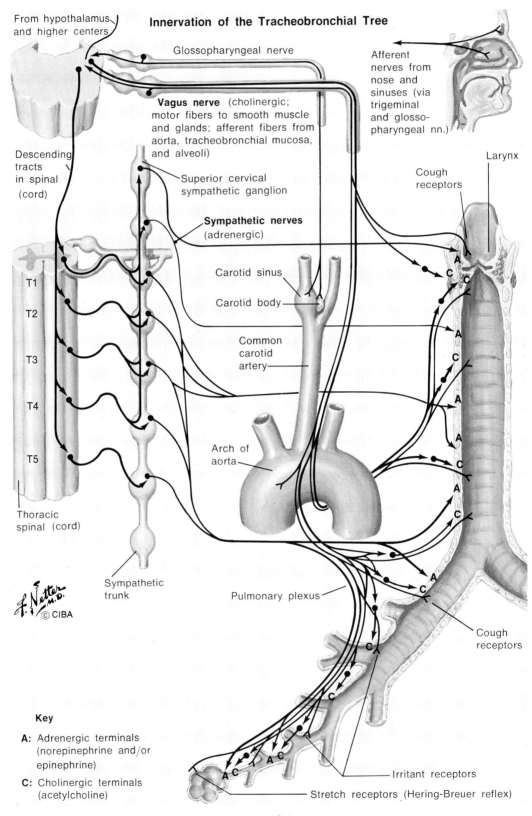

Innervation of the Tracheobronchial Tree

From hypothalamus and higher centers

Glossopharyngeal nerve

Afferent nerves from nose and sinuses (via trigeminal and glosso-pharyngeal nn.)

Vagus nerve (cholinergic; motor fibers to smooth muscle and glands; afferent fibers from aorta, tracheobronchial mucosa, and alveoli)

Descending tracts in spinal (cord)

Superior cervical sympathetic ganglion

Larynx

Cough receptors

Sympathetic nerves (adrenergic)

T1

Carotid sinus

Carotid body

T2

T3

Common carotid artery

T4

T5

Arch of aorta

Thoracic spinal (cord)

Sympathetic trunk

Pulmonary plexus

Cough receptors

Key

A: Adrenergic terminals (norepinephrine and/or epinephrine)

C: Cholinergic terminals (acetylcholine)

Irritant receptors

Stretch receptors (Hering-Breuer reflex)

Figure 9–1.

also results, and a cranially directed peristaltic wave may be stimulated in the muscular bronchi and bronchioles. Finally, when the intrathoracic pressure exceeds 100 mm Hg, the glottis suddenly opens, as the laryngeal muscles relax, and the compressed air blasts out with a velocity that can approach 500 miles per hour;[3] in fact, the tussive blast may reach 85 per cent of the speed of sound.[7] The cough may expel air at the rate of up to 6.5 l per second[3] through the narrowed airways, and this airflow can carry out mucus and foreign bodies from the middle and central airways, and may expel

them up to 12 to 15 feet beyond the mouth.

An effective reflex cough obviously requires an intact peripheral nerve supply to the abdomen, thoracic muscles, diaphragm and glottis, and the muscles of these organs must be in functioning order (Figure 9–2). The cough of a patient will be severely impaired if any component in the reflex arc is inhibited, depressed or malfunctioning. Thus, anesthesia impairs the function of the peripheral receptors, coma impairs the cough center, while paralysis, pain or weakness will prevent the effective coordinated muscular activity required in coughing. Patients with

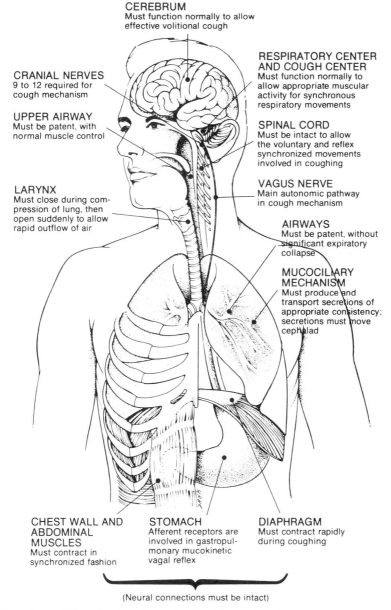

CEREBRUM
Must function normally to allow effective volitional cough

RESPIRATORY CENTER AND COUGH CENTER
Must function normally to allow appropriate muscular activity for synchronous respiratory movements

CRANIAL NERVES
9 to 12 required for cough mechanism

UPPER AIRWAY
Must be patent, with normal muscle control

SPINAL CORD
Must be intact to allow the voluntary and reflex synchronized movements involved in coughing

LARYNX
Must close during compression of lung, then open suddenly to allow rapid outflow of air

VAGUS NERVE
Main autonomic pathway in cough mechanism

AIRWAYS
Must be patent, without significant expiratory collapse

MUCOCILIARY MECHANISM
Must produce and transport secretions of appropriate consistency; secretions must move cephalad

CHEST WALL AND ABDOMINAL MUSCLES
Must contract in synchronized fashion

STOMACH
Afferent receptors are involved in gastropulmonary mucokinetic vagal reflex

DIAPHRAGM
Must contract rapidly during coughing

(Neural connections must be intact)

Figure 9–2. Interrelation of various factors involved in cough and expectoration. (After Ziment.)

obstructive respiratory disorders may possess intact afferent and efferent components, but may be unable to cough effectively because the narrowed airways do not permit an adequate velocity of airflow to be generated. Finally, glottic paralysis or intubation will interfere with the build-up of intrathoracic pressure that is required preceding the tussive blast.

ABNORMALITIES OF COUGH

The normal cough reflex is an everyday event in everyone, but frequent, symptomatic or annoying coughing is abnormal. Therapeutic intervention may be required when a patient is troubled by any type of inordinate or disturbing cough. In contrast, therapy may also be required if a patient, who is retaining secretions or a foreign body, fails to cough frequently or adequately. In some cases, the secondary complications of coughing may bring the patient to seek help; examples of such problems are poor sleep, headaches, syncope, fractured rib and other types of chest, back or abdominal pain.

There are more prescription products available for treatment of cough than for any other symptom;[8] enormous numbers of patients seek therapy for relatively minor temporary coughs, such as those self-limiting coughs that accompany colds. The huge number of prescriptions given for "cough medications" attest to the belief that physicians have in the efficacy of these drugs. Similarly, the amazing number of proprietary cough medications (over 600 in the U.S.[3, 9]) many of which are bought over the counter, demonstrate how anxiously the public attempts to cope with the problem of coughing. In contrast, there are enormous numbers of stoic individuals who casually dismiss their obviously pathologic coughs with the explanation that it is only (sic) a cigarette cough! Marked adaptation to a cough can occur, so that the patient may be unaware of the severity of the condition, although his companions may be all too conscious of it.

Patients, physicians and pharmacists actually have to cope with a sophisticated pharmacologic problem when trying to make an appropriate choice of a "cough medicine." These medications usually contain a mixture of ingredients with the following pharmacologic properties: antitussives, expectorants (mucokinetics), demulcents, antihistamines, mucosal constrictants, analgesics, anesthetics, flavoring agents and placebos. It is frequently impossible to find a rational basis for the use of some of the more exuberant concoctions that are compounded into proprietary preparations. The drug store pharmacist should be very wary of recommending a "cough medicine," since he will have to indulge in sophisticated diagnostic evaluation of a complex symptom before he can make an appropriate suggestion to a patient seeking treatment for a cough. In Table 9–2, a number of the more important

TABLE 9–2. MANAGEMENT OF COMMON TYPES OF COUGH

Type of Cough	Synonyms	Causes	Usual Treatment				
			PERIPHERAL ANTITUSSIVE	CENTRAL ANTITUSSIVE	PHYSICAL THERAPY	INTUBATION	SPECIFIC THERAPY
Ineffective	Dry, hacking, racking, irritating	1) Inflammation	+	Maybe			Soothing mist
		2) Irritants	+	+			Correct environment
		3) Tumors		+			Surgical removal
		4) Psychogenic		+			Psychotherapy
Inadequate	Nonproductive, loose, diminished	1) Weakness, debility			+	+	General support
		2) Pain		Maybe			Analgesia
		3) Poor motivation			+	Maybe	Central stimulants
Productive	Coughing with spitting	1) Infection (mainly bacterial)	+	Maybe	+		Antimicrobials
		2) Bronchorrhea		Maybe	Maybe		Depends on cause
		3) COPD	+	Maybe	+	Maybe	Bronchodilators, etc.
		4) Bronchiectasis	+	Maybe	+		Consider surgery
Complicated	Secondary	1) Bleeding (hemoptysis)	Maybe	Maybe		Maybe	Consider surgery
		2) Heart failure		+			Cardiotonic therapy
		3) Sinusitis, post-nasal drip	+	+			Mucosal constrictors
		4) Foreign body			+	+	Bronchoscopy

types of cough are classified, and appropriate general and specific treatments are suggested for consideration in the management of such coughs. The variety of problems and the range of choices involved in the selection of therapy for a cough necessitate careful analysis of the possible etiologic factors before a course of treatment can be embarked upon.[10]

The etiology of coughing includes abnormalities of both pulmonary and extrapulmonary origin.[9] Vagal and glossopharyngeal receptors can be stimulated by mechanical or chemical abnormalities in the upper airways or trachea, or lower airways and pulmonary parenchyma. Vagal stimulation can also be produced by irritation of the chest wall, pleura, diaphragm and pericardium; coughing (often accompanied by pain) may occur with diseases of these contiguous organs. The auricular branch of the vagal nerve supplies the external auditory canal, and irritation of the ear can result in coughing. Gastric irritation and abdominal distention are other causes of vagal stimulation that may be responsible for inducing a cough.[11, 12] In addition to these peripheral causes of coughing, central factors, usually of a psychogenic nature, can cause coughing; many people have a "nervous" cough, which they may attribute to a tickling sensation in the throat or more distal airways. Many other causes of coughing have been listed.[3] Thus, the search for the explanation of a cough may have to be extremely wide-ranging (see Table 9-3).

When a patient complains of a persistent cough, an attempt should be made to elucidate and then eradicate the cause. In many cases, this can eventually be achieved, but until the etiologic correction is made, symptomatic treatment of the cough may be required. When the etiology is thought to be transient, as with a viral upper respiratory tract infection, it may be reasonable to do nothing about the cough, since it will probably clear up within a short time without specific therapy. However, a cough suppressant may be useful, particularly for nocturnal use, if the cough interferes with sleep. If the cough produces sputum, it is generally advisable to avoid suppressing it, since retention of the secretions may lead to a worsening of the pulmonary status. However, if the coughing is out of proportion to the resulting expectoration, some suppressive therapy may be indicated. Whenever a patient seeks therapy for a cough, the benefits and hazards of prescribing antitussive therapy must be weighed. If antitussive drugs are thought to be unsuitable for an individual patient's cough, alternative alleviating therapy can usually be provided. There is always a process of diagnostic evaluation required in cough therapy, following which a thoughtful course of management can be instituted.

TABLE 9-3. STIMULI THAT CAUSE COUGHING

CENTRAL
　Psychogenic: anxiety, habit, tic

MAJOR AIRWAYS
　Irritation: foreign bodies, noxious vapors, chemicals, dusts
　Inflammation: pharyngitis, laryngitis, tracheitis, bronchitis
　Neoplasms: benign tumors, malignancies
　Extrinsic compression: lymphadenopathy, tumors, aneurysms, enlarged left atrium
　Allergy: asthma, anaphylaxis

PULMONARY PARENCHYMA
　Inflammation: bronchiolitis, alveolitides, pneumonias
　Vascular: pulmonary emboli, intravenous irritants, cardiac failure
　Lung disease: cystic fibrosis, bronchiectasis, tuberculosis, pertussis, measles

NONPULMONARY
　Stimulation of auricular branch of vagus nerve
　Irritation of pleura, diaphragm or pericardium
　Gastrointestinal disease: dyspepsia, abdominal distension
　Sinusitis, postnasal drip
　Elongated uvula, adenoids
　Esophageal disease, including fistula into trachea, aspiration

ANTITUSSIVE THERAPY

Most patients who seek treatment for a cough will require one or another form of antitussive therapy. Theoretically, the cough can be blocked at several different points in the reflex pathway:[3, 9] (1) peripherally, either by correcting the irritation or by blocking the receptors; (2) along the afferent arc, by blocking vagal or glossopharyngeal transmission to the hindbrain; (3) centrally, by increasing the threshold of the cough center; and (4) along the efferent arc, by blocking the activation of the expiratory muscles involved in coughing.[3] In general, antitussive measures are directed at points (1) and (3), and only in extremely rare circumstances would attempts be made to block transmission along the afferent or efferent nerves involved in the cough reflex.[10] Thus, most antitussive drugs are either peripherally-acting or centrally-acting.[11]

Adjuvant therapy for patients with coughs often ameliorates the process adequately, and thereby renders specific antitussive therapy superfluous. Adjuvant therapy includes treatment with mucokinetics (discussed in Chapters 2 and 3), bronchodilators (discussed in Chapters 3, 4 and 5), antibiotics, sedatives, analgesics and other agents. Because many proprietary "cough medicines" attempt to provide a polypharmaceutic approach to tussive therapy, in using most of these mixtures it is difficult to evaluate the role of treatment as opposed to the healing quality of time. Not surprisingly, many physicians regard cough therapy in the majority of patients as an exercise in placebology.

Evaluation of Antitussives

Although many antitussive drugs are marketed throughout the world, there is a great deal of uncertainty about the value of all but the few well-established agents. Many different techniques have been employed by investigators in their evaluation of drugs; animal experiments are usually followed by studies on induced cough in volunteers, following which the drugs are investigated in clinical practice using patients with coughs of different types.[3, 9, 10, 12] The results can be inconsistent, since animals and human volunteers who are made to cough can react very differently to antitussive drugs than do asthmatic, tuberculous, bronchitic and other patients with chronic coughs. The available information derived from different antitussive experiments consists of a mixture of data that cannot be readily compared. Moreover, the relative incidences of secondary effects and adverse reactions caused by individual drugs are similarly lacking in uniformity of reporting, and composite comparative reviews lack standards for consistency. As is so often the case in pharmacology, it is always difficult and sometimes impossible to determine a ranking order of virtues among the alternative available drugs and therapies.

Laboratory evaluation of antitussive drugs is generally carried out on both animals and normal human volunteers who are induced to cough by some irritative drug or other form of provocation. Thus, mechanical, electrical or chemical stimuli can be utilized,[10] although, more recently, experts such as Bickerman have favored inhalations of citric acid aerosol that result in a reliable and reproducible cough response.[9] Other irritating inhalants that have been employed include acetic acid, ether, acrolein, ammonia, sulfuric acid and sulfur dioxide. More physiologic stimuli have been utilized and include inhaled acetylcholine or histamine; intravenous injections of ether, paraldehyde and lobeline are also effective.[3, 10] Once coughing has been induced, the experimenter uses a suitable monitoring technique to determine the frequency and the quality of the cough, and then the evaluations are repeated after administering an antitussive drug or a placebo.

Information derived from techniques of this nature has provided the basis for the development of most of the antitussives on the market. The most effective antitussive has long been considered to be codeine; new drugs are generally compared with codeine as a standard. Other narcotics, including morphine and opium, have been standard antitussives for over 150 years; much of the recent pharmacologic effort has been directed at the development of nonnarcotic antitussives. It should be realized that the majority of the nonnarcotic cough suppressants have been developed only in the last 25 years,[3] and many of these new drugs are poorly known and lack adequate clinical experience. It is not surprising that the vast majority of physicians (including respiratory physicians, who should be particularly interested in cough therapy) have relatively little knowledge regarding antitussive drugs. In general, most physicians content themselves with learning to use four or five antitussive cough medicines, and they ignore the others.

An additional pharmacologic problem with any antitussive drug is that the exact site of action is not completely clear.[5, 10, 14] It is known that the narcotic and narcotic-like opioids act on the cough center, and perhaps serve to raise the threshold to tussive stimuli. Less is known about the mechanisms or sites of action of other drugs, although there is good evidence that some of them (particularly those with demonstrable local anesthetic action) have an effect on the peripheral receptors. Nevertheless, it is probable that most of the antitussive agents that have no sedative or psychic properties do have a direct suppressive effect on the cough center.[10] Since relatively little is understood about the mechanism whereby codeine suppresses cough — in spite of the large number of investigations that have been carried out—it is not surprising that knowledge is skimpy with respect to the less well-known antitussives. Many cough suppressants have been discovered accidentally, and the results of any individual investigator cannot always be reproduced by other workers. Thus, a considerable number of drugs have been claimed to possess antitussive properties, but many such claims cannot be evaluated, and the true properties and mechanisms of actions of such drugs await further elucidation.

In the following sections, the generally available antitussive drugs will be discussed, and an effort will be made to classify and compare them and to make recommendations regarding their use. The paucity of information and the conflicting comparative data in the literature on this subject should be kept in mind.

Peripherally Acting Antitussives

Agents that act peripherally, at the level of the cough receptors in the airway, may suffice to alleviate many types of cough. The specific qualities of such peripheral antitussives have been classified by Bickerman;[12] the following classification is an adaptation: (1) mucosal anesthetics; (2) bronchodilators; (3) mucokinetics; (4) hydrating agents; and (5) miscellaneous (see Table 9–4). This last group includes the traditional soothing, demulcent agents that have enjoyed marked popularity for many years.

Mucosal Anesthetics. It is well known that the topical application of local anesthetics to the upper respiratory tract and the major airways is a necessary requirement to allow bronchoscopy to proceed without violent coughing. Although local anesthesia is successfully used as a prelude to instrumentation of the respiratory tract, this form of therapy has not played a significant role in the treatment of the general run of coughs. In fact, local anesthetics are available as adjuncts to cough therapy by means of throat lozenges or gargles that incorporate ethoform (p-aminobenzoic acid ethyl ester)[10] or phenol. These agents are mild anesthetics, and may serve to relieve the irritation of pharyngeal receptors that is a cause of the cough that often accompanies a "sore throat." Other drug preparations with similar effects include chloroform water and compound ether spirit.[9]

It is of interest that Dautrebande[13] recommended the use of procaine hydrochloride (a local anesthetic) in his formulation of Aerolone. This product was originally used as an inhalational preparation for the treatment of bronchospasm (see Chapter 5); it may also have been of value in the treatment of certain forms of cough, such as that which commonly occurs in asthma. Patients who have a chronic cough associated with nonspecific tracheitis or bronchitis that does not yield to more conventional treatment may benefit from a short course of inhalation therapy with a mixture of a local anesthetic (such as

TABLE 9–4. PERIPHERALLY ACTING ANTITUSSIVES

Class	Examples	Clinical Use
MUCOSAL ANESTHETICS		
Topical anesthetics	Cocaine, lidocaine, tetracaine	To facilitate instrumentation
Weak anesthetics	Benzocaine, ethoform, phenol	In throat lozenges and gargles
Infiltrative anesthetics	Lidocaine	For chest-wall pain
Oral antitussives	Benzonatate, caramiphen, chlophedianol, isoaminile, oxolamine	For nonspecific cough
BRONCHODILATORS		
Sympathomimetics	Ephedrine	Bronchospasmolytic
Antitussives	Caramiphen, carbetapentane, oxeladin	Weak bronchospasmolytics
MUCOKINETICS		
Bronchomucotropics	Bromhexine	Decreases mucus viscosity
Antitussives	Caramiphen, clobutinol, noscapine	Augment bronchial secretions
HYDRATING AGENTS		
Water	Steam, aerosols, fluids	Oral, parenteral or inhalational
MISCELLANEOUS		
Demulcents	Candy, syrup	Soothe pharynx
Placebos	Many	Psychogenic relief

lidocaine 0.5–10 per cent) and a bronchodilator. Although such therapy is unconventional at present, there is reason to believe it may be useful,[13a] and nothing to suggest that it may cause any harm when administered carefully several times a day for a few days or a week. As pointed out by Eddy et al,[10] tetracaine, procaine, cocaine and other local anesthetics have been given as aerosols by various workers for the treatment of irritative coughs, and were particularly helpful in asthmatics. Some workers have even given local anesthetics intravenously in an attempt to alleviate cough,[10, 14] but there is little to recommend such an approach. Other, less important, uses of local anesthetics in the treatment of cough are discussed by Salem and Aviado.[14]

Local anesthetics and analgesics also can be used as adjunctives in the management of certain cough problems. Thus, in postoperative patients, the cough reflex is partially inhibited when the incision is disturbed by violent respiratory movements. For this reason, thoracic and upper abdominal surgical procedures are particularly susceptible to being complicated by pneumonia. The patient's ability to cough effectively will be improved by the appropriate use of analgesics, and in some cases (especially after thoracic surgery) a nerve block with a local anesthetic may considerably reduce the pain of coughing.[15]

Many antitussives that are considered to have a specific value in the treatment of cough do have local anesthetic properties, for example, isoaminile, chlophedianol, pholcodine, diphenhydramine, oxolamine, caramiphen.[10] One important local anesthetic antitussive agent is benzonatate, which is related to tetracaine. In fact, benzonatate is unique because it is the only important oral antitussive with a peripheral action. Benzonatate has been shown to act on the pulmonary stretch receptors and to inhibit the transmission of afferent vagal impulses to the cough center.[11] It is claimed that the drug depresses polysynaptic spinal reflexes, thereby inhibiting the transmission of tussal impulses along the afferent vagus[9] but it is not clear whether the local anesthetic action of benzonatate serves to prevent stimulation of the peripheral receptors in the airway. There is evidence that benzonatate also has a central antitussive effect. The drug is effective when absorbed from the bowel after oral ingestion, and it is also successful when given intravenously.[10] The properties of benzonatate suggest that it could be effective when given by aerosol and when applied topically to the respiratory mucosa; one would presume that these forms of administration would provide the most successful form of antitussive therapy with benzonatate. The drug is discussed in further detail later in this chapter.

Bronchodilators. The observations that coughs are often associated with bronchospasm, and that bronchodilators often relieve coughs, led to the Salem and Aviado hypothesis that the cough reflex is initiated by bronchospasm.[3, 11] Undoubtedly, many patients do suffer from both bronchospasm and coughing, these being common components in obstructive airways diseases. The treatment of either component is likely to benefit the other in such cases, and there is little doubt that many coughs are relieved by bronchodilator therapy. It is possible that some patients who present with only a chronic cough have a form of asthma,[19] and even though they do not wheeze or suffer from dyspnea, their pulmonary function tests may improve with bronchodilator therapy—and the cough may improve simultaneously.

Relatively little has been done to establish the specific antitussive properties of individual bronchodilators, although all would be expected to have beneficial effects. Ephedrine has been shown to have an antitussive effect in dogs, although the same property was not demonstrated by epinephrine.[10] Atropine, which is an anticholinergic drug with bronchodilator properties, would be expected to act as an antitussive, but this does not appear to be the case.[10] Several antitussive drugs (including caramiphen, carbetapentane and oxeladin) have been shown to have some bronchodilator action.[10] However, such effects are minor adjuvant benefits rather than major bronchospasmolytic successes. The role of other bronchodilators in the treatment of cough is discussed at length by Salem and Aviado.[16] At present, it appears that although there is a relationship between bronchodilator drugs and antitussives, it is not a firm one, and further efforts will be required to define the possible role of bronchodilators in the therapy of cough.

Mucokinetics. Agents that affect bronchial secretions and render them more mobile will have a favorable effect on a patient's cough. Some antitussives (including noscapine, caramiphen and clobutinol)[10] have been credited with the ability to augment bronchial secretions, although such claims are controversial. Several agents that are regarded as expectorants have been described as having antitussive properties: bromhexine, in particular, may have a true antitussive effect.[11] Other mucokinetic agents should be considered to provide an adjuvant effect in the management of cough (see Chapter 3).

Hydrating Agents. The traditional management of cough has always included hydration, either by the oral, or parenteral, or the inhalational route. Agents used in this fashion serve primarily as mucokinetics and are considered in detail in Chapters 2 and 3. As Shirkey[17] points out, however, coughs in children often result from the maintenance of a low humidity atmosphere in the home, and any simple measure designed to increase the humidity may relieve the cough without affecting mucus production. Simple vaporizers using water, with or without a mucokinetic additive, should be considered for the treatment of any irritative cough when no specific organic or psychogenic abnormality can be found. The advantage of many a "cough medicine" may rest in the glass of water that is taken four times a day to wash down the tablespoon of colored liquid; the additional hydration thereby achieved is usually extremely beneficial.

Miscellaneous. A number of peripherally acting antitussives of dubious value continue to enjoy general popularity.[17] Such cough remedies vary from cough drops, lozenges and pastilles to traditional syrups, such as can be made by dissolving two tablespoonfuls of rock candy or sugar in a cup of hot water. A more sophisticated, equally traditional, yet far more popular, remedy is made by combining sugar or honey with whiskey or rum in a glass of hot water with lemon juice. Other traditional ingredients include brown sugar, corn syrup, horehound drops, paregoric and onion juice.[17] Historically, a host of other agents have been recommended, such as goat's milk, vitriolated iron, gentian and so on. Salem and Aviado[3] list other old remedies varying from agrimony to vervain, and some newer ones, such as mist of Asperagus lucidus. Again, there is little evidence on which to base a judgement as to the efficacy of any of these assorted recommendations. However, a soothing demulcent oral medication or candy often seems to improve a cough, and the readily obtained over-the-counter antitussive syrups or lozenges that contain agents such as honey, acacia, glycerin, licorice and wild cherry, are both harmless and inexpensive for most patients, and can therefore be recommended.

The only caution to be mentioned at this point is that diabetic patients can cause a considerable disruption in their dietary control if they overindulge in those sugary cough remedies that have a soothing, demulcent effect.[18] Chalmers and Cormier list a number of antitussive preparations that are free of sugar.[20]

Centrally-Acting Antitussives

The most commonly used antitussive drugs act on the cough center to depress its sensitivity to afferent stimuli. However, these agents may also decrease a patient's perception of peripheral irritation or may help the coughing patient adapt to the abnormality. The patient is thus less reactive to the tendency to keep coughing to clear the irritation.[9, 12, 21] The most effective centrally-acting agents are narcotics, but a number of nonnarcotic drugs also have antitussive properties. The basic and standard narcotic antitussives are the opium alkaloids and their derivatives.

Narcotics. Drugs with powerful analgesic, sedative and psychic properties that have a strong tendency to produce addiction are known as narcotics. These drugs are carefully regulated as a result of the comprehensive Drug Abuse Prevention and Control Act (1970): narcotics are listed as Controlled Substances (Table 9–5). The most important narcotics are those derived from opium, which is obtained from the juice of the poppy plant, *Papaver somniferum*. Crude opium is prepared from the dehydrated gummy exudate, and more than a score of alkaloid drugs have been extracted from it. Chemically, the opium alkaloids are classified as phenanthrenes (including morphine, codeine and thebaine) and benzylisoquinolines (including papaverine and noscapine). Morphine and similar drugs are known as opioids; many derived opioids have been synthesized. One of the most important opioids (socially rather than medically) is heroin, which is diacetylmorphine.

ACTIONS OF THE OPIOIDS. The opium alkaloids are used mainly for their narcotic analgesic effects, but they have many other actions, several of which are of therapeutic benefit (Table 9–6). The opioids can cause tissues to release histamine, and perhaps other mediators, and can thus result in spasm of smooth muscle. Bronchospasm could be exacerbated, although, in practice, the sedative action supervenes and, in general, the narcotics tend to produce a decrease in

TABLE 9–5. SCHEDULES OF CONTROLLED DRUGS (NARCOTICS AND DANGEROUS DRUGS)

SCHEDULE I

Definition
Drugs with extreme psychic dependence and high abuse potential that have no accepted medical use in the United States at present

Classes of drug
Opiates, opium derivatives and hallucinogenic substances

Antitussives
Codeine-N-oxide, heroin, morphine-N-oxide, nicocodeine, nicomorphine, normethadone, pholcodine

Comment
These drugs cannot be prescribed in the United States.

SCHEDULE II

Definition
Drugs with severe psychic dependence and high abuse potential, but with limited therapeutic indications; many were formerly Class A Narcotics

Classes of drug
Opium, opiates, opium derivatives, stimulants and depressants

Antitussives
Apomorphine, codeine, dihydrocodeine, ethylmorphine, hydrocodone, hydromorphone, meperidine (pethidine), methadone, oxycodone

Comment
Must be ordered by physician on appropriate prescription form

SCHEDULE III

Definition
Drugs with limited psychic dependence and low abuse potential; drug concentrations are strictly limited to decrease possibility of addiction; drugs in this Schedule were formerly Class B Narcotics

Classes of drug
Preparations containing specified amounts of certain stimulants, depressants and narcotics

Antitussives
Codeine—not more than 1.8 gm/100 ml
Dihydrocodeinone (hydrocodone)—not more than 300 mg/100 ml
Ethylmorphine—not more than 300 mg/100 ml
Morphine—not more than 50 mg/100 ml (or 100 g)
Opium—not more than 500 mg/100 ml (or 100 g)
Paregoric—standard preparation. (In some States, paregoric is considered to be in Schedule II.)

Comment
May be ordered by physician on regular prescription form.

SCHEDULE IV

Definition
Drugs with low abuse potential, but that may induce some degree of habituation

Classes of drug
Depressants, tranquilizers and stimulants

Antitussives
No antitussives included

Comment
Require physician's prescription in most States

SCHEDULE V

Definition
Drugs with low abuse potential that can be sold over-the-counter because they are in low concentration; formerly classified as Exempt Narcotics

Classes of drug
Drug preparations containing specified amounts of narcotics (most of the drugs in Schedule V are "cough medications")

Antitussives
Codeine—not more than 200 mg/100 ml (or 100 g)
Dihydrocodeine—not more than 100 mg/100 ml (or 100 g)
Ethylmorphine—not more than 100 mg/100 ml (or 100 g)
Opium—not more than 100 mg/100 ml (or 100 g)

Comment
Drugs in this Schedule may be dispensed by a pharmacist without a prescription, provided legal requirements of age and identity of the purchaser are satisfied. No more than 240 ml of a solution containing opium or 120 ml of any other Schedule V drug solution may be purchased in a 48 hour period without a prescription.

TABLE 9-6. ACTIONS OF THE OPIOIDS

Clinically Useful

ORGAN SYSTEM	EFFECTS	CLINICAL INDICATIONS
Central nervous system	Analgesia, drowsiness, euphoria	Severe pain, preoperative, sedation
Respiratory center	Respiratory depression, relief of some forms of dyspnea	Hyperpnea (e.g., during respiratory support), cardiac "asthma"
Cough center	Increased threshold	Inappropriate cough
Intestines	Decreased motility	Diarrhea

Undesirable

ORGAN SYSTEM	EFFECTS
Emetic center	Nausea and vomiting
Stomach	Delayed emptying
Biliary tract	Spasm; may cause pain
Ureter, bladder	Spasm; may cause frequency
Bronchial muscle	Spasm; may induce asthma
Skin	Histamine release: pruritus and sweating
General	Tendency to addiction

bronchospasm. However, there is a danger of respiratory center depression; therefore opioids are usually avoided in bronchial asthma, although they can be of great value in bronchospasm due to pulmonary vascular congestion (cardiac asthma). The fear of exacerbating bronchospasm in asthmatics has led some authorities to consider that opioid antitussives should be avoided in patients who are susceptible to bronchoconstriction. This does not appear to be reasonable advice; in practice, most patients with asthma or bronchitis who develop irritating, nonproductive coughs probably receive a centrally-acting antitussive narcotic at some time without adverse consequences.

Opioid Antitussives. Although morphine and heroin can be very effective for the treatment of intractable cough, the danger of addiction precludes the use of these agents from all except perhaps dying patients who are racked by a painful cough (for example, patients with terminal lung cancer). *Heroin* (diacetylmorphine, known in the United Kingdom as diamorphine) is illegal in the U.S., but it is a popular antitussive in England, where it has long been favored in chest hospitals, such as the Brompton Hospital in London, for adjuvant therapy in terminal lung cancer. However, morphine is almost as effective, and is currently employed in the antitussive-analgesic-euphoriant mixture known as the "Brompton Cocktail" or "Mist. Euphoria": this contains morphine, cocaine, and syrup or honey, "flavored" with brandy or gin.[22] Various preparations of opium have long been used for the treatment of coughs and febrile illnesses. *Dover's powder* (named after a pirate-physician) contains ipecac and opium; it was used as a sedative-expectorant. *Brown mixture* (also known as compound opium and glycyrrhiza mixture) contains paregoric, glycyrrhiza fluidextract, antimony potassium tartrate, 10 per cent alcohol, glycerin and purified water; it still has some popularity as a tasty cough medicine.

In the United States, few such traditional mixtures survive, apart from *paregoric:* this old-fashioned preparation consists of a hydroalcoholic solution of 0.4 mg/ml opium with the addition of benzoic acid, anise and camphor (it is also known as "camphorated opium tincture," and was originally called "elixir asthmaticum" in the 18th century). This preparation, curiously enough, can be purchased as an over-the-counter anodyne in many states, although it is a controlled drug in others (Table 9-5): in some states paregoric is Schedule II, in others it is Schedule III. It can also be purchased without prescription in many states in the form of antidiarrhea mixtures that contain drugs such as bismuth subsalicylate or kaolin. It is mainly used for the treatment of diarrhea, but is also a weak antitussive. Boyd[23] claims that paregoric, unlike other narcotic antitussive drugs, increases the output of respiratory tract fluid; that is, it is a mucokinetic. Paregoric is also available in combination with an antihistamine. It is known by those who use it (often by the intravenous route) for psychedelic purposes as "blue velvet."

Codeine. This important drug was first isolated in 1832 as an impurity in the

TABLE 9-7. ADVANTAGES OF CODEINE OVER MORPHINE

Property or Effect	Morphine	Codeine
Toleration	Considerable	Moderate
Addiction potential	Considerable	Slight
Euphoria	Potent	Weak
Analgesia	Very effective	Less effective
Hypnotic	Very effective	Less effective
Respiratory depression	Potent	Weak
Risk of bronchospasm	Moderate	Slight
Constipation	Potent	Moderate
Nausea and vomiting	Potent	Moderate
Oral administration	Less effective	Very effective
Overdose hazards	Considerable	Minor

morphine derived from opium; its name is derived from the Greek for "the head of the poppy." It is the methyl ether of morphine, and although it is more toxic than morphine in many animals, it is less toxic in man. Codeine has valuable pain-relieving properties, and it can decrease bowel activity, but of more relevance is that it has long been the standard centrally-acting antitussive drug against which all other cough suppressants have to be compared. Although most of the codeine used throughout the world is employed for pain relief, there are many superior analgesics that are being used more frequently in place of codeine. However, codeine is still probably the most commonly prescribed antitussive.[10] This is a tribute to its effectiveness in suppressing cough, as well as to its useful sedative and analgesic actions. Moreover, the danger of development of dependence to codeine in practice appears to be very small, certainly much less than the well-known dangers of morphine and heroin. Codeine has not become a drug of abuse to any noticeable extent. Eddy et al., in their thorough review, report that its abuse potential is so slight that its popularity as an antitussive need not be a source of concern.[10] This safety factor can be correlated with the fact that an equal antitussive dose of codeine has only one-twentieth the psychic effect of morphine,[3, 11] and patients who take codeine are unlikely to experience the euphoriant effect. Similarly, codeine is far less effective than morphine as an analgesic when given in conventional antitussive dosages, and thus when used as an antitussive, no other potentially addictive quality is likely to accompany even prolonged use. A further advantage of codeine over morphine as an antitussive is that codeine has only one-quarter the depressant effect on respiration, and therefore it is a safer drug for patients with respiratory failure. Finally, codeine is

less likely to cause nausea, vomiting, and constipation; it may also be less likely to induce histamine release and bronchospasm in asthmatics (Table 9-7).

Other Narcotics. The opium alkaloids that have long been used for cough are the phenanthrenes morphine and codeine, and their derivatives, such as heroin, purified opium alkaloids, and paregoric. In more recent years, additional derivatives of morphine and codeine have been introduced as antitussives (Table 9-8). The most important of these agents are ethylmorphine, hydrocodone (dihydrocodeinone), hydromorphone (dihydromorphinone) and methadone. Meperidine is also of relevance, since this potent analgesic does also have an antitussive effect. Several other narcotic derivatives are used as antitussives in other countries, including dihydrocodeine, morpholinylethylmorphine (pholcodine), normethadone and oxycodone. Additional agents have received favorable reports but do not appear to be of commercial importance; codoxime and thebacon (acetyldihydrocodeinone) are the best known of these agents, whereas nicocodine and nicodicodine are of no practical value. In general, there is little to suggest that any of these agents are preferable to codeine for the suppression of most types of cough.

DISADVANTAGES OF NARCOTICS. In addition to their potent primary effects and their devastating ability to cause addiction, the more powerful opium alkaloids have many other undesirable side effects. When used as antitussives, the narcotics are generally given in smaller dosage than is required for analgesia; therefore, side effects are less of a problem when they are appropriately prescribed for coughs. Among the many side effects (Table 9-9), the more serious ones for respiratory patients are those associated with the anticholinergic-like effects and the histamine-releasing properties. Drying of the

TABLE 9–8. NARCOTIC ANTITUSSIVES

Drug	Antitussive Effect	Analgesic Effect	Sedative Effect	Respiratory Depression	Addiction Potential	Adult Dose (mg)	Duration of Effect (hrs)
Heroin* (diacetylmorphine)	++	++	++	++	++		3–4
Morphine	++	++	++	++	++	2–4	4–5
Codeine (methylmorphine)	++	+	±	+	±	5–20	4–6
Dihydrocodeine* (Paracodin, Parzone)	++	+(?)	+	+	+	10–15	4–5
Ethylmorphine (Dionin)	++	++	±	±	+	5–15	4–6
Hydrocodone (dihydrocodeinone, Codone, Dicodid, Hycodan†, Tussionex†)	++	+(?)	+	+	++	5–10	4–8
Hydromorphone (dihydromorphinone, Dilaudid)	++	+	+	+	++	0.5–1	4–5
Oxycodone (dihydrohydroxy-codeinone, Percodan†)	++	+	+	+	++	3–5	4–5
Methadone (Adanon, Amidone, Dolophine)	+	++	++	+	+	2.5–10	3–5
Normethadone* (Ticarda)	±	+	+	+	+	7.5	3–8
Morpholinylethylmorphine* (Ethnine, Pholcodine, Pholdine)	+	±	±	+	−	5–15	4–5
Meperidine (pethidine, Demerol)	±	++	+	+	+	25–50	2–4

*Not available in the United States
†These products contain additional ingredients.

mouth is common, and ciliary depression together with decreased respiratory tract fluid secretion may result in impaired mucokinesis. This can be more of a problem in those sensitive patients who develop bronchospasm as a result of the histamine release; any superimposed opioid-induced respiratory center depression can compound the problem.

The narcotics are mostly metabolized in the liver; hepatic disease may result in potentiation of the narcotic action. Endocrine deficiency and any cerebral depression can also result in an enhanced narcotic effect. The opioids act synergistically with other centrally acting depressant drugs; such drug admixtures should be avoided, if possible. Fortunately, the low dose of morphine

TABLE 9–9. PHARMACOLOGIC PROPERTIES OF MORPHINE AND OTHER POTENT NARCOTICS

THERAPEUTIC PROPERTIES

Central nervous system	Analgesia, sedation, opiate mood (euphoria, mental clouding), soporific
Medullary depression	Antitussive, respiratory depression
Gastrointestinal tract	Decreased motility (antidiarrhea)
Pulmonary circulation	Improvement in acute left ventricular failure

SIDE EFFECTS

Central nervous system	Addiction potential, drowsiness, miosis, respiratory failure
Histamine release	Bronchospasm, skin rashes, itching of nose
Antimucokinetic effects	Drying of oral and respiratory mucosae, decreased ciliary activity, depression of cough and of breathing
Idiosyncratic reactions	Delirium, agitation, convulsions, palpitations, headaches, vertigo, sweating, heavy feeling in limbs, warm feeling
Gastrointestinal tract	Nausea, vomiting, constipation
Overdose	Shock, pulmonary edema, hypothermia, coma leading to death

DRUG INTERACTIONS

Potentiation with	Anticholinergics, antihistaminics, sedatives-depressants, alcohol, muscle relaxants, antipsychotics, antidepressants

CONTRAINDICATIONS

Endocrine insufficiency	Pituitary deficiency, myxedema, Addison's disease
Cerebral disease	Head injury, delirium, cerebral depression
Liver disease	Hepatic insufficiency, delirium tremens
Respiratory disease	Respiratory failure, asthma in adults

TABLE 9-10. CLASSES OF NONNARCOTIC ANTITUSSIVE AGENTS

Class	Examples	Antitussive Value
MORPHINAN DERIVATIVES		
Opiate	Dextromethorphan	Very useful
BENZYLISOQUINOLINES		
	Noscapine	Very useful
	Papaverine	Minor value
	Narceine	Effective
	Ethylnarceine	Effective
	Hydrastinine	Effective
	Homarylamine	Effective
DIPHENYLALKYLAMINES		
Propoxyphene derivative	Levopropoxyphene	Useful
	Diphenylpiperidenopropanol	No clinical value
Diarylalkanol derivative	Chlophedianol	Useful
Thiambutene derivative	AT 327	No clinical value
PHENYLCYCLOPENTALKYLAMINES		
Cycloalkylcarboxylic acid ester	Caramiphen	Useful
Cycloalkylcarboxylic acid ester	Carbetapentane	Useful
Diethylphenylacetic acid derivative	Oxeladin	No clinical value
Oxadiazole derivative	Oxolamine	No clinical value
PHENOTHIAZENES		
Piperidino derivative	Pipazethate	Useful
Carboxylated phenothiazene	Dimethoxanate	Useful
Thioxanthene	Meprotixol	No clinical value
MISCELLANEOUS		
Dimethylamine derivative	Benzobutamine	No clinical value
Butylaminobenzoate derivative	Benzonatate	Useful
Chlorophenyl derivative	Clobutinol	Useful
Acetonitrile derivative	Isoaminile	No clinical value
Dibutyl naphthalene derivatives	Dibunates	Useful
Morpholino derivative	Melipan	No clinical value

required for antitussive action enables most patients to avoid these dangerous complications. Codeine and most of the other natural and synthetic antitussive narcotics are even safer, but whenever large amounts of any of these drugs are being used, the dangers alluded to in Table 9–9 should be kept in mind.

Nonnarcotics. A large number of nonnarcotic agents, of several chemical types, have been reported to have antitussive properties. A limited number of these are equivalent to codeine in cough-suppressing potency, but have fewer serious side effects; drugs that do not possess these dual qualities do not merit consideration. Of the agents that have gained some acceptance, either in the United States or abroad, only a few seem to be of sufficient value to justify their availability in practical therapeutics. A list of the agents that have been previously reviewed[3, 10] is presented in Table 9–10; not all of these agents are of clinical value. Several other agents have been reported,[21, 22] such as medazomide, xyloxemine, coltsfoot, hydrocotarnine and

piperidione, but they do not merit further consideration.

Although the morphinans and benzylisoquinolines are considered to be opiates, the examples listed in Table 9–10 do not have addictive properties, and are therefore not considered to be narcotics, and are not scheduled as such (see Table 9–5). These agents can be purchased without prescriptions, although there are undoubtedly people with personality problems who might develop an apparent addiction to these opioids. The rest of the agents listed do not appear to have any abuse potential.

The more important nonnarcotic centrally-acting antitussives are listed in Table 9–11. Most of these agents are able to suppress coughing as effectively as codeine when given in the appropriate dose. Many of them have some local anesthetic properties; as already discussed, benzonatate has potent anesthetic qualities. Apart from benzobutamine and oxolamine, none have significant analgesic properties, and only isoaminile and pipazethate appear to have significant de-

TABLE 9–11. NONNARCOTIC ANTITUSSIVES

Drug	Broncho-dilator	Respiratory Depression	Local Anesthetic	Analgesic	Drying Effect	Sedative	Adult Dosage
Benzobutamine	?	No	Yes	Yes	?	?	—
Benzonatate (Tessalon[1], Ventussin)	No	No**	Yes	No	No	No	100–200 mg q4–8h
Caramiphen (Taoryl, Toryn, Tuss-Ornade[2])	Yes(?)	No	Yes	No	Yes(?)*	?	10–20 mg
Carbetapentane (pentoxyverine, Reflexol, Rynatuss[2], Toclase)	Yes(?)	No	Yes	No	Yes	?	15–30 mg q6–8h
Chlophedianol (clofedanol, Detigon, Ulo[1])	No	No**	Yes	No	Yes	Yes	15–30 mg q6–8h
Clobutinol (Kat 256, Silomat)	?	No	No	No	No*	No	40 mg
Dextromethorphan (Dormethan, Methorate,	No	No**(?)	?	No	Yes	No	15–30 q4–8h
Dimethoxanate (Cothera)	?	No	Yes	No	?	No	25–50 mg
Isoaminile (Dimyril, Peracon)	Yes	Yes	Yes	No	No	No	40 mg
Levopropoxyphene (Novrad[1])	No	No	Yes	No	No(?)	?	50–100 mg q4-6h
Noscapine (narcotine, Coscopin, Nectadon, Tusscapine[1])	No	No**	No	No	No*	Yes(?)	15–30 mg q6–8h
Oxeladin (Pectamol)	Yes	No	Yes	No	?	No	15–20 mg
Oxolamine (Perebron)	Yes(?)	No	Yes	Yes	?	?	—
Pipazethate (Selvigon, Theratuss)	No	Yes	Yes	?	?	No	20–40 mg q6–8h
Sodium dibunate (Becantex, Becantyl, Linctussal)	No	No**	?	?	No	?	100 mg
Ethyl dibunate (Neodyne, Tussets)	No	No	?	?	No	?	100 mg

[1]Marketed in United States. Other preparations may have been marketed in the past.
[2]Marketed in United States as a combination preparation
*May increase mucokinesis
**May stimulate respiration

pressive action on the respiratory center. Chlophedianol and noscapine may have some sedative action, but this is dubious. Several of the agents have spasmolytic properties, and, as has already been described, a few may cause bronchodilation. Caramiphen, carbetapentane, chlophedianol and dextromethorphan have been described as causing a drying effect of the respiratory mucosa, but caramiphen has also been reported to increase mucokinesis (as have clobutinol and noscapine). All these proper-

ties are reviewed by Eddy et al,[10] and one must conclude that the side effects of these drugs are generally poorly documented and of little practical significance.

Although the nonnarcotic antitussives would appear to have advantages over the narcotic agents, few physicians use any of them apart from benzonatate and dextromethorphan. The current trend appears to be one of declining interest in most of these drugs, and it is unlikely that many of them will continue to be marketed in the United

States. Nevertheless, it is worth considering those that are currently available in the U.S.; brief descriptions will be provided in the following section.

PHARMACOLOGY OF IMPORTANT ANTITUSSIVES

Narcotic Antitussives
(Table 9–8)

Codeine

Codeine is morphine 3-methyl ether; it is a naturally occurring phenanthrene. In contrast with morphine, it is well absorbed when given by mouth; oral therapy has about two-thirds the potency of a parenterally administered dose. The usual oral dose results in effective cough suppression, but only weak analgesia and no psychic euphoriant effects. Codeine undergoes complex metabolic changes in the body, which include conversion of about 10 per cent of the administered dose into morphine. Most of its metabolic conversion seems to occur in the liver, and the major excretory route is through the kidney.

The most common side effects are sedation, drowsiness, dizziness, nausea, vomiting, constipation and dry mouth; the drug may increase the viscosity of respiratory secretions. Large doses can produce greater narcotic effects, but fatalities from overdosages are very rare.

Availability and Dosage. Since codeine is relatively insoluble in water, it is usually made available as the very soluble phosphate or the sulfate. The dose required for analgesia is about 30 mg; this has an effect similar to 300 to 600 mg of aspirin; these two drugs have synergistic actions, and can be combined for more potent analgesia. The standard antitussive dose for adults is 5 to 20 mg orally or subcutaneously; this can be repeated every three to six hours. A commonly recommended dose is 8 mg as often as every 3 hours. The usual dose for children is 1 to 1.5 mg/kg per day, divided into six doses. Shirkey recommends combining codeine with aromatic eriodictyon syrup in variable proportions to make a suitable pediatric cough suppressant of appropriate potency.[17] Many proprietary preparations of codeine are available, since the drug is often present in combination antitussive preparations. Of the over 40 such preparations listed in AMA Drug Evaluations, almost all contain codeine as the phosphate. Generic codeine products are also available for oral use and as injections. A relatively popular combination product is elixir of terpin hydrate and codeine, each 5 ml of which contains 10 mg of codeine or codeine sulfate and about 85 mg of terpin hydrate, in 35 to 42 per cent alcohol. The terpin hydrate is present as a flavoring agent, and the alcohol helps account for the popularity of this cocktail.

Hydrocodone

Although hydrocodone may be more potent than codeine, and has a greater abuse potential, it is still a valued antitussive. Nine antitussive preparations containing this drug are listed in AMA Drug Evaluations. It has not been clearly established whether the drug has analgesic properties, and since it seems to have no advantages over codeine (except perhaps a decreased tendency to cause constipation) there appears to be little reason for favoring hydrocodone.

Availability and Dosage. Hydrocodone is marketed as a generic preparation, and is incorporated (as hydrocodone bitartrate) in several proprietary mixtures, some of which are well known (Table 9–12). Most of these preparations contain various mucosal "drying agents" and mucokinetics, and some contain analgesics; they are therefore claimed to be suitable for colds accompanied by coughs. However, the logic underlying the admixture of drying agents, expectorants and cough suppressants cannot be commended for pharmacologic rationality. The thoughtful physician should be extremely selective when choosing one of these preparations, in spite of manufacturers' spirited defenses of their products.[24]

The appropriate dose of hydrocodone for adults is 5 to 10 mg; this can be repeated at four to eight hour intervals. For children, the appropriate dosage depends on age; under the age of 12 the dose should be one-half of that for adults; under the age of 2 the dose should be one-quarter of that for adults. One preparation of hydrocodone is complexed as an ion-exchange resin (Tussionex): this has a long action, and the medication need be given only every 12 hours. However, it is a relatively expensive product, and the use of this longer-acting preparation at night may result in retention of secretions with a consequent increase in dyspnea.[12] The marketed preparations containing hydrocodone are included in Schedule III (see Table 9–5), and they are ordered on a regular prescription form.

Hydromorphone

This opioid narcotic is used as an analgesic, and occasionally as an antitussive. It is much less potent than morphine, but it is a stronger analgesic than codeine, and is more likely to cause addiction. Its only advantage over codeine is that it is less likely to cause constipation. Hydromorphone is similar to hydrocodone, but is of greater value when an analgesic effect is required.

Availability and Dosage. Hydromorphone is made available as Dilaudid, and as Dilaudid Cough Syrup, which contains, in every 5 ml, 1 mg hydromorphone, 100 mg guaifenesin and 5 per cent alcohol. The adult dosage is 1 mg every three to four hours, and a proportionally lower dose is used for children. Some patients require twice the above dosage, but the danger of dependency is increased if such amounts are administered for more than a few days. The drug is a Schedule II narcotic, and therefore it is rarely prescribed.

Methadone

During the past few years, methadone has become important as a therapeutic agent for the management of narcotic addiction. Although it has an opioid effect, and can prevent or relieve narcotic-withdrawal symptoms, it lacks the morphine or heroin psychic qualities, and of itself it is less likely to be a drug of abuse. It is a very effective analgesic and sedative, and it has earned a reputation of being a valuable drug for patients with severe pain or cough associated with terminal cancer. In the United States, it has become a favored therapy for the intractable coughing associated with inoperable carcinoma of the lungs, although this has not been regarded as a primary indication for the drug.

Methadone is undoubtedly more dangerous than codeine, not only as a drug of abuse, but because it can cause severe respiratory depression if an overdose is taken. The depression of respiration can persist for 36 to 48 hours, and an overdosed patient may require respirator support. The narcotic effect can be reversed by antagonists, such as naloxone, nalorphine or levallorphan, but these have an effect that lasts only one to three hours, and repeated doses, based on careful observation, may be required.

Availability and Dosage. Methadone is a Schedule II narcotic, and can be prescribed only by a duly qualified physician using an appropriate prescription blank. It is available as Dolophine, as 5 and 10 mg tablets and as solutions for intramuscular or subcutaneous administration; the ampules contain 10 mg methadone per 1 ml. The appropriate dose in adults for cough is 2.5 to 10 mg every three to six hours as required. It is not regarded as a particularly suitable drug for children; however, Shirkey advises that if it is used its tendency to cause nausea can be averted by giving the drug as a liquid preparation poured over cracked ice or mixed with a cold carbonated beverage.[17]

Pholcodine

Although not available in the United States, Pholcodine (morpholinylethylmorphine) is regarded as an antitussive of major importance in the United Kingdom.[22] It is classified as a narcotic, but since it has little analgesic or sedative effect, it is virtually nonaddictive. The adult dosage is 5 to 15 mg, four to six times a day.

Meperidine (Pethidine)

Meperidine (known as pethidine in the United Kingdom) is generally regarded as a potent narcotic analgesic, but there is evidence that it does have antitussive properties.[12] It may be of theoretic value in asthmatic coughs, because it apparently has an atropine-like effect and may be bronchospasmolytic; however, there are reports of meperidine causing bronchospasm, and since it can undoubtedly cause respiratory depression, a safer drug should be preferred in clinical practice. Although rarely used as an antitussive, meperidine could be of particular value in a patient with severe pain and a nonproductive cough who does not require the sedative effect that morphine would cause. It is also useful postoperatively when analgesia is a major requirement, and cough suppression is needed to prevent excessive, painful coughing attacks.

Availability and Dosage. Meperidine is available in generic forms and as Demerol for both oral and parenteral administration.

Text continued on page 304

TABLE 9–12. HYDROCODONE PREPARATIONS FOR COUGHS AND COLDS*

Preparation	Basic Dose	Hydrocodone (mg)	Antihistamines (mg)	Adrenergics (mg)	Anticholinergic (mg)	Mucokinetics (mg)	Other (mg)
Citra Cough	5 ml syrup†	1.66	Pheniramine 2.5 Pyrilamine 3.3	Phenylephrine 2.5		Ascorbic acid 30 K citrate 150	
	5 ml Forte syrup	5	Pheniramine 2.5 Pyrilamine 3.33			Ascorbic acid 30 K citrate 150	Alcohol 2%
	Forte capsule	5	Methapyrilene 8.33 Pheniramine 6.25 Pyrilamine 8.33	Phenylephrine 10		Ascorbic acid 50	Phenacetin 120 Salicylamide 227 Caffeine 30
Codimal DH	5 ml liquid	1.66	Pyrilamine 8.33	Phenylephrine 5		K guaiacol-sulfonate 83.3 Na citrate 216	Alcohol 4% Citric acid 50
Dicoril†	5 ml syrup	1.66	Pyrilamine 13.33			Na citrate 167	
Expectico†	5 ml liquid	5	Chlorpheniramine 2			Guaifenesin 100 Na citrate 150	
Hycodan	5 ml syrup, tablet	5			Homatropine 1.5		
Hycomine	5 ml syrup	5		Phenylpropanolamine 25			
Hycomine Pediatric	5 ml syrup	2.5		Phenylpropanolamine 12.5			

Hycomine Compound	Tablet	5	Chlorpheniramine 2	Phenylephrine 10		Caffeine 30 Acetaminophen 250
Pseudo-Hist Expectorant	5 ml liquid	2.5	Chlorpheniramine 2	Pseudoephedrine 15	Guaifenesin 100	
S-T Forte	5 ml syrup	2.5	Pheniramine 13.33	Phenylephrine 5 Phenylpropanolamine 5	Guaifenesin 80	
Triaminic Expectorant DH	5 ml elixir	1.67	Pheniramine 6.25 Pyrilamine 6.25	Phenylpropanolamine 12.5	Chloroform 13.5† Guaifenesin 100	Alcohol 5%
Tussanil DH	5 ml liquid	1.66	Chlorphenira- mine 1.66 Pyrilamine 3.33	Phenylephrine 10 Phenylpropanolamine 5		Menthol 0.166
Tussend	5 ml syrup, tablet	5		Pseudoephedrine 60		Alcohol 5%
Tussend Expectorant	5 ml liquid	5		Pseudoephedrine 60	Guaifenesin 200	Alcohol 12.5%
Tussionex	5 ml suspension, tablet, capsule	5	Phenyltoloxamine 10			Resin complex

*These preparations, which are listed in the Physicians' Desk Reference, are classified as Schedule III narcotics, although hydrocodone itself is in Schedule II.
†Not listed in Physicians' Desk Reference, 1978.

TABLE 9–13. ANTITUSSIVE COMBINATION PREPARATIONS CONTAINING DEXTROMETHORPHAN*

Preparation	Basic Dose	Dextromethorphan (mg)	Antihistamines (mg)	Adrenergics (mg)	Mucokinetics (mg)	Other (mg)
Cerose Compound	Capsule	10	Chlorpheniramine 2	Phenylephrine 7.5	Terpin hydrate 64.8	Acetaminophen 194 / Ascorbic acid 25
Cerose-DM	5 ml liquid	10	Phenindamine 5	Phenylephrine 5	K guaiacolsulfonate 86 / Ipecac 0.01 ml / Na citrate 180	Citric acid 60 / Glycerin
Cheracol D	5 ml syrup	10			Guaifenesin 15	(Various)
Codimal DM	5 ml liquid	10	Pyrilamine 8.33	Phenylephrine 5	K guaiacolsulfonate 83.3 / Na citrate 216	Citric acid 50 / Alcohol 4%
Consotuss	5 ml syrup	15	Doxylamine 3.75			Alcohol 10%
Coryban-D	5 ml syrup	7.5		Phenylephrine 5	Guaifenesin 50	Acetaminophen 120 / Alcohol 7.5%
Dimacol	5 ml liquid, capsule	15		Pseudoephedrine 30	Guaifenesin 100	Alcohol 4.75%
Dorcol Pediatric	5 ml syrup	7.5		Phenylpropanolamine 8.75 / Pseudoephedrine 45	Guaifenesin 37.5	Alcohol 5%
Histalet DM	5 ml syrup	15	Chlorpheniramine 3			
Nilcol (Rx)	30 ml elixir, tablet	30	Chlorpheniramine 4	Phenylpropanolamine 50	Guaifenesin 200	Alcohol 10%
Novahistine DMX	5 ml liquid	10		Pseudoephedrine 30	Guaifenesin 100	Alcohol 10%
Ornacol	10 ml liquid, capsule	30		Phenylpropanolamine 25		Alcohol 8% (in liquid only)
Orthoxicol	5 ml syrup	10		Methoxyphenamine 17		
Phenergan Expectorant (Rx)	5 ml syrup	7.5	Promethazine 5		K guaiacolsulfonate 44 / Ipecac 0.17 min / Na citrate 197	Chloroform 0.25 min† / Citric acid 60
Quelidrine	5 ml syrup	10	Chlorpheniramine 2	Ephedrine 5 / Phenylephrine 5	Ammonium chloride 40 / Ipecac Fl. Ext. 0.005 ml	Alcohol 2%
Rhinex DM	5 ml syrup	7.5	Chlorpheniramine 1	Phenylpropanolamine 12.5	Guaifenesin 50 / Ammonium chloride 100	Alcohol 5%

Product	Form		Antihistamine	Decongestant		Other
Rhinosyn-DM	5 ml syrup	15	Chlorpheniramine 2	Pseudoephedrine 30		Alcohol, Glycerin, Propylene glycol
Rhinosyn Pediatric	5 ml syrup	15		Pseudoephedrine 30	Guaifenesin 100	Alcohol, Glycerin, Propylene glycol
Robitussin CF	5 ml elixir	10		Phenylpropanolamine 12.5	Guaifenesin 50	Alcohol 1.4%
Robitussin DM	5 ml elixir	15			Guaifenesin 100	Alcohol 1.4%
Rondec-DM (Rx)	1 ml drops / 5 ml syrup	4 / 15	Carbinoxamine 1 / Carbinoxamine 2.5	Pseudoephedrine 30 / Pseudoephedrine 60	Guaifenesin 20 / Guaifenesin 100	
Sorbutuss	5 ml liquid	10			Guaifenesin 100 / Ipecac Fl. Ext. 0.05 min / K citrate 85	Citric acid 35 / Sorbitol, glycerin (sugar-free)
2/G-DM	5 ml liquid	15			Guaifenesin 100	Alcohol 5%
Triaminicol	5 ml syrup	15	Pheniramine 6.25 / Pyrilamine 6.25	Phenylpropanolamine 12.5	Ammonium chloride 90	
Trind-DM	5 ml syrup	7.5		Phenylephrine 2.5	Guaifenesin 50	Acetaminophen 120 / Alcohol 15%
Tusquelin (Rx)	5 ml syrup	15	Chlorpheniramine 2	Phenylephrine 5 / Phenylpropanolamine 5	Ext. Ipecac 0.17 min / K guaiacolsulfonate 44	Alcohol 5%
Tussagesic	Tablet (slow release) / 5 ml suspension	30 / 15	Pheniramine 12.5 / Pyrilamine 12.5 / Pheniramine 6.25 / Pyrilamine 6.25	Phenylpropanolamine 25 / Phenylpropanolamine 12.5		Terpin hydrate 180 / Acetaminophen 325 / Terpin hydrate 90 / Acetaminophen 120
Tussaminic (Rx)	Tablet (slow release)	30	Pheniramine 25 / Pyrilamine 25	Phenylpropanolamine 50		Terpin hydrate 300
Tussi-Organidin DM (Rx)	5 ml elixir	10	Chlorpheniramine 2		Iodinated glycerol 30	Alcohol 15%
Unproco (Rx)	Capsule	30			Guaifenesin 200	
Vicks Formula 44	5 ml syrup	5	Doxylamine 3		Na citrate 250	Cetylpyridinium

*These products are selected for tabulation because they are described in Physicians' Desk Reference 1978 or AMA Drug Evaluations. 3rd ed. 1977. Many other products are described in Handbook of Nonprescription Drugs. 5th ed. 1977, and in Facts and Comparisons.

†Chloroform is no longer used in cough medicines.

Note: Preparations marked Rx require a prescription; all others are available over-the-counter. Manufacturers change the constituents of their products periodically.

The average adult dose is 25 to 50 mg; it can be repeated every three to four hours if need be. It should not be used as a cough suppressant for more than a few days because of the addiction potential.

Nonnarcotic Antitussives
(Table 9–11)

Benzonatate

Benzonatate (p-butylaminobenzoic acid), which is related to tetracaine, and is effective as a local anesthetic, was discovered in 1956 and has become relatively popular as an antitussive. It has been shown to inhibit afferent vagal impulses from cough receptors and stretch receptors; it also has a central antitussive action. Benzonatate does not generally appear to have a significant effect on mucokinesis, although it is claimed that it sometimes reduces the amount and consistency of sputum. Unlike narcotic agents, benzonatate has no central depressant effect on breathing, and may be a respiratory stimulant, particularly when administered intravenously. It has been claimed that benzonatate is of particular benefit in asthma, since it may result in an increase in tidal volume and cause a decrease in the patient's sense of dyspnea. This effect is attributed to an inhibition of vagal bronchoconstrictor impulses, but the physiologic significance of such claims is difficult to interpret.

Although the drug is well accepted by most patients, it can cause side effects such as a chilly sensation, headache, mild dizziness or vertigo, skin rashes or pruritus, gastrointestinal distress, a burning sensation in the eyes, and a numb feeling in the chest; hypersensitivity reactions may occur. Intravenous administration can result in a transitory increase in blood pressure. The drug should not be chewed, since it has an unpleasant taste and causes prolonged oropharyngeal anesthesia. It is probable that benzonatate would be useful for producing anesthesia if given topically into the respiratory tree prior to bronchoscopy.

In general, benzonatate appears to be safe and well tolerated, and it may be as effective as codeine in some coughs. Since no abuse potential exists, it is suitable for long-term administration. Overdosage could possibly produce central nervous system stimulation, culminating in restless tremor and possibly convulsions; profound central depression may follow.

Availability and Dosage. Benzonatate has been marketed both as capsules and tablets, and in injection form. It is best known as Tessalon perles (capsules of the liquid drug); currently, the perles contain 100 mg of drug. The adult dosage is 100 to 200 mg taken three times a day; in children, the recommended dose is 8 mg/kg per day in three divided doses. In resistant cases it may be worth giving the patient up to six doses a day for as long as the drug is tolerated. Benzonatate can be given intravenously: the suggested dose is only 5 mg, but such treatment is very rarely required.

Caramiphen

This agent is a minor cough suppressive little used in the United States, and not used in the United Kingdom; it is, apparently, used in Switzerland. The drug has local anesthetic, relaxant and anticholinergic effects and it has been reported to both increase and decrease respiratory tract secretions, and to decrease bronchospasm. It should be used with particular caution in patients with glaucoma or prostatic hypertrophy to avoid atropine-like complications. Caramiphen has erratic antitussive effects, and although it is relatively free of side effects, there seems to be little in favor of this drug.

Availability and Dosage. Caramiphen is marketed in the United States in only one preparation, Tuss-Ornade. This is a timed release capsule containing 20 mg caramiphen edisylate, with 8 mg chlorpheniramine, 2.5 mg isopropamide and 50 mg phenylpropanolamine. It is also available as a liquid; 20 ml is similar to one capsule. The preparation, which is relatively expensive, is one of many competing products used in the treatment of upper respiratory tract problems that are manifested as coughs with colds. If one chooses to use it, the adult dosage is one spansule every twelve hours or 5 to 10 ml three to four times a day. For small children weighing 15 to 25 lbs, 2.5 ml three or four times a day can be used, whereas children over 25 lbs can be given twice this amount.

Carbetapentane (Pentoxyverine)

This agent is similar to caramiphen in that it also is a cycloalkylcarboxylic acid ester. Similarly, it is a local anesthetic with atropine-like effects and limited antitussive value. It is claimed to be more potent than an equivalent dose of codeine, and it has a quicker onset of action and a longer-lasting effect. However, its long-term value has not been clearly substantiated. A minor benefit of this drug is that it may also have some bronchospasmolytic activity. Although it has few side effects, some trials have suggested that the antitussive dose is difficult to achieve without adverse anticholinergic effects and some respiratory depression.[10] Allergic reactions, particularly dermatitis, have been reported. The atropine-like effects of the drug contraindicate its use in patients with glaucoma or prostatic hypertrophy.

Availability and Dosage. Carbetapentane used to be marketed as Toclase, but at present only one systemic product in the United States contains this drug. It is present in Rynatuss, which is used in the treatment of wheezy coughs and colds. The contents of each tablet are 60 mg carbetapentane tannate, 5 mg chlorpheniramine, 10 mg ephedrine and 10 mg phenylephrine. With this particular admixture, it is difficult to attribute any definite role to the carbetapentane. Furthermore, it is relatively expensive. If one chooses to use this product, the adult dosage is 1 to 2 tablets every 12 hours. A pediatric suspension is available: 10 ml is similar in content to 1 tablet. The twelve-hourly dosage for children varies from 1.7 ml for infants under 2, to 5 to 10 ml for children over 6.

Carbetapentane has also been used in cough lozenges (for example, in Reflexol), but there is little to recommend this practice.

Chlophedianol

This agent has had its name spelled in several different ways, including clofedanol and clofedianol. It is similar in structure to the antihistamine, diphenylhydramine, and it has antihistaminic, anticholinergic and some local anesthetic properties. Thus, it may have an antimucokinetic effect. It can produce some sedation, and excessive doses may occasionally cause central excitation with hyperirritability, nightmares and hallucinations. As an antitussive, it has little to recommend it, although its effect may be somewhat longer acting than most others, and it may stimulate respiration.

Availability and Dosage. Chlophedianol has been marketed in the United States in a few preparations (Acutuss, ULO), but it

is relatively expensive and is no longer promoted. The adult dose is about 25 mg three or four times a day; for children over six years of age it can be given in a dosage of 0.5 mg/kg four times a day.

Dextromethorphan

The most important of the nonnarcotic antitussives is dextromethorphan. It is the dextro isomer of a narcotic, the codeine analog of levorphanol. Although it is an opiate, it has no analgesic or sedative effects, and it is regarded as virtually nonaddictive, although there are undoubtedly individuals who develop an exaggerated fondness for the drug. In fact, the drug is treated as a narcotic in some countries, although it is not listed in the United States Schedules of Controlled Drugs.

Dextromethorphan may have a drying effect on the respiratory mucosa, although this is debatable,[9] and it can stimulate the respiratory center, but it has no significant beneficial effects other than its antitussive properties, which are equal to those of codeine. The drug undergoes metabolic degradation in the liver; it should be avoided or used carefully in patients with hepatic insufficiency. Large doses of dextromethorphan can cause central depression and may result in reactions caused by histamine release, but the only side effects with normal doses are occasional nausea, drowsiness or dizziness.

Availability and dosage. The current popularity of dextromethorphan is illustrated by the fact that it is listed (as the hydrobromide) in over 20 combination mixtures in AMA Drug Evaluations. Some of the more commonly available are analyzed in Table 9–13; most of these are available as over-the-counter cough medicines. The drug is used in numerous preparations throughout the world, and is commonly prescribed in the United States either as dextromethorphan hydrobromide syrup, or as terpine hydrate and dextromethorphan hydrobromide elixir. The drug is also available in cough pastilles, troches and lozenges. It is frequently prescribed or purchased over-the-counter, mostly for the treatment of simple coughs and colds. Additional comprehensive listings of preparations containing dextromethorphan are readily available.[3, 18, 20, 25, 26]

The adult dose is 15 to 30 mg three to four times a day, but larger doses may be required. The dosage for children is 1 mg/kg divided into three or four doses. Although dextromethorphan hydrobromide is commonly taken as part of a combination product, it can be prescribed on its own, in the form of syrups containing 7.5 and 15 mg per 5 ml, or as 15 mg tablets.

Levopropoxyphene

The levo-isomer of the well-known analgesic propoxyphene is levopropoxyphene. Although it has local anesthetic properties, it is not an analgesic. Levopropoxyphene and dextropropoxyphene are structurally related to methadone, but neither drug is a narcotic, and they lack any real abuse potential. Levopropoxyphene is an effective antitussive, but it does not have any significant effect on respiratory tract secretions. Side effects are infrequent and usually minor; they include nausea, vomiting, dry mouth, headache, lightheadedness, dizziness, jitteriness, tremors, skin rash, urinary frequency and urgency. Overdosage causes severe tremors, agitation, vomiting and sedation. The main advantage of levopropoxyphene is that it is equally effective an antitussive as codeine, and it can safely be given chronically in the rare case when a drug is needed to suppress an annoying cough that cannot be alleviated by other measures.

Availability and Dosage. Only one preparation is marketed in the United States: this is levopropoxyphene napsylate, Novrad. It is available as 100 mg pulvules (capsules), and as a suspension containing 50 mg per 5 ml. The dosage for adults is 50 to 100 mg every four hours, and about 1 mg/kg every four hours for children. Larger doses have been given to adults without adverse effects.

Noscapine

Although noscapine (formerly called narcotine) is the second most abundant alkaloid (after morphine) in opium, it is a nonnarcotic benzylisoquinoline and is nonaddictive. It has papaverine-like spasmolytic effects in some animals, but it has no significant actions in man apart from its antitussive properties, which are comparable to those of codeine, and a tendency to cause slight sedation. Side effects include some drowsiness and nausea; allergic reactions occur rarely, and include vasomotor rhinitis and conjunctivitis. Very large doses cause central excitation and respiratory stimulation. The drug may also cause an increase in respiratory tract secretion in some patients. Noscapine is a useful antitussive, and may merit greater consideration as a treatment for many types of unwanted cough.

Availability and Dosage. Noscapine is marketed (sometimes as the hydrochloride) in a number of combination products and as the sole constituent (Table 9–14). The usual adult dose is 15 to 30 mg three or four times a day; up to 60 mg can be given safely as a single dose.[9] The drug is suitable for children over the age of six in a dosage of 7.5 to 15 mg up to four times a day. Although not many preparations are marketed, most are available without prescription.

Additional Antitissue Agents

Some additional agents have been advocated for use in the management of cough. Included among such suggestions are the following drugs:

Antihistamines. *Diphenhydramine, methaphenilene* (Diatrin)[9] and *tripelennamine* are each alleged to have antitussive properties. However, it is difficult to find convincing evidence that these agents have more specific antitussive qualities than do other antihistamines.

Neuroleptic Agents. Drugs such as *chlorpromazine* and other related *phenothiazines* are known to protect against vomiting; it has been suggested that they may have specific antitussive qualities also.[10]

Ganglion-blocking Agents. Some observers have reported that inhalations of *hexamethonium* can suppress cough. Similar reports, using the intravenous route, or related agents or a combination of both, have not been convincing; thus there is no basis for recommending such therapy.[10] Ganglionic blockade has also been used in the treatment of asthma (see Chapter 4).

Cough Lozenges. Although it is difficult to see how candy and similar demulcents can help unless a patient has pharyngitis, many such agents are made available for the treatment of cough (Table 9–15). These simple remedies are often useful when a cough is accompanied by a sore throat or a simple scratchy or tickling sensation in the throat.

Recommendations for Using Antitussive Drugs

In clinical practice, there are actually few cases in which antitussive therapy can be

Text continued on page 310

TABLE 9–14. ANTITUSSIVE PREPARATIONS CONTAINING NOSCAPINE*

Preparation	Basic Dose	Noscapine (mg)	Adrenergic (mg)	Mucokinetic (mg)	Other (mg)
Actol Expectorant	Tablet	30		Guaifenesin 200	
	5 ml syrup	30		Guaifenesin 200	Alcohol 12.5%
Conar Expectorant	5 ml liquid	15	Phenylephrine 10	Guaifenesin 100	
Conar-A	Tablet	15	Phenylephrine 10	Guaifenesin 100	
Isofil†	Tablet	30			Acetaminophen 300
Tusscapine	5 ml syrup	15			Theophylline 200
	Tablet (chewable)	15			

*These products are listed in the Physicians' Desk Reference 1978.
†Requires a prescription.

TABLE 9–15 NONPRESCRIPTION THROAT AND COUGH LOZENGES*

Preparation	Local Anesthetic	Adrenergic	Antitussive	Germicidal	Flavoring Agents
Axon	Benzocaine			Cetylpyridinium	
Baxinets	Benzocaine			Cetylpyridinium	
Cepacol Anesthetic Troches	Benzocaine			Cetylpyridinium	Aromatics
Cepacol Throat Lozenges	Benzyl alcohol			Cetylpyridinium	Aromatics
Cepastat	Phenol				Eucalyptus, menthol
Chloraseptic Lozenges	Phenol, sodium phenolate			Sodium borate, thymol	Glycerin, menthol
Chloraseptic DM Cough Control Lozenges	Phenol, sodium phenolate		Dextromethorphan		
Colrex	Benzocaine			Cetylpyridinium	
Conex	Benzocaine			Cetylpyridinium	
Histodan	Benzocaine			Cetylpyridinium	
Hold	Benzocaine		Dextromethorphan		
Lanazets	Benzocaine			Cetylpyridinium	
Listerine Cough Control	Benzocaine		Dextromethorphan		
Listerine Throat Lozenges				Hexylresorcinol, thymol	Eucalyptol, menthol, methyl salicylate
Oracin	Benzocaine				Menthol
Oradex-C	Benzocaine			Cetylpyridinium	
Robitussin-DM Cough Calmers			Dextromethorphan		Guaifenesin, alcohol
Romilar Cough Discs	Benzyl alcohol		Dextromethorphan		
SAC Throat Lozenges	Benzocaine	Phenylpropanolamine		Cetylpyridinium	Terpin hydrate
Semets	Benzocaine			Cetylpyridinium	
Silence Is Golden			Dextromethorphan		Honey
Smith Brothers Medicated Cough Drops	Benzocaine				Eucalyptol, menthol

Product					
Spec-T Antibacterial Troches	Benzocaine			Cetylpyridinium	
Spec-T Decongestant Troches	Benzocaine	Phenylephrine, phenylpropanolamine			
Spec-T Sore Throat/Cough suppressant	Benzocaine		Dextromethorphan		
Sucrets Antiseptic Throat Lozenges	Benzocaine			Hexylresorcinol	Menthol
Sucrets Cold Decongestant Formula Lozenges	Benzocaine	Phenylephrine, phenylpropanolamine			
Sucrets Cough Control Formula Lozenges	Benzocaine		Dextromethorphan		
Thantis Lozenges	Saligenin			Merodicein	
Thorzettes	Benzocaine		Dextromethorphan	Cetylpyridinium	
Thriocaine	Benzocaine			Cetylpyridinium	
Trocaine	Benzocaine			Cetylpyridinium, cetalkonium	
Trokettes	Benzocaine				
Tusscapine			Noscapine		
Tyro-Loz	Benzocaine			Tyrothricin	
Vicks Cough Silencer	Benzocaine		Dextromethorphan		Anethole, menthol, peppermint oil
Vicks Formula 44 Cough Discs	Benzocaine		Dextromethorphan		Anethole, menthol, peppermint oil
Vicks Medicated Cough Drops	Benzyl alcohol				Camphor, eucalyptol, menthol, thymol, tolu
Vicks Medi-trating	Benzocaine			Cetylpyridinium	Camphor, eucalyptus, menthol

*The information in this table is derived mainly from Handbook of Nonprescription Drugs. 5th ed., 1977. Additional products are described in Facts and Comparisons.

justified, in spite of the enormous demand for "cough medicines."[27, 28] Since the majority of marketed products are constituted to treat the complete "cough and cold syndrome," the role of cough suppressants has been difficult to define, and this lack of clear concept encourages physicians to indulge in polypharmaceutic prescribing. Not surprisingly, the F.D.A. is anxious to have many of the less-defensible preparations withdrawn from the market.[29]

In most cases in which the patient complains of a cough, the airways contain material that needs to be expelled. Most frequently, the retained material consists of viscous sputum, and what is really required is mucokinetic therapy, and not an antitussive drug (see Chapters 2 and 3). In those cases, such as carcinoma of the lung, where the cough is caused by pathologic irritation due to a nonremovable cause, a cough suppressant can be of considerable help to the patient. Similarly, each type of cough can be analyzed to provide a suitable specific form of therapy,[30] as pointed out earlier (Table 9-2). Some guidance to the management of different types of coughs is provided in Table 9-16. The relative costs of such agents should be taken into consideration, since some are indefensibly expensive. For further details consult Facts and Comparisons (see Table 1-10), which analyses most of the scores of different cough medicines that are marketed.

When a cold predominates as part of a cough and cold syndrome, it may be reasonable to combine a drying agent (such as an antihistamine) with a mucokinetic; the latter will prevent the secretions in the lower airways from becoming too viscous as a result of the drying agent's action in the upper airway. Whether a cough suppressant is desirable in such a situation is doubtful, unless used at night to prevent disturbance of sleep. In clinical practice, a physician should consider prescribing a combination mixture for use during the day, and supplementation with an extra antitussive at night. Usually, when cough control is needed, the goal should be to depress cough rather than to suppress it.[30]

In practice, it appears that codeine is the most suitable and least expensive narcotic antitussive; dextromethorphan appears to be the best nonnarcotic cough suppressant, and it can be obtained without prescription. Since most coughs and colds are self-limiting, it is probable that the majority of cough medicines that are used have little more than placebo value, and traditional remedies such as hot drinks, simple syrups and various inhalations are probably just as effective. In spite of the apparent general confidence in combination cough medicines, the weight of the evidence supports the critics of these popular nostrums.[8, 17, 18, 24, 25]

Cough Inducing Agents

The term "cough medication" is so universally identified with drugs that suppress coughing that the alternative meaning (drugs that induce coughing) is entirely overlooked. Nevertheless, it is sometimes necessary to provide treatment for patients who retain secretions, by the use of drugs that stimulate the impaired cough response. Such therapy is advantageous for many elderly, apathetic or obtunded patients with gurgling secretions in major airways, who alternatively must undergo traumatic suctioning for the removal of sputum. Unfortunately, no ideal pharmacologic approach has been developed to cope with the problem, although various tussive stimuli have been used by researchers[3, 5, 10, 21, 31] in their studies on cough. In Table 9-17, some of these agents are presented for consideration as a means of pharmacologically inducing coughing. Citric acid aerosol has attained the status of being the favored tussive stimulant of most investigators.[31, 32]

Drugs that do induce a tussive response obviously have irritative effects either peripherally in the airways or centrally on the cough center. The most popular agents are topical mucokinetics such as water or saline solutions, which can also cause stimulation of the cough receptors; in general, they are given by aerosol. The most successful means of inducing a cough response is by ultrasonic nebulization of a hypertonic salt solution; this approach should be considered initially. Intermittent positive pressure machines may be able to bring about coughing when a suitable agent is nebulized, and rapid changes in pressure help to induce a cough mechanically. Several coughing devices have been available; they impose a negative pressure phase in the breathing cycle, which may cause an effective cough. However, these are not very popular.

If aerosols and pressure devices cannot be used or are unsuccessful, intravenous therapy can be tried with agents such as paraldehyde, that act on the lung receptors, or lobeline, which acts on the respiratory

TABLE 9–16. SUGGESTED DRUG TREATMENT FOR COMPONENTS OF COUGH IN VARIOUS CONDITIONS*

Condition	Associated Factors					Suggested Therapy			
	Sputum Production	Broncho-spasm	Thoracic Pain	Disturbed Sleep	Habit	Antitussive**	Mucokinetics	Placebo	Other
Asthma	+	+++	-	+	+ or -	Dextromethorphan	Inhalations, SSKI	-	Bronchodilators
Bronchitis	+++	++	+ or -	+	-	Noscapine, dextromethorphan	Inhalations, SSKI	-	Bronchodilators, antibiotic
Bronchiectasis	+++	+	-	+	-	-	Various	-	Bronchodilators, antibiotic
Cigarette smoker	+	+	-	+	+ or ++	-	Various	Cough lozenges	Tranquilizer
Heart failure	+	++	-	++	-	Morphine, codeine	-	-	Digoxin, diuretic
Lung cancer	+	-	+++	++	-	Codeine, methadone, morphine	-	-	Specific therapy
Pneumonia	++	-	++	++	-	Codeine	Inhalations, SSKI	-	Antibiotic
Postpneumonia	+	-	+ or -	+	+ or -	Dextromethorphan benzonatate	Inhalations	Cough lozenges	-
Postsurgery	++	+ or -	+++	+++	-	Meperidine	Inhalations, SSKI	-	Adrenergic agents
Pulmonary fibrosis	-	+ or -	-	+	-	Codeine, levopropoxyphene, benzonatate	-	-	Bronchodilators
Psychogenic	-	-	-	+	+++	-	Inhalations	Cough lozenges	Sedative
Sore throat	-	-	-	+	-	-	Inhalations	Cough lozenges	Analgesic
Tracheitis	+	-	+ or ++	+	-	Codeine, dextromethorphan	Inhalations, SSKI	Cough lozenges	Antibiotic
Tuberculosis	+ or ++	-	-	+	-	-	SSKI	-	Antibiotics
Whooping cough	+	-	+ or ++	+++	- or +	Codeine, noscapine	Inhalations, SSKI	Cough lozenges	Antibiotic, sedation
Viral infection, e.g. "cold"	+ or ++	-	+	++	-	Dextromethorphan, benzonatate	Inhalations	Cough lozenges	Drying agents

*Other forms of therapy may also be needed.
**Clinical judgment is required for prescribing of antitussives. The suggestions may be appropriate for typical cases.

TABLE 9-17. DRUGS USED TO INDUCE COUGH

Agent	Clinical Value	Comment
INHALATIONAL		
Acetic acid vapor	Possible	Sometimes used to sterilize airways
Acetylcholine aerosol 1%	Possible	Causes bronchoconstriction; erratic
Acetylcysteine 10–20%	Yes	Mucolytic; may cause coughing
Acrolein gas	No	Too irritating; unstable
Ammonia gas 2–7%	Possible	Used in smelling salts; results are erratic
Ammonium hydroxide aerosol 2–3%	Possible	Used in smelling salts; results are erratic
Citric acid aerosol 2.5–25%	No	Too irritating
Ether vapor	Possible	Anesthetic effect can occur
Propylene glycol 15% or more	Yes	Standard sputum inducer
Saline 0.45–20%	Yes	Standard sputum inducer
Soap powder	No	Too irritating
Sulfur dioxide gas 0.05%	No	Too irritating
Sulfuric acid 0.5–1N	No	Too irritating
Water	Yes	Secondary sputum inducer
INTRAVENOUS INJECTION		
Chloroform 0.5–2 ml	Possible	Anesthetic effect undesirable
Doxapram 300 mg	Yes	Respiratory stimulant
Ether 0.5–2 ml	Yes	Anesthetic effect undesirable
Histamine	No	May induce bronchospasm
Lobeline 3–10 mg	No	Too many side effects
Nikethamide 2–15 ml 25% solution	Yes	Respiratory stimulant, analeptic
Paraldehyde 0-25–2 ml	Yes	Sedative; irritating to veins
Pentamethylenetetrazol 500 mg	Possible	Respiratory stimulant, epileptogenic
Prethcamide 300 mg.	Possible	Respiratory stimulant, analeptic
Trichlorethylene 0.5–2 ml	Possible	Anesthetic effect undesirable

center. Paraldehyde, ether and chloroform were each used in the past as diagnostic agents for evaluating the time taken for the blood to circulate from the point of injection through the venous system to the lungs. Although these forms of tussive therapy may not be suitable for frequent repetition, they may be of benefit when utilized on the appropriate occasion in a patient who is judged to need the induction of a bout of coughing. It is possible that tussive therapy, with its benefits, needs to be more accentuated in respiratory therapy, while antitussive therapy, with its very dubious benefits, should be allowed to subside to a more rational level.

COLDS AND RHINITIS

Anatomy and Physiology of the Nose

The nose constitutes the initial part of the respiratory tract, and it possesses anatomic and pathophysiologic features that closely resemble those found in the lower airways. The external anatomy of the nose is based upon the bony and cartilaginous skeleton; the muscles associated with the nasal structure are of only minor physiologic significance. The two nostrils, or nares, open into elongated triangular cavities separated by the nasal septum. Each cavity is encroached upon from the lateral wall by three curled turbinate bones (conchae) that are covered by vascularized mucous membrane. The function of the turbinates is to increase the area of contact for the respired air threefold, thereby improving the moisturizing of the inspirate and the filtering of foreign materials.[33]

Surrounding the nasal passages are the accessory air spaces, or paranasal sinuses; the lateral sinuses drain into the nose through orifices situated in the middle meatus between the inferior and middle turbinates. The role of the sinuses is not entirely clear, although they primarily serve to lighten the skull and protect the brain. The sinuses do not participate in respiratory function, and although they are frequently diseased in patients who have lower airway problems, most respiratory physicians do not regard the sinuses as being in their primary area of interest.

The inner nose is lined by ciliated epithelium, which contains goblet cells, and beneath which is a heavy endowment of mucous glands; the activities of the mucociliary mechanism of the nose are similar to those of the tracheobronchial tree.[34] The mucociliary flow is generally in the posterior direction, and the secretions are carried into the nasopharynx where they are swallowed without there being conscious awareness of the phenomenon; over 500 ml of thin mucus may be produced and cleared each day. When excessive secretions are formed, especially in disease, part of the mucociliary clearance is directed anteriorly, and the material leaves the nose through the nostrils. The paranasal sinuses are also lined by ciliated mucus-producing epithelium, and the mucus that is secreted drains into the nose, leaving the sinuses filled with air.

The nose serves to air condition the respired gases that pass through it, and it is capable of supplying about two-thirds of the humidification that is acquired by the air in its passage along the respiratory tract. The efficiency of the nose as a humidifying organ depends upon the rich vascular supply in the nasal mucosa. The arterial blood is derived from the ethmoidal branches of the ophthalmic artery, the sphenopalatine and other branches of the maxillary artery, and from branches of the facial artery. The supplying vessels form a rich subepithelial plexus of arterioles, and these drain into venous plexuses; those around the inferior turbinate have a cavernous quality and the mucosa behaves like erectile tissue.[35] The large amount of blood that may be diverted into these plexuses can result in considerable engorgement of the nasal mucosa, which leads to marked narrowing of the nasal passages. These changes are usually manifested as a stuffy feeling in the nose, and obstruction to free airflow.

The nasal mucosa is liberally endowed with autonomic nerves, which supply the afferent receptors in the mucosa and subserve efferent vasomotor and secretory functions. The sympathetic supply originates from the lower cervical and upper thoracic spinal cord; the nerves synapse in the stellate ganglion, then reach the nose along the petrosal canal in the vidian nerve. The parasympathetic supply is provided by the maxillary division of the fifth cranial nerve; the fibers are derived from the superior salivatory nucleus and synapse in the sphenopalatine ganglion. The parasympathetic fibers join those of the sympathetic supply to form the vidian nerve, which enters the posterior part of the nose and is distributed through the mucosa to supply afferent receptors and the mucous glands and blood vessels. Somatic sensory nerves originate in the nose and travel along ophthalmic and maxillary divisions of the trigeminal nerve to the medulla oblongata.

The mucociliary mechanism of the nose ensures that most of the larger particles suspended in its inspired air are filtered out. The nasal mucosa is also able to remove many soluble contaminating vapors and gases, thereby protecting the lower respiratory tract.[33] The efficiency of the nose is enhanced by the narrowing and the increased mucosal surface area that result from the turbinate bones. Further protection is provided by the sneeze reflex, which closely resembles the cough reflex; the expiratory maneuver during sneezing involves depression of the uvula, which thereby diverts most of the exhaled air through the nose rather than the mouth. Sneezing is a more forceful process than coughing, and it is less subject to voluntary control. Unlike coughing, repetitive sneezing must be regarded as a relatively useless clearance mechanism and therefore therapeutic measures designed to suppress the sneeze are more often justified than is antitussive therapy.

Secretory Disorders of the Upper Respiratory Tract

The important disorders of the upper respiratory tract of relevance in respiratory pharmacology are those conditions associated with excessive or abnormal secretions of the nose and sinuses. Irritation, by chemical irritants or as a result of allergy, and infection underlie most of the important conditions associated with altered nasal and sinus secretions. The most common disorder of the nose is *rhinitis,* which is manifested by a sense of discomfort in the nose, and by the production of excessive secretions. The mucoid discharge may cause sneezing or a "running nose," or may cause postnasal congestion and "drip", which tend to cause the patient to sniff and hawk in an effort to clear the nasal passages. The nasal mucosa usually becomes markedly engorged in such circumstances, and this results in difficulty in breathing through the nose. The degree of engorgement is increased in response to various exacerbating factors, such as temperature change, position and emotion. Often when the patient lies down, the engorgement of the affected nasal erectile tissue increases; similarly, if a patient lies on one side, the dependent nostril may become more obstructed.[34, 35]

The nose is the commonest target organ in allergic reactions, and it is estimated that

TABLE 9–18. CAUSES AND TREATMENT OF RHINITIS

Condition	Causes	Treatment Topical Vasocon-strictor	Antihist-amine	Anti-biotic	Other
Allergic rhinitis (Hay fever)	Hypersensitivity	Maybe	Yes	No	Desensitization, glucocorticoid, cromolyn
Acute rhinitis (Coryza)	Infection (often viral)	Yes	Maybe	Maybe	Analgesic
Vasomotor rhinitis (Perennial)	Autonomic imbalance	Yes	Yes	No	Glucocorticoid, anticholinergics
Postnasal drip	Cigarette smoking, irritation	No	Maybe	Maybe	Eliminate irritation, irrigate
Sinusitis	Infection, poor drainage	Maybe	No	Yes	Analgesics, irrigate, surgery
Nasal polyps	Allergy, infection	Maybe	Maybe	Maybe	Desensitization, glucocorticoid, cromolyn, surgery
Rhinitis medicamentosa	Excessive use of vasoconstrictors	Discontinue	Discontinue	No	Glucocorticoid
"Endocrine" rhinitis	Hypothyroidism, pregnancy	Maybe	Maybe	No	Treat underlying condition

over 13 million Americans suffer from seasonal *allergic rhinitis* (hay fever).[36] In the vast majority of cases, the allergen is a plant pollen, or a mold, or animal protein (usually derived from fur, hair or feathers), and is only rarely related to hay; similarly, very few patients actually suffer from fever. Although hay fever is poorly named, it is an extremely real and annoying disease, causing difficulty in breathing, repetitive sneezing and nasal discharge; usually, there is also conjunctivitis, and a sensation of itching around the nose and eyelids, which often involves other areas, such as the palate and the skin of the upper back. The symptoms of allergic rhinitis are caused mainly by histamine, which is released from sensitized mast cells and basophils by IgE antibodies (reagin).[36, 37] The mechanism is similar to that involved in allergic asthma (see Chapter 4), and many allergic rhinitis patients also suffer from asthma.

Allergic rhinitis has to be distinguished from other forms of rhinitis (Table 9–18); the most frequent cause of a similar syndrome is the *common cold* (coryza), which is often associated with constitutional symptoms and a cough, but which is not usually accompanied by the itching that characterizes allergic rhinitis. Most colds are probably caused by viruses, but in susceptible patients secondary bacterial infection may supervene; over 150 viruses and many bacteria have been implicated. Patients who are susceptible to

asthma readily develop bronchospasm as a secondary complication of an upper respiratory tract infection.

Other causes of rhinitis are described in Table 9–18. The most common form, which needs to be distinguished from allergic rhinitis, is *vasomotor rhinitis* (Table 9–19). This latter condition is not fully understood, but is believed to result from an imbalance in the autonomic nervous activity of the nasal mucosa. The condition can be exacerbated by emotion, but the nose of these patients is, to express it simplistically, oversensitive, and rhinitis may be exacerbated by changes in the weather or the ambient temperature, or by alterations in the general health of the patient. The condition is often confused with allergic rhinitis, but since vasomotor rhinitis does not require specific immunologic therapy, it is important to differentiate the condition, and to avoid the error of treating it with the conventional desensitization injection therapy that may be appropriate treatment for seasonal allergic rhinitis.[18, 36–38] In extreme cases, the condition can be alleviated surgically by sectioning the vidian nerve.[39]

The physician who deals with nasal disease is often confronted by a patient who has persistent or worsening rhinitis in spite of taking a number of the topical agents readily available for the treatment of rhinitis. The patient may, in fact, be suffering from the effect of the drugs, which allow rebound

TABLE 9-19. COMPARISON OF MAJOR FORMS OF RHINITIS

	Allergic	Vasomotor	Infectious
Provoking factors	Pollens, animal danders, molds	Smoke, dust, alcohol, temperature change	Viral infection, sinusitis, foreign body
Seasonal dependency	Yes	Affected by weather change	More in winter
Recognition of allergen (grass, etc.)	Frequently	No	No
Other allergies	Common	Unusual	Coincidental
Family history of allergy	Usual	Coincidental	Coincidental
Rhinorrhea	Watery	Mucoid	Purulent
Paroxysmal sneezing	Usual	Unusual	Rare
Nasal, ocular, palatine itching	Yes	Uncommon	Rarely
Pharyngitis, etc.	Rare	Rare	Common
Conjunctivitis	Common	No	Occasional
Nasal eosinophils	Usual	Rare	No
Fever, systemic symptoms	No	No	Yes
Short attacks	Can occur	Characteristic	No
Persistence of symptoms	Maybe	Yes	No
Appearance of nasal mucosa	Edematous, pale	Hyperemic	Swollen, red
Nasal polyps	Occasionally	Occasionally	Maybe
Skin test reactivity	Almost always	Coincidental	No
IgE mediated	Yes	No	No
Steroid responsive	Yes	No	No

congestion after the initial decongesting action, and which may have a direct irritative effect. This iatrogenic form of nasal congestion is known as "rebound congestion" or *rhinitis medicamentosa,* and it usually responds to withdrawal of the topical decongestant therapy.[35]

Sinusitis is another common disease which may present with rhinitis; simple acute cases may be difficult to differentiate from rhinitis of other types, but infection often supervenes and causes facial pain, swelling, fever and malaise. Although the basic treatment of the problem may require antibiotics or surgical drainage, symptomatic relief may be obtained from simple drainage procedure, or from irrigation; decongestant therapy may also be helpful. It is possible that careful positive pressure instillation of drugs into the nose could be of benefit in some cases of sinusitis. Chronic sinusitis should be considered as a possible underlying problem in patients with asthma, since correction of the sinus condition may lead to an improvement in the asthma.[39] In contrast, there are some patients with chronic sinusitis whose condition improves only after the effective treatment of associated problems such as bronchiectasis.

Various forms of rhinitis and sinusitis may be associated with the development of *polyps.*[39, 40] These mucosal outgrowths may exacerbate the underlying condition, and full relief of the disease complex may require polypectomy. Some cases of polyps are related to infection, whereas others appear to develop as a manifestation of allergy. Polyps are common in children with cystic fibrosis, and they may also be found in association with asthma. There is a curious interrelationship between aspirin sensitivity and asthma: severe asthma attacks may be provoked by aspirin in patients who have polyps. In many of these patients, unfortunately, polypectomy does not improve the asthma, and might even result in a worsening of the condition.

Other problems related to disorders in nasal and paranasal mucosal problems exist; the general population resorts to a tremendous amount of self-therapy with an extraordinary array of folk remedies and over-the-counter preparations in addition to prescribed medications for the treatment of "colds" and nasal congestion. One of the grossest errors in therapeutics is the attempt to "treat" the dripping nose that so often occurs in people exposed to a cold environment: the dripping fluid is a normal physical outcome of warm, humidified exhaled air condensing its moisture when it contacts the chilled nasal passages, and it does not represent abnormal mucosal secretion.[35] Of course, true vasomotor rhinitis may complicate the problem; nevertheless, the patient would be well advised to either tolerate the inconvenience or prevent it by warming the nose or the inspired air, rather than resorting to rhinologic medications.

DECONGESTANT THERAPY

The main decongestants used are of two groups: (1) antihistamines, and (2) alpha-adrenergic sympathomimetics. The antihistamines are particularly indicated when a true allergy exists, as may be suggested by symptoms of itching or by skin tests (Table 9–19). These two classes of agents will be discussed in the following sections.

Antihistamines

Knowledge about histamine has accumulated since its synthesis in 1907; it is an imidazole, and is also known as β-imidazolylethylamine. Since 1966, it has been recognized that the body contains two types of receptors that are stimulated by histamine; most of the reactions involved in allergy are mediated by H_1 receptors, whereas gastric secretion and some other histamine mediated reactions are dependent on the activation of H_2 receptors. The classic antihistamine drugs are essentially inhibitors of H_1 receptors, and these agents are of particular therapeutic value for the treatment of nasal allergy;[41] the drugs that will be discussed in this section are all antagonists of histamine at the H_1 receptors.

The first antihistamine compounds were synthesized in 1937, and the first agent to find a role in therapeutics was phenbenzamine (Antergan); subsequently, more suitable drugs were introduced, including pyrilamine (Neo-Antergan), which is still of value today.[42] Although the antihistamines are primarily of importance because of their ability to antagonize the actions of histamine, which are listed in Table 9–20, they do have a number of additional properties,[43] many of which are of importance in the treatment of conditions that do not involve histamine (Table 9–21).

Over the years, well over fifty antihistamines have been introduced into clinical practice, and perhaps half of these are relatively popular at present. Most of them are substituted ethylamines with the same general formula (Fig. 9–3), which are arbitrarily classified on the basis of their structure; several classes are generally recognized[42] (Table 9–22). The main agents of therapeutic importance are described in Table 9–23, and additional details are provided below.

Ethanolamines (aminoalkyl ethers, or aminoethyl ethers). These are based on the structure -O-C-C-N$<$ (see Figure 9–3), and the prototype is *diphenhydramine*. The antihistamines in this class are moderately potent H_1 blockers; they also possess anticholinergic activity. Many patients experience significant sedation and drowsiness when taking drugs of this class, although individual variation between drugs and between patients is marked. Ethanolamine effects are short lasting; the drugs are generally given up to four times a day. Of the compounds listed in Table 9–23, *carbinoxamine* produces the least side effects, with relatively little sedation; its more potent levo-isomer, *rotoxamine,* has similar qualities. Although these agents are effective in the treatment of allergy, several are of greater clinical value in the management of nausea, motion sickness and vertigo. They are particularly useful when sedation is a desired outcome of the treatment, and therefore they are often reserved for use at bedtime, in patients who are troubled by their symptoms during sleep.

Ethylenediamines. Ethylenediamines are derivatives based on the structure $>$N-C-C-N$<$ (see Fig. 9–3); the prototype is *pyrilamine*. Agents in this class are of value for the treatment of rhinitis, but are not antiemetics; indeed, many of them

TABLE 9–20. HISTAMINE

PRODUCTION SITES OF HISTAMINE
Mast cells, basophils, epidermis, respiratory tract, gastrointestinal tract, central nervous system

AGENTS PROVOKING RELEASE OF HISTAMINE
Antigen-antibody reactions, trauma, irritation, opium derivatives, other alkaloids, l-tubocurarine, diamidine, dyes, antibiotics, endotoxins, proteolytic enzymes, venoms, surface-active agents; also released at gastric and nervous system nerve endings

ACTIONS OF HISTAMINE
Vasodilation, increased capillary permeability, tissue edema, smooth muscle constriction, bronchospasm, sneezing, rhinorrhea, whealing, pain, urticaria, itching, anaphylaxis, gastric secretion

TABLE 9–21. ACTIONS OF ANTIHISTAMINES

Therapeutic Properties	Possible Clinical Indications
1. Antagonism of histamine-mediated allergic diseases:	
Of the respiratory tract	Rhinitis, sinusitis, bronchospasm
Of the skin	Urticaria, itching, whealing
Of general nature	Drug reactions, anaphylaxis
In other organs	Headache
2. Anticholinergic effects:	
Drying of mucous membranes	Rhinorrhea
Central effect	Sedation, nausea, vomiting, motion sickness, vertigo, Parkinsonism
3. Local anesthetic effect	Not of clinical value
4. Quinidine-like action	Arrhythmias

TABLE 9–22. MAJOR CLASSES OF ANTIHISTAMINES

Class	Antihistaminic Activity	Sedative Effects	Anticholinergic Activity	Antiemetic Effects	Gastrointestinal Side Effects	Duration of Effects	Examples of Agents in Addition to Those Listed in Table 9–23
ETHANOLAMINES (Amino alkyl ethers)	+ to ++	++ to +++	+++	++ to +++	+	3–6 hrs	
ETHYLENEDIAMINES	+ to ++	+ to ++	−	−	+++	3–6 hrs	Mepyramine, methaphenilene, thenylpyramine, thonzylamine
ALKYLAMINES (Propylamines)	++ to +++	+ to ++	++	−	+	4–12 hrs	
PIPERAZINES	++ to +++	+ to +++	+	+++	+	4–24 hrs	Buclizine, cinnarizine, chlorcyclizine, cyclizine, meclizine
PHENOTHIAZINES	+ to +++	+++	+++	++++	−	4–24 hrs	Isothipendyl, methdilazine, oxomemazine, parathiazine (pyrathiazine)
PIPERIDINES	++	+ to ++	++	−	+	6–8 hrs	Thenalidine

tend to produce nausea and even vomiting in sensitive patients. These agents cause relatively little sedation, although curiously enough some of them, such as *methapyrilene* and *pyrilamine,* are used in over-the-counter sleeping pills (such as Dormin, Nytol, Sleep-Eze and Sominex) in spite of the fact that studies have shown them to be no more effective for insomnia than placebos.[18] The ethylenediamines have relatively little anticholinergic activity, and overall their incidence of side effects is acceptably low. Several agents in this class are no longer promoted, probably because they have relatively poor potency when compared to their more established competitors.

Alkylamines (propylamines). Alkylamines are agents that have the basic structure -C-C-C-N< (Fig. 9–3). The prototype of this class is *chlorpheniramine,* which is clearly the most popular general antihistamine. The alkylamines are very potent in small dosage, and they cause only little or moderate sedation and induce few other disturbing side effects in most patients. However, some of these drugs do cause a higher incidence of sedation, while others, in contrast, cause central excitation. A few cases of toxic psychosis have been attributed to *pheniramine,* which, nevertheless, remains a curiously popular and inappropriately valued drug, particularly in combination preparations, in which it is often combined with pyrilamine—an indefensible choice, since the pairing of these drugs seems to offer no advantages. *Pyrrobutamine* and *triprolidine* are relatively long-acting general antihistamines alleged to have a low incidence of side effects; they are moderately popular for the treatment of rhinitis.

Piperazines. Piperazines are agents that contain the piperazine nucleus (Figure 9–3); the prototype of this class is *chlorcyclizine.* Although these agents do have antihistaminic properties, their main value is as antiemetics, and most of the piperazines are not promoted for the treatment of rhinitis or nasal congestion.

The most important antihistaminic piperazine is *hydroxyzine,* a potent sedative and tranquilizer and an effective antiemetic. It has proved to be useful in the management of bronchospasm, where its properties potentiate other bronchodilators; it is incorporated for this purpose in Marax (see Chapters 4 and 5). The drug is ideal for the sedation of an anxious asthmatic patient who is not retaining carbon dioxide, and it is the drug of choice for preoperative sedation of patients with chronic obstructive lung disease. It is of considerable value in the treatment of pruritus, but it is of only moderate benefit in the management of allergic rhinitis; it may be more suitable for vasomotor rhinitis.

Phenothiazines. Phenothiazines are characterized by the phenothiazine nucleus (Fig. 9–3), and these agents are generally regarded as major tranquilizers. However, a number of phenothiazines do possess antihistaminic properties, but the ones that are commonly available are usually employed as antipruritics or sedatives rather than for rhinitis. *Promethazine,* which is a potent phenothiazine, has many useful properties, and is credited with antitussive qualities as well as sedative and antiemetic actions. As a consequence of its many therapeutic uses, promethazine is a widely prescribed antihistaminic, and it is available as a component of an expectorant medication (Table 9–13), although it is rarely used in cold remedies. The phenothiazines have variable durations of effectiveness, and a single dose of promethazine, for example, may exert antihistaminic action for up to 24 hours, although it is more usual to administer the drug every four to six hours for symptomatic therapy. Promethazine has been described as the most potent antagonist of histamine discovered,[42] but it does have a relatively high incidence of side effects.

Piperidines. Piperidines are agents that contain the piperidine nucleus (Fig. 9–3). The most important drug in this group is *cyproheptadine,* which has antiserotonin as well as antihistaminic properties. It is mainly of value as an antipruritic, but is of use in the treatment of rhinitis. Rather surprisingly, it has not been found to be of marked value in adult asthma, although it is often useful in childhood asthma. One advantage of the drug is that it may stimulate the appetite, particularly in underweight children, and it has been found to offer therapeutic advantages to asthmatics with poor appetites.

Phenindamine is of interest because it is the only important antihistamine that causes central stimulation rather than sedation. The drug has been used in combination preparations with more potent antihistamines in order to decrease their sedative effects while increasing their antihistaminic potency.

Miscellaneous Antihistamines

Various antihistamines have been described apart from those discussed above, and alternative preparations are available in

Text continued on page 323.

TABLE 9–23. MAJOR ANTIHISTAMINES

Agent	Brand Names	Dosage Forms Available	Sedative Effects	Main Clinical Uses	Side Effects	Usual Oral Dosage Adult	Usual Oral Dosage Child
ETHANOLAMINES							
Bromodiphenhydramine	Ambenyl,* Ambodryl	Elixir 3.75 mg/5 ml Capsule 25 mg	+++	General antihistamine	Anticholinergic effects	25–50 mg tid	—
Carbinoxamine	Clistin, Rondec	Elixir 4 mg/5ml Tablet 4 mg Long-acting tablets 8 and 12 mg	++	General antihistamine	Low incidence of side effects	4–8 mg tid or qid	2–4 mg tid or qid (0.4 mg/kg/24 hours in divided doses)
Dimenhydrinate	Dramamine, Meni-D*	Liquid 12.5 mg/4ml Tablet 50 mg Injection 50 mg/ml Suppository 100 mg	+++	Antiemetic, for motion sickness	Can mask effect of ototoxic antibiotics. Hypertension, EKG changes.	50–100 mg q4h	5 mg/kg/24 hours in 4 doses; up to 300 mg/24 hours in divided doses
Diphenhydramine	Ambenyl,* Benadryl, Benylin,* etc.	Capsules 25 and 50 mg Elixir 12.5 mg/5ml Injections 10 and 50 mg/ml	+++	General antihistamine; agent of choice for administration by injection	Anticholinergic effects; drowsiness may diminish with continued use.	25–50 mg tid or qid	10–20 mg tid or qid, or 5 mg/kg/24 hours in divided doses
Doxylamine (Decapryn)	Bendectin*	Syrup 6.25 mg/ml Tablets 12.5 and 25 mg	+++	Sedative and antiemetic	Low incidence of side effects	12.5–25 mg qid or 50 mg h s	2 mg/kg/24 hours in 4–6 doses
Phenyltoloxamine	Naldecon,* Sinutab*	Only available in combination products	+++	Rhinitis	Drowsiness	—	—
Rotoxamine	Twiston	Long-acting tablet 4 mg	++	(l-isomer of carbinoxamine)	Low incidence	2–4 mg tid or qid	1–2 mg tid or qid
ETHYLENEDIAMINES							
Antazoline	Antastan. Antistine. Vasocon-A	Tablet 100 mg	+	Topical ophthalmic decongestant	Very few	50–100 mg tid or qid	—
Chloromethapyrilene (Chlorothenylpyramine)	Chlorothen, Tagathen	Tablets 25 and 50 mg	+	General antihistamine	Nausea, vomiting	25–50 mg tid or qid	—
Methapyrilene	Allergin, Hista–Clopane,* Histadyl, Semikon	Capsules 25 and 50 mg Syrup (fumarate) 30 mg/5 ml Injection 20 mg/ml	++	General antihistamine; suitable for topical and parenteral use	Dizziness, headache; clopane tends to counteract side effects.	25–50 mg 4–5 times/day	0.88–1.32 mg/kg 4–6 times/day, up to 300 mg/24 hours.

Drug	Trade names	Preparations		Indications	Side effects	Adult dose	Child dose
Pyrilamine	Anthisan, Histalet,* Histalon. Neo-Antergan, etc.	Tablets 25 and 50 mg	+	Mainly for rhinitis	Relatively few; nausea, vomiting	25–50 mg qid	12.5–15 mg 3–4 times/day (for children 6–12)
Thenyldiamine	NTZ.,* Thenfadil	Nasal solution and spray	++	Mainly for rhinitis	Slight sedation	Use spray several times a day.	
Tripelennamine	PBZ-SR. Pyribenzamine, Stanzamine	Tablets 25 and 50 mg Long-acting tablets 50 and 100 mg Elixir (Citrate) 30 mg/4 ml Injections 25 mg/ml	++	General antihistamine	Citrate is more palatable than hydrochloride salt; may cause nausea.	25–100 mg 1–3 times/day; up to 600 mg a day can be given	25–50 mg 3–4 times/day; infants: 10–20 mg as needed
ALKYLAMINES							
Brompheniramine	Brocon,* Dimetane, Dimetapp*	Tablet 4 mg Extentabs 8 and 12 mg Elixir 2 mg/5ml Injections 10 and 100 mg/ml	+	Mainly for rhinitis	Anticholinergic effects, drowsiness	4–8 mg 3–4 times/day, or 1 Extentab q 8–12 h	2–4 mg 3–4 times/day, or 1 Extentab q12h; children under 3: 0.44 mg/kg/day in divided doses
Chlorpheniramine	Allerbid, Antagonate, Chlor-trimeton, Histaspan, Teldrin, etc.	Tablet 4 mg Long-acting tablets and capsules 8 and 12 mg Syrup 2 mg/5 ml Injections 10 and 100 mg/ml	+	General antihistamine	Slight drowsiness or dizziness, anticholinergic effects or sweating	2–4 mg qid, or 1 long-acting preparation q 12 h	0.35 mg/kg/24 hours, in 4 divided doses
Dexbrompheniramine	Disomer, Disophrol* Drixoral*	Tablet 2 mg Repeat-action tablets 4 and 6 mg Syrup 2 mg/5ml	+	Similar to brompheniramine, but twice as potent	Anticholinergic effects, drowsiness	2–4 mg 3–4 times/day. or 1 repeat-action tablet q 8–12 h	0.17 mg/kg/24 hours in 3–4 divided doses, or 1 repeat-action 4 mg tablet q 12 h
Dexchlorpheniramine	Polaramine	Tablet 2 mg Repetabs 4 and 6 mg Syrup 2 mg/5ml	+	Similar to chlorpheniramine, but twice as potent	Similar to chlorpheniramine	1–2 mg 3–4 times/day, or 1 Repetab q 8–12 h	5 mg/kg/24 hours in 4 divided doses; up to 300 mg/day
Dimethindene (Dimethpyrindene)	Forhistal, Triten	Tablet 1 mg Delayed release tablet 2.5 mg Syrup 1 mg/5ml	++	Pruritus, rhinitis; long-acting general antihistamine	Drowsiness	1–2 mg 1–3 times/day, or a 2.5 mg tablet 1–2 times/day	Same dose as for adult for children over 6.
Pheniramine	Trimeton,* Triaminic,* Tussagesic,* etc.	Tablet 40 mg	++	Relatively obsolete general antihistamine	Similar to chlorpheniramine; toxic psychosis	20–40 mg 2–3 times/day	Used only in combination preparations

*Combination preparations

Table continued on the following page

TABLE 9-23. MAJOR ANTIHISTAMINES (Continued)

Agent	Brand Names	Uncombined Dosage Forms Available	Sedative Effects	Main Clinical Uses	Side Effects	Usual Oral Dosage Adult	Usual Oral Dosage Child
Pyrrobutamine	Co-Pyronil,* Pyronil	Tablet 15 mg	+	Long-acting general antihistamine	Minimal	15–30 mg 2–3 times/day	0.3 mg/kg twice a day
Triprolidine	Actidil, Actifed*	Tablet 2.5 mg Syrup 1.25 mg/5ml	+	Long-acting potent antihistamine; has no taste	Minimal; may cause central excitation	2.5 mg 2–3 times/day	0.6–2.5 mg 2–3 times/day
PIPERAZINES							
Hydroxyzine	Atarax, Vistaril	Tablets 10,25,50 and 100 mg Capsules 25,50 and 100 mg Suspensions 25 mg/5ml Syrup 10 mg/5ml Injections 50 and 100 mg in 2 ml	+++	Antihistamine, sedative, antiemetic, ataractic; useful in asthma.	Drowsiness	25–100 mg 3–4 times per day	2 mg/kg/24 hours in 4 divided doses
PHENOTHIAZINES							
Methdilazine	Tacaryl	Tablets 4 and 8 mg Syrup 4 mg/5ml	—	Antipruritic, general antihistamine	Drowsiness, dizziness, nausea, headache, rash, dry mucosae	8 mg 2–4 times/day	0.3 mg/kg/24 hours in 2 divided doses
Promethazine	Phenergan, Remsed, Zipan	Tablets 12.5, 25 and 50 mg Syrups 6.25 and 25 mg/5ml Suppositories 25 and 50 mg Injections 25 and 50 mg/ml	+++	Sedative, antiemetic, potent antihistamine. Potentiates analgesics and antitussives.	Drowsiness, infrequent anticholinergic effects, extrapyramidal reactions, jaundice, hypotension, photosensitivity	12.5–50 mg up to 4 times a day	0.5 mg/kg/dose as needed, e.g. full dose at night, ¼ dose in morning or p.r.n.
Trimeprazine	Temaril	Tablets 2.5 mg Spansules 5 mg Syrup 2.5 mg/5ml	++	Antipruritic	Drowsiness, nausea, anticholinergic effects, extrapyramidal reactions, jaundice	2.5–10 mg qid; up to 80 mg per day	3.75–7.5 mg per day in 3 divided doses
PIPERIDINES							
Cyproheptadine	Periactin	Tablet 4 mg Syrup 2 mg/5ml	+	Pruritus, general antihistamine, antiserotonin, appetite stimulation	Drowsiness, anticholinergic effects, headache, nausea, rash	4 mg tid; up to 32 mg per day	0.25 mg/kg/24 hours in 2 to 4 divided doses
Diphenylpyraline	Diafen,* Hispril, Histryl	Tablet 2 mg Spansule 5 mg	+	General antihistamine	Drowsiness, headache, dizziness, dry mouth, nausea	2 mg q 4 h or 5 mg q 12 h	1–2 mg 2–4 times/day. Not for children under 6
Phenindamine	Histalet,* Nolamine,* Thephorin	Tablet 25 mg	—	General antihistamine	Central stimulation, convulsions	25 mg 1–4 times/day	

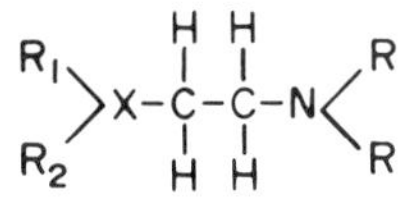

GENERAL STRUCTURE OF
ANTIHISTAMINES

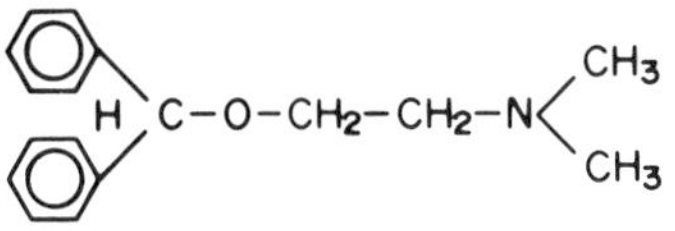

1. ETHANOLAMINE (DIPHENHYDRAMINE)

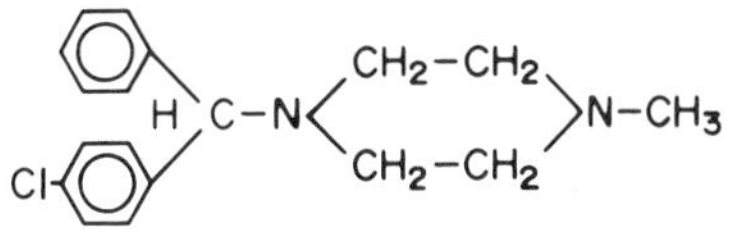

4. PIPERAZINE (CHLORCYCLIZINE)

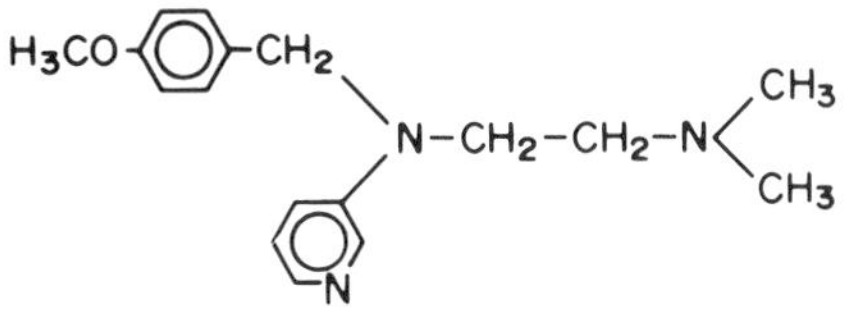

2. ETHYLENEDIAMINE (PYRILAMINE)

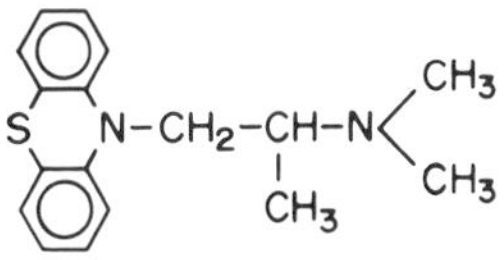

5. PHENOTHIAZINE (PROMETHAZINE)

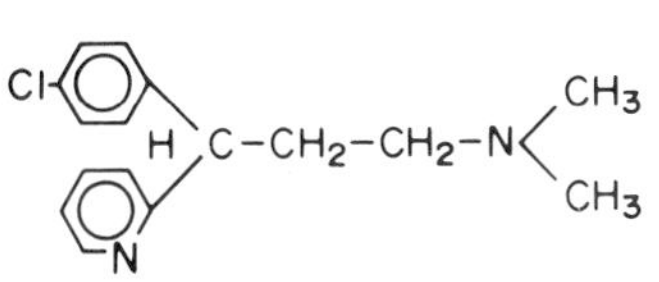

3. ALKYLAMINE (CHLORPHENIRAMINE)

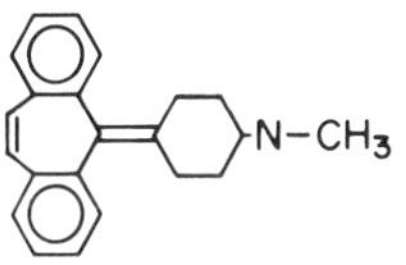

6. PIPERIDINE (CYPROHEPTADINE)

Figure 9–3.

other countries, for example, bamipine, clemizole, deptropine, dimethothiazine, embramine, halopyramine, mebhydrolin, thiazinamium, tolpropamine and trimethobenzamide.[22] More recently, a European agent, clemastine, has been investigated in the United States by plethysmography, and it has been shown to be an effective nasal mucosal decongestant with certain advantages.[44] However, it is generally agreed that there are more than enough antihistamines available already, and any additional agent would have to have quite outstanding properties to justify its manufacture and promotion for the treatment of rhinitis.

General Pharmacology of the Antihistamines

In general, the antihistamines are well absorbed when taken by mouth, and their effects appear within 15 to 30 minutes. Hydroxylation and glucuronidation occur in the liver, and the metabolites are excreted in the urine. Barbiturates may induce the production of hepatic enzymes that lead to breakdown of antihistamines, but in practice these two classes of drugs potentiate rather than antagonize their respective central actions. Caution is advised when giving antihistamines to patients with hepatic insufficiency, since drug accumulation may occur.

The main actions of the antihistamines have been tabulated in Table 9–21. Their adverse properties, effects and drug interactions are summarized in Table 9–24. All patients receiving antihistamines should be cautioned about the possibility of adverse effects: this is of particular importance with respect to those agents with potent sedative effects, since they may interfere with driving skills and with the ability to carry out precise work. The atropine-like drying effects can be unpleasant for patients, since they may result in a dry mouth and an uncomfortable nose. Moreover, in patients with excessive lower respiratory secretions, mucokinesis may be impaired, and the pulmonary status may deteriorate. Although antihistamines may be expected to be of value in allergic asthma, many patients worsen when given these drugs, and, in general, antihistamines are therefore not recommended in the treatment

TABLE 9-24. ANTIHISTAMINES

MAIN ACTIONS
  Immunologic   — Antiallergy properties
  Anticholinergic   — atropine-like and antiParkinsonism effects
  Central depressant— sedative, soporific and antiemetic effects
  Local anesthetic — and antipruritic actions
  Quinidine-like   — on the heart

MAIN CLINICAL INDICATIONS
  Urticaria, angiodermatitis
  General allergy
  Allergic rhinitis, seasonal conjunctivitis
  Nausea, vomiting, motion sickness
  Insomnia, anxiety, Parkinsonism

POSSIBLE ADVERSE EFFECTS
  Nonspecific   — Nausea, vomiting, diarrhea, chills
  Nervous system— Oversedation, excitation, disorientation, delirium, insomnia, tremors, vertigo, irritability,
                    convulsions; blurred vision, dry mouth, urinary retention, tachycardia, constipation.
  Mucosae   — Dry mouth, inspissated secretions
  Skin   — Dry, warm skin, photosensitivity, rashes
  Other   — Hyperthermia, nephrosis, agranulocytosis, anaphylaxis

ADVERSE DRUG INTERACTIONS
  Potentiation of sedatives, tranquilizers, depressants, narcotics, anesthetics, phenothiazines
  Potentiation of pressor effect of epinephrine, and of hypotensive effects and side effects of rauwolfia alkaloids
  Potentiation of anticholinergics
  Potentiated by monoamine oxidase inhibitors; combination potentiates catecholamines
  Antagonism of anticholinesterases
  Enzyme induction may increase metabolic breakdown of hormones (e.g., glucocorticoids), phenytoin, phenyl-
    butazone and anticoagulants

CONTRAINDICATIONS
  Patients with major seizure disorders
  Hepatic insufficiency
  Patients who must avoid sedation (except phenindamine)
  Glaucoma (especially ethanolamines and phenothiazines)

EFFECTS OF OVERDOSAGE
  Atropine-like effects:
  Dryness of mouth and respiratory tract
  Pyrexia
  Dilated pupils
  Convulsions, hallucinations
  Coma, respiratory depression

of most asthmatics, and they are contraindicated in severe asthma and in status asthmaticus. However, mild asthma, especially in children, may respond well to antihistamines, perhaps as a result of their sedative effects, which are not accompanied by marked respiratory center depression. Chlorpheniramine has been credited with benefitting the asthma of patients who are being treated with the drug for concomitant nasal allergy.[45] Although diphenhydramine, promethazine, chlorpheniramine and pyrilamine, in particular, have been credited with antitussive properties — which have resulted in their incorporation in some "cough medicines" (see Tables 9–12 and 9–13) — their drying effect on the respiratory mucosa may actually be deleterious.[12, 30]

The antihistamines are used in hundreds of proprietary combination preparations, and unfortunately all too many of these lack a rational basis.[40] Frequently, antihistamines from different classes are combined with each other in the hope that the more desirable properties of each will be expressed while the less desirable effects will be suppressed; there is little evidence that such a result is attainable,[45] and in many cases the choice of constituents lacks a clear pharmacologic basis. However, phenindamine may be a rational addition since it can cause central stimulation, and thus counteract the sedative effects of other antihistamines. Similarly, the gastrointestinal side effects of an ethylenediamine (for example, pyrilamine or tripelennamine) may be counteracted by the antiemetic action of an ethanolamine (such as phenyltoloxamine). Curiously enough, manufacturers more frequently choose to use an alkylamine as a

TABLE 9–25. SOME TOPICAL NASAL DECONGESTANTS

Brand Names	Sympathomimetic	Antihistamine	Other*
Afrin Nasal Spray/Drops	Oxymetazoline 0.05%		A,S
Alconefrin Drops	Phenylephrine 0.16–0.5%		
Allerest Nasal Spray	Phenylephrine 0.5%	Methapyrilene 0.2%	A,S
Anti-B Nasal Spray	Phenylephrine		
Benzedrex Inhaler	Propylhexedrine		
Biomydrin Spray	Phenylephrine 0.25%		Thonzonium
Clopane Drops (Rx)	Cyclopentamine 0.5%		
Contac Nasal Mist	Phenylephrine 0.5%	Methapyrilene 0.2%	A
Coricidin Nasal Mist	Phenylephrine 0.5%	Chlorpheniramine 0.3%	
Coryban-D Nasal Spray	Phenylephrine 0.5%		A
Dristan Nasal Mist	Phenylephrine	Pheniramine	A,F
Duration Spray	Oxymetazoline 0.05%		
Forthane Inhaler	Methylhexaneamine		F
Gluco-Fedrin Drops	Ephedrine 1%		A,F,S
Hydra Spray	Phenylephrine 0.25%	Methapyrilene 0.2%	A,S
I-Sedrin Plain Drops	Ephedrine 1%		A,S
Isophrin Nasal Drops/Spray	Phenylephrine 1/8–1%		
Naso Mist Spray	Phenylephrine 0.5%	Methapyrilene 0.15%	A
Neo-Synephrine Spray, Drops, Jelly	Phenylephrine 1/8–1%		A(spray)
NTZ Drops/Spray	Phenylephrine 0.5%	Thenyldiamine 1%	A
Otrivin (Rx)	Xylometazoline 0.05%		
Privine Drops, Spray	Naphazoline 0.05%		A
Sine-Off Spray	Phenylpropanolamine	Chlorpheniramine	
Sine-Off Once-A-Day Spray	Xylometazoline 0.1%		F
Sinex-L.A. Spray	Xylometazoline 0.1%		A
Sinutab Decongestant Sinus Spray	Phenylephrine 0.5%		Thonzonium
Soltice Spray	Phenylephrine 0.25%	Methapyrilene 0.1%	
Super-Anahist Spray	Phenylephrine 0.25%		A,F
Triaminicin Spray	Phenylpropanolamine 0.75% Phenylephrine 0.25%	Pheniramine 0.125% Pyrilamine 0.125%	A
Tuamine Inhaler	Tuaminoheptane 1%		F
Tyrohist Spray	Phenylephrine 0.25%	Pyrilamine 0.15%	A
Tyzine Solution (Rx)	Tetrahydrozoline 0.1%		
Vasoxyl (Rx)	Methoxamine 0.5%		
Va-Tro-Nol Drops	Ephedrine 0.35%	Methapyrilene 0.15%	A,F
Vicks Inhaler	L-desoxyephedrine		F
Vicks Sinex Spray	Phenylephrine 0.5%	Methapyrilene 0.12%	A,F
4-Way Nasal Spray	Phenylephrine 0.5% Phenylpropanolamine 0.5% Naphazoline 0.05%	Pyrilamine 0.2%	

*A = Antiseptics
 F = Aromatic flavoring agents
 S = Stabilizers, buffers, etc.

Note — These preparations are available as over-the-counter products, except those marked Rx, which require a prescription. Other products are marketed, but those listed are representative.

member of an antihistamine pair, with little obvious benefit to be discerned.

Care should always be taken to adjust the dose of a preparation, and the timing of its administration, to the needs of each patient.[46] In general, long-acting preparations are not recommended, and parenteral administration is rarely indicated other than for sedation. Topical administration into the nose by sprays, drops, jellies, tampons or pledgets may be useful in various forms of rhinitis — particularly allergic rhinitis — and preparations are marketed for topical use that contain chlorpheniramine, methapyrilene, pheniramine, phenyltoloxamine, pyrilamine or thenyldiamine (see Table 9–25).

Recommendations for Antihistamine Therapy

In respiratory therapy, most antihistamines other than the piperazines are of primary value in the control of upper respiratory tract allergic manifestations. Oral and topical antihistamines alone or in combination preparations are of symptomatic benefit in seasonal and perennial allergic rhinitis, but their use should be restricted to not more than a few days at a time for exacerbations of the disease. Whether or not the antihistamines should be used to prevent allergic rhinitis depends upon the individual patient; certainly, prophylactic therapy can be successful.[45] Topical antihistamines should be used with great selectivity, since overuse can irritate the nasal mucosa and produce the chronic irritation that characterizes rhinitis medicamentosa. Continued use of an antihistamine tends to be associated with a decreased effect because tolerance develops; some authorities advise stopping the drug for a few days every three or four weeks, or changing periodically to a different class of antihistamine.[42] Agents with a sedative effect are most useful at night, and they may help suppress annoying coughing; however, if the nocturnal cough is a symptom of asthma, bronchodilator therapy may be more appropriate. Hydroxyzine has a special value as an adjuvant in the management of asthma, whereas cyproheptadine may be of particular benefit for the undersized asthmatic child who requires an appetite stimulator.

Although antihistamines are often used in the treatment of the common cold, there is very little controlled evidence to support this practice. A drying effect may be produced temporarily, but this may actually increase the nasal discomfort. At present, there are no good studies of the effects of antihistamines on nasal secretions and nasal mucociliary clearance;[35] they may have an adverse effect on the natural history of viral coryza. Most studies suggest that antihistamines are of only little benefit in this all too common disease, although they may provide initial symptomatic relief.

The antihistamines do appear to potentiate the adrenergic mucosal decongestant drugs, and in practice most physicians become familiar with a few proprietary combination preparations of these two types of drug, which they prescribe for various forms of rhinitis. There is evidence that some antihistamines, including chlorpheniramine and tripelennamine, have cocaine-like effects on sympathetic nerve terminals thereby potentiating the effect of norepinephrine;[35] this may be considered as evidence of a rational basis for claims that the antihistamines act synergistically with sympathomimetic mucosal decongestants. Although

the two classes of drugs can be used interchangeably in rhinitis, they do differ in their pharmacologic actions, as will become evident in the ensuing discussion on adrenergic decongestants.

Alpha-adrenergic Sympathomimetic Drugs

A large number of synthetic catecholamine derivatives possess significant alpha-adrenergic stimulating properties with absent, or relatively minor, beta-adrenergic properties. Drugs that are pure stimulators of alpha receptors produce vasoconstriction of blood vessels in mucosae and in the skin; they have no other significant direct properties, although secondary and reflex consequences may be manifested in the intact organism. The common therapeutic application of alpha-adrenergic agents is almost limited to the treatment of the respiratory tract mucous membranes. These drugs are usually classified as nasal decongestants or as mucosal constrictants.

Many of the drugs considered to fall into the category of nasal decongestants do possess some beta-activity, which may result in an adverse effect on the mucosa. It is possible that some of these drugs cause initial mucosal vascular constriction, as a consequence of rapid alpha-receptor stimulation, followed by vascular dilation when the effects of beta-receptor stimulation begin to predominate. Because of this possibility, drugs such as epinephrine, which are potent beta-stimulators as well as alpha-stimulators, are not favored for the treatment of mucosal congestion, since the short-lived decongestion is followed by "rebound" congestion.

The decongestants are of two types:[47, 48] those that have only a direct stimulating effect on alpha-receptors, and those that also act indirectly by causing the release of stored norepinephrine from sympathetic nerve endings. The norepinephrine is responsible for direct stimulation of both alpha- and beta-receptors, and the decongestant drug is therefore classified as an indirect alpha- and beta-stimulator. Further discussion of the actions of drugs on the adrenergic receptors is provided in Chapter 4.

At present, four classes of alpha-adrenergic decongestant drugs are recognized (Table 9–26). Members of each of these classes are available as proprietary preparations, mainly for topical use. Some of the related agents are used principally as pressor agents, since they have potent vasoconstrictor effects on the general vasculature, and they are less suited for the treatment of the respiratory mucosa.

Arylalkylamines (β-phenylethylamines). These agents have one of several structures (see Figure 9-4), and most of them have some beta-activity. *Ephedrine, pseudoephedrine* and *epinephrine* are major beta-2 receptor agonists, and they are generally used as bronchodilators. However, it is worth recalling that the traditional Chinese name for ephedrine means "yellow astringent," and was presumably an acknowledgement of the vasoconstrictor properties of the drug. Pseudoephedrine is very similar to ephedrine in action, although it is generally considered to be mainly a nasal decongestant; this categorization is incorrect, since the drug is also a bronchodilator.

The most important of all the nasal decongestants is *phenylephrine*, which is a potent direct stimulator of alpha-receptors. It is used mainly as a nasal decongestant, and is available in topical and in oral preparations, although the latter result in erratic effects.[40] It is a popular constituent in many combination preparations used in the treatment of colds. Although it is a potent drug, it is available without prescription. Phenylephrine is also incorporated with some aerosol bronchodilators (see Chapter 4), and it can be given on its own, by aerosolization, into the lung. Such a form of therapy may be useful for tracheitis, bronchitis or laryngitis, and is particularly indicated for the treatment of postintubation mucosal congestion. The recommended dose is 0.5 ml of 1 per cent solution; this can be added to a bronchodilator or diluted in 1 to 3 ml saline.

The second most popular decongestant for use in combination preparations is *phenylpropanolamine*. This agent has both direct and indirect alpha-effects, and very slight indirect beta-effects; the latter have not been regarded as of sufficient potency to justify using the drug as a bronchodilator. Although phenylpropanolamine is occasionally used as a topical decongestant, it is mainly employed as a constituent in oral combination cold remedies.

Methamphetamine (also known as desoxyephedrine) has replaced amphetamine, which used to be popular for the alleviation of nasal congestion. It is much less susceptible to drug abuse than is amphetamine, and it has few significant side effects when used appropriately. Methamphetamine has a low vapor pressure, and it is incorporated with aromatic volatile agents in nasal dispensers;

inhalation of the volatilized fumes results in a penetrating form of topical therapy, suitable for the treatment of nasal and sinus congestion.

Additional arylalkylamine decongestants are available, but are rarely used in clinical practice. These include hydroxyamphetamine (Paredrine) and phenylpropylmethylamine (Vonedrine). *Mephentermine* sulfate (Wyamine) is mainly used as a systemic pressor agent, but the base is volatile and has been used as a decongestant inhalant; the sulfate could also be used as a 0.5 per cent topical solution on the nasal mucosa. Metaraminol, marketed as the bitartrate (Aramine, Pressonex), and methoxamine, marketed as the hydrochloride (Vasoxyl), are additional alpha-adrenergic agents that are mostly used systemically for their pressor effects. However, *methoxamine* is available as a nasal decongestant.

Cycloalkylamines (Figure 9-4). The important decongestant agents in this group have both direct and indirect alpha effects, with minor beta effects. *Cyclopentamine* is used in similar fashion to phenylephrine as a nasal decongestant, and as a companion to isoproterenol for the aerosol therapy of bronchospasm (Aerolone). It is also used in combination with antihistamines for the treatment of rhinitis and other allergies. *Propylhexedrine* is a volatile drug used in inhalers in similar fashion to methamphetamine.

Alkylamines (Figure 9-4). The agents in this group are very similar to the cycloalkylamines. *Methylhexaneamine* (methylhexamine) and the more popular *tuaminoheptane* are both volatile, and are marketed in inhalers. In addition, tuaminoheptane sulfate is a liquid, and is made available as a solution for topical application. An additional agent in this group, methylaminoheptane (Oenethyl), is of less value, and this preparation is not promoted.

Imidazolines (Figure 9-4). The agents in this group are all direct-acting alpha-receptor stimulators. They are used as solutions and sprays, and are relatively popular. *Naphazoline* has been subjected to the most clinical evaluation, and it has gained some adverse publicity. In particular, instillation of the drug into the nose may be followed by absorption and consequent cerebral depression in children. However, the same problems can probably occur with the other imidazolines, *oxymetazoline, tetrahydrozoline* and *xylometazoline*. None of these agents should be given to young children.

Text continued on page 331

TABLE 9–26. PROPERTIES OF NASAL DECONGESTANTS

Agent	Examples of Brand Names	Adrenergic Receptor Stimulation α	β	Direct (D) or Indirect (I)	Mode of Administration Topical	Oral	Comment
ARYLALKYLAMINES (β-Phenylethylamines)							
Ephedrine and derivatives		++	++	D,I	Solutions 1–3% Sprays 1%	Tablets 25, 50 mg	Oral bronchodilator; not used as an aerosol bronchodilator
Epinephrine	Adrenalin	++	++	D	Solution 1%		Short acting; mainly a bronchodilator
Methamphetamine (desoxyephedrine)	Vicks Inhaler	++	±	D,I	Combined with aromatics for inhalation		Volatile inhalant unlikely to be drug of abuse
Methoxamine	Vasoxyl	++	–	D	Solution 0.5%, 1%		Mostly used as a pressor agent
Phenylephrine	Neo-Synephrine	++	–	D	Sprays 0.25%, 0.5% Jelly 0.5% Solutions 0.125%, 0.25%, 1%	Tablets 10 mg	Most popular topical vasoconstrictor; used in combination bronchodilator aerosols also
Phenylpropanolamine	Propadrine	++	±	D,I	Combination sprays 0.5–1%	Capsules 25, 50 mg Elixir 20 mg/ml	Most popular oral decongestant
Pseudoephedrine	Sudafed	++	++	D,I		Tablets 30, 60 mg Syrup 30 mg/5 ml	Popular oral decongestant and bronchodilator
CYCLOALKYLAMINES							
Cyclopentamine	Clopane	++	±	D,I	Solutions 0.5%, 1% Spray 0.5%		Useful vasoconstrictor; used in combination bronchodilator aerosol

Propylhexedrine	Benzedrex, Dristan	++	±	D,I	Combined with aromatics for inhalation	Volatile; little central stimulation
ALKYLAMINES						
Methylhexaneamine (methylhexamine)	Forthane	++	±	D,I	Combined with aromatics for inhalation	Volatile; less popular preparation.
Tuaminoheptane	Tuamine	++	±	D,I	Combined with aromatics for inhalation Solution (sulfate) 1%	Base is volatile, whereas the sulfate is used as a solution
IMIDAZOLINES						
Naphazoline	Privine	++	−	D	Solution 0.05% Spray 0.05%	Overdosage has caused deep sleep and coma in children; initially, may cause stinging sensation; marked "rebound" congestion may occur.
Oxymetazoline	Afrin	++	−	D	Solution 0.05% Spray 0.05%	Relatively long action; could cause central depression in children
Tetrahydrozoline	Tyzine	++	−	D	Solution 0.05, 1% Spray 0.1%	Overdosage has caused coma and hypothermia in children; may cause "rebound" congestion.
Xylometazoline	Otrivin	++	−	D	Solution 0.05, 1% Spray 0.05, 1%	Could cause central depression in children

1. ARYLALKYLAMINES

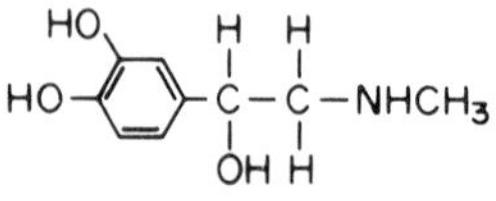

EPINEPHRINE

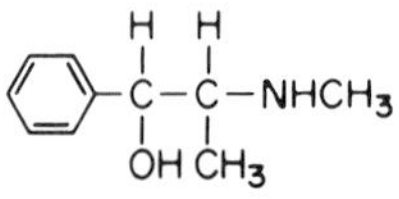

EPHEDRINE

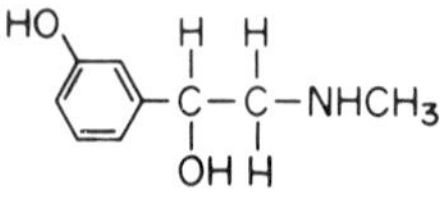

PHENYLEPHRINE

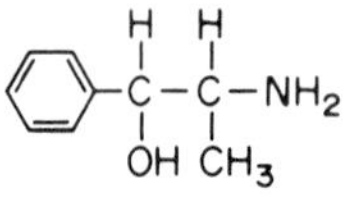

PHENYLPROPANOLAMINE

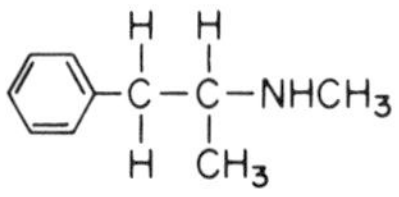

METHAMPHETAMINE

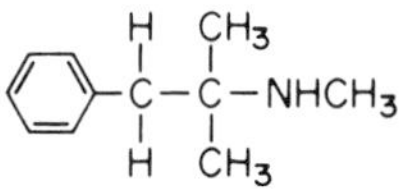

MEPHENTERMINE

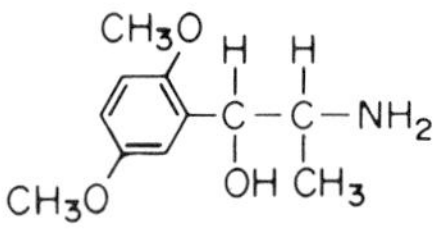

METHOXAMINE

2. CYCLOALKYLAMINES

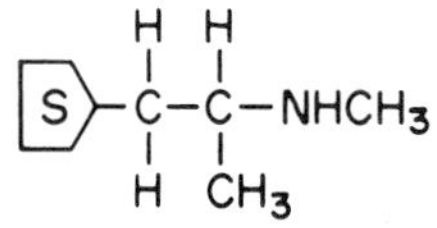

CYCLOPENTAMINE

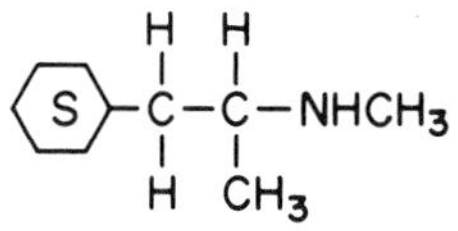

PROPYLHEXEDRINE

3. ALKYLAMINES

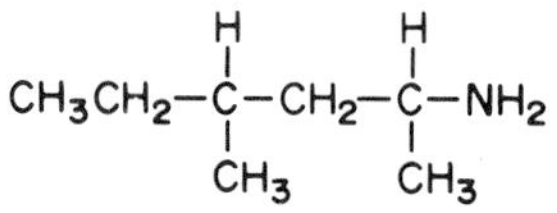

METHYLHEXANEAMINE

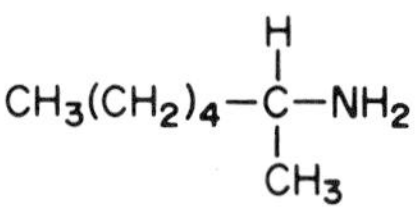

TUAMINOHEPTANE

4. IMIDAZOLINES

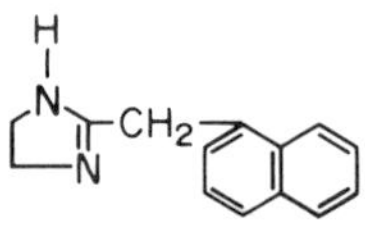

NAPHAZOLINE

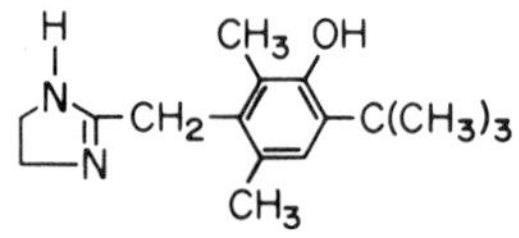

OXYMETAZOLINE

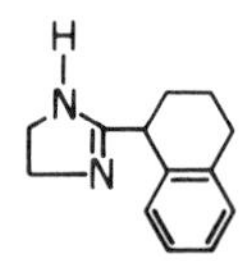

TETRAHYDROZOLINE

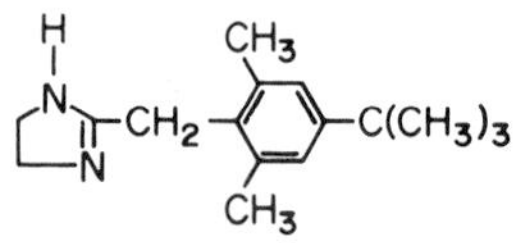

XYLOMETAZOLINE

Figure 9–4.

Naphazoline and tetrahydrozoline, allegedly, have a marked propensity to cause rebound congestion, which may result in symptomatic worsening of the nasal symptoms in susceptible patients. A further problem with the imidazolines is that they can cause cardiac irregularities that are presumed to be secondary to coronary artery vasoconstriction.[40] Some manufacturers claim that these agents are long lasting, and require only one administration a day; however, there are no objective data to suggest the imidazolines are significantly longer acting than other decongestants.

General Pharmacology of Alpha-Adrenergic Sympathomimetic Drugs
(Table 9–27)

The mucosal decongestants are characterized by their vasoconstrictive properties. When given orally or parenterally, these agents cause generalized vasoconstriction to some degree, and the nasal mucosa is not affected preferentially. When given topically into the nose, the local mucosa is the primary site of action, but part of the administered dose may be swallowed and absorbed, and part may enter the circulation directly. Thus, systemic effects may occur even when topical therapy is employed: the incidence of these undesired effects can probably be lessened by using appropriate amounts of the volatile agents by means of nasal inhalers.

The effects of the mucosal decongestants on the nasal mucosa are similar to those of the topical antihistamines, but the alpha-adrenergic agents act more rapidly. Unfor-

tunately, many decongestant drugs result in a subsequent increase in mucosal congestion after the initial decongestant effect; this "rebound" may be a physiologic result of the relative ischemia that the mucosa is subjected to by the drug, but it may, in part, be a consequence of the weak beta-adrenergic properties that many sympathomimetic decongestant drugs possess, as pointed out earlier. However, the contribution of the beta-adrenergic vasodilator effect cannot be considered an important factor in most cases, since drugs such as phenylephrine and the imidazolines lack beta effects but are reputed to cause marked rebound congestion.

When alpha-adrenergic agents are used repeatedly, their effectiveness tends to decline over the course of a few days, and the rebound phenomenon may become more exaggerated and appear more rapidly. The decongestant effect that the patient seeks gradually wanes as tachyphylaxis develops; overuse of topical drugs is a frequent response of the poorly educated patient. The tachyphylactic outcome may be more pronounced in drugs that have an indirect adrenergic effect, since they manifest their decongestant action by means of the norepinephrine they release from storage granules. One would therefore expect more of a problem with agents whose action is indirect, but there is no evidence to suggest that tachyphylaxis is less likely with a direct-acting agent such as phenylephrine.

The alpha-adrenergic side effects are numerous and are more likely to occur with oral administration of the drugs. The main adverse reactions are similar to those pro-

TABLE 9–27. SYMPATHOMIMETIC DECONGESTANTS

PRIMARY EFFECTS
    Alpha effects—Mucosal vasoconstriction, decreased mucosal congestion and secretion.
    Beta effects—Mucosal vasodilation, weak bronchodilation, central stimulation, cardiac stimulation.

POSSIBLE ADVERSE EFFECTS
    Topical—Nasal stinging, dryness and irritation, rebound congestion, tachyphylaxis, rhinitis medicamentosa, possibility of systemic absorption, infection due to contamination.
    Systemic—Tachycardia, arrhythmias, hypertension, nervousness, central stimulation, nausea, dizziness. Imidazolines may also cause hypertension followed by hypotension, bradycardia, sweating, drowsiness, deep sleep, and coma (especially in children).

DRUG POTENTIATIONS
    Other sympathomimetics, bronchodilators, monoamine oxidase inhibitors, thyroid derivatives, antihistamines, anticholinergics.

CONTRAINDICATIONS
    Known sensitivity, hypertension, cardiac ischemia, arrhythmias, tremulousness, hyperthyroidism, diabetes, cerebral depression. Imidazolines should not be given to small children. Decongestants may exacerbate glaucoma and prostatism. Avoid in patients who are taking tricyclic antidepressants.

TABLE 9–28. DOSAGES OF ORAL DECONGESTANTS

Product	CNS Stimulation	Adult Dosage	Pediatric Dosage
Ephedrine	+++	15–50 mg q 3–4 h	3 mg/kg/24 hr in 4–6 doses
Phenylephrine*	±	10 mg tid	Children aged 6–12: 5 mg tid
Phenylpropanolamine	+	25–50 mg q 3–6 h	Children aged 8–12: 20–25 mg tid
Pseudoephedrine	++	30–60 mg q 6–8 h	1 mg/kg q 6 h

*Relatively ineffective by oral route.

duced by the sympathomimetic bronchodilators (Chapter 5): dizziness, nervousness, insomnia, tremors, palpitations, pallor, sweating, urinary retention, frequency, dry mouth, headache, vomiting, and rashes. The drugs can exacerbate hypertension, and can cause arrhythmias. Particular care is needed if patients have underlying diseases that may be exacerbated, for example, hypertension, myocardial ischemia, arrhythmias, hyperthyroidism, mental instability, glaucoma, prostatic hypertrophy. The side effects associated with topical use include initial burning or stinging sensations in the nose and subsequent dryness of the mucosa. In severe cases the ensuing nasal irritation may be worse than the initial congestion that prompted the use of the drug; an unsophisticated patient may try to obtain "stronger" over-the-counter decongestants to try to conquer the apparently progressive disease that causes nasal torment. The eventual outcome of such mismanagement is rhinitis medicamentosa, which responds to withdrawal of all topical therapy (Table 9–18).

Side effects may be a particular problem in children; the potentially dangerous imidazolines should be avoided in small children and infants, as well as in adults with unstable cardiovascular or nervous system disorders. When using sprays or drops, the patient should always be cautioned to use, at first, not more than the minimal dose, and to increase this to the optimum by careful trial; usually no more than three or four sprays or drops are required in each nostril at one time, and repeat treatments should not be carried out more often than every six hours. The topical treatments should generally be administered with the patient in the upright or leaning forward position, so that any excess medication will run out of the nose. Although the volatile inhalants can be used more often, it is wise to discourage use of the manufacturer's maximum dosage (which may be as much as a treatment every hour), and to limit

TABLE 9–29. USE OF TOPICAL NASAL DECONGESTANTS

VOLATILE INHALANTS
Inhale deeply into each nostril in turn while occluding the other nostril. Repeat if necessary after 2–3 minutes, and again if required. Limit treatments to not more than three such inhalations per hour, for a few days at most.

NASAL SPRAY
Spray deep into each nostril, and blow the nose after a few minutes. Repeat again if necessary after five minutes. Up to four such treatments may be taken every 4–6 hours. Limit such therapy to the minimum, and discontinue after a few days.

NASAL DROPS
Sinus Therapy. Insert 1–3 drops into the nostril with head tilted back or to side; repeat in other nostril. Avoid swallowing drops if possible, e.g. by leaning forward following treatment, or by spitting out medication entering pharynx.
Eustachian Therapy. Instil 2–3 drops into nostril while lying supine; head may be turned slightly toward affected side. Position should be maintained for 5 minutes.
Other. Alternative forms of administration should be carried out under the supervision of an otorhinologist.

GENERAL PRINCIPLES
Use lowest concentrations and lowest dosages initially.
Use infrequently, as needed, rather than routinely.
Limit treatments to a few days at a time.
Use with particular care in children.
Prefer volatile agents, when suitable for the individual patient.
Prefer single entity pharmacologic preparations over combination products.

topical treatments to three or four a day. Nasal droppers should be kept clean to avoid bacterial infection. Oral drug therapy should be used sparingly (dosages are provided in Table 9–28), and an attempt should be made to determine if an oral or inhalational preparation is more suitable for each individual patient. In all cases, the essential advice is that treatments be carried out as infrequently as the patient can readily tolerate, and to try to limit courses of therapy to three or four days. For treatment details, see Table 9–29.

Combination Antihistamine and Sympathomimetic Preparations

Numerous combination preparations are available for topical use (Table 9–25) and for oral use; both over-the-counter (Table 9–30) and prescription preparations (Table 9–31) are marketed in abundance.[18, 25, 26, 49, 50] It is not possible to list all the preparations, but the ones that are tabulated offer a reference for most of the more frequently utilized products. Recommendations cannot readily be offered, and the major consideration should probably be the relative cost of competing brands.[49] Generic products in uncombined forms are obviously more desirable on this basis; the thoughtful physician may find it difficult to justify the use of any combination preparation for the treatment of colds or rhinitis. However, there are undoubtedly many patients who claim benefits from proprietary cold remedies, and in most cases the nonprescription items should be favored, since they are less expensive and are probably just as effective. In terms of pharmacologic reality, it is difficult to see any meaningful difference between the average prescription preparations and the popular over-the-counter products.

Certain additional classes of drugs are often present in combination preparations:[49]

Antitussives. These have already been described, and some are listed in Tables 9–12, 9–13 and 9–14.

Analgesics. *Aspirin* is suitable for most patients, but *acetaminophen* is an effective and generally safer alternative. There is no sound reason for preferring other analgesics such as *salicylamide*, and there is no rational pharmacologic basis for using more than one type of analgesic in a combination product.

Mucokinetics. Although guaifenesin is often provided by manufacturers, other agents may be better (see Chapter 3).

Drying Agents. The addition of anticholinergic muscarinic agents such as *atropine, homatropine,* or *isopropamide* seems to be unnecessary in a combination product that already has an antihistamine/sympathomimetic; the additional drying effect is unlikely to be significant. Theoretically, anticholinergic drugs may be helpful in vasomotor rhinitis, but convincing proof of this is lacking.

Caffeine. Caffeine is sometimes added to counteract the sedative effect of the antihistamine. The amount included is unlikely to have any therapeutic value. Other methylxanthines such as *papaverine* are of dubious value in combination cold remedies.

Antacids. Antacids such as *aluminum hydroxide* and *magnesium hydroxide* are generally provided in suboptimal amounts when they are incorporated in cold remedies, and there is little to justify such an addition to a combination preparation.

Antibiotics. Antibiotics are sometimes incorporated in topical nasal products; this practice is mentioned only in order to condemn it.

Ascorbic acid. Ascorbic acid is a controversial agent believed by many faithful partakers to offer both prophylactic and therapeutic properties in the mystique of cold prevention and treatment. The dosages claimed to be of value are much greater than the normal dietary needs, and the evidence to support such massive dosages is not persuasive. One major problem is that although everyone thinks they know what a "cold" is, the entity is difficult to distinguish from other forms of rhinitis. Since vasomotor rhinitis may have a psychic basis in many patients, a placebo in which faith is invested may have benefits, and the misguided patient may consider the drug has had an effect on the propensity to catch or the ability to handle a viral "cold." Since ascorbic acid has been shown to have antihistaminic and mucolytic properties (Chapter 3), one might expect vitamin C to have an effect on the respiratory mucosa. However, considering the already described difficulty in demonstrating that the common antihistamines and mucolytics are of any benefit in the common cold, it is hardly surprising that one cannot find an acceptable pharmacologic explanation for the role of vitamin C in this mysterious ailment. To indulge in a flight of fancy, there may be more rational grounds for nebulizing small amounts of ascorbic acid into the nose rather than taking large amounts orally. Unfortunately, the present

TABLE 9–30. NONPRESCRIPTION PREPARATIONS FOR COLDS AND SINUSITIS†

Brand Names	Antihistamine (mg)	Decongestant (mg)	Analgesic (mg)	Other (mg)
Alka-Seltzer Plus Cold Tablet	Chlorpheniramine 2	Phenylpropanolamine 24	Aspirin 324	
Allerest Time Capsule	Methapyrilene 10 Pyrilamine 15	Phenylpropanolamine 50		
Allerest Regular Tablet	Chlorpheniramine 2	Phenylpropanolamine 18.7		
Bayer Children's Cold Tablet		Phenylpropanolamine 3.13	Aspirin 81	
Chlortrimeton Decongestant Tablet	Chlorpheniramine 4	Pseudoephedrine 60		
Citra Capsule	Methapyrilene 8.33 Pheniramine 6.25 Pyrilamine 8.33	Phenylephrine 10	Phenacetin 120 Salicylamide 227	Ascorbic acid 50 Caffeine 30
Congesprin Tablet		Phenylephrine 1.25	Aspirin 81	
Contac Time Capsule	Chlorpheniramine 4	Phenylpropanolamine 50		Belladonna 0.2
Coricidin Tablet	Chlorpheniramine 2		Aspirin 325	
Coricidin-D Tablet	Chlorpheniramine 0.5	Pseudoephedrine 7.5	Acetaminophen 120	Alcohol 7%
Coryban-D Capsule	Chlorpheniramine 2	Phenylpropanolamine 12.5	Aspirin 325	
Co-Tylenol Liquid/5 ml	Chlorpheniramine 2	Phenylpropanolamine 25		Caffeine 30
Co-Tylenol Tablet	Chlorpheniramine 2	Pseudoephedrine 30	Acetaminophen 325	
Demazin Repetab*	Chlorpheniramine 4	Phenylephrine 20		
Demazin Syrup/5 ml	Chlorpheniramine 1	Phenylephrine 2.5		Alcohol 7.5%
Dristan Tablet	Chlorpheniramine 2	Phenylephrine 5	Aspirin	Caffeine. Al(OH)$_3$. MgCO$_3$
Duadacin Capsule	Chlorpheniramine 1 Pyrilamine 12.5	Phenylephrine 5	Acetaminophen 120 Salicylamide 200	Ascorbic acid 50 Caffeine 30
Fedahist Tablet	Chlorpheniramine 4	Pseudoephedrine 60		
Fedahist Syrup/5 ml	Chlorpheniramine 2	Pseudoephedrine 30		
Fedrazil Tablet	Chlorcyclizine 25	Pseudoephedrine 30		
4-Way Cold Tablet		Phenylephrine 5	Aspirin 325	Mg(OH)$_2$ 125 Phenolphth- alein 15
Guistrey Fortis Tablet	Chlorpheniramine 1	Phenylephrine 10		Guaifenesin 100
Neo-Synephrine Compound Cold Tablet	Thenyldiamine 7.5	Phenylephrine 5	Acetaminophen 150	Caffeine 15
Novafed A Liquid/5 ml	Chlorpheniramine 2	Pseudoephedrine 30		Alcohol 5%
Novahistine Elixir/5 ml	Chlorpheniramine 2	Phenylpropanolamine 18.75		Alcohol 5%
Novahistine Tablet	Chlorpheniramine 2	Phenylpropanolamine 18.75		
Ornex Capsule		Phenylpropanolamine 18	Acetaminophen 325	
Rhinex Tablet	Chlorpheniramine 1.25	Phenylephrine 2.5	Aspirin 150	Al(OH)$_3$, Mg(OH)$_2$
Rhinosyn Syrup/5 ml	Chlorpheniramine 4	Pseudoephedrine 60		
Rhinosyn Pediatric Syrup/5 ml	Chlorpheniramine 2	Pseudoephedrine 30		
Sinarest Tablet	Chlorpheniramine 1	Phenylephrine 5	Acetaminophen 300	Caffeine 30
Sinulin Tablet	Chlorpheniramine 2	Phenylpropanolamine 37.5	Acetaminophen 325 Salicylamide 250	Homatropine 0.75
Sinutab Tablet	Phenyltoloxamine 22	Phenylpropanolamine 25	Acetaminophen 325	
Sinutab II Tablet		Phenylpropanolamine 25	Acetaminophen 325	
Triaminic Syrup/5 ml	Pheniramine 6.25 Pyrilamine 6.25	Phenylpropanolamine 12.5		
Triaminicin Allergy Tablet	Chlorpheniramine 4	Phenylpropanolamine 37.5		
Triaminicin Tablet	Chlorpheniramine 2	Phenylpropanolamine 25	Aspirin 450	Caffeine 30
Ursinus Tablet	Pheniramine 12.5 Pyrilamine 12.5	Phenylpropanolamine 25	Aspirin 300	

†These products are selected because they are listed either in Physicians' Desk Reference, 1978 or in Med. Lett. Drugs Therap. 17:89–92, 1975. Many others are listed in Handbook of Nonprescription Drugs, 5th ed. 1977, Ch. 8. Manufacturers change constituents in preparations from time to time.

*Long-acting preparation.

grounds for using vitamin C in any form can hardly be considered rational.

Additional Agents Used for Rhinitis

Cromolyn Sodium. In Europe, topical therapy with cromolyn is used in the prophylaxis of allergic rhinitis (see Chapter 8). Various preparations are available outside the United States, including a 2 per cent solution (such as Rynacrom). The drug can be extremely effective, particularly in patients with high IgE levels and in those with positive skin tests.[51] However, the effect of the drug can be disappointing, even in patients with clear pollen-related hay fever type problems. Nevertheless, cromolyn would be worth trying in selected patients with troublesome nasal allergy. Whether or not cromolyn could prevent colds is worth further studies, since the drug has recently been shown to inhibit virus-induced cytopathic effects.[52]

Glucocorticoids. Both topical and systemic steroid therapy can be of value in the treatment of rhinitis of various types (Table 9–18). For many years, dexamethasone sodium phosphate has been available as an intranasal spray (Turbinaire Decadron Phosphate), and it can help about three-quarters of the patients who get only partial relief from antihistamines and decongestants. The spray should be used for only a few days or weeks at a time for severe symptoms. One regimen that has been suggested[38] is as follows: initially, two sprays in each nostril three times a day, with reduction to two treatments and then one treatment a day as the condition improves; further weaning should occur, and eventually one spray in each nostril at bedtime may suffice. This type of regimen may be required by severely symptomatic patients throughout the pollen season, but continued therapy can produce systemic side effects, and may cause local damage such as an atrophic nasal mucosa or nasal septal perforation. More recently, an investigational topical steroid, *flunisolide*,[53] has been found useful in hay fever; this preparation apparently causes less local and systemic side effects.

Some patients with allergic rhinitis and some with severe rhinitis medicamentosa gain relief from systemic steroid therapy.[38] In patients who are severely troubled by symptoms that do not respond adequately to or worsen with other drugs, oral *prednisone* can be given in a single daily dose of 20 to 25 mg. The dose should be reduced over the next few days to 10 to 15 mg per day, and further weaning continued, or a switch made to alternate-day therapy if symptoms exacerbate. Some authorities have recommended a single injection of a long-acting steroid to help a patient through the hay fever season, but such an approach is of disputed value.

Some asthmatic patients who are weaned from steroid therapy as the asthma improves may develop withdrawal symptoms of rhinitis (Chapter 7). In such cases, topical nasal steroid therapy may be required. As further knowledge is gained, it is possible that topical agents such as *beclomethasone dipropionate*,[54, 55] and *triamcinolone acetonide* (see Chapter 7) may find a use in the topical therapy of rhinitis as well as asthma. Drugs of this type may provide the most reliable and safest forms of antiinflammatory treatment for the reactive respiratory mucosa.

Summary of the Treatment of Nasal Congestion and Rhinitis

In most patients, the symptoms of nasal obstruction, sneezing and excessive secretions are temporary and may improve readily enough without treatment. However, persistent or frequently recurring symptoms usually deserve drug therapy for a strictly limited period of time; chronic treatment is undesirable and may actually perpetuate the symptoms.[35, 40] General symptomatic measures often suffice when the symptoms appear to be part of a viral "upper respiratory tract infection": adequate fluids, humidification of the ambient atmosphere, avoidance of rapid temperature changes, and analgesics or antipyretics should be tried for a few days in troublesome cases. If symptoms are sufficiently annoying, nasal decongestant therapy can be utilized.

For the management of persistent rhinitis, the simple over-the-counter single pharmacologic ingredient products are the most suitable. Volatile inhalants and nasal sprays are preferrable to nasal drops, and all forms of topical treatment are preferred to oral or systemic dosage when the treatment is used in the correct fashion, that is, strictly when needed, for a minimal number of days. The basic agents are the alpha-adrenergic decongestants, which can be of value in all forms of rhinitis, as well as in sinusitis. They are also valuable, particularly when admin-

TABLE 9–31. PRESCRIPTION PREPARATIONS FOR COLDS AND SINUSITIS†

Brand Names	Antihistamine (mg)	Decongestant (mg)	Analgesic (mg)	Other (mg)**
Actifed Tablet	Triprolidine 2.5	Pseudoephedrine 60		
Actifed Syrup/5 ml	Triprolidine 1.25	Pseudoephedrine 30		
Codimal-L. A. Capsule*	Chlorpheniramine 8	Pseudoephedrine 120		
Colrex Compound Capsule	Chlorpheniramine 2	Phenylephrine 10	Codeine 16 Acetaminophen 300	Ascorbic acid 100
Corilin Infant Liquid/1 ml	Chlorpheniramine 0.75		Aminoacetic acid 25 Na salicylate 80	
Coriforte Capsule	Chlorpheniramine 4		Phenacetin 130 Salicylamide 190	Ascorbic acid 50 Caffeine 30
Deconamine Tablet	Chlorpheniramine 4	Pseudoephedrine 60		
Deconamine Elixir/5 ml	Chlorpheniramine 2	Pseudoephedrine 30		Alcohol 15%
Deconamine SR Capsule*	Chlorpheniramine 8	Pseudoephedrine 120		
Dimetapp Extentabs*	Brompheniramine 12	Phenylephrine 15 Phenylpropanol- amine 15		
Dimetapp Elixir/5 ml	Brompheniramine 4	Phenylephrine 5 Phenylpropanol- amine 5		Alcohol 2.3%
Disophrol Chronotab*	Dexbrompheniramine 6	Pseudoephedrine 120		
Disophrol Tablet	Dexbrompheniramine 2	Pseudoephedrine 60		
Drixoral Tablet*	Dexbrompheniramine 6	Pseudoephedrine 120		
Emprazil Tablet		Pseudoephedrine 20	Aspirin 200 Phenacetin 150	Caffeine 30
Extendryl Tablet/5 ml Syrup	Chlorpheniramine 2	Phenylephrine 10		Methoscopolamine 1.25
Extendryl Capsule*	Chlorpheniramine 8	Phenylephrine 20		Methoscopolamine 2.5
Fedahist Capsule*	Chlorpheniramine 10	Pseudoephedrine 65		
Histabid Duracap*	Chlorpheniramine 8	Phenylpropanolamine 75		
Histalet Forte Tablet*	Chlorpheniramine 4 Pyrilamine 25	Phenylephrine 10 Phenylpropanolamine 50		
Histalet Syrup/5 ml	Chlorpheniramine 3	Pseudoephedrine 45		
Histospan-D Capsule*	Chlorpheniramine 8	Phenylephrine 20		Methoscopolamine 2.5
Isoclor Tablet	Chlorpheniramine 4	Pseudoephedrine 25		
Isoclor Liquid/5 ml	Chlorpheniramine 2	Pseudoephedrine 12.5		
Isoclor Trimesule*	Chlorpheniramine 10	Pseudoephedrine 65		
Kronohist Kroncocaps*	Chlorpheniramine 4 Pyrilamine 25	Phenylpropanolamine 50		
MSC Triaminic Tablet	Preniramine 25 Pyrilamine 25	Phenylpropanolamine 50		Methoscopolamine 4

Product	Antihistamine	Sympathomimetic	Analgesic	Anticholinergic
Naldecon Tablet	Chlorpheniramine 5 Phenyltoloxamine 15	Phenylephrine 10 Phenylpropanolamine 40		
Naldecon Syrup /5 ml	Chlorpheniramine 2.5 Phenyltoloxamine 7.5	Phenylephrine 5 Phenylpropanolamine 20		
Naldecon Pediatric Syrup/5 ml	Chlorpheniramine 0.5 Phenyltoloxamine 2	Phenylephrine 1.25 Phenylpropanolamine 5		
Napril Plateau Caps*	Chlorpheniramine 4 Pyrilamine 25	Phenylpropanolamine 25		Methoscopolamine 2.5
Narine Gyrocaps*	Chlorpheniramine 8	Phenylephrine 20		
Neotep Granucaps*	Chlorpheniramine 9	Phenylephrine 21		
Nolamine Tablet	Chlorpheniramine 4 Phenindamine 24	Phenylpropanolamine 50		
Novafed A Capsule*	Chlorpheniramine 8	Pseudoephedrine 120		
Oraminic Spancap*	Chlorpheniramine 8	Phenylpropanolamine 50		
Ornade Spansule*	Chlorpheniramine 8	Phenylpropanolamine 50		Atropine 0.3 Isopropamide 2.5
Pseudo-Hist Liquid/5 ml	Chlorpheniramine 2	Pseudoephedrine 15		
Pseudo-Hist Capsule*	Chlorpheniramine 10	Pseudoephedrine 65		
Rhinex D Lay Tablet*	Chlorpheniramine 4	Phenylpropanolamine 60		
Rondec Tablet/5 ml Syrup	Carbinoxamine 4	Pseudoephedrine 60	Acetaminophen 300 Salicylamide 300	
Rondec Drops/1 ml	Carbinoxamine 2	Pseudoephedrine 25		
Rynatan Tablet	Chlorpheniramine 8 Pyrilamine 25	Phenylephrine 25		
Rynatan Suspension/5 ml	Chlorpheniramine 2 Pyrilamine 12.5	Phenylephrine 5		
Singlet Tablet*	Chlorpheniramine 8	Phenylephrine 40	Acetaminophen 500	
Sinovan Timed Capsule*	Chlorpheniramine 20	Phenylephrine 20		
Sinubid Tablet	Phenyltoloxamine 66	Phenylpropanolamine 100	Acetaminophen 300 Phenacetin 300	Methoscopolamine 2.5
Sudachlor T.D. Capsule*	Chlorpheniramine 10	Pseudoephedrine 65		
Triaminic JR Juvelet	Pheniramine 12.5 Pyrilamine 12.5	Phenylpropanolamine 25		
Triaminic Infant Drops/ 1 ml	Pheniramine 10 Pyrilamine 10	Phenylpropanolamine 20		
Triaminic Tablet	Pheniramine 25 Pyrilamine 25	Phenylpropanolamine 50		

†These products are selected because they are described in Physicians' Desk Reference, 1978.
*Long-acting preparation.
**Atropine, isopropamide and methoscopolamine are anticholinergic agents which are used for their drying action on mucous membranes.

istered topically, for shrinking the mucosa to facilitate instrumentation of the nose, and for helping prevent barotrauma to the ears and sinuses in susceptible patients who are at risk when undergoing changes in altitude or ambient pressure. Relatively few patients ever need other pharmacologic types of decongestants or alternative means of administration; however, antihistamines are useful if extranasal symptoms are present, in which case oral administration is required.

Extreme cases of rhinitis of the hay fever type demand more vigorous measures. If possible, the patient should avoid the allergen, or if a specific recurrent exposure is unavoidable, a course of desensitization injection therapy may be required. Decongestant medications may offer substantial symptomatic relief when given for a few days at the height of the illness; in some cases a longer course of drug therapy may be demanded by the patient who finds the untreated symptoms intolerable. Antihistamines offer the next therapeutic approach, and their systemic use may be particularly helpful at night. In patients with intolerable symptoms that do not respond to simpler methods of treatment, steroid therapy may be justified: short courses of topical therapy are preferable, but the need for longer courses may justify alternate-day oral therapy. When intranasal cromolyn is available, it may provide valuable long-term prophylactic therapy for allergic rhinitis of the hay fever type.

Most of the other treatments of coughs and colds, which are both too readily available and all too often recommended, serve to reveal that irrational pharmacologic principles and public faith in medications seek each other out and unite in a triumphal display of placebo effectiveness.

REFERENCES

1. Murray, J. F.: The Normal Lung. The Basis for Diagnosis and Treatment of Pulmonary Disease. Philadelphia, W. B. Saunders Company, 1976.
2. Widdicombe, J. G.: Reflex control of breathing. In MTP International Review of Science. Physiology Series 1. Vol. 2: Respiratory Physiology. J. G. Widdicombe (Ed.). London, Butterworths and Co., Ltd. 1974. Ch. 10.
3. Salem, H. and Aviado, D. M.: The cough reflex in health and disease. In International Encyclopedia of Pharmacology and Therapeutics. Section 27: Antitussive Agents. Vols. 1 and 2. H.
4. Chou, D. T. and Wang, S. C.: Studies on the localization of central cough mechanism; site of action of antitussive drugs. J. Pharmacol. Exp. Ther. 194:499–505, 1975.
5. Bucher, K.: Antitussive drugs. Physiol. Pharmacol. 11:175–200, 1965.
6. Comroe, J. H., Jr.: Physiology of Respiration. Chicago, Yearbook Medical Publishers Incorporated. 2nd ed., 1974.
7. Newhouse, M., Sanchis, J. and Bienenstock, J.: Lung defense mechanisms. N. Engl. J. Med. 295:990–998, 1976.
8. Burack, R. and Fox, F. J.: The New Handbook of Prescription Drugs. New York, Ballantine Books, 1975.
9. Bickerman, H.: Clinical pharmacology of antitussive drugs. Clin. Pharmacol. Ther. 3:353–368, 1962.
10. Eddy, N. B., Friebel, H., Hahn, K.-J. and Halbach, H.: Codeine and its Alternatives for Pain and Cough Relief. Geneva, World Health Organization, 1970.
11. Aviado, D. M.: Kranz and Carr's Pharmacologic Principles Of Medical Practice. Baltimore, The Williams and Wilkins Company, 8th ed., 1972.
12. Bickerman, H.: Antitussive drugs, in Drugs of Choice 1974–1975. W. Modell (Ed.). St. Louis, The C. V. Mosby Company, 1974. Ch. 27.
13. Dautrebande, L.: Microaerosols: Physiology, Pharmacology, Therapeutics. New York, Academic Press, 1962.
13a. Howard, P., Cayton, R. M., Brennan, S. R. and Anderson, P. B.: Lignocaine aerosol and persistent cough. Br. J. Dis. Chest 71:19–24, 1977.
14. Salem, H. and Aviado, D. M.: Local anesthetics. In International Encyclopedia of Pharmacology and Therapeutics. Section 27: Antitussive Agents, Vol. 3. H. Salem and D. M. Aviado (Eds.). Oxford, Pergamon Press, 1970.
15. Byrd, R. B. and Burns, J. R.: Cough dynamics in the post-thoracotomy state. Chest 67:654–657, 1975.
16. Salem, H. and Aviado, D. M.: Bronchodilators. Ch. 13, Ref. 14.
17. Shirkey, H. C.: Coughs and hiccups. In Pediatric Therapy. H. C. Shirkey (Ed.). St. Louis, The C. V. Mosby Company, 4th ed., 1972.
18. Graedon, J.: The People's Pharmacy. New York, St. Martin's Press, 1976.
19. McFadden, E. R., Jr.: Exertional dyspnea and cough as preludes to acute attack of bronchial asthma. N. Engl. J. Med. 292:555–558, 1975.
20. Chalmers, R. K. and Cormier, J. F.: Antitussives. In Handbook of Non-Prescription Drugs. G. B. Griffenhagen and L. L. Hawkins (Eds.). Washington, American Pharmaceutical Association, 4th ed. 1973, pp. 15–25.
21. Brunk, S. F.: The evaluation of antitussive agents. J. Clin. Pharmacol. 13:305–308, 1973.
22. Blacow, N. W. (Ed.): Martindale: The Extra Pharmacopoeia. London, The Pharmaceutical Press, 26th ed., 1972.
23. Boyd, E. M.: Antitussives, antiemetics, and dermatomucosal agents. In Drill's Pharmacology in Medicine. J. R. DiPalma (Ed.). New York,

Salem and D. M. Aviado (Eds.). Oxford, Pergamon Press, 1970.

McGraw-Hill Book Company, 4th ed., 1971. Ch. 49.

24. Notes and Comments: Cough mixtures. Br. Med. J. 3:633, Sept. 1970.

25. diCyan, E. and Hessman, L.: Without Prescription. New York, Simon and Schuster, Inc. 1972, pp. 47–56.

26. Levin, R. H.: Upper respiratory infections. *In* Clinical Pharmacy and Therapeutics. E. T. Herfindal and J. L. Hirschman (Eds.). Baltimore, The Williams and Wilkins Company, 1975.

27. Editorial: Cough suppressants for children. Br. Med. J. 2:493, Aug., 1976.

28. Cough remedies. Med. Lett. Drug Ther. 13:9–11, 1971.

29. Editorial: Antitussives in jeopardy, J.A.M.A. 224: 621, 1973.

30. Calvert, J. C.: Cough: differential diagnosis and treatment. Drug. Intell. Clin. Pharm. 10:640–650, 1976.

31. Kasé, Y.: Evaluation of antitussive agents. *In* Selected Pharmacological Testing Methods. A. Burger (Ed.). New York, Marcel Dekker, Inc., 1968, Vol. 3, Ch. 12.

32. Bickerman, H. A.: Evaluation of antitussive drugs: clinical and challenge techniques. *In* Evaluation of Gastrointestinal, Pulmonary, Antiinflammatory, and Immunological Agents. F. A. McMahon (Ed.). Futura Publishing Company, 1974. Ch. 11.

33. Lough, M., Boat, T. and Doershuk, C. F.: The nose. Respiratory Care 20:844–848, 1975.

34. Proctor, D. F.: The upper airways. I: Nasal physiology and defence of the lungs. Am. Rev. Respir. Dis. 115:97–129, 1977.

35. Proctor, D. F. and Adams, G. K.: Physiology and pharmacology of nasal function and mucus secretion. Pharmac. Ther. B. 2:493–509, 1976.

36. Norman, P. S.: Allergic rhinitis and sinusitis. Postgrad. Med. 54:94–100, Nov., 1973.

37. Mendelson, L. M., Nyhan, W. L. and Hamburger, R. H.: Allergic rhinitis. Calif. Med. 117:37–44, 1972.

38. Symposium: Easing the miseries of hay fever. Patient Care 10:54–77, Jun., 1976.

39. Chasin, W. D.: The upper respiratory passages (nose, throat and sinuses) in bronchial asthma. *In* Bronchial Asthma: Mechanisms and Therapeutics. E. B. Weiss and M. S. Segal (Eds.). Boston, Little, Brown and Company, 1976. Ch. 32.

40. Torsney, P. J.: Allergic rhinitis and otologic allergy. Semin. in Drug Treat. 2:403–412, 1973.

41. Bevan, M. A.: Histamine. N. Engl. J. Med. 294: 30–36, 320–325, 1976.

42. Schacter, M. (Ed.): Histamine And Antihistamines. Section 74 International Encyclopedia Of Pharmacology And Therapeutics. Oxford, Pergamon Press, 1973.

43. Anon: Antihistamines. Brit. Med. J. 1:217–219, Jan., 1970.

44. Thomas, J. S., Heurich, A. E., Ralph, J. W., Crane, R. and Shepherd, D. A.: Double-blind controlled study of clemastine fumarate, chlorpheniramine and placebo in patients with seasonal allergic rhinitis. Ann. Allergy 38:169–174, 1977.

45. Karlin, J. M.: The use of antihistamines in allergic disease. Ped. Clin. N. Amer. 22:157–162, 1975.

46. Douglas, H., Bertino, M. and Toy, H. S.: Those stubborn ear/nose infections: which Rx is best? Current Prescribing, Feb. 1977, pp. 82–96.

47. Aviado, D. M.: Sympathomimetic Drugs. Springfield, Ill., Charles C Thomas, 1970.

48. Salem, H. and Aviado, D. M.: Topical nasal decongestant preparations available in the United States. Rev. Allergy 25:271–277, 1971.

49. Anon: Oral cold remedies. Med. Lett. Drugs Therap. 17:89–92, 1975.

50. Cormier, J. F. and Bryant, B. G.: Cold and allergy products. *In* Handbook of Nonprescription Drugs. Washington, American Pharmaceutical Association, 5th ed. 1977, Ch. 8.

51. Cohan, R. H., Bloom, F. L., Rhoades, R. B., Wittig, H. J. and Haugh, L. D.: Treatment of perennial allergic rhinitis with cromolyn sodium. J. Allergy Clin. Immunol. 58:121–128, 1976.

52. Penttinen, K., Aarnio, A. and Hovi, T.: Disodium cromoglycate can inhibit virus-induced cytopathic effects in vitro. Br. Med. J. 1:82, Jan., 1977.

53. Turkeltaub, P. C., Norman, P. S. and Crepea, S.: Treatment of ragweed hay fever with an intranasal spray containing flunisolide, a new synthetic corticosteroid. J. Allergy Clin. Immunol. 58:597–606, 1976.

54. Editorial: Intranasal beclomethasone: wonder drug or hazard. Br. Med. J. 2:1522–1523, Dec. 1976.

55. Brown, H. M.: Intranasal beclomethasone. Br. Med. J. 1:376–377, Jan. 1977.

CHAPTER
10
ANTIMICROBIAL THERAPY

Antibiotic and antifungal agents make up a major class of drugs used in the treatment of respiratory diseases. These drugs are, of course, used for the treatment of infections that arise in all organs of the body; therefore, only those features most relevant to the respiratory tract will be discussed here.

Antimicrobial drugs are used in respiratory medicine to prevent an infection from developing, as well as to treat an established disease. Certain antibiotics, such as tetracycline and ampicillin, are employed, prophylactically or therapeutically, to such a considerable extent in the management of chronic obstructive pulmonary disease that they can almost be considered primary respiratory agents. It is rather disturbing to find, however, that much of this usage of antibiotics is not based on clear bacteriologic principles.[1, 2] The most important causative organisms responsible for the low-grade infection of the respiratory mucosa in chronic obstructive disease are generally believed to be *Diplococcus pneumoniae* (pneumococcus) and *Haemophilus influenzae.*[1, 3, 4] Yet, it is common experience that routine culture of the infected sputum of most bronchitics fails to grow out these specific organisms; usually, the bacteriology laboratory reports "normal oropharyngeal flora," which implies a mixture of streptococci, neisseriae, anaerobes and perhaps also pneumococcus and *H. influenzae.* Nevertheless, the fundamental studies of May in England spearheaded the belief that these latter two organisms are the prime pathogens in bronchitis in the United Kingdom, and presumably in the United States.[2, 5]

There is often difficulty in establishing the cause of an acute pulmonary infection, such as in pneumonia, since the sputum expectorated through the mouth becomes contaminated and yields a confusing mixture of bacteria on culture. Indeed, many physicians recognize that sputum cultures may be of little value, unless the presence of an unusual organism is a strong possibility.[6] More precise diagnosis usually entails the obtaining of sputum by a procedure such as transtracheal aspiration, bronchoscopy, endotracheal intubation or transpulmonary aspiration; blood cultures may also be of help. Preliminary information, which can be extremely accurate, can be obtained prior to the culture report by gram-staining a suitable specimen of sputum, and thereby determining the morphologic characteristics of any predominant organisms associated with inflammatory cells. In the case of suspected tuberculosis a careful acid-fast stain is mandatory, since this can reliably provide a diagnosis weeks before the bacteriologic cultures become available. The diagnoses of other pneumonias may require more sophisticated techniques, such as bronchoscopy or lung biopsy. The range of organisms that most frequently affect the respiratory tract, causing various diseases, is tabulated in Table 10–1.

Because of the difficulties in obtaining reliable sequential studies of infections in the tracheobronchial tree and in the pulmonary parenchyma, accurate information regarding the value of different antibiotic agents, the appropriate dosages and the best modes of administration is not readily available.[7] As a

TABLE 10–1. MAJOR RESPIRATORY PATHOGENS

Organism	Associated Diseases	Comment
GRAM-POSITIVE BACTERIA		
Group A *Streptococcus*	Pharyngitis, tonsillitis, sinusitis, otitis	May be present in aspiration pneumonias
Staphylococcus aureus	Sinusitis, otitis, pneumonia, lung abscess, empyema, cystic fibrosis	Many species are now penicillin-resistant
Diplococcus pneumoniae	Sinusitis, otitis, bronchitis, pneumonia, empyema	Main cause of pneumonia
GRAM-NEGATIVE BACTERIA		
Haemophilus influenzae	Epiglottitis, bronchitis, bronchiolitis, pneumonia, acute otitis in children	Accompanies *D. pneumoniae* in bronchitis
Pseudomonas aeruginosa	Pneumonia, lung abscess, empyema, cystic fibrosis	Common in debilitated patients
Klebsiella pneumoniae	Pneumonia, lung abscess, empyema, bronchiectasis	Uncommon cause of pneumonia presently
Escherichia coli *Proteus* species *Serratia marcescens* *Enterobacter aerogenes*	Pneumonia, lung abscess, empyema, bronchiectasis, cystic fibrosis	Opportunistic-infections. Can be introduced by contaminated inhalation therapy equipment.
ANAEROBIC BACTERIA		
Bacteroides species *Streptococcus* species Others	Sinusitis, otitis, aspiration pneumonia, lung abscess, empyema	Cause foul-smelling pus; usually present in mixed infection
MYCOPLASMA AND VIRUSES		
Mycoplasma pneumoniae	Pneumonia	Common in young adults and children
Adenoviruses	Common cold, pharyngitis, bronchiolitis, bronchitis, croup, pneumonia	One of commonest group of respiratory viruses
Respiratory syncytial virus	Bronchiolitis, pneumonia	Occurs in children
Influenza viruses	Rhinitis, pharyngitis, laryngotracheitis, pneumonia	Cause influenza syndromes
Parainfluenza		
Rhinovirus, Coronavirus, etc.	Common cold	Probably major causes of colds
MYCOBACTERIA		
Mycobacterium tuberculosis	Tuberculosis syndromes	Can cause similar diseases of lungs and other organs
Atypical mycobacteria	Tuberculosis-like syndromes	
FUNGI		
Coccidioides immitis	Coccidioidomycosis	Tend to develop in normal hosts as primary infections
Histoplasma capsulatum	Histoplasmosis	
Blastomyces dermatitidis	Blastomycosis	
Sporotrichum schenkii	Sporotrichosis	
Actinomyces israelii	Actinomycosis	
Aspergillus fumigatus	Aspergillosis	Tend to develop in abnormal hosts as opportunistic infections
Candida species	Candidiasis (moniliasis)	
Cryptococcus neoformans	Cryptococcosis	
Nocardia species	Nocardiosis	
PARASITES (Protozoa)		
Pneumocystis carinii	Pneumonia	Develops in immunosuppressed hosts and in infants
Toxoplasma gondii		Seen mainly in immunologically abnormal infants

consequence, the medical literature is replete with claims that inhalational administration of antimicrobial agents is beneficial, whereas most clinical practitioners today do not favor this mode of therapy.[8, 9] However, it is worth considering, in some detail, the existing information on inhalational therapy with antimicrobial agents.

INHALATIONAL ADMINISTRATION OF ANTIMICROBIAL DRUGS

Antibacterial aerosol therapy was first used in 1942 by Barach and his colleagues, and was later adopted with enthusiasm by Prigal.[9] Over the next few years, aerosols of penicillin, streptomycin, tyrothricin, tetracyclines, polymyxins, bacitracin, chloramphenicol, sulfonamides and other antimicrobial agents were recommended for the treatment of a variety of pulmonary infections,[8, 10, 11] and claims were even made that inhalation of these drugs constituted the optimal route of administration in many patients.[9, 12]

Since the 1950s, careful studies have been undertaken to elucidate the means by which antibiotic therapy can affect pulmonary infection. Many of these studies have been carried out on children with cystic fibrosis, which is the only situation for which there is any remaining enthusiasm for antibiotic inhalational therapy.[13] Studies in patients with chronic bronchitis, pneumonia, bronchiectasis, lung abscess and opportunistic infections have not led to any general support for the use of nebulized antibiotic therapy in the management of these diseases.

Disadvantages of Aerosol Therapy with Antimicrobial Agents
(Table 10-2)

A major problem with all nebulized antimicrobial agents is that they can cause reactive bronchospasm. A further difficulty is that large volumes of the diluted drug may need to be given, and the treatment is often tiring and distressing to the patient. Furthermore, it is difficult to get the agent to the site of active disease, since the proximal airways are usually full of the infected mucoid or purulent secretions. Moreover, topical antibiotics could be removed relatively rapidly by the mucociliary escalator and by coughing, or by binding with DNA or protein in the sputum, or by enzyme inactivation. It has been suggested that improved distal deposi-

TABLE 10-2. DISADVANTAGES OF AEROSOL ADMINISTRATION OF ANTIMICROBIAL DRUGS

1. Bronchospasm is common complication.
2. Agent may not reach infected site.
3. Drug may be inactivated in mucus.
4. Systemic side effects can occur.
5. Ambient air becomes contaminated by drug.
6. Nosocomial problems and superinfections can result.
7. Optimal technique of delivery not established.
8. Prolonged nebulization sessions may be needed.
9. Dosages of aerosolized drugs not established.
10. Proof of efficacy has not been established.

tion and better toleration of an antimicrobial agent are obtained by administering it with an ultrasonic nebulizer, and using adjuvant drugs such as bronchodilators, mucolytics (for example, acetylcysteine or pancreatic dornase) or wetting agents (such as Alevaire), in addition to IPPB and postural drainage.[9] The role of these ancillary measures is likely to be more successful than that of the antimicrobial drug; these additional respiratory therapy modalities constitute major factors in the treatment of pulmonary infection and emphasize the need for improved drainage of secretions out of the tracheobronchial tree.

A consequence of these disadvantages is that the antimicrobial dosage recommendations that have been offered by different workers show a considerable variation, and the dose selected may vary over one hundredfold. Of course, the dose of the drug measured into a nebulizer bears little relationship to the amount actually deposited in the lung, since little more than 10 per cent of the original dose remains in the tracheobronchial tree (see Chapter 1). Correct inspiratory patterns, rebreathing of the nebulization mixture and other techniques designed to improve the delivery of the drug may be of importance, but no standard method of optimal administration has been devised.

More recent studies have been carried out with selected drugs in special circumstances. Thus, Feeley et al.[14] have used aerosolized polymyxin in the management of patients on a respiratory-surgical intensive care unit to prevent the development of *Pseudomonas aeruginosa* pneumonia. The routine use of this form of prophylactic therapy was found to be self-defeating, since it led to an increased incidence of pneumonias caused by organisms resistant to polymyxin. A major problem accompanying the general utilization of aerosolized antibiotics in a ward unit is that the air becomes contaminated with the drug, and resistant organisms may be selectively favored in the environment, thereby resulting in an increased risk of nosocomial infections resulting from the iatrogenically created opportunistic hazard. A further problem is that both the patients and the staff may become sensitized to the aerosolized antibiotics in the environment; this is a particular concern with drugs such as penicillin, which are notorious for causing sensitization. Currently, it is felt that the topical use of penicillin and its derivatives is contraindicated both in dermatology and in respiratory therapy, since unpleasant or severe allergic reactions may be induced in patients and personnel who are exposed to the drugs. Feeley and colleagues point out that aerosolized antibiotic prophylaxis, with polymyxin, can be justified in special circumstances: the drug is given only to patients when the active threat of an outbreak of *Pseudomonas* infections exists in the ward unit, and individual patient aerosolization treatments are continued for five days after the index patients have been cleared of the infection or have left the unit.[15]

Indications for Aerosolized Antimicrobial Therapy

There are very few acceptable uses for aerosol administration of antimicrobial agents (Table 10–3); these can be categorized as follows:

To Eliminate Colonization. Patients with impaired mucociliary clearance and antibac-

TABLE 10–3. INDICATIONS FOR AEROSOLIZATION OF ANTIMICROBIAL AGENTS*

1. To eliminate organism colonizing (as opposed to infecting) respiratory tract
2. To treat low-grade infection in patient with chronic, recurrent infectious exacerbations in respiratory tract.
3. As an adjunct to systemic therapy when the latter is unsuccessful
4. When alternative routes are not available
5. When toxic reactions preclude systemic therapy with an indicated antimicrobial
6. For topical therapy with an agent that is not suitable for systemic administration (such as bacitracin, neomycin, nystatin)

*Agents should be chosen that are effective, poorly absorbed through the lung, nonirritating and nonallergenic.

terial lung defenses are susceptible to becoming passive hosts to a variety of potential pathogens. *Pseudomonas* and the *Klebsiella-Enterobacter* groups of enteric organisms are the common offenders among the gram-negative organisms, and the *Staphylococcus* is the main gram-positive invader. These organisms behave as opportunists, and may colonize a patient's respiratory mucosa without initially causing any inflammatory changes in the parenchyma. The patient may produce purulent sputum, in which a predominant opportunist may be recognized on Gram's stain or culture, but there will be no evidence of pulmonary infection on chest radiograms, and the patient will be afebrile with a normal peripheral blood white count. In such circumstances, it is correct to diagnose respiratory tract *colonization* rather than infection.[16] If the patient or other patients on the unit are at risk of becoming infected by the colonizing organism, it may be appropriate to use nebulization therapy with a selected antibiotic to suppress the bacteria. Thus, polymyxin would be suitable for *Pseudomonas*, gentamicin or perhaps amikacin or tobramycin for both *Pseudomonas* and other gram-negative organisms, while bacitracin or neomycin could be suitable for *Staphylococcus* species.

The sensitivities of the organisms, as determined by the bacteriology laboratory, should be taken as a guide to therapy.

To Treat Chronic Infection. Patients with chronic airway diseases such as cystic fibrosis may always demonstrate low-grade infection. At times, when the bacteria become invasive, systemic antibiotic therapy is required. At other times the mucus becomes more viscous and purulent, and although symptoms may become exacerbated there may be little evidence of parenchymal invasion, and systemic therapy will be deemed unnecessary. In such circumstances, a course of aerosol therapy with an appropriate antibiotic would be indicated. Although there are still enthusiasts for this form of management, there appears to be declining faith in its value, and it can be recommended only if carried out as a careful trial on patients who are under evaluative supervision in a hospital.

As a Therapeutic Alternative. Certain patients who develop pulmonary infections may present contraindications to conventional antibiotic administration. Thus, the presence of deteriorating renal function may militate against giving parenteral injections of nephrotoxic agents such as gentamicin or amphotericin. Similarly, a patient with greatly decreased body mass and sclerosed peripheral veins may present an insurmountable obstacle to the delivery of intramuscular or intravenous drugs, whereas the respiratory tract is always available as a portal. In circumstances such as these, a trial of aerosol antimicrobial therapy can be justified.

Administration of Antimicrobial Aerosols

When a decision is made to administer antimicrobial therapy by means of nebulization, a dosage should be selected from among the ranges presented in Table 10-4. In all cases, the patient should receive bronchodilator therapy, either prior to or accompanying the antimicrobial aerosol. The actual amount of antimicrobial solution to be administered is variable; most workers recommend 2 to 10 ml for each session. Treatments can be repeated every two to eight hours, according to the severity of the problem. Some experts choose to add a mucolytic agent: 100,000 units of pancreatic dornase or 3 to 10 ml of 20 per cent acetylcysteine are favored by Miller[9] (for further details of these drugs refer to Chapter 3).

It is advisable to administer the initial treatment under the careful supervision of a respiratory therapist, who should be aware of the possibility of a bronchospastic reac-

TABLE 10-4. ANTIMICROBIAL AGENTS THAT HAVE BEEN GIVEN BY NEBULIZATION

Drug	Range of Dosage*	Comments
Amphotericin*	1–20 mg	Has been used to treat coccidioidomycosis, and lung infections with *Candida, Aspergillus,* etc.; dose has to be built up
Ampicillin	125–250 mg	Should not be used, because of danger of inducing hypersensitivity
Bacitracin*	5,000–200,000 u	Used for sensitive (e.g. staphylococcal) infections in cystic fibrosis
Carbenicillin	125–1,000 mg	Has been used for *Pseudomonas* and other gram-negative respiratory tract infections
Cephaloridine	125–250 mg	Not recommended; value of aerosol therapy not demonstrated
Cephalothin	125–250 mg	Not recommended; value of aerosol therapy not demonstrated
Chloramphenicol	50–400 mg	Not recommended; value of aerosol therapy not demonstrated
Colistin*	2–300 mg (100 mg†)	Used for elimination of sensitive gram-negative organisms; similar to polymyxin, but less likely to cause bronchospasm
Erythromycin	20–100 mg	Not recommended, although formerly utilized
Framycetin	25 mg	Has been used in cystic fibrosis; no longer available in U.S.
Gentamicin	5–120 mg	Has been used for sensitive gram-negative infections, such as *Pseudomonas*
Kanamycin*	25–500 mg (250 mg†)	Relatively safe and well tolerated; has mucokinetic effect; is active against most gram-negative bacteria, except *Pseudomonas* and *Bacteroides;* some organisms (e.g., *E. coli, Staphylococcus* and mycobacteria) rapidly develop resistance
Methicillin	125–250 mg	Not recommended, because of danger of inducing hypersensitivity
Neomycin*	25–400 mg (50 mg†)	Similar spectrum to kanamycin, and more popular for topical therapy; more toxic than kanamycin when given systemically
Nystatin*	25,000 u	Has been used in the treatment of pulmonary aspergillosis
Oxytetracycline	50 mg	Rarely used; experience in aerosol administration is limited
Penicillin	100,000 u	Not recommended, although it was popular in former years; risk of allergy and hypersensitivity reactions is too great
Polymyxin*	5–50 mg (50 mg†)	Useful for prophylaxis and for elimination of gram-negative organisms colonizing respiratory tract; resistance develops only slowly, but superinfection may occur; can cause severe bronchospasm in asthmatics; not effective against *Proteus* species
Streptomycin	50 mg	No longer used by aerosolization
Sulfonamides		Rarely used now; some sulfonamides may have a mucolytic effect
Tobramycin	50 mg	Similar to gentamicin
Vancomycin		Inadequate information available, although it may be suitable for nebulization

*These drugs may be the safest and most effective for nebulization therapy.
†Usual dosage for adults
Note: Usually, the drug is dissolved in 2 ml saline; treatments are given 2–4 times a day. A bronchodilator should be added.

tion in a susceptible patient. The initial treatment should use a test dose of the antibiotic, and if the drug is well tolerated subsequent treatments should rapidly build the dosage toward the upper end of the range listed in Table 10–4. The danger of severe bronchospasm is particularly great in asthmatics, and the polymyxins, which may release histamine, should be given with great care to such patients;[17] however, other agents may be equally hazardous in some patients. Most antibiotics can probably be absorbed across the blood-bronchial barrier into the systemic circulation following nebulization, and generalized toxic or allergic reactions may occur in susceptible patients. An awareness of the toxic properties of individual nebulized antibiotics is therefore a necessity.

Instillation Therapy With Antimicrobial Agents

More success may be obtained in the treatment of respiratory infections when an antibiotic is instilled in relative bulk into the lungs. The easiest method of instillation is by injecting a bolus of solution down an endotracheal tube in an intubated or tracheostomized patient.[18-20] An alternative route can be provided by placing a small transtracheal catheter through the cricothyroid membrane, and taping it in place for the duration of therapy; there has been some enthusiasm for this form of therapy,[21, 22] although there is little evidence that many respiratory physicians subscribe to the practice. A more risky technique is to insert a transthoracic catheter between the ribs into the lung: this technique has been reported on favorably in the treatment of lung abscess, since it allows large amounts of antibiotic therapy to be delivered to the infected site.[23] The hazards of this form of management appear to be unacceptably high compared with the dubious benefits that can be expected.

The value of administering antibiotics such as gentamicin or polymyxin down an endotracheal tube in the management of bronchitis and other pulmonary infections may merit further evaluation.[24] The rationale for this form of therapy is sometimes presented in a confusing fashion: it is claimed that topical therapy with gentamicin results in a high antimicrobial drug level in the sputum, whereas oral or parenteral therapy may produce a negligible level.[22, 24, 25] This reasoning may not be appropriate, since the antimicrobial levels in the parenchyma and the submucosa and in the distally impacted infected sputum, which may not be accessible to sampling, may be more relevant. The ultimate question is this: does topical therapy work better and with less toxicity than oral or parenteral therapy? At present, no adequate comparative studies seem to have been carried out to answer such concerns.

Oral and Parenteral Antimicrobial Therapy

Many workers have attempted to determine whether adequate antibiotic penetration of the blood-bronchus barrier is obtained with systemic antimicrobial therapy. The literature has been summarized and analyzed by Pennington, who emphasizes the unpredictability and variability of results obtained for the various antibiotics in different animals or human subjects.[26] Many complex factors govern the entry of drugs

TABLE 10–5. VARIABLES ASSOCIATED WITH IMPROVED ANTIMICROBIAL PENETRATION OF BLOOD-BRONCHIAL BARRIER

Factor	Enhanced Penetration	Examples
MOLECULAR PROPERTIES		
Molecular weight	High molecular weight	Erythromycin, polymyxins, vancomycin
Size of molecule	Very small size	Isoniazid, cycloserine
Solubility in lipids	Lipophilic agents	Chloramphenicol, doxycycline, sulfonamides
Dissociation constant (pKa)	Different from 7.40	Cloxacillin, cephalosporins
Protein binding	Low binding	Isoniazid, kanamycin
Mucus binding	High binding	Tetracyclines, gentamicin
Transport	Active transport	Doxycycline, ampicillin, tobramycin, sulfonamides, trimethoprim
GENERAL FACTORS		
Serum concentration	High concentration	Intravenous dosage
Disease of barrier	Infection	Pneumonia
Blood vessel permeability	Rupture of blood vessel	Hemorrhagic bronchitis
Metabolism/excretion	Slow inactivation of drug	Renal insufficiency

into the infected areas of the lung (Table 10–5). An interesting finding is that larger molecules (such as gentamicin, polymyxin and erythromycin) penetrate the blood-bronchial barrier more readily than do smaller molecules (such as the penicillins and the cephalosporins).[26, 27] However, it is uncertain whether this finding is universally applicable. In many cases, the concentration of an antibiotic found in the respiratory secretions following conventional dosages would appear to be inadequate to kill the infecting bacteria. In the case of anaerobic or pneumococcal infections, however, the minimal inhibitory concentration required to eliminate the very susceptible causative bacteria is so low that penicillin suffices. It is, of course, common experience that penicillins and cephalosporins are extremely effective in treating susceptible pulmonary infections, and one may conclude that a trial of therapy is more relevant than the complexities of theory conjured up by the reported concentrations that antibiotics achieve in the sputum. However, in severe infections, with a great quantity of purulence in an architecturally disordered lung, it is prudent to strive for a relatively high penetration of antibiotic by administering the drug in the maximal range of dosages. Thus, while pneumococcal pneumonia in an otherwise healthy young adult may respond adequately to 600,000 units of penicillin twice a day, the same infection in a debilitated elderly patient with emphysema merits up to ten times this total amount per day in divided dosage. Similarly, when there is a large infectious burden, such as occurs with poorly draining lung abscesses, even greater doses of penicillin are indicated. A drug such as penicillin, which is inexpensive and as readily tolerated in large dosage as in smaller doses, should be given in generous amounts in cases of doubt; large dose therapy with this drug has few documented disadvantages, and fears that an increased incidence of superinfection may be induced appear to be unfounded.

When the more toxic or expensive agents such as carbenicillin, gentamicin or amphotericin are required, it is evident that further studies are required to establish the optimal dosages and modes of administration for various disease states in patients of different ages, and with specific impairments of lung architecture and host defenses. These considerations cannot be authoritatively responded to at the present state of our knowledge. However, some general guidelines for antibiotic therapy in common infections of the lungs are discussed below.

ANTIMICROBIAL TREATMENT OF RESPIRATORY TRACT INFECTIONS

The more important groups of respiratory infections will be discussed with respect to their antimicrobial therapy (see Table 10–6).

Bronchitis. Chronic bronchitis is a disease of impaired mucokinesis, bronchospasm and infection. The treatment of the first two components of this triad has been thoroughly discussed in earlier chapters. Unfortunately, far less is known about the infectious component, and much of the information we have is derived from empirical experience. The role of *Diplococcus pneumoniae* and *Haemophilus influenzae* has been described earlier, and therapeutic efforts are generally directed at these two bacteria. Various antibiotics have been reported to be effective: tetracycline, ampicillin and erythromycin have received the most favorable recommendations. Doses vary from 250 mg to 500 mg or more, and treatment is usually given orally, one to four times a day; a course may last from five to fifteen days or longer. Judgment must be exercised by the individual clinician, but it should be recognized that prolonged therapy is of dubious benefit.[5, 28] In recent years, the combination of sulfamethoxazole with trimethoprim has become very popular in the United Kingdom;[29] this preparation is recommended for trial in patients who have purulent secretions. There is an increasing incidence of *H. influenzae* resistance to ampicillin, and this antibiotic may not always be successful in patients infected with such an organism.

When a patient's chronic bronchitis becomes exacerbated, it is usually necessary to change the antibiotic, and to use larger doses at least for a few days; if the patient is toxic, intravenous therapy for at least 24 to 48 hours is usually desirable. Ampicillin (up to 1 gm four times a day) or a cephalosporin (for example, cefazolin, cephalexin or cephradine, 1 gm four times a day) is also of value. Amoxicillin is favored by some workers, who feel it achieves a better serum and sputum concentration than does the parent compound, ampicillin;[30] 250 mg every eight hours is suggested. Many other antibiotics have also been used; of these, there is adequate evidence to suggest that doxycycline would be one of the better alternative agents.[31]

Asthma. When an asthmatic develops infected sputum, treatment as described above for bronchitis is usually effective. Alternatively, one of the macrolide antibiotics (erythromycin or troleandomycin) could be used, particularly when the patient's exacerbation necessitates an increase in glucocorticoid therapy.[32] The macrolides appear to potentiate the action of steroids by interfering with their metabolic degradation; erythromycin estolate is apparently more effective than other derivatives (see Chapter 4).

Pneumonias. The majority of pneumonias in most patient populations are caused by the pneumococcus,[1, 33] and the majority of pneumococcal pneumonias respond to penicillin. Relatively low doses are effective, but much larger dosage regimens can and should be employed in very sick patients. If a patient is allergic to penicillin, then an erythromycin, clindamycin or chloramphenicol can be used; the tetracyclines are still effective against most pneumococci, but resistant organisms are prevalent in certain areas. Many pneumococcal lobar pneumonias respond so readily to antibiotics that a single injection of a long-acting penicillin may suffice, and the patient can be managed on an out-patient basis.[34]

For nonpneumococcal pneumonias, gram-staining and bacteriology laboratory culture reports should provide a guide to therapy.[35] A staphylococcal pneumonia should initially be treated with a penicillinase-resistant penicillin, such as methicillin; if the laboratory finds that the organism does not produce penicillinase and that it is sensitive to penicillin, a change to penicillin should be made. For patients allergic to penicillin, a cephalosporin can be used.

In the treatment of gram-negative pneumonias, each hospital should adopt guidelines as to the appropriate selection of antibiotics. Gentamicin is a favored choice, but other antibiotics are suitable; a cephalosporin may be added for its synergistic effect. In very sick patients, a combination of antibiotics is generally advisable; carbenicillin is a useful synergist in such cases.

A particularly important pneumonia is the type described as aspiration or decubitus pneumonia. It occurs as a result of vomiting, but it also may arise in a patient whose cough reflex is impaired due to debility, narcotizing

drugs or alcohol. It should be remembered that contaminated inhalation therapy equipment can cause a pneumonia of this type, in which gram-negative organisms tend to predominate. Aspiration pneumonias acquired outside the hospital are generally caused by the oropharyngeal flora, consisting largely of anaerobic bacteria.[36] Fortunately, these are all sensitive to penicillin, which is the drug of choice: it is used in the same way as for pneumococcal pneumonia. Clindamycin and chloramphenicol are both excellent alternatives, since they are very effective against anaerobes and other oropharyngeal flora. If a patient or the environment has been exposed to antibiotics, a resistant organism may be involved in the infection. Therefore, hospital-acquired aspiration pneumonias should receive a broader spectrum of antibiotic coverage; in such cases gentamicin or another aminoglycoside could be added to the regimen, particularly if Gram's stain of the respiratory secretions suggests gram-negative infection.[37]

As discussed earlier, inhalational antibiotics can be used to prevent hospital-acquired aspiration pneumonias.[14] Polymyxin or colistimethate is perhaps the best prophylactic agent.

Empyema. Sometimes a pneumonia is complicated by an empyema; this serious infection requires surgical drainage as well as antibiotic therapy. The appropriate antimicrobial agent, based on bacteriologic studies, should be given intravenously in the same or larger dose than is given for uncomplicated pneumonia; therapy may have to be continued for several weeks.[37, 38] Although some surgeons favor the instillation of antibiotics into an empyema, with or without pancreatic dornase, this practice is currently not in favor.

Lung Abscess. Most lung abscesses arise as a complication of an aspiration pneumonia, or are secondary to an inhaled foreign body or a malignancy. Bronchoscopy and surgical drainage are sometimes indicated, but antibiotic therapy and postural drainage offer a very successful basic regimen.[39] Many lung abscesses are caused by oral flora; this is likely to be the case if the expectorated pus has a foul odor, since this is the signature of the anaerobic bacteria.[38] In such cases, large dose penicillin therapy is generally required, and intravenous administration may need to be continued for four to six weeks; clindamycin is a suitable alternative to penicillin. If other specific organisms

TABLE 10-6. ANTIBIOTIC REGIMENS FOR VARIOUS PULMONARY INFECTIONS

Disease	Antibiotics of Choice	Dosage*	Comments
Bronchitis			
Prophylaxis	Tetracycline or erythromycin Trimethoprim — sulfa- methoxazole	250–500 mg 2–4 times/day 2 tablets q. 12 h.	Courses should be given for 5–15 days when sputum changes, suggestive of infection, appear.
Exacerbation	Ampicillin A cephalosporin	500–1,000 mg q. 4–6 h. 500–1,000 mg q. 4–6 h.	A bactericidal agent should be given to treat an exacerbation.
Asthma			
With infection	Erythromycin (Ilosone) Ampicillin	500 mg q. 6 h. 0.5–2 gm q. 6 h.	Ilosone potentiates glucocorticoids. Doses can be reduced when patient improves.
Pneumonias			
Pneumococcal	Procaine penicillin G Penicillin V	600,000 U. I.M. 9.12 h. 250–1,000 mg q 4–6 h. P.O.	Larger doses in debilitated, toxic patients with abnormal lung architecture are advisable.
Staphylococcal	Methicillin	2 gm q. 4 h.	Other penicillinase-resistant penicillins could be used.
Aspiration	Cefazolin Penicillin Clindamycin	1 gm q. 6 h. 2,000.000 U. q. 6 h. 600 mg q. 6 h.	Other cephalosporins could be used. Large doses intravenously are usually required for several weeks. Add gentamicin initially if infection is hospital-acquired.
Gram-negative	Gentamicin Amikacin	3–5 mg/kg/day I.M. or I.V. 15 mg/kg/day I.M. or I.V.	Tobramycin is an alternative. Sensitivities should be used as a guide to therapy.
Prophylaxis	Polymyxin or colistin (aerosol)	5–50 mg in 2 ml saline q. 4 h.	Aerosol therapy should be used for only a few days.
Empyema			
Specific	As indicated by sensitivities	Large doses	Several weeks of treatment and surgical drainage are required.
Lung abscess			
Putrid	Penicillin Clindamycin Chloramphenicol	4,000.000 U. q. 6 h. 900 mg q. 6 h. 0.5–1 gm q. 6 h.	Long-term therapy and drainage procedures are required. Chloramphenicol should not be given for more than 2 weeks, and peripheral blood indices should be monitored. Gentamicin ± carbenicillin may be indicated for gram-negative infections.
Specific	As indicated by sensitivities	Large doses	

Bronchiectasis			
Mixed	Penicillin	Variable doses	Acute exacerbations should be treated as pneumonia.
Specific	As indicated by sensitivities	Variable doses	
Cystic fibrosis			
Colonization	Bacitracin or neomycin inhalation	See Table 10–4	Aerosol, oral or parenteral administration should be used depending on severity of the condition.
Specific	As indicated by sensitivities	Variable doses	
Mycoplasma			
Pneumonia	Erythromycin	500 mg q.i.d.	Not more than 5 days treatment is usually required.
	Tetracycline	500 mg q.i.d.	
Fungal			
Aspergillosis			The optimal intravenous dose has to be built
Coccidioidomycosis	Amphotericin B	1 mg/kg 3 times/week	up, and then is continued until a total of about
Histoplasmosis			2 gm has been given. Nebulization therapy is of dubious benefit.
Moniliasis	Amphotericin	1 mg/kg 3 times/week	A relatively short course of therapy may suffice, e.g., 2–4 weeks.
(candidiasis)	5-Flucytosine	50–150 mg/kg/day	Nystatin may be useful when given by nebulization.
	Nystatin	500,000 U. b.i.d.	
Parasitic			
Pneumocystis	Pentamidine isethionate	4 mg/kg/day	Intramuscular administration for 14 days may suffice.
	Trimethoprim-sulfamethoxazole	4 tablets q.i.d.	Oral administration for 14 days.
Mycobacterial			
Tuberculosis			
uncomplicated	Isoniazid	300 mg q. a.m.	Treatment should be continued for 1–2 years.
	Ethambutol	15 mg/kg q. a.m.	Treatment may be stopped after activity of disease is completely arrested.
complicated	Add streptomycin	1 gm q. a.m.	Dosage may be reduced to 3 per week after a few weeks, and stopped when activity of disease is completely arrested.
retreatment	Use rifampin as part of regimen	10 mg/kg q. a.m.	Treatment is continued until disease is completely controlled.
resistant	Use other agents	See Tables 10–7 and 10–18	Long-term therapy may be needed.
atypical	Isoniazid and several other agents	300–600 mg q. a.m. Individualize	Long-term individualized therapy is needed.

*Oral or aerosol administration can be used for prophylaxis. Oral therapy may suffice for mild infections, but parenteral administration is advisable in more severe infections for at least first few days.

Note: all antibiotics require a physician's prescription for oral, parenteral or inhalational administration.

are causative, long-term, high-dose therapy with the appropriate antibiotic will be required.

Bronchiectasis. Patients with bronchiectasis are similar to those with bronchitis; they generally have low-grade infections that are susceptible to exacerbations. In most cases penicillin will suffice, but when gram-negative or other resistant organisms predominate an alternative antibiotic will need to be selected. Inhalational therapy with antibiotics is sometimes useful, but other forms of respiratory therapy and postural drainage are more valuable.

Cystic Fibrosis. Children with cystic fibrosis fluctuate between colonization and invasive infection of their respiratory tracts, and they are particularly susceptible to *Pseudomonas* and *Staphylococcus* infections. Huang[13, 40] and others advocate the use of systemic and aerosolized antibiotics for the treatment of these patients; the appropriate agent is determined by the particular organism recovered. The dosages to employ and the length of a course of therapy must be carefully chosen by the clinician.

Mycoplasma Pneumonia. The incidence of *Mycoplasma pneumoniae* pneumonia is relatively high in young adults.[33] Milder infections do not require antibiotic therapy, but more severe infections should be treated orally or parenterally. Only erythromycin and tetracycline are of value; one of these agents can be given for a few days.[41]

Fungal Infection. The main fungal infections of the lungs are caused by *Coccidioides immitis* (coccidioidomycosis), *Histoplasma capsulatum* (histoplasmosis) or *Candida* species (candidiasis, moniliasis, thrush); less common invaders are *Blastomyces dermatitidis* (blastomycosis), *Aspergillus fumigatus* (aspergillosis) and *Cryptococcus neoformans* (cryptococcosis).[42, 44] The agent of choice for these diseases is amphotericin B, which must be given intravenously.[44] Some success may occasionally be achieved by giving this very unpleasant drug by aerosolization,[45] but this cannot be recommended until more definitive information has been gathered. The course of intravenous amphotericin that is required is usually 1.6 to 2 gm, at least; often, larger doses are needed. Since only 50 mg can be given three times a week to the average patient, more than 10 weeks of therapy are usually mandated.

More recently, 5-fluorocytosine has been found to be of value in the treatment of candidiasis and cryptococcosis,[46] but it is unlikely to be of major value in coccidioidomycosis. Since this drug is given orally and has fewer side effects than amphotericin, it is to be hoped that it, or an equally benign antimycotic drug, will prove to be a suitable alternative to amphotericin. Other antifungal agents include the older nonspecific agents, such as saturated solution of potassium iodide: when given by mouth it is still the standard treatment for sporotrichosis; the nebulized drug may also be effective. An alternative agent, used for treating North American blastomycosis, is intravenous 2-hydroxystilbamidine.[47]

Parasitic Diseases. Several parasites can affect the lungs, but the most important in the U.S. is *Pneumocystis carinii*, a protozoan that infects immunosuppressed hosts. The standard therapy is the relatively toxic intramuscular preparation pentamidine isethionate, but pyrimethamine and sulfadiazine are used as an alternative. More recently, success has been obtained with large doses of the combination of trimethoprim (960 to 1200 mg per day) and sulfamethoxazole (4800 to 6000 mg per day); a special intravenous preparation may be required.[48]

Tuberculosis. The treatment of all forms of tuberculosis is based on isoniazid (INH); various other agents are added to the regimen as indicated by the clinical situation and the bacteriologic data.[49, 50] Certain general principles can be summarized here (see Table 10–7):

1. INH is given to an adult in a single daily dose of 300 mg a day; somewhat smaller doses may be given to children, who tolerate the drug well. INH therapy is usually continued for 12 months to two years for active disease, and prophylactic pyridoxine (vitamin B_6, 10 mg once or twice a day) is given to patients susceptible to peripheral neuritis. The other major problems to be aware of are the hypersensitivity reactions, including hepatitis.

2. Ethambutol is the usual choice of a second drug for active disease, and it is usually continued for 18 months to two years; patients who respond very rapidly to therapy could probably stop this drug before discontinuing the INH after the conventional 12 months to two years. This drug is relatively well tolerated, but patients should be monitored for color vision changes and optic neuritis.

3. Streptomycin injections are added for more severe infections. Initially, one injection a day is given, but after a few weeks,

TABLE 10-7. USUAL COURSES OF THERAPY FOR PULMONARY TUBERCULOSIS IN ADULT

Regimen	Type of Infection	Drug	Daily	Intermittent	Duration	Comments
A	Minimal infection, PPD conversion, serious exposure to tuberculosis, no mycobacteria in sputum	isoniazid (NIH)	5–10 mg/kg P.O. (300 mg q.a.m.)		1 year in most cases	Prophylactic INH should be given to patients at risk of developing overt tuberculosis, unless risk of therapy is greater.
B	Active disease, culture positive	INH + ethambutol or rifampin	300 mg q.a.m. P.O. / 15 mg/kg q.a.m. P.O. / 600 mg q.a.m. P.O.	15 mg/kg twice/wk. (P.O. or I.M.) / 50 mg/kg twice/wk. (P.O.) / Not recommended	1½–2 years. / 1½–2 years / 6–12 months	Isoniazid and ethambutol are usually continued long after full recovery has occurred. PAS could be used with INH for children. The addition of rifampin to isoniazid may decrease the time for full recovery.
C	Active cavitary or widespread disease	Regimen B + streptomycin	1 gm I.M. (for first few weeks)	1 gm I.M. (up to 3 times/week)	1½–2 years / 3–6 months	Streptomycin is given daily for first 2–6 weeks, then three times a week (or two times a week in patients over 55) until three successive mycobacterial cultures are negative.
D	Relapse, resistant bacilli, intolerance of first-line drugs	Regimen B + pyrazinamide and/or ethionamide or another second-line drug.	See Table 10–18	Intermittent regimen not established	Usually treatment is required for 2 years or more	If a regimen fails, two new drugs should be added. The second-line drugs are more toxic, and it may be difficult to guarantee that treatment is taken unless the patient is kept under supervision.
E	Unreliable patient, who has failed on previous therapy, with severe cavitary or widespread destructive disease	Regimen B + an injectable agent: streptomycin or kanamycin or capreomycin or (viomycin)	As in Regimen C / 15 mg/kg I.M. / 1 gm I.M. / 1 gm I.M.	15 mg/kg I.M. / 1 gm I.M. / 1 gm I.M. } 2 or 3 times a week	Usually treatment is required for 2 years or more, and oral agents may need to be continued indefinitely.	Injectables are given as for streptomycin i.e. daily for first 2–6 weeks, then three times a week in younger patients and twice a week in older patients, provided response is adequate. Viomycin is rarely indicated.
F	Life-threatening disease or severely toxic patient; involvement of meninges, pericardium or peritoneum	Regimen C or E + a glucocorticoid, e.g., prednisone	Large doses, e.g., 60 mg/day		1–2 weeks, then wean over next 4 weeks	Initially, steroid therapy may be life-saving.

provided there is a satisfactory response, three times a week therapy can usually be adopted and continued until the patient's sputum is culture-negative. Younger patients tolerate 1 gm injections, but older patients may develop vestibular damage (affecting balance) or auditory impairment, or renal damage, unless the dose is reduced to 0.5 gm. The patient must be monitored for the appearance of these possible problems.

4. Rifampin is advisable for use in re-treatment regimens, or if a resistant organism is involved. Usually, this drug is combined with isoniazid and either ethambutol or streptomycin, and it is stopped when criteria for discontinuing these latter agents have been met. Rifampin can cause liver and renal damage, particularly if given intermittently.

5. The second-line agents are used mainly in difficult retreatment problems, or when the patient is allergic to the first-line drugs.[51] They are all more toxic than the first-line drugs, and skill is required for their correct use.

6. If a patient is doing poorly on a drug regimen, a "failing" drug should be replaced by two additional ones. In most cases of this type it is advisable to use one injectable agent in the combination.

7. In recent years, short courses of intensive therapy (for example, for six months)[52] and intermittent courses of larger doses of drugs (for example, twice weekly administration)[53] have shown considerable promise during the majority of many careful trials. Before too long, it is likely that some of these modified courses will be authorized as standard therapy.

8. Toxic complications must be looked for while patients are on antituberculosis therapy. These are sometimes subtle, such as optic neuritis developing on ethambutol, which is recognized only if color vision is routinely tested.

9. Atypical mycobacterial infections are similar to tuberculosis, but are generally more indolent and resistant to therapy. Infections with *M. intracellulare* may be resistant to all drugs but cycloserine in vitro.[51] Regimens employing multiple anti-tuberculosis drugs are sometimes required, and in extreme cases most of the oral drugs are given simultaneously. Higher dosages and prolonged therapy are occasionally necessitated by progressive resistant disease. The other common atypical disease, caused by *M. kansasii,* often responds well to standard therapy of isoniazid with ethambu-

tol or streptomycin, with the addition of rifampin.[51]

10. Aerosol antituberculosis therapy has been tried, but has no place in modern therapeutics.

Upper Respiratory Tract Infections. Various bacteria can cause otitis, sinusitis, pharyngitis, laryngitis, tracheitis and tracheobronchitis. Viruses can cause these diseases (Table 10–1), and in children they can also cause epiglottitis and bronchiolitis, although these conditions are often the result of *H. influenzae* infection. The treatment of these diseases is, in part, specific, using an appropriate antibiotic (based on experience or on cultures), and, in part, symptomatic, using cough and cold medications (mainly decongestants and demulcents), as discussed in Chapter 9.

When a poorly draining cavity is infected, as occurs with the sinuses and ear, secondary invaders may eventually appear; chronic infections in these upper respiratory sites often include gram-negative bacteria in their resident flora. Ampicillin and erythromycin are usually the best antibiotics for upper respiratory bacterial infections, with penicillin, clindamycin, a tetracycline and cephalexin serving as alternatives. If these agents do not suffice, and a gram-negative organism is present, broad-spectrum coverage may be necessitated.[54]

It is important to consider chronic sinus infection as a possible covert etiologic cause of lower respiratory disease, and in some patients with asthma, bronchitis or bronchiectasis marked improvement eventually occurs once the upper respiratory component is effectively treated. Surgical drainage or irrigation procedures may be required, and in some stubborn sinus infections more radical drainage may have to be produced by a suitable operative procedure.

Mechanisms of Actions of Antimicrobial Agents

Most antimicrobial drugs interfere at specific points in the metabolism of susceptible microorganisms. The majority of agents that have been discovered have activity in animal metabolic processes; for this reason, they may be equally, or more, toxic to the host than to the infecting organisms. Of the many thousands of antimicrobial agents that have been isolated, only a few score are sufficiently effective and nontoxic to justify their use in therapeutics. The antimicrobial mechanisms of the commonly used agents can be classified as follows:[55]

Inhibitors of Bacterial Cell Wall Formation. The replication of bacteria involves the synthesis of peptidoglycan subunits, and many antibiotics interfere with the linking of these subunits in the cell wall. As a consequence, the bacteria lose osmotic stability, and they disintegrate in body tissues. Agents that act in this fashion include the *penicillins,* the *cephalosporins, bacitracin, vancomycin* and *cycloserine.*

Agents That Damage Bacterial Cell Membranes. The cell membrane on the inner side of the cell wall is a semipermeable barrier membrane whose integrity is essential for cellular function. Surface-active agents and many antibiotics bind to the membrane and render it leaky, allowing essential molecules to escape from the cell. The drugs in this category include the *polypeptides,* the antifungal *polyenes* and many antibacterial sterilizing agents.

Agents That Interfere With Protein Synthesis. Intracellular ribosomes in microorganisms are responsible for the synthesis of vital proteins. Several agents bind to ribosomal subunits and interfere with their ability to function. In this group are the *aminoglycosides, chloramphenicol,* the *macrolides,* the *tetracyclines* and the *lincomycins,* and perhaps *viomycin.*

Agents That Inhibit Nucleotide Formation or Metabolism. Some of the antituberculosis drugs appear to interfere with nucleotide function. *Rifampin* inhibits RNA-polymerase, and blocks ribonucleic acid formation. *Isoniazid* is believed to depress DNA synthesis, whereas ethambutol depresses RNA synthesis. The exact mechanisms of action of *para-aminosalicylic acid, pyrazinamide* and *ethionamide* are not known.

Antimetabolites. *Sulfonamides* inhibit the synthesis of dihydrofolic acid in sensitive microorganisms by competitively blocking the incorporation of the essential precursor, para-aminobenzoic acid (PABA), into the molecule, which is a precursor of folic acid. In the presence of excess PABA, which occurs for instance in pus, sulfonamides are not able to function optimally. *Trimethoprim* and *pyrimethamine* are inhibitors of dehydrofolate reductase, and thereby also inhibit folic acid synthesis by susceptible microorganisms; they also potentiate the action of sulfonamides against certain bacteria and protozoa.

PHARMACOLOGY OF INDIVIDUAL ANTIMICROBIAL AGENTS

Penicillins
(Tables 10–8 and 10–9)

The penicillins continue to provide adequate therapy in pneumococcal pneumonia, aspiration pneumonia acquired in a nonhospitalized patient (who is unlikely to have an opportunistic gram-negative infection), and in putrid lung abscesses caused by the normal oropharyngeal flora that includes *Bacteroides* species and other anaerobes. The broader spectrum derivatives, such as ampicillin and the similar amoxicillin and hetacillin, are suitable for the treatment of exacerbations of bronchitis, since they are usually effective against the two major causative organisms, the pneumococcus and *H. influenzae.* The penicillinase-resistant derivatives (methicillin, oxacillin, cloxacillin, dicloxacillin and nafcillin) are indicated for treatment of infection caused by a *Staphylococcus* that produces this enzyme. These drugs are less effective against other gram-positive organisms, and if anaerobes, *Streptococci* or other susceptible bacteria are also believed to be present, concomitant penicillin therapy may also be required. The broad-spectrum agents carbenicillin and ticarcillin are effective against *Pseudomonas,* and they are often given with an aminoglycoside for treating a gram-negative pneumonia. Large doses of these expensive penicillin agents are required; therefore, they should never be used when simpler penicillins would suffice.

The penicillins should no longer be considered suitable for nebulization therapy, since they are rarely indicated even when liberal guidelines are utilized. Moreover, they may cause asthma, rashes and other hypersensitivity reactions. Some workers favor nebulizing carbenicillin for the treatment of susceptible pulmonary infections,[56] but it is doubtful that this practice can be justified. The relatively low molecular weight of the penicillins may suggest that they do not cross the blood-bronchus barrier very readily, but the vast and favorable clinical experience of oral and systemic therapy tends to refute this theoretic justification for giving the penicillins by inhalation.

Penicillin Preparations. Numerous variations of penicillin have been produced and marketed,[57] but only the most important ones need be considered, since the additional agents offer no significant advantages.

TABLE 10–8.   THE PENICILLINS

Preparation	Routes ORAL I.M. I.V.			Approximate Daily Dosage for Adults*	Major Indications
Penicillin (See Table 10–9)	+	+	+	600,000–10,000,000 U or 1–4 gm (P.O.)	Pneumococcal pneumonia, aspiration pneumonia, lung abscess; not effective against *H. influenzae*
Amoxicillin (Amoxil, Larotid, Polymox, Robamox, Sumox, Trimox)	+			0.75–1.5 gm†	Similar to ampicillin, but may be better absorbed, and may have fewer side effects.
Ampicillin (Amcill, Omnipen, Penbritin, etc.)	+	+	+	1–4 gm	Bronchitis, chronic obstructive disease (for prophylaxis or treatment of exacerbation); very effective against *H. influenzae*, usually
Carbenicillin (Geopen, Pyopen) (Geocillin)	+	+	+	30–40 gm	Severe gram-negative or anaerobic infections; not effective against *Klebsiella;* effective against *Pseudomonas* and *H. influenzae*
Cloxacillin (Cloxapen, Tegopen)	+			3–6 gm	For penicillin-resistant *Staphylococcus*
Dicloxacillin (Dycill, Dynapen, Pathocil, Veracillin)	+			2–6 gm	For penicillin-resistant *Staphylococcus*
Hetacillin (Versapen)	+			0.9–4.5 gm	Similar to ampicillin
Methicillin (Azapen, Celbenin, Staphcillin)		+	+	4–12 gm	For penicillin-resistant *Staphylococcus*
Nafcillin, (Nafcil, Unipen)	+	+	+	1–6 gm	For penicillin-resistant *Staphylococcus*
Oxacillin (Bactocil, Prostaphlin)	+	+	+	1–6 gm	For penicillin-resistant *Staphylococcus*
Ticarcillin (Ticar)		+	+	3–20 gm	Similar to carbenicillin

*Divided doses are usually administered 4–6 times a day.
†Amoxicillin is usually given in 3 divided doses a day.

TABLE 10–9.   SIMPLE PENICILLINS AND DERIVATIVES

Preparation	Brand Names	Route ORAL I.M. I.V.			Number of Doses Per Day	Comment
Penicillin G crystalline (Na and K preparations)	Pentids, Pfizerpen G, etc.	+	+	+	4–6	Standard product; oral absorption unreliable
procaine	Bicillin, Crysticillin, Duracillin, Wycillin		+		1–2	Long-acting
benzathine	Bicillin, Permapen	(+)	+	(+)	1 or less	Very long-acting
Phenoxymethyl penicillin penicillin V	Pen·Vee, V-Cillin	+			4–6	Well absorbed by mouth
hydrabamine penicillin V	Compocillin-V	+			4–6	Well absorbed by mouth
potassium penicillin V	Compocillin-VK, Ledercillin VK, Pen·Vee K, V-Cillin K, etc.	+			4–6	Well absorbed by mouth
Phenoxyethyl penicillin phenethicillin	Maxipen, Syncillin	+			3–6	Well absorbed by mouth

PENICILLIN AND CLOSE CONGENERS. The first penicillin to be introduced into therapeutics was *penicillin G*, and this preparation is still one of the most useful.[58] It is marketed as both the sodium salt and the potassium salt, although the latter is more effective; other salts, such as the aluminum preparation, are rarely used currently. Penicillin G can be taken orally, but since it is not stable in an acid environment, it is not reliably absorbed; intramuscular and intravenous administration of aqueous preparations of the crystalline drug are more suitable for acute or serious infections.

Longer-acting depot preparations have been manufactured for intramuscular injection; the most important of these are *procaine penicillin G* (which can result in measurable blood levels for up to a week) and *benzathine penicillin G* (which may result in a therapeutic blood level lasting 10 to 20 days). An injection of procaine penicillin can be given to a patient with moderate susceptible disease (such as pneumococcal pneumonia) according to different regimens; thus, one injection may constitute adequate therapy in less severe disease, but, more commonly, twice-daily administration is required for a few days. Benzathine penicillin is not often used in the treatment of respiratory diseases, but it may be worth further evaluation: one injection could provide adequate therapy for selected patients with penicillin-sensitive infections.

A less potent derivative of penicillin G is *penicillin V* (phenoxymethyl penicillin). This preparation is better absorbed when given by mouth with meals, and results in a serum level that is 3 to 5 times that achieved by an equal oral dose of penicillin G. However, if penicillin G is taken on an empty stomach, it can achieve similar concentrations, and, since it is less expensive and more active, its use should generally be preferred to that of penicillin V.

Phenethicillin (phenoxyethyl penicillin) is another semisynthetic derivative suitable only for oral administration. It is comparable to penicillin V, and does not offer any noteworthy advantages.

AMPICILLIN. Ampicillin is an important semisynthetic derivative, which has, however, probably gained more popularity than it deserves. It has a wider spectrum than that of penicillin, being effective against many gram-negative organisms, including *H. influenzae*. In general, other more potent antibiotics are preferred for the treatment of most gram-negative pulmonary infections,

and the respiratory role of ampicillin may best be restricted to the treatment of bronchitis, exacerbations of chronic obstructive disease, and the management of the less severe pneumonias. The drug is reliably absorbed when given by mouth, and it can also be given parenterally. In severe pulmonary infections, 1 gm should be given every six hours; this large a dose may not be tolerated by mouth, and parenteral administration will usually be required.

A major advantage of ampicillin is that it is less protein bound than the other penicillins, and it seems to be very effective in pulmonary infections, in spite of evidence that it does not enter the sputum reliably or in adequate amounts.[5, 26, 59]

Two recently developed modifications of ampicillin have been marketed. *Amoxicillin* is very similar to ampicillin, but it is better absorbed and may produce higher serum levels after oral administration. There are claims that it is more effectively distributed into the lungs,[30] but this is a dubious benefit. It does, however, offer the advantage of a lower incidence of gastrointestinal and dermatologic side effects.[60] *Hetacillin* is a derivative that is rapidly hydrolyzed in the body to release ampicillin and acetone. It is doubtful that this product offers any advantages over the less expensive ampicillin.

PENICILLINASE-RESISTANT PENICILLINS. Over the course of the years since penicillin was introduced, some susceptible bacteria have developed resistance. The most important organism to have thus adapted is *Staphylococcus aureus*, many species of which are currently resistant; the incidence of resistance is higher in the hospital environment, but penicillin resistance is becoming more common in community strains of Staphylococci. The bacteria, in common with many other nonsusceptible species, produce the enzyme penicillinase, which hydrolyzes and thereby inactivates the simpler penicillins. To cope with this problem, the pharmaceutical industry has synthesized a number of penicillinase-resistant derivatives. The important agents are *methicillin, nafcillin,* and the isoxazole derivatives, *oxacillin, cloxacillin, dicloxacillin* and *flucloxacillin.*[57, 61] These agents are similar in their properties, but differ in their routes of administration and absorption: thus, oxacillin is less reliably absorbed when given orally than are the other preparations; it should always be given on an empty stomach. Each of these derivatives can be used for susceptible infections: the choice of one should be based on familiarity with the agent and suitability for administration to the individual patient.

CARBENICILLIN. This semisynthetic penicillin is similar to ampicillin, but it is effective against *P. aeruginosa* and indole-positive *Proteus.* However, very large amounts of the drug are required, and these can be given only intravenously; a course of therapy is relatively expensive. Carbenicillin is rarely used on its own; more often, it is combined with a drug such as gentamicin for its synergistic action on gram-negative bacteria (each drug should be given separately to avoid inactivation of the carbenicillin). The coverage against anaerobes that carbenicillin may provide constitutes a useful extension of therapy in the management of an undiagnosed serious infection. Carbenicillin does not cross the blood-bronchial barrier as effectively as gentamicin,[62] although the clinical significance of this is unclear at present.

A recent derivative, *indanyl carbenicillin,* is suitable for oral administration; it is converted into carbenicillin in the body. It is of value only for treating low-level urinary tract infections caused by *Pseudomonas,* and it should not be given for infections in other sites, since it does not achieve a high enough blood level to be effective.

TICARCILLIN. Recently this semisynthetic penicillin was marketed as an alternative to carbenicillin. Ticarcillin appears to be more effective than carbenicillin against all susceptible organisms except *Staphylococcus epidermidis* and enterococci. Some strains of *Pseudomonas* may develop resistance fairly rapidly, and it is therefore advisable to use ticarcillin in conjunction with synergistic agents such as gentamicin. This new antibiotic is available for administration only by systemic injection, and it is effective in the treatment of susceptible acute and chronic respiratory tract infections, particularly those caused by gram-negative organisms. It appears to have advantages over carbenicillin, the most important being that it is effective in lower dosage.

The addition of the uricosuric agent *probenecid* (Benemid) should be considered when using penicillin therapy, since this agent interferes with the excretion of the antibiotic and results in higher and more prolonged blood levels. This can be of value when using an oral penicillin or when giving an expensive drug such as carbenicillin. Probenecid in a dose of 250 to 500 mg 2 to 4 times a day can result in a doubling or tripling of the serum level of the penicillin. The main disadvantages of probenecid are that it can cause gastrointestinal intolerance and that it may occasionally result in hypersensitivity reactions, such as rashes, which may be mistaken for penicillin reactions.

Adverse Effects of Penicillins. None of the penicillins have serious pharmacologic toxicity when given in the usual doses, and, in general, these antibiotics are relatively safe. However, a major disadvantage is that susceptible individuals can manifest hypersensitivity reactions, which vary from mild skin rashes to potentially fatal anaphylactic reactions. Since the overall extent of the use of the penicillins is considerable, serious reactions are not rare, and measures must always be taken to prevent them. The main requirement of the physician is to enquire if there is a history of penicillin allergy before prescribing the drug, and when a patient is given an initial parenteral injection, he should be kept under observation for half an hour. The physician should be prepared for emergency treatment if an allergic reaction appears: 0.5 ml epinephrine 1:1000 I.M., I.V. or even by direct injection into the heart, with other resuscitative measures, may be required.

The hazard of severe hypersensitivity reactions is markedly decreased if an oral agent is used; in contrast, the danger of a prolonged reaction is increased when a depot intramuscular preparation is given. For these reasons, physicians should be reluctant to give an ambulatory office or clinic patient a "shot" of penicillin followed by oral therapy: in general, if it is considered that a course of oral therapy will be effective, the initial injection is probably not justified. However, when parenteral therapy is judged to be necessary, it should not be withheld if suitable monitoring of the patient can be provided. Similar concerns about hypersensitivity reactions, as well as lack of proof of effectiveness, have led to the abandonment of topical therapy with the penicillins, both in dermatologic and respiratory therapy.

Cephalosporins
(Table 10–10)

Cephalothin was the first of this increasingly large family of agents to be introduced and it rapidly found two major indications: as an alternative to penicillin, and as a synergistic agent to use with aminoglycosides in the treatment of some gram-negative infections, particularly *Klebsiella.* In general, the cephalosporins appear to be overused, and

TABLE 10–10. THE CEPHALOSPORINS

Preparation	ORAL	Routes I.M.	I.V.	Approximate Daily Dosage For Adults GM/DAY	Comments
Cefazolin (Ancef, Kefzol)		+	+	1–6	Relatively more effective for anaerobes, *E. coli* and *Klebsiella;* suitable for intramuscular administration
Cephalexin (Keflex)	+			1–4	Well absorbed by mouth, on an empty stomach; relatively low potency
Cephacetrile (Celospor)		+	+	2–12	Similar to cephalothin; investigational
Cephaloridine (Loridine)		+	+	1.5–4	Nephrotoxic; rarely used currently
Cephalothin (Keflin)		+	+	2–12	Basic cephalosporin; must be given intramuscularly (painful) or intravenously (venosclerotic)
Cephapirin (Cephadyl)		+	+	4–12	Similar to cephalothin
Cephradine (Anspor, Velosef)	+	+	+	1–8	Only cephalosporin suitable for both oral and parenteral administration

The cephalosporins are rarely regarded as first-line drugs; they are the primary alternatives to penicillin for gram-positive infections. and are often used with other broad-spectrum agents in the treatment of gram-negative infections. Doses are usually administered 4 times a day.

they should not be regarded as primary agents for the treatment of any pulmonary infection.[58, 63]

The newer cephalosporins are now displacing the original agents, cephalothin and cephaloridine. Cephradine is particularly useful, since it can readily be given orally as well as intramuscularly or intravenously; cephalexin is the only other oral cephalosporin suitable for the treatment of pulmonary disease. For systemic therapy, cefazolin appears to be the current favorite of many clinicians.

Although the cephalosporins have a relatively low molecular weight, which would suggest that they penetrate the blood-bronchus barrier poorly, there is little clinical evidence to suggest that this consideration is relevant. At present, one cannot recommend any of the cephalosporins as inhalational agents.

Cephalosporin Preparations. A rather bewildering number of cephalosporins has appeared on the market, and it is difficult to establish clear guidelines for the use of each one.[63]

CEPHALOTHIN. Cephalothin was the first cephalosporin to be introduced into therapeutics, and it continues to be the standard. It is not well absorbed when given by mouth, but it is very effective when administered parenterally. The parenteral preparations have the serious disadvantage of being irritating: intramuscular injections are relatively painful, and intravenous administration can cause phlebitis.

CEPHALORIDINE. Cephaloridine was introduced as a less irritating derivative, which is more acceptable for both intramuscular and intravenous injection. Although it is a very effective antimicrobial, it has the serious disadvantage of being nephrotoxic, and it is therefore currently losing favor.

CEFAZOLIN. Cefazolin is at present the most popular cephalosporin in many hospitals. It produces higher and more sustained serum levels than cephalothin, and it is not irritating when given by intramuscular or intravenous injection. Although it is one of the most potent cephalosporins for most susceptible microorganisms, it is less effective than its congeners against penicillin-resistant *Staphylococcus.*[60]

CEPHAPIRIN. Cephapirin is one of the newest cephalosporins for parenteral administration. However, it appears to be more irritating than cefazolin, causing pain on intramuscular injection and phlebitis with intravenous administration. If offers no advantages, and it cannot be recommended as a primary choice for any respiratory infection.

CEPHACETRILE. This parenterally administered agent is similar to cephapirin and offers no advantages. At present it is an investigational agent, and there appears to be little reason to market it.

CEPHALEXIN. This important product was the first of the synthesized cephalosporins to be suitable for oral administration, and it is made available only as oral preparations. It is less potent than the other cephalosporins, and some organisms are relatively resistant to it. Because of this, it cannot be recommended without reservation, although it is apparently effective in the treatment of many cases of otitis and pharyngitis. It is less likely to be useful in the treatment of lower respiratory tract infections. Its poor reliability in *H. influenzae* infections, particularly in those of children, makes it a relatively unsuitable choice for respiratory infections in which this bacterium plays a role.

CEPHRADINE. Cephradine is the only available cephalosporin that can be administered both orally and parenterally. It is somewhat less potent than the other parenteral cephalosporins, and it is comparable to cephalexin. Although it is an alternative agent to cephalexin for oral administration, it is not as suitable as cefazolin for parenteral therapy.

CEPHALOGLYCIN. Cephaloglycin is an oral drug that is poorly absorbed; since it becomes concentrated in the urine, it has been promoted for the treatment of urinary tract infections. It has no place in the management of respiratory infections.

In summary, the best cephalosporin for intramuscular administration is cefazolin. This agent is also the best for intravenous use, while cephalothin is an alternative. For oral administration, cephalexin or cephradine should be considered.

Adverse Effects of Cephalosporins. The cephalosporins are generally used as alternatives to the penicillins, particularly if a patient is allergic to penicillin. Since the cephalosporin nucleus is similar to that of penicillin, the cephalosporins can produce similar toxic effects including rashes, fever and other hypersensitivity reactions, including a positive Coombs test with or without hemolysis. Serious reactions, such as anaphylaxis, are rare, and cross-reactivity with penicillin is not a major concern; nevertheless, if a patient has previously had a very severe reaction to penicillin (such as anaphylaxis or exfoliative dermatitis), it is advisable not to expose the patient to a cephalosporin.

Other toxic reactions are similar to those seen with many other antibiotics, and include gastrointestinal disturbances (particularly diarrhea, which is less frequently a problem with cephalexin), depression of bone marrow, hemolytic anemia, minor (chemical) hepatitis, which is usually transient, and various neurologic symptoms.

Tetracyclines
(Table 10–11)

The large number of available tetracyclines should not distract one from the fact that tetracycline itself is the best of these agents for most purposes. The use of tetracycline in the prophylaxis and treatment of bronchitis has been long established, and is based on the ability of this antibiotic to kill the pneumococcus and *H. influenzae.* Theoretically, ampicillin would be better than tetracycline in a severe infection, because the former is bactericidal whereas the latter is bacteriostatic; in practice, there is

TABLE 10–11. THE TETRACYCLINES

Preparation	Usual Adult Dosage (ORAL OR I.V.)	Comments
Tetracycline (Achromycin V, etc.)	250–500 mg q.i.d.	Standard drug for bronchitis, and for *Mycoplasma* infections
Chlortetracycline (Aureomycin)	250–500 mg q.i.d.	Rarely used; similar to tetracycline
Demeclocycline (Declomycin)	300 mg q. 12 h.	Rarely used; may cause photosensitivity and nephrogenic diabetes insipidus
Doxycycline (oral) (Doxychel, Doxy II, Vibramycin)	100–200 mg q. 12–24 h.	More active against anaerobes than most other tetracyclines; does not accumulate in renal failure
Doxycycline hyclate (I.V.) (Vibramycin)	100 mg q. 12 h.	Useful long-acting drug; once a day dosage suffices after first few days
Methacycline (Rondomycin)	150 mg q.i.d.	Rarely used, but effective; moderately long-acting
Minocycline (Minocin, Vectrin)	100 mg q. 12 h.	Similar to doxycycline, but may cause vestibular disturbance
Oxytetracycline (Terramycin, etc.)	250–500 mg q.i.d.	Similar to tetracycline
Rolitetracycline (Syntetrin)	350–700 mg q. 12 h.	Rarely used product for intramuscular administration; not available in U.S.

little to suggest that tetracycline is any less suitable.

The longer-acting tetracyclines (such as doxycycline) are useful, since they permit therapy to be given only twice a day; moreover, their degree of absorption may be better. Doxycycline has been shown to penetrate the blood-bronchus barrier in small but adequate amounts to reach a bacteriostatic or even bactericidal level in the sputum. The sputum levels attained after a few days of therapy may approach 50 per cent of the serum level, but results are variable.[31, 64] Clinical experience has shown this agent to be useful, in a dosage of 100 to 200 mg twice a day, for the management of the tracheobronchitis, with annoying cough that often follows, and lingers on, after a viral respiratory infection. At present doxycycline can be regarded as a drug of choice in the treatment of bronchitis.[65]

The tetracyclines are usually given orally; their parenteral use is less popular. When given by mouth, they should be taken before food, and without calcium, to avoid decreased absorption of the drug as a result of chelation in the bowel.

The tetracyclines have relatively low molecular weights, although doxycycline hyclate is exceptional in having a weight over 1000. However, there is little evidence that any of these antibiotics need be given by nebulization; in fact, there are no significant reports of this use of the tetracyclines.

Tetracycline Preparations. There are two major classes of tetracyclines: the short-acting preparations and the longer-acting derivatives.

SHORTER-ACTING TETRACYCLINES. The prototype drug is *tetracycline,* which is the most commonly used congener. It can be given orally (on an empty stomach, for better absorption), or by intramuscular or intravenous injection; however, intramuscular administration can be very painful and should rarely be employed. *Chlortetracycline* was introduced prior to tetracycline, but it is less commonly used at present. *Oxytetracycline* is similar to both the preceding congeners, and may offer some advantages: it causes less diarrhea and it is less likely to stain the teeth in young children during the development phase of the permanent dentition. *Methacycline* is similar to oxytetracycline in structure; it is less well absorbed from the bowel than are the other short-acting tetracyclines, and it has a longer half-life because it is excreted slowly. Methacycline has been reported to be as effective

as ampicillin in the treatment of exacerbations of chronic bronchitis.[66] This preparation is, in fact, a relatively long-acting tetracycline, but since it appears to offer no advantages, it is not often used, and it cannot be recommended.

LONGER-ACTING TETRACYCLINES. The most popular of these preparations is probably *doxycycline.* It is well absorbed when given by mouth, and it has a long serum half-life. It need be given only once or twice a day in relatively low dosage. Further advantages include its low toxicity and its safety in patients with renal insufficiency. It does not chelate as readily as do tetracycline and its similar congeners, and can therefore be given with food. Doxycycline has a higher degree of lipid solubility than other tetracyclines, and it is more highly protein bound; it is speculated that it may be actively transported into the respiratory secretions.[31, 64] Doxycycline is available for oral administration as a monohydrate, as a calcium salt, and as doxycycline hyclate; the latter is suitable for intravenous administration, and its higher molecular weight may result in increased penetration through the blood-bronchus barrier. Once a day dosage suffices for lesser infections, but twice a day administration is needed for acute infections for at least the first few days.

MINOCYCLINE. Minocycline is similar to doxycycline in that it is absorbed well when given with food, and it penetrates well into the sputum. This preparation may be effective against *Nocardia* infections, whereas other tetracyclines are not. It has been shown to be as effective as ampicillin or doxycycline in the treatment of infectious exacerbations in chronic obstructive pulmonary disease.[67] It may be less long-acting than doxycycline, and it may be safe in patients with renal insufficiency. Minocycline has a serious toxic potential in that it can cause transient vestibular disturbance, resulting in dizziness and ataxia; for this reason, high doses should be avoided. Although it can be given intravenously, there appears to be no advantage to this route if the patient can take the drug orally.

DEMECLOCYCLINE. Demeclocycline is less desirable as an antibiotic than the other longer-acting tetracyclines, since it is more frequently the cause of photosensitivity skin reactions. This agent can produce a nephrogenic diabetes insipidus, a property put to clinical use in the treatment of inappropriate antidiuretic hormone secretion, a syndrome that may complicate diseases such as severe pneumonia or cancer of the lung.

ROLITETRACYCLINE. Rolitetracycline is a more soluble form of tetracycline, and is the only one truly suitable for intramuscular administration, since it is less irritating than the other derivatives. It can also be given intravenously, but it has no therapeutic advantages over the other long-acting tetracyclines. This preparation is used in some countries, but it is not promoted in the U.S.

Adverse Effects of Tetracyclines. In general, these popular agents are well tolerated, even when given in daily therapy for weeks or months. Allergic reactions are uncommon and are rarely serious. The most frequent side effects are gastrointestinal intolerance, particularly nausea and diarrhea. Minor hepatic disturbance can occur, but pregnant women are at greater risk and are susceptible to severe hepatic damage, particularly with intravenous doses in excess of 2 gm per day. In any case, tetracyclines should not be given to pregnant women (nor to children under age 8) because of the discoloration and growth disturbances of the child's permanent dentition that can result.

The tetracyclines have an antianabolic effect, and may worsen azotemia in patients with renal insufficiency; they should not be given to patients with renal failure. However, doxycycline is excreted into the bowel, and this derivative appears to be safe in such circumstances. The tetracyclines rarely cause bone marrow depression; other serious side effects are very rare. A major problem in many women, however, is a tendency to develop vulvovaginitis while on tetracycline therapy; this is a greater risk in diabetic women.

Aminoglycosides
(Table 10–12)

Antibiotics in this group are also known as *aminocyclitols*. These agents have a broad spectrum of action, mainly against gram-negative bacteria. They are toxic drugs, with the capability of causing severe damage to the ear (affecting hearing or balance, or both) and the kidney. These considerations are important factors in favor of administering the aminoglycosides by nebulization rather than by parenteral injection. Furthermore, several of these agents (such as gentamicin and neomycin) have proved useful for topical therapy of infections of the skin; the evidence is that they are not absorbed to a significant degree when applied topically to the skin or a mucous membrane.

Kanamycin had been subjected to more careful aerosol studies than any other aminoglycoside. It is poorly absorbed, well tolerated and safe when nebulized into the lung, although it does accumulate in lung tissue with repeated administration. Unlike polymyxin, it does not cause any increase in airway resistance.[68–70] A further advantage of kanamycin is that it appears to precipitate with DNA in purulent sputum, thereby decreasing its viscosity, and it may thereby improve airway mechanics by improving mucokinesis. Since kanamycin is rarely used parenterally at present, it may be appropriate to reserve its use in respiratory therapy to

TABLE 10–12. THE AMINOGLYCOSIDES

Preparation	ORAL	Routes I.M.	I.V.	TOPICAL	Approximate Dosage For Adults	Comments
Amikacin (Amikin)		+	+		7.5 mg/kg q 12 h*	Similar to gentamicin; useful alternative
Gentamicin (Garamycin)		+	+	+	1–1.7 mg/kg q 8 h	Standard agent for treating *Pseudomonas* and other gram-negative infections, and *Staphylococcus*; not effective against anaerobes
Kanamycin (Kantrex)	(+)	+	+			Rarely used now; may be useful in aerosol therapy
Neomycin (Mycifradin)	+			+		Only used topically; it is the most toxic aminoglycoside; ineffective against *Pseudomonas*
Streptomycin		+			0.5–2 gm/day in 1 or 2 divided doses	Rarely used, except in treatment of tuberculosis; bacteria develop resistance rapidly
Tobramycin (Nebcin)		+			1–1.7 mg/kg q 8 h	Alternative to gentamicin; may be more effective against *Pseudomonas*

*Total daily amount can be given in two or three divided doses.

the nebulization treatment of colonization or early infection by susceptible gram-negative bacteria and *Staphylococcus* species.

Neomycin is similar to kanamycin, but more toxic; it has never been considered suitable for parenteral therapy, but it has a long history of topical usage. It may be of particular value in the aerosol treatment of cystic fibrosis, in which it has been reported successful in eliminating *Staphylococcus* and other susceptible organisms.

The other aminoglycosides are relatively rarely used in aerosol therapy, but the evidence suggests that gentamicin[24] and tobramycin[71] may be effective and safe in the elimination of early infections or colonization by *Pseudomonas,* or other susceptible gram-negative bacteria, and *Staphylococcus.* Evaluation of amikacin is inadequate at present but it will probably prove to be a valuable drug.[40] These agents are relatively heavy molecules, and they appear to penetrate the blood-bronchial barrier successfully. This would suggest that nebulization therapy is less necessary for these antibiotics, and at present their value in aerosol therapeutics has not been determined. Some investigators have reported unfavorably on aerosolized gentamicin, although better results were obtained in the treatment of *Pseudomonas* infections by combining gentamicin with carbenicillin.[56] Unfortunately, aerosolized gentamicin may cause marked bronchospasm in susceptible patients, probably as a nonspecific response to irritant effects of the drug vehicle.[71a]

Streptomycin was formerly used by some workers in the aerosol therapy of tuberculosis. However, this form of administration is not credited at the present time, and it is no longer advocated, although streptomycin remains a major antituberculosis drug when given by intramuscular injection. A further disadvantage with this antibiotic is that resistance is built up by susceptible organisms quite rapidly when the drug is used alone.

Aminoglycoside Preparations. The aminoglycosides are potent and toxic drugs, and are used only in hospitalized patients with serious infections. New aminoglycosides are introduced periodically, and some of the older ones have become less useful as a result.

GENTAMICIN. Gentamicin is currently the most important antibiotic in this group. It is suitable for both intramuscular and intravenous administration; topical dermatologic preparations are available as creams and ointments, and the parenteral prepara-

tion of the drug can be used topically in aerosol therapy. For very serious infections, a dose of 5 mg/kg a day is used, but 3 mg/kg suffices for infections that are not life threatening. In less serious infections, and for urinary tract infections, a total daily dose of 1 mg/kg is usually employed. It is of interest that the serum level achieved is related to the hematocrit, and if this is below 30 per cent, the 1 mg/kg dosage is likely to produce a serum level similar to that achieved with a 5 mg/kg dosage in patients with a hematocrit over 45 per cent.

KANAMYCIN. Kanamycin is an older agent, and is now of waning interest. The drug is best suited for intramuscular use; the intravenous route is used only in seriously ill patients. It is more toxic than gentamicin, and can cause severe deafness, particularly if given in excessive dosage to a patient with renal insufficiency. Since it has a narrower spectrum of activity than gentamicin, kanamycin is rarely the drug of choice. However, it may be reasonable to reserve this aminoglycoside for aerosolization in appropriate cases, and an extension of existing studies on this use of the drug would be justified.

TOBRAMYCIN. Tobramycin is similar to gentamicin, but it is more effective against some strains of *P. aeruginosa.* It can be given by the intramuscular or intravenous route, and the dosage ranges used are similar to those for gentamicin. The drug should be used when bacterial sensitivity studies suggest that it would be more effective than gentamicin.[72]

AMIKACIN. This new agent is similar to gentamicin, and it should be used for the treatment of those gram-negative organisms that are found to be more susceptible to it: occasional organisms remain sensitive to amikacin when they are resistant to the other aminoglycosides.[72] The drug is given both by the intramuscular and intravenous routes; the dosage is similar to that for kanamycin, and is larger than that for gentamicin or tobramycin. It appears that amikacin is comparable to gentamicin in both effectiveness and toxicity, and parenteral administration is successful in the treatment of gram-negative pulmonary infections.[73]

NETILMICIN. Netilmicin is an investigational drug, which will probably be marketed as an additional alternative to gentamicin.[72] Similar agents, such as sisomicin, can also be expected in the next few years.

NEOMYCIN. Neomycin is the most toxic aminoglycoside, and it is used only topically.

It is available as creams and ointments, while oral tablets are used for sterilizing the bowel. The powder preparation that is marketed can be dissolved in saline for use as an aerosol.

STREPTOMYCIN. Streptomycin is used mainly in the treatment of tuberculosis, but it is also of value in the therapy of pneumonic and bubonic plague, and for tularemia. It is occasionally used with penicillin in the treatment of some pneumonias (for example, those caused by *H. influenzae* or *K. pneumoniae*), and the combination is the treatment of choice for enterococcal endocarditis. Although streptomycin has been used as an aerosol drug, there are no current indications for this, and since the topical drug can induce hypersensitivity, aerosolization has been virtually abandoned.

Adverse Effects of Aminoglycosides. These toxic drugs are especially damaging to the ear and the kidney. Otic damage may be predominantly auditory (for example, from neomycin, kanamycin) or vestibular (for example, from streptomycin), but hearing loss, tinnitus, and impaired balance can all occur as an outcome of the use of any of these agents. Other major toxic side effects are less common, but include hypersensitivity, blood cell element damage, and mild hepatitis. Of more interest and significance is that the aminoglycosides can cause neuromuscular blockade resulting in paralysis, which may seriously impair breathing and may even result in apnea.[74, 75] The mechanism underlying this phenomenon differs from that of curare, and it appears to be caused by competitive blockade. Kanamycin, however, may resemble the polymyxins and cause a noncompetitive blockade. The effect of the aminoglycosides is usually intensified when a patient is receiving a concomitant general anesthetic or a mus-

cle relaxing agent, and postoperative respiratory failure can then occur. The block is sometimes reversed by giving adequate amounts of an intravenous calcium preparation (such as 200 mg of 10 per cent calcium gluconate); in other cases, the intravenous administration of neostigmine (1 mg) or edrophonium (1–10 mg) may be effective. In addition to the aminoglycosides, a similar neuromuscular phenomenon may occur with bacitracin, the polymyxins, the tetracyclines[74] and clindamycin. For further discussion of neuromuscular block, see Chapter 11.

Polymyxins
(Table 10–13)

The polymyxin antibiotics are polypeptides, and they have some relationship to the aminoglycosides. The only important agents in this class are polymyxin B and polymyxin E (colistin and colistimethate). Although they have spectrums of antibacterial activity similar to that of gentamicin, they are less effective in practice, and they have fallen into virtual disuse for parenteral therapy. However, they are of value as topical agents, and they have been used successfully as respiratory aerosols.[76-78]

Polymyxin B has been the subject of the most study, and, as was explained earlier in this chapter, aerosolization has been particularly useful for eliminating *Pseudomonas* and other gram-negative bacteria that colonize the respiratory tract.[14] The main disadvantage of polymyxin is that it can increase airway resistance, and it may result in severe bronchospasm in susceptible subjects,[17] probably as a result of histamine release. Colistimethate and colistin are similar to polymyxin B, but are less irritating and do

TABLE 10–13. THE POLYPEPTIDE ANTIBIOTICS

Preparation	ORAL	Route I.M.	I.V.	TOPICAL	Usual Daily Dosage for Adults†	Comment
POLYMYXIN E						
Colistimethate sodium (Coly-Mycin M)		+	+		2.5–5 mg/kg	For parenteral therapy; less toxic than polymyxin B.
Colistin sulfate (Coly-Mycin S)	+			+	3–5 mg/kg	Used in topical therapy for bowel infections; it is only slightly absorbed. This preparation may be more suitable for nebulization therapy.
POLYMYXIN B						
Polymyxin B sulfate (Aerosporin)		+	+	+	1.5–2.5 mg/kg	More painful than colistimethate on I.M. injection.
BACITRACIN				+	See Table 10–4	Too toxic for parenteral use, but well tolerated when given topically.

†Usually given in 3 divided doses.

not appear to release histamine,[76] although some patients tolerate them poorly.[56] Although few comparative studies have been carried out, it is probable that one of these forms of polymyxin E would be preferable to polymyxin B in aerosol therapy. Colistimethate has been reported on favorably for the aerosol suppression of gram-negative colonization in the lungs.[76, 78]

Polymyxin Preparations

At present, the polymyxins are of declining importance, and only a few antibiotics in this class are available.

POLYMYXIN B. Polymyxin B is available as a topical dermatologic and ophthalmic antibiotic, and it is marketed for intramuscular and intravenous use. The intramuscular injection of this drug can produce a relatively long-lasting muscle pain; therefore, polymyxin B should not be given by this route. A solution of the powder in saline (1–10 mg/ml) can be used for aerosolization.

POLYMYXIN E. Two preparations are available. *Colistimethate* is the sulfomethyl derivative of colistin, and its sodium salt may be given intramuscularly or intravenously. The intramuscular preparation does not cause pain, and is therefore preferable to polymyxin B. *Colistin,* as the sulfate, is used as an oral preparation for the topical treatment of bacterial enteritis.

The high molecular weight of colistimethate (about 1750) suggests that this drug would penetrate well into the respiratory mucosa. However, there is little experimental data to suggest that this drug has any particular value in the treatment of respiratory infections. Nevertheless, since the drug is relatively well tolerated on administration and has no more serious toxicity than gentamicin when used in appropriate dosage, colistimethate may be a reasonable alternative to the aminoglycosides for parenteral therapy of gram-negative pulmonary infections. Colistimethate aerosol can eradicate colonizing gram-negative organisms; the drug is well tolerated and not absorbed.[76, 78] The aerosol is safer than that of polymyxin, and it should probably replace the latter drug.

BACITRACIN. Bacitracin is also a polymyxin. This agent was formerly a useful antibiotic for the treatment of penicillin-resistant staphylococci. It has a high molecular weight (1400), and it has been used as an aerosol, as well as a topical dermatologic and mucosal antibiotic; it is too nephrotoxic for parenteral use. It is effective against gram-positive cocci and *Clostridia,* but unlike the other polymyxins, it is not effective against gram-negative bacteria. The drug currently is not readily available for aerosol use, and thus it can no longer be regarded as a respiratory drug.

Adverse Effects of Polymyxins. Although the polymyxins resemble the aminoglycosides in their nephrotoxicity, and in their property of causing neuromuscular blockade, they do not have ototoxic side effects. Furthermore, the nephrotoxicity can usually be detected early enough (by urine analysis, and from blood urea or creatinine determinations) to enable administration of the drug to be discontinued and thereby allow full renal recovery. Polymyxin is more toxic than colistimethate, and it should be abandoned as a parenteral drug.

It should be recognized that colistimethate is much less nephrotoxic than polymyxin B. The other toxic effects of colistimethate are annoying or even hazardous, but they are not permanent. Such effects include the neurotoxic symptoms of irritability, drowsiness, circumoral paresthesias, numbness of the extremities, peripheral neuropathy and blurring of vision. Neuromuscular block, clinically similar to that of the aminoglycosides, may occur, particularly in the presence of muscle-relaxing agents; this serious effect may be reversed by calcium, whereas neostigmine and edrophonium may be ineffective.[79] It is of interest that polymyxin B is the most potent antibiotic neuroblocking agent.[80] When used carefully with avoidance of excessive dosage colistimethate is a potent, useful drug that can be relatively safe, and it is therefore still worth consideration as an alternative to the aminoglycosides. Greater safety may be attained by basing the dose of the drug on the surface area or the square root of the body weight of the patient.[81]

Macrolides
(Table 10–14)

The macrolide antibiotics are structurally based on a lactone ring; they have relatively large molecular weights and appear to distribute well into organs such as the lungs. They are usually considered to be less effective in the treatment of most serious infections caused by susceptible bacteria, and they are primarily regarded as alternatives to penicillins.

The erythromycins are the main macrolide antibiotics. These agents are effective

TABLE 10–14. THE MACROLIDES

Preparation	Route ORAL	I.M.	I.V.	RECTAL	Comments
ERYTHROMYCINS*					
Erythromycin (base) (E-mycin, Erythrocin, Ilotycin, Robimycin, RP-Mycin)	+			+	Standard preparation; usually well tolerated; active against most gram-positive bacteria, *H. influenzae* and *Mycoplasma*
Erythromycin estolate (Ilosone)	+				This preparation is the best absorbed when given orally. It can cause a hypersensitivity cholestatic jaundice after 10 days' administration; potentiates glucocorticoids in asthma
Erythromycin ethylsuccinate (E.E.S., Erythrocin, Pediamycin)	+	+			Parenteral form may be useful for systemic therapy
Erythromycin gluceptate (Ilotycin gluceptate)			+		Parenteral product, rarely used
Erythromycin lactobionate (Erythrocin Lactobionate)			+		Parenteral product, rarely used
Erythromycin stearate (Bristamycin, Erypar, Ethril, Pfizer-E, SK-Erythromycin)	+				Similar to erythromycin
TROLEANDOMYCIN†					
Triacetyloleandomycin (TAO)	+				Similar to the erythromycins; rarely used now; potentiates glucocorticoids in asthma; the drug can be hepatotoxic

*Usual dose of the erythromycins is 1–4 gm. per day, in divided doses, in adults.
†Usual dose of TAO is 1–2 gm per day, in divided doses, in adults.

against most gram-positive bacteria, *H. influenzae* and many anaerobes; furthermore, they are active against *Mycoplasma*. They are therefore often of value in the treatment of pneumonias of differing etiologies, including the atypical pneumonia caused by *Mycoplasma pneumoniae* (the PPLO or Eaton agent). Aerosolized erythromycin was formerly one of the agents used by some workers for the treatment of bronchitis, but it is no longer in favor.[82] Various preparations of erythromycin have been synthesized, but most of them are poorly absorbed when given by mouth. The value of the oral, and perhaps even the parenteral, erythromycins should be given greater recognition than has been customary; they are undoubtedly very useful for treating pulmonary infections.

The other major macrolides are the oleandomycins, of which only troleandomycin is currently used. This oral agent is similar to erythromycin in its spectrum of activity, but it is less potent and more toxic, and is therefore rarely used.

ERYTHROMYCINS. Of the many erythromycin derivatives, the most interesting is *erythromycin estolate*. This is the only derivative that is well absorbed when given by mouth, particularly if given before meals. It is of special value in the treatment of susceptible infections in asthmatic patients on steroid therapy, because the estolate appears to interfere with glucocorticoid metabolism, thereby potentiating the steroid effect (see Chapter 4). Unfortunately, patients may develop a hypersensitivity to this drug, resulting in a cholestatic jaundice. However, this serious side effect is uncommon, and has appeared mainly in patients who have received the drug for more than 10 days, or who have had repeated courses within a few months.

The other erythromycin preparations are less effective when given by mouth, and most of them are used only for parenteral administration. Since they are rarely regarded as first-line drugs, the injectable derivatives of erythromycin are not often used in practice. However, they are valuable alternatives to the parenteral tetracyclines for the treatment of *Mycoplasma* pneumonia in a severely ill patient who cannot tolerate oral medications.

TROLEANDOMYCIN. Troleandomycin is similar to erythromycin estolate: it is given by mouth, it potentiates the effect of glucocorticoids in asthma,[32] and it is hepatotoxic.

Adverse Effects of Macrolides. The erythromycins rarely cause serious side effects, other than the hypersensitivity jaundice associated with the estolate. The estolate may also cause right upper quadrant abdominal discomfort or colic without the condition necessarily progressing to jaundice. The other derivatives may also cause abdominal discomfort, but nausea, vomiting and diarrhea are more usual manifestations, and these occur particularly after large doses. Troleandomycin causes similar problems, and also causes a toxic, reversible hepatitis, and is more likely to cause anaphylactic reactions.

In general, the macrolide of choice is oral erythromycin base, since this is well tolerated and effective. The estolate may be given if more assured absorption is of particular importance, or for the treatment of infection in an asthmatic. The intramuscular erythromycins are rarely used, because they can be very painful on injection. The intravenous preparations are more acceptable but should be administered slowly, to avoid causing irritation of the vein.

Lincomycins
(Table 10–15)

There are two antibiotics in this group: *lincomycin,* which is now obsolete, and its more recent derivative, *clindamycin,* which is similar but more potent. Currently, clindamycin is regarded as an alternative to penicillin for the treatment of gram-positive infections, although some strains of *Staphylococcus* are resistant to it. The lincomycins are extremely effective against almost all anaerobic bacteria, including *Bacteroides fragilis,* which is notably resistant to penicillin, but they are not effective against gram-negative organisms.

CLINDAMYCIN. Clindamycin is available for oral, intramuscular and intravenous administration; the intramuscular injection can be painful and intravenous infusion may result in phlebitis. It does not appear to have been given as an aerosol, or by instillation into an infected site. Such methods of administration are not justified, however, since the drug crosses the blood-bronchial barrier adequately.[26]

Clindamycin is one of the major drugs of value in the therapy of aspiration pneumonia, lung abscess and empyema when these conditions are caused by mixed oropharyngeal flora or by specific anaerobes.[38]

LINCOMYCIN. Lincomycin is also available for oral, intramuscular and intravenous administration; it is less painful than clindamycin on injection. Larger doses of this less potent agent are required, and it offers no therapeutic advantages over clindamycin.

Adverse Effects of Lincomycins. These agents cause only occasional rashes and rarely result in hypersensitivity reactions. However, cholestatic jaundice may occasionally occur. Other uncommon side effects include leucopenia, purpura, eosinophilia, dizziness, headache and myalgia. Rapid intravenous injection, particularly of lincomycin, can cause hypotension, cardiac arrhythmias, and even cardiac arrest. Clindamycin can cause neuromuscular blockade, and should be given with care in the presence of other neuromuscular blocking agents such as the aminoglycosides.

The most disturbing side effect caused by these drugs is diarrhea, which, in the case of clindamycin, may progress to a severe pseudomembranous colitis that can be fatal. If diarrhea develops, immediate cessation of antibiotic therapy may result in improvement. There is some evidence that established colitis may respond to the drug cholestyramine.[83] As many as 21 per cent of patients receiving clindamycin manifest diarrhea and may show evidence of colitis. Since fatal complications may ensue, particularly in debilitated adults, clindamycin has to be regarded as a potentially hazardous drug. A further serious disadvantage of this useful antibiotic is that it is relatively expensive.

Chloramphenicol
(Table 10–16)

This antibiotic is effective against a large spectrum of gram-positive and gram-negative bacteria, and is the specific agent for treating serious *Salmonella* infections. It is extremely potent against anaerobic bacteria, particularly the *Bacteroides* species. The drug diffuses well into the lungs, and can be of value in the treatment of aspiration pneumonias, lung abscess and empyema resulting from mixed oropharyngeal flora or from anaerobes. It is also effective in bronchitis and some other specific respiratory infections, but it is not active against *Pseudomonas.* Chloramphenicol is a valuable alternative to ampicillin for the treatment of *H. influenzae* infections.

The oral preparation is generally used, since it is absorbed well. Administration by the intramuscular route causes pain and comparatively poor serum levels; therefore, the drug is rarely given by this means. Chloramphenicol can be given intravenously, but this route is not commonly employed. Although topical dermatologic and mucosal preparations are available, the drug is not favored for aerosolization or instillation into the lungs.

Adverse Effects. The main disadvantage of chloramphenicol is that it can cause an

TABLE 10–15.   THE LINCOMYCINS

Preparation	ORAL	Routes I.M.	I.V.	Usual Adult Dose	Comments
Lincomycin (Lincocin)	+			500–750 mg q.i.d.	Virtually succeeded by
		+	+	600–1000 mg q. 6–12 h.	clindamycin, which is more potent
Clindamycin (Cleocin)	+			150–450 mg q.i.d.	Effective against most
		+	+	300–1200 mg q. 6–8 h.	*Staphylococcus* species and anaerobes, and some gram-negative infections; may cause a severe enterocolitis

TABLE 10–16.   CHLORAMPHENICOL

BRAND NAMES	Chloromycetin, Amphicol, Mychel
ANTIBACTERIAL SPECTRUM	1. Most gram-positive bacteria 2. Most gram-negative bacteria except *Pseudomonas;* very effective against *H. influenzae* and *Salmonella* species 3. Most anaerobic bacteria

TOXIC EFFECTS	1. Hematologic — include:
	  (a) Dose-dependent anemia
	  (b) Hypersensitivity aplastic anemia/agranulocytosis
	  (c) Hemolysis in G-6-PD deficient patients
	2. Neonatal "gray-baby" syndrome
	3. Gastrointestinal disturbances
	4. Optic neuritis, peripheral neuropathy, encephalopathy

PRECAUTIONS	1. Do not use unnecessarily 2. Avoid giving over 20 gm during a course, if possible 3. Monitor peripheral blood, and serum iron and iron-binding capacity
ADULT DOSAGE	250–500 mg qid P.O., I.V. (use up to 50 mg/kg/day maximum for few days)

idiosyncratic or hypersensitivity depression of the marrow, resulting in agranulocytosis or aplastic anemia. These complications can be fatal, but fortunately they are rare, and although chloramphenicol has acquired a sinister reputation, other antibiotics such as clindamycin may be associated with a comparable or higher incidence of fatal complications.[84] In distinction to the idiosyncratic effect on the marrow, chloramphenicol universally causes a dose-dependent hematopoietic depression, and a course of about 20 gm of the drug can result in anemia with characteristic vacuolation of red and white cells. The two hematologic dangers described necessitate caution in using chloramphenicol, and a course of therapy should rarely be permitted to exceed two weeks. Every few days a peripheral blood examination should be carried out, and an elevation in serum iron can be looked for in suspicious cases, since this may be an early sign of marrow depression. The development of a sore throat may presage the appearance of agranulocytosis.

Another serious complication of chloramphenicol is seen in neonates, who may develop a dose-related shock-like state ("gray-baby syndrome"). Allergic rashes may occur, but serious anaphylactic reactions are rare. Gastrointestinal disorders may be induced, and mild headache, fever, depression or confusion can appear. Rarely, optic neuritis with papilledema and peripheral neuropathy appear as complications. The drug is excreted by the liver, and the presence of hepatic disease predisposes the patient to toxic complications.

Since chloramphenicol has the potential for so many complications, some of which are life threatening or inevitably fatal, the drug cannot be regarded as a first-line agent. However, it is a valuable secondary choice in appropriate circumstances, and its retention as a general antibiotic is justified as long as it is utilized cautiously and knowledgeably.

Vancomycin

This toxic drug has a spectrum similar to that of penicillin against aerobic gram-positive organisms. It is essentially reserved for use in the patient allergic to penicillin, or for treatment of those few species of *Staphylococcus* that are resistant to both penicillin and the penicillinase-resistant penicillins; it is also a useful agent for the management of staphylococcal shunt infections in patients on hemodialysis.

The drug is generally administered by the intravenous route; the usual adult dose is 1 gm twice a day. It can be given orally to treat staphylococcal enteritis; it is absorbed unreliably, and the oral route is unsatisfactory for therapy of respiratory infections. Intravenous administration readily achieves an adequate serum level.

The major toxic effects of vancomycin are similar to those of kanamycin; the drug is nephrotoxic, and it is ototoxic. Chills, fever, rashes and anaphylaxis are not rare. A practical disadvantage of the drug is its tendency to cause thrombophlebitis. All these considerations suggest that vancomycin may best be reserved for aerosol use in the management of respiratory infections; however, there is little recent experience on this potentially valuable use of the drug (see Table 10–4).

Sulfonamides
(Table 10–17)

The sulfonamides are considered to be synthetic chemotherapeutic agents, distinct from the naturally occurring antibiotics and similar agents that can be synthesized. The chemotherapeutic era was initiated by the introduction of the sulfonamides in the 1930s, and although these drugs have had a diminishing role in therapeutics, they are still of value. A major advantage of the sulfonamides is that they are very inexpensive, and they are valued in countries the economies of which are not able to welcome each new high-costing antibiotic.

At present, less than 30 sulfonamides are used therapeutically, and in practice each physician need be familiar only with three or four of them. The various preparations have different lengths of action, and they can be classified as short-acting, intermediate-acting, long-acting, ultra–long-acting, and topical agents.[85, 86] Although they are mainly used for the treatment of urinary tract infections, they are also of value in the management of otitis, tonsillitis, pharyngitis and bronchitis. The sulfonamides can reach relatively high concentrations in the sputum, for example, 3.76 mcg/ml.[26]

The sulfonamides are effective for the treatment of respiratory infections caused by streptococci, the pneumococcus and *H. influenzae,* but they are not so effective for conditions in which anaerobes are involved.

TABLE 10–17. IMPORTANT SULFONAMIDES

Preparation	Usual Daily Dosage For Adults	Comments
Sulfadiazine	0.5–1 gm q6h P.O.; 30–50 mg/kg q6h I.V.	Short-acting; relatively insoluble
Sulfisoxazole (Gantrisin, Soxomide)	1–2 gm q6h P.O.; 1–2 gm q6h I.V., S.C.	Short-acting; safest sulfonamide; mainly used for urinary tract infections
Sulfamethoxazole (Gantanol)	1 gm 2–3 times/day P.O.	Medium-acting; similar to sulfisoxazole
Sulfamethoxazole 400 mg + Trimethoprim 80 mg (Bactrim, Septra) — per tablet or 10 ml	2 tablets or 20 ml; 2–3 times/day P.O.	Combination is very effective in bronchitis, and has been used in the treatment of *Pneumocystis* infections

Although the sulfonamides are inferior to the commonly used antibiotics, their usefulness has recently been extended by the addition of the antimetabolic agent *trimethoprim.* This agent results in a synergistic enhancement of sulfonamide activity, and the combination is very effective in the treatment of acute and chronic bronchitis, and is also of value in the therapy of nocardiosis.

The sulfonamides have been given by nebulization in the past, but there is no evidence that they are currently used in this fashion. Another declining use for these agents is as secondary choices for the treatment of South American blastomycosis and histoplasmosis; they can also be used in combination with pyrimethamine for the treatment of *Pneumocystis carinii* infection.

Major Sulfonamide Preparations. *Sulfadiazine* and *sulfisoxazole* are the short-acting preparations that are most useful for the treatment of respiratory tract infections.

Sulfamethoxazole is an intermediate-acting agent that is also of value; currently, this sulfonamide has been selected for marketing in combination with trimethoprim (as Bactrim and Septra). The combination preparation may well become a selection of choice for the treatment of bronchitis and for infectious exacerbations of chronic obstructive pulmonary disease.[87, 88]

Adverse Effects of the Sulfonamides. Unfortunately, the sulfonamides may cause numerous side effects, some of which are dangerous. However, the three agents discussed above are safer than the many other preparations. Anorexia, nausea and vomiting are relatively common, and various rashes are even more frequent, occurring in 5 to 10 per cent of patients; rashes may be caused by photosensitivity and patients should be cautioned to avoid undue exposure to the sun. Fever may occur in 3 per cent of patients,

but other hypersensitivity reactions are less common; however, they include pulmonary infiltrates with eosinophilia, and asthma. Bone marrow depression, hemolytic anemia and other hematologic side effects must be watched for. Neurologic complications include headaches, lassitude, depression, ataxia, convulsions, psychosis and peripheral neuropathy; these unpleasant reactions are, fortunately, very uncommon. Patients should be instructed to ingest a large amount of fluid, since crystallization of sulfonamides can occur in the urinary tract of a dehydrated patient, particularly if the urine is acid. Hypersensitivity renal complications are additional rare side effects.

Trimethoprim has pharmacokinetic properties and side effects similar to those of sulfamethoxazole, the drug with which it is combined. An additional problem with trimethoprim is that prolonged administration may cause folate deficiency, and this could theoretically produce teratogenic effects in a pregnant woman. The combination sulfamethoxazole-trimethoprim is known as cotrimoxazole in many countries.

Antituberculosis Drugs
(Table 10–18)

The first important antituberculosis drug to be discovered was streptomycin in 1944. Soon afterwards, para-aminosalicylic acid was introduced, whereas isoniazid (INH) did not become available until 1954. Since that time many other agents have been discovered, but only two other agents have proved to be major antituberculosis drugs—first, ethambutol in 1961, and, most recently, rifampin (1966). In the early days of the chemotherapy of tuberculosis, it was found that during the treatment of a patient with

TABLE 10–18.   DRUGS USED IN THE TREATMENT OF TUBERCULOSIS

Agent	Total Daily Dosage (mg/kg)	Number of Divided Doses a Day	Usual Adult Daily Dose	Route		Major Toxic Effects			Other Possible Toxicity
				ORAL	I.M.	LIVER	KIDNEY	EAR	
FIRST-LINE DRUGS									
Isoniazid (INH) (Hyzyd, Niconyl, Nydrazid)	5–10	1	300 mg	+	(+)	+			Peripheral neuritis, severe hepatitis, restlessness, psychosis, hypersensitivity (e.g., rashes, arteritis, systemic lupus erythematosus), anemia, vitamin B_6 (pyridoxine) deficiency
Ethambutol (Myambutol)	15(–25)	1	1.1 gm	+					Optic neuritis, peripheral neuritis, allergy, nausea, confusion, gout
Rifampin (Rifadin, Rimactane)	10–20	1	600 mg	+		+	(+)		Hypersensitivity, hemolysis, purpura, red urine, leucopenia, decreased effect of oral anticoagulants
Streptomycin	15–20	1	1 gm (max.)*		+		+	+	Rashes, fever, paresthesias, hypersensitivity, neuromuscular blockade, optic neuritis
SECOND-LINE DRUGS									
Pyrazinamide (Pyrazinamide)	15–30	3–4	2 gm	+		+			Fever, hyperuricemia, gout, photosensitivity
Ethionamide (Trecator)	10–30	3–4	1 gm (max.)	+		+			Anorexia, nausea, hypersensitivity, peripheral neuropathy, optic neuritis, skin rashes, gynecomastia, hypothyroidism
Cycloserine (Seromycin)	10–20	3–4	1 gm	+			+		Psychosis, convulsions, depression, malabsorption, rash, peripheral neuropathy
Capreomycin (Capastat)	15–30	1	1 gm (max.)*		+		+	+	Hypokalemia, allergy, neuromuscular blockade
Viomycin (Viocin)	15–30	1	500 mg*		+		+	+	Electrolyte imbalance, neuromuscular blockade; more toxic than capreomycin
Para-aminosalicylic acid (PAS) (Pamisyl, Parasal, Rezipas)	150–200	3–4	10–12 gm	+		+			Nausea, vomiting, malabsorption, hypokalemia, acidosis, goiter, hypersensitivity, rashes, jaundice, vasculitis
Kanamycin (Kantrex)	15–30	1–2	1 gm (max.)*		+		+	+	Neuromuscular blockade, rash, fever, peripheral neuritis

*The parenteral drugs are usually given in a dosage of 1 gm 2 to 4 times a week; smaller daily doses could be given.

active disease, the causative organism *Mycobacterium tuberculosis* rapidly developed resistance if only one agent was used; as a result of this finding, double drug therapy soon became established. In more advanced cases, such as cavitary pulmonary tuberculosis, experience revealed that the addition of a third drug for at least the first few weeks of therapy resulted in a more favorable outcome. The mycobacterium grows very slowly: it probably divides not more than once a day, whereas most pyogenic organisms replicate themselves over 40 times a day. In similar fashion, the bacteriology laboratory can grow out most pathogenic bacteria within one day, whereas most pathogenic mycobacteria take about 40 times as long to produce identifiable growth. These findings can be translated into practical therapeutics: the antibiotic therapy of most uncomplicated pneumonias is accomplished in one to two weeks, whereas the complete treatment of active tuberculosis requires one to two years. These traditional concepts have undergone modification in the last decade, since careful trials have shown that shorter courses for six to nine months often suffice for the treatment of uncomplicated tuberculosis. The addition of rifampin to the armamentarium has been of added benefit, because this drug helps bring about more rapid control of the infection.

The essence of good therapy in tuberculosis is to use the appropriate drugs for a prolonged period without any improper interruptions in their administration.[89] However, good results can be obtained with intermittent therapy using large doses of drugs twice a week; this form of treatment is of value for unreliable outpatients who can readily be given their twice weekly medications under supervision. Some details of the various regimens that can be used were discussed earlier, and the options available are presented in Table 10–7.

The treatment of a new case of tuberculosis is relatively straightforward, whereas management failures, relapses and new patients with unreliable past drug exposure can present formidable challenges.[89] The selection of the initial drug regimen in such patients should be based on the concept of overtreatment rather than allowing the possibility of inadequate drug coverage; rifampin often occupies a cornerstone in such retreatment schedules. The onset of drug intolerance or allergy when using the more toxic second-line agents may also tax the ingenuity of the physician, and considerable familiarity with the pharmacology and therapeutics of tuberculosis is required for a successful outcome in these challenging situations. Similar difficulties and therapeutic requirements are common to the atypical mycobacterial diseases.

First-Line Antituberculosis Drugs (Table 10–18). At present, isoniazid, ethambutol, rifampin and streptomycin are regarded as the most potent and effective agents; one or more of these drugs are utilized in the management of virtually every case of tuberculosis or atypical mycobacterial disease.

ISONIAZID (INH). This agent is the hydrazide of isonicotinic acid; it is a relatively simple molecule with a molecular weight of only 137. Apart from its spectacular antimycobacterial properties, it has no other antimicrobial actions or additional therapeutic values. The drug is usually administered as a single daily dose by mouth, either in tablet form or as a syrup; an intramuscular preparation containing 100 mg/ml is available.

The drug is well absorbed following oral administration, and it has a variable half life, which is dependent on a patient's genetically determined metabolic phenotype.[90] Isoniazid is primarily metabolized by acetylation to acetylisoniazid; other metabolites include acetylhydrazine, hydrazones and isonicotinic acid. These enzymic conversions occur mainly in the liver, with the amount of available enzyme, acetylase, being genetically determined; accordingly, acetylation is slow in autosomal homozygous recessives, and rapid in either homozygous dominants or heterozygotes. Generous inherent endowments of hepatic acetylase are more common among Eskimo and Asiatic people, with over 90 per cent of such populations being capable of rapid acetylation of INH. In European and American populations, only about 50 per cent of people are rapid inactivators.[55] Children and diabetics are often found to be more rapid acetylators than are normal adults of the same population. The slow acetylators are likely to become noninfectious on INH therapy sooner than are rapid acetylators, since the former maintain therapeutic levels of the active drug for a longer period each day. However, these differences have not been found to be of practical importance with regard to either the total dosage or the method of timing each dose for individual patients or different racial groups.

Although slow acetylation may offer a

therapeutic advantage, it also renders the patient more susceptible to side effects that are dose dependent. The most important of such problems are neurologic, including peripheral neuropathy.[91] This is the most serious of the more common complications, and it can occur in up to 2 per cent of all patients taking INH. The syndrome is more likely to appear in malnourished or alcoholic patients, or in individuals with underlying neurologic disease. Symptoms may first appear within a few weeks of starting therapy, and pyridoxine 10 to 20 mg daily can be given to prevent this complication in susceptible individuals; higher doses of pyridoxine may be required to treat the established disease, which may only partially respond, even with months of therapy.

Acute overdosage of INH can cause coma, seizures, hyperpyrexia and hyperglycemia. Lactic acidosis may also occur following excessive dosage.[92] Other complications associated with drug excess, particularly in slow acetylators, include pellagra-like symptoms, central nervous system overstimulation or depression, and psychosis. However, it should be borne in mind that many of these symptoms were originally reported in sick patients confined to sanitaria, and it is probable that INH has been unfairly blamed for a number of complications that were actually caused by other factors.

One of the most troublesome problems with INH is the potential of the drug to cause hepatic damage.[90] Many patients develop abnormalities of liver function while taking INH, but these are transitory, and intervention is not required. However, in some cases a syndrome similar to viral hepatitis appears, which may be ushered in by malaise and abdominal discomfort, following which jaundice appears; in a minority of cases progressive liver damage follows, which can be fatal. Although this syndrome had been thought to be a hypersensitivity response, it is not accompanied by serologic markers of allergy, and therefore it is more likely to be a toxic reaction in susceptible patients. There is evidence that the hepatotoxin is derived from acetylated INH, and in keeping with this is the finding that INH-induced hepatitis is more common in rapid acetylators. The hepatocellular damage may appear anytime during the first year of INH therapy, but it occurs most frequently in the first three months. Individuals under the age of 20 are rarely affected, but the complication becomes more frequent in patients over the

age of 35. The problem is most common in the elderly, and alcoholism or preexisting liver disease predisposes the patient to hepatitis; in alcoholic patients over the age of 50, there may be an incidence of hepatitis in excess of 2.3 per cent. In general, INH-hepatitis need not be actively sought, but all patients should be warned to report any untoward symptoms that may suggest the onset of this complication; early withdrawal of the drug is usually associated with a favorable outcome, although the problem of managing the patient's tuberculosis without the benefit of INH then has to be met.

True hypersensitivity to INH does occur occasionally;[91] reactions include fever, rashes, hematologic reactions, vasculitis, lupus erythematosus or the appearance of L. E. cells in the blood. A specific problem with INH therapy may be encountered in epileptic patients, because INH is an inhibitor of phenytoin (Dilantin) metabolism, and the dosage of this drug has to be reduced to prevent phenytoin intoxication. This problem is more common in slow acetylators. Isoniazid can induce an anemia, the mechanism of which is not entirely explained, which responds to pyridoxine therapy. Although some physicians routinely administer pyridoxine with INH, this is unnecessary. In general, pyridoxine (vitamin B_6) should be given in a dose of 10 mg per 100 mg INH per day only to those patients at particular risk of developing neurologic complications or to patients on high doses of INH, while twice this dosage, or even more, of the vitamin can be given to treat established neuropathy or anemia.

Although serious INH-induced toxicity is not too common, occurring in less than 5 per cent of all patients on doses of 10 mg/kg or less, it is still a sufficient enough threat to necessitate restraint in the use of this drug. More stringent criteria should be adopted in the prophylactic use of the drug in patients with minimal or suspected tuberculosis. Until recently, it was common to give a year's course of INH to any patient who had undergone conversion of the tuberculin skin test, but, at present, treatment is not advised for older converters or for those with liver disease. There is less risk in using INH prophylaxis in healthy patients under the age of 35, and no serious risk for teenagers and children; thus, less stringent criteria for giving INH are adopted in these patients, particularly since INH is very well tolerated in most children even when given in relatively large doses. There is still some controversy as to whether INH should be given to patients with either old tuberculosis or a positive tuberculin skin test when they develop an additional risk factor such as a malignancy, unstable diabetes, gastrectomy or silicosis, or when they are started on a course of immunosuppressive or glucocorticoid therapy. The best approach for the physician is to judge each situation as a unique problem, and to balance the patient's risk of INH complications against risks to the individual and community incurred by withholding treatment. When in doubt, the essential requirement is to keep the patient under frequent surveillance, whether INH is utilized or not.

ETHAMBUTOL (EMB). Ethambutol is a potent and generally well tolerated drug with few side effects. The most serious problem is optic nerve damage, which is initially manifested by loss of red-green color vision discrimination; if drug therapy is not discontinued, this can proceed to optic atrophy with loss of visual acuity and eventual loss of vision. These severe complications arise only if larger doses of the drug are given, or if excretion of the drug is impaired as a consequence of renal insufficiency. When the drug was first introduced, it was advised that EMB be given in a daily dosage of 25 mg/kg for the first few weeks, and then reduced to 15 mg/kg a day. More recently, the recommendations have been to administer the lower dosage from the start; as a result, optic complications and other side effects have been largely eliminated. It may be advisable to use the higher dose in some retreatment schedules, and such patients should be carefully monitored for visual problems, and for other possible side effects, which include skin rashes, fever, dizziness, hallucinations, gastrointestinal disturbances and gout. Although the FDA has not permitted EMB to be recommended for the treatment of children under 13 years of age, there is little to suggest that it cannot be given equally safely in young children, but monitoring for color vision and visual acuity changes is difficult; thus, there may be an increased risk in such patients.

Ethambutol can be used alone in the treatment of minimal disease when INH is contraindicated, but, in general, it should be utilized only in combination therapy. The drug has no value other than its antituberculosis properties. Ethambutol is made available only as 100 mg and 400 mg tablets.

RIFAMPIN. This agent is an antibiotic that inhibits most gram-positive bacteria and many gram-negative organisms, including *Pseudomonas.* It has been found to be very effective in meningococcal meningitis, and it can eliminate *Neisseria meningitidis* from carriers. The drug is also effective against some viruses, and it may potentiate the antifungal effect of amphotericin B. However, the only important use for this versatile antibiotic is the treatment of tuberculosis.

Rifampin is available only as 300 mg capsules; combinations of preparations of rifampin and INH are marketed also (Rifamate, Rimactazid), but these preparations are probably best avoided. Rifampin is reasonably well tolerated by most patients, but it can cause a number of serious side effects. A major problem is hepatotoxicity, which can present a diagnostic and management dilemma in patients who are taking concomitant INH and other hepatotoxic drugs. Rifampin may make the liver more susceptible to INH-induced toxicity, although this has not been established with certainty. The problem of hepatitis usually arises in the first few weeks of therapy, and may amount to nothing more than chemical abnormalities; the liver returns to normal when the dose of rifampin is temporarily reduced, following which the original dose can be tentatively reintroduced. If more severe liver damage develops, the drug should be discontinued. Some patients may develop renal failure in addition to hepatic dysfunction; this serious complication is more likely to occur if the drug is taken on an intermittent basis.[93] These hypersensitivity reactions may be accompanied by rashes, fever and thrombocytopenia; antibodies to rifampin can be detected in many of the patients. In spite of these serious complications, many patients can be successfully treated with intermittent rifampin therapy, although hypersensitivity reactions might be expected in up to 5 per cent of them. Intermittent rifampin therapy should be permitted only when knowledgeable and careful monitoring of the patient is possible.

Other complications due to rifampin are less serious. Pains in the legs, joints or abdomen are occasionally experienced. A small percentage of patients develop rashes, and all patients are likely to notice that their tears, saliva, urine and other secretions are colored reddish-orange by rifampin metabolites. Rifampin can interfere with the effectiveness of oral contraceptives, and the drug impairs the effectiveness of coumarin-type anticoagulants, the dosage of which may then need to be increased. Improved bioavailability of the drug is assured by giving it one hour before or two hours after a meal.

STREPTOMYCIN. Streptomycin has already been described as one of the aminoglycosides. It is currently of less importance in tuberculosis therapy, having been displaced by ethambutol and rifampin. Nevertheless, it is a valuable agent when used in combination therapy, and when "sentencing" a patient to a course of this injectable drug, that individual must be kept under close surveillance during the period of treatment; this is of importance in the successful management of recalcitrant or unreliable patients. A derivative of streptomycin, dihydrostreptomycin, was formerly used in the hope of reducing the toxic effects of the antibiotic; however, it became evident that this derivative has severe ototoxicity, and the drug has been abandoned.

Second-Line Antituberculosis Drugs (Table 10–18). Many agents have some activity against mycobacteria, but a limited number are favored in the U.S. Nevertheless, it should be realized that the following antimicrobials may have some antimycobacterial capability: cephaloridine; chloramphenicol; kanamycin, gentamicin and other aminoglycosides; and the tetracyclines.[94] In other countries, additional inexpensive, but relatively weak, antimycobacterial drugs are of importance: among these are thiacetazone (amithiozone) and other thiosemicarbazones, and prothionamide, which is related to ethionamide.[95]

In the U.S., the second-line drugs are pyrazinamide, ethionamide, cycloserine, capreomycin, viomycin and para-aminosalicylic acid. Kanamycin is often regarded as a less effective alternative to streptomycin. The second-line agents should rarely, if ever, be given without the accompaniment of one or more first-line drugs.

PYRAZINAMIDE. Pyrazinamide is a synthetic derivative of nicotinamide, and it is one of the more effective second-line agents. The drug is marketed as 500 mg tablets that are available for dispensation only by hospitals and tuberculosis clinics. The drug has not been shown to be safe in children, and it should be excluded from pediatric regimens, if feasible.

Pyrazinamide often causes gastrointestinal disturbances, and it tends to cause dose-related hepatic toxicity: liver function tests should be obtained every month during therapy, and if the SGOT value doubles, the drug should probably be discontinued. Pyrazinamide always causes hyperuricemia; susceptible patients may develop gout, which may be controlled by uricosuric agents. The only other common reaction to pyrazinamide is photosensitivity. In fact, the toxicity of this drug may have been overstated in the past, but its propensity to cause liver damage is a problem when it is given with other hepatotoxic agents such as INH, and the drug cannot be recommended for patients with underlying liver disease. Pyrazinamide is not regarded as effective in the treatment of atypical mycobacteria, but it is sometimes added to multiple drug regimens. It is, however, favored as one of the drugs for use in short-term therapy of tuberculosis. Clearly, pyrazinamide is a valuable antituberculosis drug that is reasonably safe in spite of its hepatotoxicity.

ETHIONAMIDE. Ethionamide is similar in many respects to pyrazinamide; it is also related to INH, being a synthetic derivative of isonicotinic acid. Ethionamide has about one-tenth the activity of INH, but is less well tolerated, with up to 30 per cent of patients having to discontinue the drug, mainly because of gastrointestinal side effects.

The drug has an objectionable taste, and often causes anorexia, salivation, nausea, vomiting and diarrhea; in some cases, it is better tolerated by administering it with food in three divided doses, whereas, in other patients, it may be better to give it as one dose at night with a sedative. Other toxic effects include hepatitis, peripheral neuritis, optic neuritis, depression, impotence, phototoxicity, rashes, thrombocytopenia, gynecomastia, stomatitis, difficulty in managing diabetes, and hypothyroidism. Thus, ethionamide combines the adverse properties of isoniazid with some of its own, and it is a difficult drug to use in practice. It may also increase the toxic effects of pyrazinamide, and of cycloserine; it should probably not be used in conjunction with the latter drug, because convulsions may be provoked. In spite of these objections to its use, it has been successful, particularly in retreatment programs, and in some short-course therapy regimens in Asia and Africa.

CYCLOSERINE. Cycloserine is an antibiotic, which is effective against *E. coli*, and some other gram-negative and gram-positive bacteria. It is concentrated in the urine and can be used for treating susceptible urinary tract infections—including those caused by mycobacteria. Cycloserine is a useful antituberculosis agent when combined with one or more first-line drugs, and it may be of particular value in the treatment of atypical mycobacterial disease.[51] Although tolerated well by most patients, the drug can cause severe neurologic toxicity: the problems include twitching, which may progress to convulsions, coma, vertigo, psychotic disturbances, loss of memory and minor personality changes. Some common side effects are less serious, such as nausea and diarrhea; of greater concern are liver damage, a malabsorption syndrome, folate deficiency, and peripheral neuropathy, which are uncommon complications.

Cycloserine can be given only orally, and it should be initiated in a dose of 250 mg two or three times a day. If this is well tolerated, the dose can be increased after a few days to a maximum of 1 gm per day (10 to 20 mg/kg). In some cases, a lower dose given once a day has been adequate. The drug should be given with caution when used in combination with INH, since the neurotoxic effects of each may be potentiated. Cycloserine is contraindicated in alcoholics, epileptics and mentally disturbed patients; similarly, it should not be given to patients receiving other epileptogenic drugs, or agents such as glucocorticoids that may also induce psychoses.

CAPREOMYCIN. Capreomycin is an antibiotic that is related to viomycin. It is almost as potent as streptomycin and it is more potent than kanamycin. Since it is also injectable, it can be considered as an alternative to streptomycin for a patient whose mycobacteria are resistant to that drug. Unlike streptomycin, capreomycin is of no practical value for the elimination of any other microorganisms.

The main toxic effect of capreomycin is its nephrotoxicity: it is more dangerous in this respect than the aminoglycosides. However, it has comparatively little ototoxicity, and it can generally be given safely for several months. As with streptomycin, initial daily intramuscular injections are reduced to twice or three times a week after the first few weeks of effective therapy are accomplished. If signs of renal toxicity appear, complete recovery will occur when capreomycin therapy is discontinued.

Other side effects do occur. Some hepatic toxicity can be expected, but this is not a practical problem in the vast majority of cases. Hypersensitivity reactions, such as fever and rash, are rare, but eosinophilia is not uncommon. Tinnitus, vertigo and headaches are occasional problems, and hypokalemia may appear during a course of therapy. Neuromuscular blockade can occur, but only when large intravenous doses are given: however, the drug is not recommended for administration by this route. Capreomycin should be avoided in patients with renal damage, and should not be given to elderly patients if possible; concomitant therapy with other nephrotoxic or ototoxic drugs should be avoided.

VIOMYCIN. Viomycin is an antibiotic that is less effective than capreomycin, and it has been rendered of less practical value by the introduction of the latter agent. Viomycin has to be given in larger doses, and is more nephrotoxic and ototoxic; organ damage may not be completely reversible when the drug is discontinued. Hypersensitivity reactions are rare, but rashes may occur. Electrolyte disturbances sometimes appear during the course of therapy. When given with a curariform drug, neuromuscular blockade is potentiated.

Viomycin has a very limited role in the management of any form of tuberculosis, but as an injectable agent it is occasionally useful in a retreatment program. It should not be given with other ototoxic or nephrotoxic drugs, and it should be avoided in the elderly and in patients with renal impairment.

PARA-AMINOSALICYLIC ACID (PAS). This was originally considered to be a first-line drug, but it is used only rarely now that ethambutol and rifampin are available. This drug is also known as aminosalicylic acid; calcium, potassium and sodium aminosalicylates as well as other PAS preparations have been marketed (resin forms, or with the addition of ascorbic acid). The drug has to be given in large doses amounting to 200 to 300 mg/kg a day, and tablets of 0.5 and 1 gm are available; other formulations have been marketed including sachets, granules, liquids and so on. The salt derivatives have to be given in even larger doses, since their PAS content amounts to only 70 to 80 per cent; comparatively large quantities of calcium, potassium or sodium are contained in the daily dosages. These alternatives to PAS are sometimes tolerated, in appropriate dosages, by patients who are intolerant of PAS itself. Some combination tablets have been marketed that contain INH and various PAS products.

The problems with PAS are that it is very unpleasant to take and it has numerous disturbing or dangerous side effects.[92] It was well known that when PAS was a first-line drug, as many as 50 per cent of sanitarium patients did not actually take the PAS that was dispensed to them. The drug can cause severe anorexia and nausea, with vomiting, abdominal cramps, diarrhea and malabsorption; these side effects preclude continued treatment with PAS in about 15 per cent of patients. At least 4 per cent of patients develop hypersensitivity reactions usually between the second and seventh weeks. These include fever, rash, pruritus and even exfoliative dermatitis; pulmonary infiltrates with eosinophilia; an infectious mononucleosis-like syndrome; hepatic damage, varying from jaundice to acute fatal liver failure; goiter; encephalopathy; myocarditis; hematologic disturbances; and, rarely, lupus erythematosus. True anaphylaxis is rare; nevertheless, the drug is undoubtedly dangerous. A further problem with PAS is that it has salicylate properties, and it could provoke asthma in patients who are allergic to aspirin; it can also prolong the prothrombin time and potentiate anticoagulants.

Although PAS is rarely used for the treatment of adults in the U.S., it may be more acceptable to other ethnic groups, and it still has a role in Asia and Africa. It may also be useful for some children with advanced tuberculosis who may tolerate the drug relatively well. Some adult patients may be more accepting of PAS if it is administered only once a day in a dose of about 6 gm, and this reduced dose may be effective when combined with adequate first-line drugs. However, with the declining status of PAS as a major antituberculosis drug, it may not be possible to gain adequate controlled experience of its value in adjusted dosage when combined with the orthodox drug regimens advocated in Table 10–7.

Antifungal Drugs
(Table 10–19)

A limited number of antifungal agents are of value in the treatment of the pulmonary mycoses; these drugs can be categorized as either polyene antibiotics or synthetic agents.

Polyene Antibiotics. The major polyenes are amphotericin B and nystatin; candicidin, hamycin, pimaricin and trichomycin are investigational. Only amphotericin B and nystatin are of relevance in respiratory therapeutics.

AMPHOTERICIN B. Amphotericin B is the most potent antifungal antibiotic, and it is the only one available for parenteral use; invasive mycotic infections require parenteral therapy. Amphotericin is the only suitable drug for major pulmonary infections such as blastomycosis, candidiasis, coccidioidomycosis, cryptococcosis, histoplasmosis and mucormycosis.[96]

Amphotericin is poorly soluble in water, and it is marketed as a bile-salt complex that forms a colloidal suspension in dextrose-water solutions; the suspension loses stability after 24 hours, but a fresh solution does not require protection (for example, from light) if administered within the next few hours.[97] The drug does not penetrate tissue barriers well, and after intravenous administration it fails to get into the nervous system in adequate amounts, and therefore has to be given intrathecally. Although it does not appear to cross the blood-bronchial barrier adequately,[26] the relevance of this is questionable, since intravenous therapy is effective in the treatment of pulmonary infections. Furthermore, there is no evidence to suggest that inhalational administration can eliminate true tissue infection, although the aerosolized drug can suppress colonization.[45] Endocavitary infusion of amphotericin may be of benefit in selected patients.[21]

The toxicity of amphotericin makes this drug the most unpleasant of the antimicrobial agents that are in common use. The solution tends to cause thrombophlebitis with sclerosis of veins, and the finding of an entry route in an individual patient on prolonged therapy can become a major problem. Initial treatments should be given in small peripheral veins utilizing a small, thin needle; the addition of a small amount of heparin (for example, 10 mg) may prevent sclerosis of the veins. Acute toxic symptoms include a febrile reaction, which may be severe; accompanying chills, sweating, anorexia, vomiting, headache, delirium and hypotension are not uncommon. This reaction can often be ameliorated by prior prophylaxis with an antihistamine or a sedative, or by aspirin; 25 to 50 mg hydrocortisone should be infused with the amphotericin if simpler measures do not prevent the toxic reaction. It is a common practice to give a patient a small test dose of 0.5 to 1 mg amphotericin in a slow drip over several hours when initiating therapy, but this cautious approach may be ill founded, since it is unlikely to prove any more acceptable, and, paradoxically, can even result in more severe reactions.[98] Present recommendations are to initiate treatment with a dose that amounts to 0.25 mg/kg

TABLE 10-19. MAJOR ANTIFUNGAL AGENTS FOR RESPIRATORY MYCOSES

Agent	Route Oral	I.V.	Aerosol	Usual Daily Dosage For Adults	Toxicity	Comments
POLYENE ANTIBIOTICS Amphotericin B (Fungizone)		+	(+)	1 mg/kg three times a week. Dissolve in 5% dextrose solution (0.1 mg/ml); infuse over 1–6 hours.	Acute: febrile reaction. hypotension, shock; nausea, vomiting, vertigo, seizures, coma; rashes, phlebitis. Chronic: renal impairment, anemia, hypokalemia, neuropathies	Dose has to be built up initially using daily infusions; acute reactions may be alleviated by antihistamine, aspirin or glucocorticoid.
Nystatin (Mycostatin, Nilstat)	+ (topical)		(+)	500,000–1,000,000 units t.i.d.	Nausea, vomiting.	No value in treating systemic infection; oral drug is used to treat oropharyngeal thrush; aerosol may suppress colonization by *Candida*.
SYNTHETIC Flucytosine (Ancobon)	+			150 mg/kg in 4 divided doses	Nausea, vomiting, diarrhea, rash, anemia, leukopenia. thrombocytopenia, headache, drowsiness, vertigo, hallucinations, slight liver impairment, slight renal impairment	Use with particular care in presence of liver or renal disease, or marrow depression.
Hydroxystilbamidine isethionate		+		225 mg in 200 ml 5% dextrose or normal saline over 2–3 hours	Anorexia, nausea, vomiting, headache, chills, hypotension, tachycardia, dizziness, flushing, syncope, salivation, sweating, twitching, edema of eyelids, incontinence, liver impairment.	I.M. dose possible, but painful.

body weight, and to give the infusion over three to four hours. If this amount is well accepted, the dosage can be built up in daily treatments over the next 7 to 14 days to the standard maintenance dose of 1 mg/kg, up to a maximum of 50 mg a day in adults; the maintenance dosage in children is usually taken to be 0.5 mg/kg a day. Most patients find that the adverse acute reaction becomes progressively less severe, and after a few days or weeks the drug may not cause any acute reaction. Particular precautions should be taken to prepare the amphotericin solution according to the manufacturer's directions.

Once the maintenance dose is reached, it is usual to give that dose three times a week, taking four hours or less to infuse the drug; in many patients, greater acceptance is achieved if the infusion is given over the course of just one hour. The frequency of treatments is determined by the toxicity of amphotericin, with the nephrotoxicity being the common limiting factor. Most patients develop renal irritation, which results in cylinduria and white cells in the urine; the serum creatinine should be monitored twice a week but the blood urea nitrogen is a less meaningful parameter. Most physicians are sufficiently concerned by the marked rise in serum creatinine that sometimes occurs the day after a dose of amphotericin to withhold the next dose until the creatinine returns to normal, which may take three or four days. Renal tubular acidosis and eventually nephrocalcinosis may appear, but it is important to recognize that renal function usually returns close to normal within six months of the completing of a course of the amphotericin that had caused nephrotoxic damage.[98] It has been suggested that concomitant administration of sodium bicarbonate or mannitol may mitigate nephrotoxicity, but these agents are unlikely to make any significant difference.[97, 98]

Other side effects of chronic therapy must be expected. Hypokalemia occurs in about 25 per cent of patients as a consequence of renal loss, and potassium chloride supplementation is required. Amphotericin tends to result in a decrease in erythrocyte production, and progressive anemia is usual, but treatment for this is not indicated unless the patient becomes symptomatic; in some cases, hemolysis may complicate the picture.

In most pulmonary mycoses that require amphotericin, a total dose of at least 1.5 gm is required.[47, 97] If the disease is not suffi-ciently controlled, a course of two to three gm should be aimed for; a few patients require larger doses, with an occasional unlucky victim needing up to 4 gm of the drug. Unfortunately, no reliable laboratory assays for amphotericin serum levels have been established, and correlating dosage with minimum inhibitory concentrations (as is possible for most antibiotics used to treat bacterial infections) is not feasible. Undoubtedly, there is a great need to find a more benign and effective drug than amphotericin B, but none is available at present. However, it is possible that other drugs, including rifampin, could be used synergistically with amphotericin in some fungal infections, thereby permitting a lower dosage of amphotericin to be given.[99] New developments of this type would be important advances if successful.

NYSTATIN. Nystatin is similar to amphotericin in its action, but it is too toxic for parenteral administration.[97] It is therefore used only topically for the treatment and prophylaxis of dermatologic and mucosal mycotic infections, particularly those caused by *Candida* species. Oral tablets, of 500,000 units, can be given several times a day to prevent candidiasis from developing in the oropharynx; this of value in some immuno-suppressed patients who are receiving broad-spectrum antibiotics. Topical therapy is also indicated for the thrush-like condition that can develop in asthmatics using aero-solized glucocorticoid therapy. Oral suspensions are available also, and they may provide better topical therapy than the tablet preparations.

Nystatin, like amphotericin, has been given by aerosol to suppress *Candida* colonization of the respiratory tract. Although the fungus can be eliminated, there is no evidence that invasive candidiasis can be controlled, and aerosolization of either nystatin or amphotericin[100] cannot be regarded as a means for treating an established mycotic pulmonary infection. The oral and aerosol preparations are generally well tolerated.

Synthetic Antifungal Drugs. Many synthetic drugs have been used in the treatment of mycotic infections, but only a few are of value for respiratory fungal diseases.[101]

FLUCYTOSINE (5-FLUOROCYTOSINE). This drug is of low toxicity and is effective when given orally, since it is well absorbed from the gastrointestinal tract. The drug is able to cross the blood-bronchial barrier adequately, whereas amphotericin does not.[26] It has been effective in the treatment of visceral candidiasis, cryptococcal meningitis, chromomycosis and torulopsosis.[101a] There is some evidence to suggest that flucytosine can be regarded as a secondary alternative to amphotericin for invasive infections of the lung by *Candida* and *Cryptococcus*.[101] The drug may also be of value when given in combination with amphotericin to permit a lower total dosage of the latter in the treatment of other diseases, but information in this respect is inadequate at present.[98]

Flucytosine is made available as 250 and 500 mg capsules, and is given in a dosage of 50 to 150 mg/kg per day in four divided doses. Its major side effects are nausea, vomiting, diarrhea and reversible alterations in liver function tests. The drug may also cause rashes and hematologic changes; less frequently, renal impairment and central nervous system problems occur. The drug should be given with extreme caution to patients with underlying renal insufficiency.

2-HYDROXYSTILBAMIDINE ISETHIONATE. This is an older drug that is of value only in the therapy of blastomycosis.[96, 101] It is less effective than amphotericin, but it is also less toxic. The drug is given intravenously as an infusion of 225 mg in 200 ml of 5 per cent dextrose or normal saline, taking 30 minutes for the procedure. Daily treatment is given and a total dosage of about 8 gm or more is required.

Hydroxystilbamidine produces liver toxicity, which may be severe; liver function tests should be monitored weekly during therapy. Other side effects are also severe: flushing, dizziness, and hypotension may culminate in syncope; salivation, sweating, lethargy, twitching, edema of the eyelids and urinary incontinence are additional possibilities. Occasional patients develop shaking chills, fever, malaise, nausea and vomiting – a reaction similar to that which occurs more often and more severely with amphotericin.

POTASSIUM IODIDE. Potassium iodide is still one of the best agents for the treatment of pulmonary sporotrichosis.[96, 101] A saturated solution (SSKI) is given orally in a dosage of up to 12 ml per day for several weeks or months. Problems associated with the use of SSKI have been discussed in detail in Chapter 3.

CLOTRIMAZOLE. This is an investigational oral agent that may be of value in the treatment of candidiasis and aspergillosis.[101] Gastrointestinal side effects are a problem; it is unlikely that the therapeutic:toxic ratio will be sufficiently favorable for this drug.

MICONAZOLE. This is an investigational agent similar to clotrimazole in that it is an imidazole derivative. It can be given both orally and intravenously, and, apart from diarrhea, side effects are infrequent. Preliminary experience suggests that it may be of use in some pulmonary mycoses, and it may eventually become a secondary alternative to amphotericin when the latter drug cannot be used.[102]

DI-IODOHYDROXYQUINOLINE. This is an antiamebic agent reported to be of value in the treatment of pulmonary aspergillosis, which may be associated with asthma.[103] Further investigations of this drug would be of interest.

Antiparasitic Drugs

The only important antiparasitic agents for use in the U.S. in the treatment of respiratory diseases are diethylcarbamazine and pentamidine. Diethylcarbamazine is an antifilarial agent, but it is of interest also as a prophylactic agent in certain forms of asthma: this topic is discussed in Chapter 4.

PENTAMIDINE ISETHIONATE. This is used in the treatment of *Pneumocystis carinii*, an opportunistic protozoan that can cause a severe pneumonia in immunosuppressed patients. This toxic agent is not generally available, and experience in its use should be a requirement for physicians who choose to employ the drug. Pentamide isethionate is given intramuscularly in a daily dosage of 4 mg/kg; the total daily dose for a patient should not exceed 56 mg. Adverse effects may be expected in about half the patients;[104] these effects include impaired renal function, liver dysfunction, hypoglycemia, hematologic abnormalities, pain or abscess at site of injection, hypotension, rashes and hypocalcemia. The toxicity of pentamidine has caused clinicians to seek alternative therapies, including the combination of a sulfonamide with pyrimethamine, or the combination of sulfamethoxazole-trimethoprim (cotrimoxazole).

Special Considerations in Antimicrobial Therapy

The appropriate use of antimicrobial drugs is dependent on the information provided by the microbiology laboratory; individual hospitals and clinics generate specific results that may differ markedly from standard recommendations. Thus, the sensitivity of a specific organism to various agents cannot be

TABLE 10–20. RECOMMENDED ANTIBIOTICS FOR THE TREATMENT OF ORGANISMS INFECTING THE RESPIRATORY TRACT*

Organism	First Choice	Second Choice	Others
GRAM-POSITIVE			
Diplococcus pneumoniae (pneumococcus)	Penicillin	Erythromycin	A cephalosporin, clindamycin, chloramphenicol, a tetracycline
Staphycoccus aureus non-penicillinase producer	Penicillin	A cephalosporin	Erythromycin, clindamycin, vancomycin, gentamicin
penicillinase producer	Any penicillinase-resistant penicillin	A cephalosporin	Clindamycin, erythromycin, vancomycin, kanamycin
Streptococcus pyogenes	Penicillin	Erythromycin	Clindamycin, a cephalosporin
GRAM-NEGATIVE			
Haemophilus influenzae	Ampicillin, amoxicillin	A tetracycline	Chloramphenicol, a sulfonamide (± trimethoprim)
Enterobacter (Aerobacter)	Gentamicin	Amikacin, tobramycin	Colistin, polymyxin, kanamycin, chloramphenicol, a tetracycline, carbenicillin
Escherichia coli	Ampicillin	Gentamicin	A cephalosporin, amikacin, kanamycin, polymyxin, chloramphenicol
Klebsiella pneumoniae	Gentamicin (± a cephalosporin)	Amikacin or tobramycin (± a cephalosporin)	Kanamycin, a tetracycline, a cephalosporin, chloramphenicol
Proteus mirabilis	Ampicillin	Kanamycin	A cephalosporin, gentamicin, chloramphenicol
Other Proteus species	Gentamicin	Tobramycin	Kanamycin, carbenicillin, a tetracycline, chloramphenicol
Pseudomonas aeruginosa	Tobramycin (± carbenicillin)	Gentamicin (± carbenicillin)	Amikacin, colistin, polymyxin
Serratia marcescens	Gentamicin	Kanamycin, amikacin	Sulfamethoxazole-trimethoprim, chloramphenicol, carbenicillin
ANAEROBES (oropharyngeal)			
Bacteroides	Penicillin	Clindamycin	Chloramphenicol, a tetracycline, ampicillin, carbenicillin
Streptococcus species	Penicillin	Clindamycin	Erythromycin, a tetracycline
MYCOPLASMA			
M. pneumoniae	Erythromycin	A tetracycline	None

*These recommendations are only guidelines; in all cases, laboratory studies are required as a basis for definitive antimicrobial therapy.

N.B. *Legionnaire's disease,* which is caused by an unclassified organism, should be treated with an erythromycin or a tetracycline.

obtained with reliability from a book; therefore, the recommendations provided in this chapter and summarized in Table 10–20 must be recognized as having general applicability rather than specific relevance.

Precision in antimicrobial usage can be achieved in difficult cases of infection by obtaining serum levels of a drug following its administration to a specific patient. This information is of particular value when the absorption, metabolism or excretion of the drug is abnormal; in renal insufficiency, such information may be vitally important, since many antimicrobials accumulate when their renal excretion is impaired, and toxic effects may be precipitated unless the dosage is adjusted. Many guidelines have been provided that offer general recommendations for such dosage changes in renal insufficiency, and additional recommendations are available for dosages when the patient is on maintenance dialysis.[105] Adjustments in dosage are not so important in other metabolic derangements, although liver disease is a major indication for caution in the use of most antimicrobials.

Dosages of antimicrobial agents should be adjusted in children; current recommendations for standard dosages of the common drugs are presented in Table 10–21. Pregnant women and nursing mothers also require special consideration, since a number of agents can cross the placenta and harm the fetus, or enter breast milk and thereby harm the newborn infant.[106] Some of the major dangers of antibiotic therapy in pregnant or nursing women are presented in Table 10–22.

Ideally, a precise knowledge of the pharmacokinetic properties of individual antimicrobial drugs would be of assistance in planning optimal therapy. Unfortunately, our understanding of how to use such information in the treatment of respiratory infections is very limited, and the relevance of molecular weights and dissociation constants, for example, requires further clarification. However, in case some of this information

Text continued on page 383

TABLE 10–21. ANTIBIOTIC DOSAGES FOR CHILDREN

Drug	Total Daily Dosage mg/kg/24 hr	Usual Number of Doses Per Day	Route Oral	Route I.M.	Route I.V.
PENICILLINS					
Amoxicillin	20–40	3	+		
Ampicillin	50–400	4	+	+	+
Carbenicillin	50–500	4–6		+	+
Cloxacillin	50–100	4	+		
Dicloxacillin	12.5–25	4	+		
Hetacillin	22–45	4	+	+	+
Methicillin	100	4		+	+
Nafcillin	25–120	3–6	+	+	+
Oxacillin	50	4	+	+	+
Penicillin G	25,000–400,000 U/kg	2–6	+	+	
Penicillin V	25,000–50,000 U/kg	4	+		
CEPHALOSPORINS					
Cefazolin*	25–50	3–4		+	+
Cephalexin	25–100	4	+		
Cephaloridine*	30–100	3–4		+	+
Cephalothin	80–225	4–6		+	+
Cephapirin	40–80	4		+	+
Cephradine	25–100	4	+		+
MACROLIDES, ETC.					
Erythromycin	30–100	4–6	+		
Lincomycin*	10–20	2–4	+	+	
Clindamycin	8–25	3–4	+	+	+
Chloramphenicol	25–50	4	+		+
TETRACYCLINES‡					
Chlortetracycline	10–50	2–4	+		
Demeclocycline	10	2–4	+		
Doxycycline	2.2–4.4	2	+		+
Methacycline	12	2–4	+		
Minocycline	4	2	+		
Oxytetracycline	10–50	2–4	+		
Roliotetracycline	15–20	2		+	+
Tetracycline	10–50	2–4	+	+	+

Drug	mg/kg/24 hr	Doses/24 hr			
AMINOGLYCOSIDES					
Amikacin	15	2–3		+	+
Gentamicin	3–7.5	3		+	+
Kanamycin	6–15	2		+	
Neomycin†	50–90	4–6	+		
Tobramycin	3–5	2–4		+	
POLYMYXINS					
Colistimethate	2.5–5	2–4		+	+
Colistin sulfate	3–5	3	+		
Polymyxin B	1.5–2.5	4		+	+
ANTITUBERCULOSIS DRUGS					
Cycloserine†	10	2	+		
Ethambutol	15–25	1	+		
Ethionamide	12–15	3	+		
Isoniazid	10(–30)	1–2	+	+	
Para-aminosalicylic acid	300	3	+		
Rifampin	10–20	1	+		
Streptomycin	20	1		+	
Viomycin†	40	1		+	
SULFONAMIDES					
Sulfadiazine	100	3–4	+		+
Sulfisoxazole	100	3–4	+	+	+
Sulfamethoxazole	60	2	+		
Sulfamethoxazole } Trimethoprim	40 / 8	2 / 2	+		
ANTIFUNGAL DRUGS					
Amphotericin B	1–1.5	1			+
Nystatin	400,000–2,000,000 Units	4	+		
Flucytosine	50–150	4	+		

NOTE: (1) Information for this table is derived mainly from Shirkey, H. S.: Pediatric Drug Handbook. Philadelphia, W. B. Saunders Company, 1977.

(2) In all cases of doubt, manufacturers' literature should be consulted. For older or heavier children, adult dosage recommendations should be followed.

*Should not be used in infants until further evidence of safety is available.

†Safety and optimum dosage, especially in younger children, have not been officially established.

‡Tetracyclines should not be given to children under the age of 8, since permanent dentition may be damaged.

TABLE 10–22. DANGERS OF ANTIMICROBIAL DRUGS ADMINISTERED TO MOTHER

Drugs	Harmful to Fetus During Pregnancy	Harmful to Breast-Fed Infant
PENICILLINS		
Ampicillin	No	No
Penicillin G	No	No
Methicillin	No	No
CEPHALOSPORINS		
Cefazolin	Probably not	Probably not
Cephalexin	No	No
Cephalothin	No	No
TETRACYCLINES	Dental damage and other malformations	Dental damage
AMINOGLYCOSIDES		
Amikacin	Unknown	Unknown
Gentamicin	Possible ototoxicity	No
Kanamycin	Possible ototoxicity	No
Streptomycin	High risk of ototoxicity and other malformations	No
Tobramycin	Unknown	Unknown
MISCELLANEOUS		
Colistin	No	No
Erythromycin	No	No
Clindamycin	No	No
Chloramphenicol	Can cause fetal death	Could cause "gray-baby syndrome"
Vancomycin	Uncertain	Uncertain
Sulfonamides	Cause kernicterus, liver atrophy, anemia	Cause hyperbilirubinemia
ANTITUBERCULOSIS AGENTS		
Isoniazid	May cause encephalopathy and retarded psychomotor activity of newborn	No
Ethambutol	Uncertain	Probably not
Rifampin	Uncertain	Probably not
Pyrazinamide	Uncertain	Probably not
Ethionamide	May cause malformations	Probably not
Cycloserine	Uncertain	Probably not
Capreomycin	Uncertain	Probably not
PAS	Uncertain	Probably not

TABLE 10–23. PHARMACOKINETIC DATA ON MAJOR ANTIMICROBIAL DRUGS*

Agent	Molecular Weight	pKa	Dose	Serum Level That Might Be Achieved (mcg/ml)	Sputum Level That Might Be Achieved (mcg/ml)	Typical MIC Required (mcg/ml)
Penicillins						
Penicillin G	356		1,000,000 U I.M.	12		1
Penicillin V	350		250 mg P.O.	2		4
Amoxicillin	365		1 gm P.O.	17	1	0.8
Ampicillin	349	2.5, 7.2	1 gm P.O.	17	1	0.8
Carbenicillin	378		4 gm I.V.	47	5	2.5–50
Cloxacillin	436	2.7	250 mg P.O.	6	1.6	0.5
Methicillin	420	3.0	500 mg I.M.	16	1.0	2
Nafcillin	414		500 mg I.V.	11		1
Cephalosporins						
Cefazolin	476	2.3	500 mg I.M.	45		8
Cephalexin	347	4.5	500 mg P.O.	20	0.32	16
Cephalothin	396	2.5	500 mg I.M.	10		8
Tetracyclines						
Tetracycline	444	8.3	250 mg P.O.	4	0.8	3
Doxycycline	444	3.4, 7.7, 9.7	100 mg P.O.	3	1.5	1.6
—hyclate	1026		100 mg I.V.	4	3	1.6
Aminoglycosides						
Amikacin	781		500 mg I.M.	20		12
Gentamicin	425		120 mg I.M.	10	6.0	8
Kanamycin	484	7.2	15 mg/kg I.M.	30		12
Streptomycin	744		500 mg I.M.	15		8
Tobramycin	467		80 mg I.M.	4	6	8
Erythromycin						
—base	734	8.8	250 mg P.O.	1.3	0.55	2.5
—estolate	1056		250 mg P.O.	3		2.5
Chloramphenicol	445	5.5	1 gm P.O.	12		5
Clindamycin	425	6.9	300 mg P.O.	5	2.7	2
Vancomycin	3293		500 mg I.V.	40	2.5	33
Colistimethate	1750		2.5 mg/kg I.M.	7		5
Sulfonamides	250 (approx)	4.9–6.4	1 gm P.O.	50–100		50
Trimethoprim	290		80 mg P.O.	3	6	1
Antifungals						
Amphotericin B	924		1 mg/kg I.V.	4		0.9
Flucytosine	129		2 gm P.O.	40		4

*This information is incomplete at the present time. The serum and sputum levels and the minimum inhibitory concentrations (MIC) may be variable, and the above information provides only a general indication of typical levels. The significance of the dissociation constants (pKa) requires further pharmacokinetic evaluation.

may be helpful, these pharmacokinetic properties for the most important agents are presented in Table 10–23: for further details, consult a standard pharmacology text and see Reference 107. Also presented in this table are the serum and sputum concentrations that may be obtained with typical dosages of the individual drugs (for further details consult References 5, 26, 94, 95, 108–110, 113). An attempt has been made to include the range of minimum inhibitory concentrations (M.I.C.) required in the serum for each antimicrobial if it is to be effective against organisms considered to be susceptible to it; these ranges are of general interest, and they should not be regarded as strictly appropriate for individual situations. When it is thought that a knowledge of the M.I.C. of an organism infecting a particular patient could be helpful, the clinician should seek help from the local microbiology laboratory. In the vast majority of cases, empirical standardized dosages of antimicrobials can be used successfully to treat most infections, but in problem cases the help of a sophisticated laboratory is inestimable. Obviously, antiinfectious therapy is a constantly evolving field, and current information will always be needed to supplement that provided here.

In this chapter, an attempt has been made to survey antimicrobial therapy in relation to the treatment and prophylaxis of infections of the respiratory tract. The literature on this subject is enormous, and further details can be obtained from any standard pharmacology textbook, and from the following selected references: 55, 84, 94, 108–113.

REFERENCES

1. Crofton, J.: The chemotherapy of bacterial respiratory infections. Am. Rev. Respir. Dis. 101:841–859, 1970.
2. Burrows, B. and Nevin, W.: Antibiotic management in patients with chronic bronchitis and emphysema. Ann. Intern. Med. 77:993–995, 1972.
3. Editorial: Antimicrobial treatment of chronic bronchitis. Lancet 1:505–506, 1975.
4. Smith, C. B., Golden, C. A., Kanner, R. E. and Renzetti, A. T.: *Haemophilus influenza* and *Haemophilus parainfluenzae* in chronic obstructive pulmonary disease. Lancet 2:1253–1255, 1976.
5. May, J. R.: Chemotherapy of Chronic Bronchitis and Allied Disorders. London, The English Universities Press Ltd., 1968.
6. Barrett-Connor, E.: The nonvalue of sputum culture in the diagnosis of pneumococcal pneumonia. Am. Rev. Respir. Dis. 103:845–848, 1971.
7. Hallett, W. Y.: Infection: the real culprit in chronic bronchitis and emphysema? Med. Clin. North Am. 57:735–750, 1973.
8. Dautrebande, L.: Physiological and pharmacological characteristics of liquid aerosols. Physiol. Rev. 32:214–276, 1952.
9. Miller, W. F.: Antibiotic aerosols. *In* Antimicrobial Therapy. B. M. Kagan (Ed.). Philadelphia, W. B. Saunders Company, 2nd ed., 1974. Ch. 43.
10. Friedman, L. G.: Chronic bronchitis and bronchiectasis. *In* Therapeutics in Internal Medicine, F. A. Kyser (Ed.). New York, Paul B. Hoeber Inc., 2nd ed., 1953, pp. 393–399.
11. Kanig, J. L.: Pharmaceutical aerosols. J. Pharmaceut. Sci. 52:513–535, 1963.
12. Abramson, H. A.: Principles and practice of aerosol therapy of the lungs and bronchi. Ann. Allergy 4:440, 1946.
13. Huang, N. N.: Antibiotic therapy. *In* Guide to Drug Therapy in Patients With Cystic Fibrosis. Atlanta, The National Cystic Fibrosis Research Foundation, 1972, pp. 7–25.
14. Feeley, T. W., du Moulin, G. C., Hedley-White, J., Bushnell, L. S., Gilbert, J. P. and Feingold, D. S.: Aerosol polymyxin and pneumonia in seriously ill patients. N. Engl. J. Med. 293:471–475, 1975.
15. Feeley, T. W. et al.: Prevention of gram-negative pneumonia. N. Engl. J. Med. 293:1263, 1975.
16. Johanson, W. G., Pierce, A. K., Sanford, J. P. and Thomas, G. D.: Nosocomial respiratory infections with gram-negative bacilli: the significance of colonization of the respiratory tract. Ann. Intern. Med. 77:701–706, 1972.
17. Marschke, G. and Sarauw, A.: Danger of polymyxin B inhalation. Ann. Intern. Med. 74:296–297, 1971.
18. Klastersky, J., Huysmans, E., Weerts, D., Hensgens, C. and Daneau, D.: Endotracheally administered gentamicin for the prevention of infections of the respiratory tract in patients with tracheostomy: a double-blind study. Chest 65:650–654, 1974.
19. Klastersky, J., Hensgens, C., Noterman, J., Mouawad, E. and Meunier-Carpentier, F.: Endotracheal antibiotics for the prevention of tracheobronchial infections in tracheotomized unconscious patients. Chest 68:302–306, 1975.
20. Ramirez-R., J. and O'Neill, E. F.: Endobronchial polymyxin B: experimental observations in chronic bronchitis. Chest 58:352–357, 1970.
21. Aslam, P. A., Larkin, J., Eastridge, C. E. and Hughes, F. A.: Endocavitary infusion through percutaneous endobronchial catheter. Chest 57:94–96, 1970.
22. Odio, W., Van Laer, E. and Klastersky, J.: Concentrations of gentamicin in bronchial secretions after intramuscular and endotracheal administration. J. Clin. Pharmacol. 15:518–524, 1975.
23. Newsom, S. W. B., Milstein, B. B. and Stark, J. E.: Local chemotherapy for *Pseudomonas* lung abscess. Lancet 2:530–531, 1974.
24. Klastersky, J., Geuning, C., Mouawad, E. and Daneau, D.: Endotracheal gentamicin in bronchial infections in patients with tracheostomy. Chest 61:117–120, 1972.
25. Lake, K. B., Van Dyke, J. J. and Rumsfeld, J. A.: Combined topical pulmonary and systemic gentamicin: the question of safety. Chest 68:62–64, 1975.
26. Pennington, J. E.: Kinetics of penetration and clearance of antibiotics in respiratory secretions. *In* Immunologic and Infectious Reactions in the Lung. C. H. Kirkpatrick and H. Y. Reynolds (Eds.). New York, Marcel Dekker, Inc., 1976, Ch. 17.
27. Wong, G. A., Peirce, T. H., Goldstein, E. and Hoeprich, P. D.: Penetration of antimicrobial agents into bronchial secretions. Am. J. Med. 59:219–223, 1975.
28. Stott, N. C. H. and West, R. R.: Randomised controlled trial of antibiotics in patients with cough and purulent sputum. Br. Med. J. 2:556–559, Sept., 1976.
29. Editorial: Chemotherapy of bronchitis. Br. Med. J. 1:125–126, Jan., 1970.
30. Ingold, A.: Sputum and serum levels of amoxicillin in chronic bronchial infections. Brit. J. Dis. Chest 69:211–216, 1975.
31. Hartnett, B. J. S. and Marlin, G. E.: Doxycycline in serum and bronchial secretions. Thorax 31:144–148, 1976.
32. Itkin, I. H. and Menzel, M. L.: The use of macrolide antibiotic substances in the treatment of asthma. J. Allergy 45:146–162, 1970.
33. Fekety, F. R., Caldwell, J., Gump, D., Johnson, J. E., Maxson, W., Mulholland, J. and Thoburn, R.: Bacteria, viruses and mycoplasmas in acute pneumonia in adults. Am. Rev. Respir. Dis. 104:499–507, 1971.
34. Sutton, D. R., Wicks, A. C. B. and Davidson, L.: One-day treatment for lobar pneumonia. Thorax 25:241–244, 1970.
35. Rahal, J. R.: A quick review of pneumonia therapy. Hosp. Physician, Sept., 1974, pp. 54–61.
36. Bartlett, J. G., Gorbach, S. L. and Finegold, S. M.: The bacteriology of aspiration pneumonia. Am. J. Med. 56:202–207, 1974.
37. Bartlett, J. G.: Treatment of postoperative pulmonary infections. Surg. Clin. North Am. 55:1355–1360, 1975.
38. Bartlett, J. G. and Finegold, S. M.: Anaerobic

infections of the lung and pleural space. Am. Rev. Respir. Dis. 110:56–77, 1974.

39. Lung abscess — Medical Staff Conference, University of California, San Francisco. West. J. Med. 124:476–482, Jun., 1976.

40. Huang, N. N., Laraya–Cuasay, L. R., Yasmin, N., Keith, H. H., Borden, M. and Cundy, K. R.: Clinical experience with amikacin in patients with cystic fibrosis. Am. J. Med. U.S. Amikacin Conference, 1977, pp. 186–195.

41. Cherry, J. D. and Welliver, R. C.: *Mycoplasma pneumoniae* infections of adults and children. West. J. Med. 125:47–55, July, 1976.

42. Codish, S. D. and Tobias, J. S.: Managing systemic mycoses in the compromised host. J.A.M.A. 235:2132–2134, 1976.

43. Young, L. S.: Antifungal agents: a ready reference to antimicrobial therapy. Hosp. Physician Sept., 1974, pp. 75–77.

44. Sarosi, G. A., Parker, J. D., Doto, I. L. and Tosh, F. E.: Chronic pulmonary coccidioidomycosis. N. Engl. J. Med. 283:325–329, 1970.

45. Eisenberg, R. S. and Oatway, W. H.: Nebulization of amphotericin B. Am. Rev. Respir. Dis. 103:289–292, 1971.

46. Harder, E. J. and Hermans, P. E.: Treatment of fungal infections with flucytosine. Arch. Intern. Med. 135:231–237, 1975.

47. Bennett, J. E.: The treatment of systemic mycoses. Rational Drug Therapy, Vol. 7, #4, April, 1973.

48. Lau, W. K. and Young, L. S.: Trimethoprim-sulfamethoxazole treatment of *Pneumocystis carinii* pneumonia in adults. N. Engl. J. Med. 295:716–718, 1976.

49. Byrd, R. B., Kaplan, P. D. and Gracey, D. R.: Treatment of pulmonary tuberculosis. Chest 66:560–567, 1974.

50. Barlow, P. B.: Treatment of tuberculosis. Basics of RD (published by the American Thoracic Society), Vol. 5, #1, Sept., 1976.

51. Bailey, W. C., Raleigh, J. W. and Turner, J. A. P.: Treatment of mycobacterial disease. (An official statement of the American Thoracic Society.) Am. Rev. Respir. Dis. 115:185–187, 1977.

52. Fox, W. and Mitchison, D. A.: Short-course chemotherapy for pulmonary tuberculosis. Am. Rev. Respir. Dis. 111:325–353, 1975.

53. Hudson, L. D. and Sbarbaro, J. A.: Twice weekly tuberculosis chemotherapy. J.A.M.A. 223:139–143, 1973.

54. Bartlett, J. G. and Gorbach, S. L.: Bacterial infections: initial therapy guidelines. Hosp. Physician, March 1974, pp. 27–47.

55. Thompson, J. H.: Chapters 52–61. In Essentials of Pharmacology. J. A. Bevan (Ed.). Hagerstown, Maryland, Harper and Row, 2nd ed., 1976.

56. Pines, A., Raafat, H., Siddiqui, S. M. and Greenfield, J. S. B.: Treatment of severe Pseudomonas infection of the bronchi. Brit. Med. J. 1:663–665, March, 1970.

57. Wang, R. I. H. and Garthwaite, S. M.: The clinical pharmacology of antibiotics II: Semisynthetic penicillins. Drug Therapy, Sept., 1974, pp. 87–99.

58. Garrod, L. P.: Choice among penicillins and cephalosporins. Brit. Med. J. 3:96–100, July, 1974.

59. Stewart, S. M., Fisher, M., Young, J. E. and Lutz, W.: Ampicillin levels in sputum, serum, and saliva. Thorax 25:304–311, 1970.

60. Weinstein, A. J.: Newer antibiotics: guidelines for use. Postgrad. Med. 60:75–80, Oct., 1976.

61. Barza, M. and Weinstein, L.: Pharmacokinetics of the penicillins in man. Clin. Pharmacokinetics. 1:297–308, 1976.

62. Pennington, J. E. and Reynolds, H. Y.: Concentrations of gentamicin and carbenicillin in bronchial secretions. J. Infect. Dis. 128:63–68, 1973.

63. Editorial: Cephalosporins, present and future. Lancet 2:364–365, 1973.

64. Johnson, A. J., MacArthur, C., Chadwick, M. V. and Wingfield, H. J.: Gastrointestinal absorption and sputum penetration of doxycycline. Am. Rev. Respir. Dis. 115, #4 Pt. 2:125, 1977.

65. Aitchison, W. R. C., Grant, I. W. B. and Gould, J. C.: Treatment of acute exacerbations in chronic bronchitis. Br. J. Clin. Pract. 22:343–345, 1968.

66. Chodosh, S., Baigelman, W. and Medici, T. C.: Methacycline compared with ampicillin in acute bacterial exacerbations of chronic bronchitis. Chest 69:587–592, 1976.

67. Ellithorpe, D. B., Gonzalez, R. and Mogabgab, W. J.: Antibiotic treatment of acute bronchial infections superimposed on chronic obstructive pulmonary disease. Curr. Therap. Res. 20:121–129, 1976.

68. Ayres, S. M., Griesbach, J. and Gianelli, S.: A study of bronchial irritation and systemic absorption of aerosolized kanamycin. Curr. Therap. Res. 14:153–157, 1972.

69. Dickie, K. J. and deGroot, W. J.: Ventilatory effects of aerosolized kanamycin and polymyxin. Chest 63:694–697, 1973.

70. Lifschitz, M. I. and Denning, C. R.: Safety of kanamycin aerosol. Clin. Pharmacol. Therap. 12:91–95, 1971.

71. Hoff, G. E., Schiotz, P. O. and Paulsen, J.: Tobramycin treatment of Pseudomonas aeruginosa infections in cystic fibrosis. Scand. J. Infect. Dis. 6:333–337, 1974.

71a. Dally, M. B., Kurrle, S. and Breslin, A. B. X.: Ventilatory effects of aerosol gentamicin. Thorax 33:54–56, 1978.

72. Rahal, J. J.: How to choose the newest aminoglycosides. Current Prescribing, Aug. 1977, pp. 30–35.

73. Bartlett, J. G.: Amikacin treatment of pulmonary infections involving gentamicin-resistant gram-negative bacilli. Am. J. Med. U.S. Amikacin Conference, 1977, pp. 151–154.

74. Pittinger, C. B., Eryasa, Y. and Adamson, R.: Antibiotic-induced paralysis. Anesth. Analg. 49:487–501, 1970.

75. Wright, E. A. and McQuillen, M. P.: Antibiotic-induced neuromuscular blockade. Ann. N.Y. Acad. Sci. 183:358–368, 1971.

76. Burns, M. W.: Indirect pathogenicity of gram-negative bacilli in the bronchi: the value of colistin aerosol. Brit. J. Dis. Chest 68:95–102, 1974.

77. Greenfield, S., Teres, D., Bushnell, L. S., Hedley-Whyte, J. and Feingold, D. S.: Prevention of gram-negative bacillary pneumonia using aerosol polymyxin as prophylaxis. J. Clin. Invest. 52:2935–2940, 1973.

78. Rose, H. D., Pendharker, M. B., Snider, G. L. and

Kory, R. C.: Evaluation of sodium colistimethate aerosol in gram-negative infections of the respiratory tract. J. Clin. Pharmacol. 10:274–281, 1970.

79. Lee, C., Chen, D. and Nagel, E. L.: Neuromuscular block by antibiotics: polymyxin B. Anesth. Analg. 56:373–377, 1977.

80. Lindesmith, L. A., Baines, R. D., Bigelow, D. B. and Petty, T. L.: Reversible respiratory paralysis associated with polymyxin therapy. Ann. Intern. Med. 68:318–327, 1968.

81. Koch-Weser, J., Sidel, V. W., Federman, E. B., Kanarek, P., Finer, D. C. and Eaton, A. E.: Adverse effects of colistimethate. Ann. Intern. Med. 72:857–868, 1970.

82. Waterman, D. H., Domm, S. E. and Rogers, W. K.: Total care of the chronic bronchitis patient. Dis. Chest 53:457–461, 1968.

83. Keusch, G. T. and Present, D. H.: Summary of a workshop on clindamycin colitis. J. Infect. Dis. 133:578–587, 1976.

84. Ziment, I., Barrett, P. V. D., Beall, G. N. et al.: Complications of antibiotic therapy. Calif. Med. 117:24–48, Nov., 1972.

85. Ziment, I.: Sulfonamides and urinary tract antibacterial agents. In Antimicrobial Therapy. B. M. Kagan (Ed.). Philadelphia, W. B. Saunders Company, 2nd ed., 1974, Ch. 12.

86. Ziment, I.: Sulfonamides et al.: A ready reference to antimicrobial therapy. Hosp. Physician. June, 1974, pp. 28–36.

87. Finland, M.: Combinations of antimicrobial drugs: trimethoprim-sulfamethoxazole. N. Engl. J. Med. 291:624–627, 1974.

88. Schiffman, D. O.: Evaluation of an anti-infective combination: trimethoprim-sulfamethoxazole (Bactrim, Septra). J.A.M.A. 231:635–637, 1975.

89. Moulding, T. and Davidson, P. T.: Tuberculosis I: drug therapy. Drug Therapy, Jan., 1974, pp. 79–88.

90. Mitchell, J. R., Zimmerman, H. J., Ishak, K. G., Thorgeirsson, U. P., Timbrell, J. A., Snodgrass, W. R. and Nelson, S. D.: Isoniazid liver injury: clinical spectrum, pathology, and probable pathogenesis. Ann. Intern. Med. 84:181–192, 1976.

91. Goldman, A. L. and Braman, S. S.: Isoniazid: a review with emphasis on adverse effects. Chest 62:71–77, 1972.

92. Neff, T. A. and Coan, B. J.: Incidence of drug intolerance to antituberculosis chemotherapy. Chest 56:10–12, 1969.

93. Poole, G., Stradling, P. and Worlledge, S.: Potentially serious side effects of high-dose twice-weekly rifampicin. Br. Med. J. 3:343–347, Aug., 1971.

94. Barker, B. M. and Prescott, F.: Antimicrobial Agents in Medicine. Oxford, Blackwell Scientific Publications, 1973.

95. Kucers, A. and Bennett, N. M.: The Use of Antibiotics. Philadelphia, J. B. Lippincott Company, 2nd ed., 1975.

96. Busey, J. F.: Modern concepts in the diagnosis and management of the pulmonary mycoses. American Thoracic Society, Clinical Notes on Respiratory Diseases. Vol. 14, #4, Spring, 1976.

97. Bennett, J. E.: Chemotherapy of systemic mycoses, I. N. Engl. J. Med. 290:30–31, 1974.

98. Einstein, H. E.: Coccidioidomycosis. In Management of Fungus Diseases of the Lungs. H. A. Buechner (Ed.). Springfield, Charles C Thomas, 1971, Ch. 4. (Supplemented by personal communication.)

99. Medoff, G. and Kobayashi, G. S.: Amphotericin B: Old drug, new therapy. J.A.M.A. 232: 619–620, 1975.

100. Oehling, A., Giron, M. and Subira, M. L.: Aerosol chemotherapy in bronchopulmonary candidiasis. Respiration 32:179–184, 1975.

101. Bennett, J. E.: Chemotherapy of systemic mycoses, II. N. Engl. J. Med. 290:320–321, 1974.

101a. Utz, J. P., Kravetz, H. M., Einstein, H. E., Campbell, G. D. and Buechner, H. A.: Chemotherapeutic agents for the pulmonary mycoses. Chest 60:260–262, 1971.

102. Editorial: Miconazole: a new antimycotic drug. Br. Med. J. 2:347, Aug., 1977.

103. Horsfield, K., Nicholls, A., Cumming, G., Hume, M. and Prowse, K.: Treatment of pulmonary aspergillosis with di-iodohydroxyquinoline. Thorax 32:250–253, 1977.

104. Hughes, W. T.: Treatment of Pneumocystis carinii pneumonitis. N. Engl. J. Med. 295:726–727, 1976.

105. Ziment, I. and Koppel, M. H. J.: Antimicrobials when kidneys can't cope. Current Prescribing, Aug., 1976, pp. 32–43.

106. Cherry, J. D.: Antimicrobials in pregnancy: what are the risks? Current Prescribing, March, 1976, pp. 35–38.

107. Ritschel, W. A.: Handbook of Basic Pharmacokinetics. Hamilton, Ill., Drug Intelligence Publications, Inc., 1976.

108. Sanford, J. P.: Guide to Antimicrobial Therapy 1977 (available from author, P.O. Box 34456, West Bethesda, MD 20034).

109. Braude, A. I.: Antimicrobial Therapy. Philadelphia, W. B. Saunders Company, 1976.

110. McCabe, W. R.: Chemotherapeutic and antibiotic agents. In Communicable and Infectious Diseases. F. H. Top and P. F. Werhle (Eds.). St. Louis, The C. V. Mosby Company, 8th ed., 1976, Ch. 5.

111. Finegold, S. M. and Hewitt, W. L.: Antibiotics: a ready reference to antimicrobial chemotherapy. Hosp. Physician, April, 1974, pp. 26–46.

112. Handbook of Antimicrobial Therapy. New Rochelle, N.Y., The Medical Letter on Drugs and Therapy, 1976.

113. Special series on antimicrobial agents. Mayo Clin. Proc. Vol. 52:#10 and 11, 1977.

11

AGENTS THAT AFFECT RESPIRATION

The process of breathing can be affected by drugs that act on the nervous controlling mechanisms, and by agents that act peripherally on the muscles involved in respiratory movements. Stimulation of respiration can be effected pharmacologically, although this approach is used relatively rarely, in deference to the greater success and reliability of mechanical methods coupled with adjunctive drug therapy designed to relieve associated problems such as bronchospasm, mucus impaction and infection. Respiratory stimulants have been in and out of vogue; currently, some of these analeptic agents may be commencing a limited recouping of former popularity.

A more common pharmacologic concern is that of respiratory depression: this can be a specific desired outcome of therapy, but it is all too often an unwanted side effect of treatment with drugs that have central depressant properties. Respiratory depression is a possible outcome of antitussive therapy, and is a danger in narcotic therapy. The use of primary analgesic or psychotherapeutic drugs is associated with the possibility of respiratory depression, particularly in patients who have underlying respiratory insufficiency; overdosage of such drugs often culminates in death from respiratory depression. Therapeutically planned respiratory depression is, of course, a concomitant of general anesthesia; occasionally, a patient requiring ventilatory support is subjected to

a general anesthetic or paralyzing drugs as part of the management of a difficult situation.

Discussion of various drugs that cause respiratory stimulation or depression constitutes the basis for this chapter.

RESPIRATORY STIMULANTS

Control of Respiration

Normal breathing is an automatic rhythmic function the control of which depends upon a complex regulatory set of nuclei scattered throughout the brainstem. The overall complex is known as the respiratory center; associated nuclei subserve various specialized functions, and are recognized as the cough center, sneeze center, and so on. It is known that the vomiting center is closely associated with these respiratory control nuclei, and it is postulated that a mucokinetic center also exists in this area of the hindbrain (see Chapter 2). The various centers receive afferent inputs from other central tracts in the brain, and from the IXth and Xth cranial nerves and other autonomic nerves. Localized chemoreceptor regions, mainly located on the ventrolateral surfaces of the medulla, are thought to be stimulated by the carbon dioxide content of the blood (which leads to changes in the acidity of the cerebrospinal fluid), and specifically by the acidity of the cerebrospinal fluid. Increases in $PaCO_2$ or, more specifically, decreases in CSF pH result in marked stimulation of the chemosensitive regions, whereas relative inhibition of respiration results from changes of $PaCO_2$ or pH in the opposite direction.[1-3]

The activity of the respiratory center is also markedly affected by incoming impulses that originate with the peripheral respiratory chemoreceptors. The most important of these are located in the carotid bodies,[2] whereas secondary chemoreceptors are found in the aortic bodies. They can be very sensitive to decreases in PaO_2, and are also stimulated by an increase in $PaCO_2$ (probably as a result of the corresponding fall in pH), but this stimulus is less effective than that provided by severe hypoxemia. These chemoreceptors can also be artificially stimulated by intravenously administered drugs. Agents that have been used experimentally include sodium cyanide (which causes intracellular hypoxia), lobeline, nicotine, acetylcholine, DMPP, anticholinesterases (such as physostigmine), ATP, veratridine, paraverine, potassium ions, serotonin, sulfides, phenyldiguanide and piperidine.[3] Relatively toxic doses of these agents may be required, and they cannot be regarded as therapeutic respiratory stimulants.

When the peripheral chemoreceptors are stimulated, afferent impulses are generated and reach the respiratory centers by means of the glossopharyngeal nerves from the carotid bodies and the vagus nerves from the aortic bodies; carotid body activity is also thought to be involved in the mechanism of asthma.[4] Decreased afferent outflow from the chemoreceptor bodies results from the negative or sedative effect of hyperoxemia on the carotid and aortic body sensory cells; in certain patients with reduced CO_2 chemosensitivity who are chronically hypoxic, hyperoxia, which abolishes the chemoreceptor response to the low PaO_2, can reduce the respiratory drive to levels that result in ventilatory failure. The effect of the increase in PaO_2 during oxygen therapy can overcome the stimulatory effect of an increase in $PaCO_2$; in such patients the elevated PaO_2 will abolish normal ventilation, even though the $PaCO_2$ might rise to high levels. It should be noted that the full explanation of this effect of oxygen has not yet been determined.[5]

The afferent stimulatory input into the respiratory center has an effect similar to that resulting from direct chemical stimulation of the medulla caused by a fall in pH. The result in each case is a corresponding increase in efferent output through the phrenic and intercostal nerves to the respiratory muscles, which respond with an increase in the frequency and depth of breathing. In a hypoventilating patient, such a response results in a restoration of blood gases toward normal with a subsequent improvement in the patient's clinical status.

Use of Respiratory Stimulants

For many years, physicians have sought to provide a pharmacologic stimulus that would result directly or indirectly in an increased output from the respiratory center. To some extent, irritant physical and psychic stimuli (for example, pain, IPPB, verbal exhortation) can achieve this outcome in a nonspecific fashion; the stimulus may result in central nervous system excitation, and the respiratory center participates in this response. Numerous pharmacologic agents have a similar effect, in that they can cause central excitation with secondary respiratory center activation. Agents of this type are referred to as *analeptics;* characteristically, they cause dose-dependent degrees of central stimulation that may culminate in convulsions.

Unfortunately, most analeptic agents that have been used to cause respiratory stimulation have a marked toxic potential, and any respiratory benefits may be outweighed by adverse central excitation. Moreover, the analeptic effect is transient, lasting only 5 to 10 minutes following an intravenous bolus; the benefits of such respiratory stimulation are unlikely to have any persistent therapeutic value. Analeptics were used extensively in former years in several situations: to reverse drug-induced (for example, barbiturate) narcosis, to help overcome the effects of alcoholic intoxication, and to hasten recovery from general anesthesia. They were also occasionally used by workers in the treatment of myxedema, Cheyne-Stokes breathing and in shock, but their value in such circumstances has never been satisfactorily demonstrated. Although few physicians use the available analeptics for such purposes currently, there would be a place for a safe, effective agent in the management of selected narcotized patients. However, their use in patients with chronic respiratory failure will remain dubious, since analeptics can work only as respiratory stimulants by causing an increase both in the work of breathing and in oxygen consumption, which may be intolerable to patients with abnormal respiratory mechanics. Thus, in respiratory failure, analeptic therapy can be utilized only for effecting a transient response; if such a brief result can be of value, then the use of a suitable agent can be condoned.

In practice, few respiratory physicians use analeptic stimulation under any circumstances.[6] Some enthusiasts claim that these drugs can be given to an acutely decompensated patient with chronic obstructive pulmonary disease to produce an increase in ventilation, which is achieved by a larger tidal volume and a slower respiratory rate.[7] Such an effect may be manifested by a sustained fall in $PaCO_2$, and to this extent analeptic therapy may be as effective as IPPB. Supporters of analeptic use claim that the central arousal and the respiratory center stimulation that these agents produce, when given as a rapid intravenous dose, result in a decrease in narcosis of a patient with respiratory failure, and that this response may be accompanied by the induction of a forceful cough. Thus, analeptics may act as tussive agents (see Table 9–17).

Skeptics who oppose the use of analeptics in the general management of respiratory failure are willing to admit there may be an occasional indication for their administration. Thus, when a worsening of respiratory failure has been precipitated or aggravated by injudicious use of oxygen or hypnotics, respiratory stimulants may be of value.[8] More recently, a multicenter trial of one of the best respiratory stimulants, doxapram, resulted in the conclusion that intravenous administration of the drug over the course of two hours could be effective in preventing a rise in the $PaCO_2$ of a patient with acutely decompensated chronic respiratory failure who was started on oxygen therapy.[9] Thus, it is fair to say that pharmacologic respiratory stimulants may be of value in certain patients and may serve as an alternative to or an adjunct to IPPB and other forms of respiratory augmentation. However, it is unlikely that any benefit can be expected after the first day of therapy, and there is little to suggest that chronic administration of these drugs offers any therapeutic advantages.[10]

Classes of Respiratory Stimulants
(Table 11–1)

Various agents can stimulate respiration either by direct or indirect effects on the respiratory center; in some cases, the phar-macokinetic mechanism has not been determined.[11] Physiologically, both hypoxemia and acidemia, including an increase in carbon dioxide tension, serve as respiratory stimulants, and in practice intravenous *acids* or *carbon dioxide* inhalation can be administered to produce a measurable respiratory response. *Sympathomimetic agents* have a nonspecific central excitatory effect, and can cause respiratory center stimulation; the nonbronchodilator psychoactive drugs are more potent in this respect. The *methylxanthines* also have a central action and can cause respiratory center stimulation. It should be noted that the basic liquid *ethylenediamine*, which is used as a solvent for theophylline in aminophylline, is also a respiratory center stimulant, with the particular property of being able to correct Cheyne-Stokes breathing (see Chapter 6).

Other agents, through their property of causing respiratory tract irritation, can stimulate breathing. Thus, various inhalational agents, such as ammonia, ether, and hypertonic and other aerosols, cause nonspecific nasal or tracheobronchial irritation, which results in gasping, coughing or sneezing through the activation of protective respiratory reflexes. Again, mechanical stimulation of the respiratory tract can produce a similar nonspecific reaction.

The largest class of respiratory stimulants are the analeptics, which will be discussed in detail below. Another class of important agents are various hormones, which will also be discussed in detail. Additional miscellaneous respiratory stimulants that merit consideration will also be discussed.

Analeptics. The term analeptic means "restorative"; drugs in this class are regarded as capable of exciting, or restoring to normal, cerebral and medullary functions. The analeptics of current interest have been divided into the following chemical classifications.[11, 12]

TETRAZOLES. These are related to one of the oldest analeptics, *camphor*. The only important therapeutic member of this class is *pentylenetetrazol*.

AROMATIC ACID AMIDES. The well-known and still useful member of this class is *nikethamide*. *Ethamivan* was formerly popular, but is rarely used currently.

GLUTARIMIDES. Glutarimide is a heterocyclic ring compound resembling barbituric acid; members of this class were thought to be specific competing antagonists of the barbiturates. *Bemegride* was the major drug in

TABLE 11-1. RESPIRATORY STIMULANTS

Class of Agent	Examples	Adult Dosage
Analeptics	See Table 11-2	
Hormones	Progesterone	100–200 mg/day I.M.
	Medroxyprogesterone	20 mg 3–4 times/day sublingual
	Estrogen (e.g. estradiol)	1–2 mg/day P.O.
	ACTH, adrenal hormones	No definite dosages
	Thyroid hormones	Dosages depend on thyroid status
	Insulin	Experimental
Methylxanthines	Caffeine	5–10 mg/kg 1–3 times/day P.O. or I.V.
	Theophylline	200–300 mg q6h P.O.
	(Ethylenediamine in amino-phylline)	250–400 mg q6h I.V. as aminophylline
Adrenergic and related agents	Ephedrine	25–50 mg P.O., S.C., I.M. or I.V.
	Amphetamine	2.5–15 mg q.i.d. P.O.
	Dextroamphetamine	10–20 mg q.i.d. P.O. or I.M.
	Methylphenidate	5–20 mg q.i.d. P.O.
	Levarterenol	1–2 mg/500 ml solute, I.V. infusion
Salicylates	Acetylsalicylic acid	6–8 gm I.V. over 1 hour (may be toxic,
	Sodium salicylate	and is therefore not advised)
Acids and acid salts	Carbon dioxide	5–10% CO_2 inhalation as required
	Hydrochloric acid	Experimental
	Ammonium chloride	1–2 gm q.i.d. P.O.
Peripheral chemo-receptor stimulants	Nicotine	Experimental
	Sodium cyanide	Experimental
Irritants	Ether	Light anesthesia
	Ammonia	Inhalation of fumes
Narcotic antagonists	Nalorphine	5–10 mg I.V.; up to 3 doses
	Levallorphan	1 mg I.V., then repeat 0.5 mg doses up to 3 mg
	Naloxone	0.1–0.4 mg S.C., I.M. or I.V. as needed
Carbonic anhydrase inhibitors	Acetazolamide	250–500 mg I.V. or P.O.
	Dichlorphenamide	50–100 mg b.i.d. P.O.

this class, and although it was once popular as a barbiturate antagonist, it is no longer used.

THIAZOLES.   Agents in this class may also be narcotic drug antagonists but they are no longer employed for this purpose. The marketed drug in this class was *amiphenazole*.

ALIPHATIC ACID AMIDES.   A mixture of two aliphatic acid dimethylamides has been marketed as *prethcamide*. Although it has not been used in the U.S., this agent has been reported on favorably in other countries.

BENZOPYRANONES   (chromones). The most important member of this series was *dimefline*, but the drug is no longer used, and will not be discussed further.

DIHYDROOXAZINEDIONES.   *Diethadione* was used as an analeptic, but it may cause toxic stimulation, and it is not used therapeutically.

BENZYLAMINES.   In this group is *fominoben*, which also has antitussive properties.

It has not been found to be of practical value, however.

PYRROLIDINONES.   One of the most potent compounds in this class is *doxapram*. This is one of the newest and most useful of the respiratory analeptic agents.

DILACTONES.   *Picrotoxin* is a naturally occurring analeptic that consists of picrotoxinin (which is active) and picrotin (which is inert). It is one of the most active central stimulants, and has little value as a specific respiratory stimulant.

PIPERIDINES.   *Lobeline* is a substituted piperidine, and is a traditional antiasthma remedy (see Chapter 4). It possesses analeptic properties that are of experimental rather than therapeutic interest. Piperidine itself is a stimulator of peripheral chemoreceptors.[3]

Additional former analeptics include camphor, strychnine and phthalic diethylamide (Neospiran);[6] none of these can be regarded as suitable respiratory stimulants. Other investigational analeptics have been described, including aethimizol, taloximine, DNPMT, PEY-1401, imidazole, DH-524 and SaH 41-178.[11]

Properties and Side Effects of Analeptics. The analeptic agents which stimulate the respiratory center all cause central excitation; the safest agents are those that have a relatively greater effect on respiration. Agents that readily cause central arousal are more likely to result in twitching; this may rapidly proceed to convulsions. The analeptic agents can cause an increase in the metabolic rate and may result in an increase in the oxygen debt of a respiratory patient.

Other central effects that may occur include restlessness, agitation, tremor, rigidity, disorientation, confusion, euphoria, hallucinations, dizziness, sweating, pyrexia paresthesiae, mydriasis, pilomotor erection and headaches. Respiratory manifestations of analeptic therapy may include coughing, sneezing, hyperventilation, dyspnea, laryngospasm, bronchospasm and hiccup. High doses of most analeptics cause hypertension, whereas lower doses may cause hypotension; other cardiovascular side effects may include bradycardia, extrasystoles, premature ventricular contractions, arrhythmias and chest discomfort. Additional problems are salivation, sour taste, nausea, vomiting, gastritis, defecation, urinary retention or incontinence, rashes (amiphenazole and prethcamide) and pruritus (doxapram). Analeptics are contraindicated in patients susceptible to seizures, or in those with blood pressure problems; they probably should not be used in asthmatics.

Individual Analeptic Agents (see Table 11–2). Several of the above agents may be of use in respiratory therapeutics.

DOXAPRAM. Doxapram is a pyrrolidinone derivative, and is currently the safest and best accepted of the respiratory stimulants, since it stimulates respiration more than it activates the cortical or spinal neurons.[11, 13] The drug is available only as a 2 per cent solution for intravenous use, and it may be given as a bolus of 140 mg,[14] or as a continuous infusion of 2 to 2.8 mg per minute for up to two hours;[9] tablet preparations have been used in some studies. The drug may be useful in acute respiratory failure, to prevent a rise of $PaCO_2$ with oxygen therapy.[9] It may also be of value postoperatively when given in combination with morphine or other analgesics that can depress respiration; the doxapram encourages deep breathing and coughing, and thereby can contribute to a decreased incidence of postoperative lung complications.[14] Doxapram may also be of value in initiating respiration in the newborn; it has been given both intravenously and lingually.[11] It can also be used to stimulate a sigh or to stimulate respiration postoperatively.[13]

Doxapram is safer and more effective than other respiratory stimulants; it is said to have a therapeutic:toxic ratio of 70:1,[6] although experience casts doubt on this claim. In view of its expense and short-lived effect, its role in respiratory therapeutics cannot be regarded as important.[15, 16] However, the undoubted effectiveness of the drug may justify further evaluation of its practical potential in the management of selected cases of respiratory failure, such as the hypoventilation syndromes.[16] Doxapram stimulates the carotid bodies as well as the medulla, and it can be a useful investigational tool for evaluating peripheral chemoreceptor function.

ETHAMIVAN (N,N-diethylvanillamide, vanillic diethylamide). Ethamivan has been available as tablets and solutions. Although it had been regarded as a useful form of therapy for respiratory depression,[17] it is rarely used currently. The intravenous dose recommended was 100 mg given over 20 to 30 seconds, followed by doses with 50 mg increments, if necessary, every 10 minutes; treatment is stopped if twitching or other side effects appear. Oral treatment was formerly available with tablets: as much as 320 mg every four hours was advocated for milder chronic respiratory failure,[17] but its alleged success must be regarded as dubious.

LOBELINE. This ancient drug (Chapter 1) is an alkaloid obtained from the leaves of *Lobelia inflata* (Indian tobacco). It has properties similar to those of nicotine but is much less potent; it has been used as a nicotine substitute (for example, in Nikoban) in programs (of doubtful value) designed to wean smokers from cigarettes. The drug in large doses can cause vomiting, diarrhea and diuresis, in addition to vasomotor, medullary and respiratory depression. Therapeutically, it is of little value, although it is still used in some herbal treatments for asthma. Thus, it is present in cigarettes and powders for burning, and the inhaled drug may have a bronchodilator and respiratory stimulant ef-

TABLE 11–2. ANALEPTIC AGENTS USED AS RESPIRATORY STIMULANTS

Agent	Availability	Sites of Action*	Usual Dosage‡	Possible Side Effects	Comment
Amiphenazole (Daptazole)		Medulla	100–400 mg I.V. or P.O. or 10 mg/min I.V.	Nausea, vomiting, rashes, insomnia, twitching, bone marrow depression	Was used as a barbiturate antagonist
Bemegride (Megimide)		CNS	50–1500 mg I.V.	Retching, nausea, twitching, hypertension or hypotension, convulsions	Was used as a barbiturate antagonist
Doxapram (Dopram†, Doxapril, Stimulexin)	20 mg/ml solutions	(1) Medulla (2) Carotid bodies	0.5–2 mg/kg up to 300 mg I.V. or P.O. or 1–5 mg/min I.V.; a total of up to 3 gm may be given I.V. during a course of treatment	Coughing, nausea, vomiting, sweating, pruritus, restlessness, hypertension, tachycardia, arrhythmias, tremors, rigidity, convulsions, laryngospasm, feeling of warmth, flushing	Safest and most effective respiratory stimulant; should be used according to manufacturer's instructions
Ethamivan (Emivan, Vandid)	(1) 20 mg/ml solution (2) 20 mg tablets	(1) CNS (2) Medulla (3) Carotid bodies	0.5–1.5 mg/kg up to 400 mg I.V. or 20–320 mg P.O.	Irritability, sneezing, gasping, laryngospasm, pruritus, twitching, convulsions, vasoconstriction, hypotension followed by hypertension.	Obsolete respiratory stimulant
Lobeline (Nikoban†)		Carotid bodies	3–10 mg I.V., I.M. or P.O.	Nausea, vomiting, diarrhea, coughing, mucokinesis, bronchodilation, tremors, dizziness, diaphoresis, paresis, headache, tachycardia, hypotension, coma	Was used in the treatment of asthma and as a mucokinetic agent; used as a nicotine substitute

Drug	Preparation	Site of action*	Dosage‡	Side effects	Comments
Nikethamide (Aminocordine, Anacardone, Cardiamide, Cormed, Coramine†, Nikorin, etc.)	25% solutions	(1) CNS (2) Carotid bodies	50–750 mg I.V. or I.M. or 20 mg/min I.V.	Sweating, nausea, vomiting, itching at back of nose, coughing, flushing, twitching, convulsions, anxiety, CNS depression, increase or decrease in blood pressure	Potent general and respiratory stimulant
Pentylenetetrazol (Analeptone†, Cardiazol Leptazol, Metrazol†)	(1) 100–200 mg/5 ml (2) 100 mg tablets	(1) CNS (2) Medulla	50 mg–2 gm parenteral or 100–300 mg P.O.	Convulsions, respiratory depression, increase in blood pressure	Potent central analeptic; more readily available than other analeptics
Picrotoxin (Cocculin)		Brainstem	3–6 mg I.V.	Sweating, nausea, vomiting, coughing, flushing, twitching, convulsions, anxiety, CNS depression, hypertension, arrhythmias	Potent central analeptic
Prethcamide (Micoren)	75 mg/ml	CNS	225–450 mg I.V. or P.O., or 20 mg/min. I.V.	Headache, paresthesiae, restlessness, excitement, twitching, tremors, flushing, dyspnea, coughing, nausea, vomiting, rashes	Effective respiratory stimulant

*CNS = nonspecific central nervous system sites of action
†Available in U.S.A.
‡Dosages may be given as needed, for example every 4 hours, or as a continuous infusion.

fect. The oral tincture is an emetic expectorant that is virtually obsolete. The intravenous preparation is also becoming obsolete as a respiratory stimulant.

NIKETHAMIDE (N,N-diethylnicotinamide). Some physicians regard this drug as a valuable respiratory stimulant. It can be given intravenously in a dosage of 20 mg/kg over the course of 15 minutes every two hours, for up to seven doses; repeat therapy can be administered after 12 hours.[7] Other workers prefer to give the drug as a continuous infusion. Nikethamide is regarded as one of the most effective analeptics; central and cardiac side effects can be expected if overzealous dosages are administered to stimulate respiration. The drug has a similar structure to that of ethamivan; it is converted in the body to nicotinamide.

PENTYLENETETRAZOL (pentetrazol). Pentylenetetrazol is an effective analeptic; it is no longer regarded as a respiratory stimulant, since it can cause twitching or convulsions.[13] It is available for oral as well as subcutaneous, intramuscular and intravenous administration, and has been used as a convulsant for the treatment of depression. The drug is used in several oral combination forms with various vitamins as a "stimulant" for geriatric patients.

PICROTOXIN. Picrotoxin is extracted from the berries of an East Indian shrub known as "fishberries," so named because, when thrown into the water, they can kill fish that eat them. The drug is a very potent analeptic, and it causes cardiovascular stimulation, which may be manifested as arrhythmias. When given intravenously, there is a long latency period (of 3 to 17 minutes, depending on the dose) before respiratory stimulation appears,[11] and the resulting breathing may be irregular. It is therefore a poor choice for use as a respiratory stimulant.

PRETHCAMIDE. Prethcamide can be given orally or intravenously. In the short-term, the drug may be an effective and safe respiratory stimulant. At present, this agent has not been utilized in the U.S., although it is still in favor in the United Kingdom.[18]

Hormones. Various hormones have been credited with the ability to stimulate respiration.[19] *Thyroid hormones* stimulate metabolism, and result in increased oxygen demands; this causes a corresponding increase in respiration. In contrast, one of the features of myxedema and other forms of hypothyroidism is relative hypoventilation, which can lead to respiratory failure.[20] Eupnea is restored in these patients when thyroid replacement therapy is initiated.

Other hormones that affect metabolism can result in respiratory stimulation (see Table 11–1): *catecholamines, insulin, ACTH, adrenal hormones* and *estrogen* have each been credited with this property.[21] However, the only important hormones with therapeutic value as respiratory stimulants are the *progestational agents*. It has long been known that hyperventilation occurs during pregnancy; studies have demonstrated that progesterone can cause an increase in minute ventilation and a fall in $PaCO_2$. This hormone also causes a slight rise in basal body temperature, but this contributes only a small part to the stimulation of respiration. Progesterone has been found to be an effective respiratory stimulant in certain classes of patients, including those with emphysema, hypoventilation due to obesity, and some cases of idiopathic alveolar hypoventilation. It appears that progesterone lowers the threshold of the respiratory center and increases its excitability, but the precise mechanism involved has not been determined.[21] Estrogen may have a similar effect on the respiratory center, but part of the effect of this hormone is caused by its stimulation of the metabolic rate of the body.

PROGESTERONE (Tables 11–1 and 11–3). Progesterone is a natural hormone produced by the corpus luteum and the placenta. Possible, but relatively rare, progestational side effects include the following: breast tenderness or galactorrhea, nervousness, insomnia, somnolence, dizziness, depression, thrombophlebitis, pulmonary embolus, pruritus, urticaria, general rash, anaphylaxis, acne, alopecia, hirsutism, nausea, cholestatic jaundice, headache, hyperpyrexia and menstrual irregularities. The preparation in oil, and to a greater degree the aqueous preparations, in dosages as large as 100 mg, may be painful on intramuscular injection; large doses may result in some catabolic effect and a transient increase in sodium and chloride excretion. It is available as generic preparations and as brand products (Table 11–3); the solutions are for intramuscular injection only. The recommended dosage is 100 to 200 mg I.M., and daily treatment can be given for many months, both to men and women. Patients with hypoventilation syndromes should show a response within hours, or at most within three days. The drug is unlikely to be beneficial in chronic obstructive airway disease; it is probably most

TABLE 11-3. PROGESTATIONAL HORMONES USED AS RESPIRATORY STIMULANTS*

Hormone	Brand Names	Tablets (mg)	Injections (mg/ml)
Progesterone	Progesterone in oil (various)		25, 50, 100
	Progesterone, aqueous (various)		25, 50, 100
	Lipo-Lutin (in oil)		50
	Proluton (in oil)		50
Medroxyprogesterone acetate	AMEN	10	
	Depo-Provera		100, 400
	Provera	2.5, 10	

*Numerous other progesterone-like agents are available, but they do not appear to have been used as respiratory stimulants.

effective in the obesity hypoventilation (pickwickian) syndrome,[22] and it may help reduce obesity in such patients.[22, 23] According to its advocates, the drug is usually well tolerated;[21] however, one may well wonder whether the pain on injection is responsible for much of the analeptic effect that is claimed for this drug.

MEDROXYPROGESTERONE. This is a synthetic progestational agent that has similar properties to progesterone, and it can be used as an alternative. The advantage of this agent is that it can be given orally or sublingually; a dose of 10 to 20 mg three or four times a day has been used. Intramuscular medroxyprogesterone acetate can also be given once a day.[23] The main side effect of prolonged therapy is impotency in males,[22] but other side effects, similar to those of progesterone, may occur.

Methylxanthines. *Theophylline* and its derivatives can stimulate the respiratory center, and since other favorable cardiopulmonary responses are produced (Chapter 6), these drugs may have a far more beneficial effect in respiratory failure than the analeptic agents. As already discussed, the ethylenediamine in aminophylline also has a stimulatory and regularizing effect on respiratory center function.

CAFFEINE. Caffeine is the xanthine with the greatest analeptic effect, and it is still regarded by some physicians as an effective respiratory stimulant. It is probably most useful for the treatment of apnea in premature neonates;[24] it is less likely to be of value in older patients, but some physicians use it in the management of barbiturate-induced narcosis. For parenteral (as well as oral) administraton, caffeine is made more water soluble by combination with sodium benzoate; caffeine itself or in citrated form is available for oral use (Table 11-4). The respiratory stimulant dose is equivalent to 5 to 10 mg/kg of caffeine orally or intravenously, up to a maximum of 500 mg, given one to three times a day. The analeptic dosage for adults is 200 mg of caffeine, 300 mg of citrated caffeine, or 500 mg of caffeine and sodium benzoate.

Adrenergic Agents. The sympathomimetic adrenergic-receptor stimulating agents have been considered in detail in Chapters 4 and 5. Agents that possess selective beta-2 function are valuable bronchodilators, whereas agents with more alpha-activity serve as pressor agents (some of these were discussed in Chapter 9). Both groups of drugs may have central stimulatory effects. Noncatecholamine sympathomimetic agents, such as amphetamine, have much more potent central stimulatory properties. Some of these drugs can serve as analeptics. *Ephedrine, amphetamine, dextroamphetamine* and *levarterenol* all have such properties. Some authors regard them as being respiratory stimulants; however, this action is completely nonspecific, and is simply a reflection of the central stimulation that they cause.

METHYLPHENIDATE (Ritalin). Methylphenidate is of particular interest, although it is not a catecholamine-like drug; it is a piperidine derivative, which has a structural relationship to amphetamine. Methylphenidate also has some properties in common with amphetamine: thus, it is a central stimulant, but it has more effect on mental than on motor function. Like amphetamine, dextroamphetamine and ephedrine, this agent has been used in the treatment of narcolepsy. Methylphenidate has probably

TABLE 11-4. AMPHETAMINE AND CAFFEINE PREPARATIONS

Product	Tablets (mg)	Timed-Release Capsules (mg)	Elixirs (mg/ml)	Injections (mg/ml)
AMPHETAMINE PRODUCTS*				
Amphetamine HCl	5,10,15	15		20
Amphetamine sulfate (Benzedrine, generic)	5,10	15		
Dextroamphetamine HCl (Daro)	5	15		
Dextroamphetamine sulfate (Curban, Dexedrine, generic)	5	5,10,15	1	
Dextroamphetamine tannate (Obotan)		5,7.5†		
Methamphetamine HCl (Desoxyn, Fetamin, Obedrin-LA)	2.5,5,10	5,10,15		
CAFFEINE PRODUCTS				
Caffeine		100,250		
Citrated caffeine	65			
Caffeine and sodium benzoate				250,500*

*Require prescription
†Equivalent dose of base

been more successful than the other adrenergic agents when used as a respiratory stimulant.[6] Thus, 10 mg q.i.d. of the drug has been reported to be of value in the management of alveolar hypoventilation.[25] In practice, 10 to 20 mg doses should be tried on a lethargic, hypoventilating patient, such as an individual who has just been weaned from ventilatory support given for the management of respiratory failure. Additional doses can be given as required, but no more than four doses a day are advised, since severe agitation and seizures or psychosis may be induced, although the more usual side effects are nervousness, insomnia and anorexia. Other possible adverse problems include dizziness, dyskinesis, nausea, abdominal pain, rash, hypertension, hypotension, headache, tachycardia and arrhythmias. However, careful use of this stimulatory drug may be of value in selected hypoventilating, sleepy, patients who need to be aroused into a more cooperative state to partake of routine respiratory therapy. It should be noted that the drug increases respiratory rate, but might not result in an augmented effective alveolar ventilation.[13]

Acetylsalicylic Acid (aspirin). Acetysalicylic acid is generally regarded as an antipyretic and analgesic. However, relatively large doses of this drug have marked, and complex, effects on respiration. Therapeutic doses result in uncoupling of oxidative phosphorylation, and thereby increase oxygen consumption and CO_2 production. The CO_2 stimulates respiration, resulting in an increase in the depth of breathing; if the respiratory center is narcotized, however, the $PaCO_2$ increases and a respiratory acidosis develops. A second action of aspirin results from direct stimulation of the medulla, causing both an increase in the rate and depth of breathing. Larger doses of aspirin given acutely can result in this action predominating, thereby producing a respiratory alkalosis. Serious overdosage with aspirin causes respiratory center depression, and the patient will manifest a severe respiratory acidosis: pulmonary edema can also occur, and vasomotor collapse is likely, which results in an associated metabolic acidosis.

Although aspirin can be considered to be a respiratory stimulant, its effects are complex, and numerous toxic manifestations may occur. Other severe side effects of large doses of aspirin may also appear: these include the syndrome of salicylism, characterized by headache, dizziness, ringing in the ears (tinnitus), impaired hearing, impaired vision, confusion, lassitude, nausea, vomiting and diarrhea. Other salicylate complications include a hemorrhagic tendency, gastrointestinal bleeding, rashes and encephalopathy. Since the respiratory stimulant dose of aspirin is about 6 to 8 gm, whereas the therapeutic antipyretic dose is 0.325 to 1 gm, this drug is not of practical value in the management of depressed respiration.

Narcotic Antagonists (Table 11–5). Not infrequently, a sedative or analgesic drug is given to a patient with chronic lung disease, and causes respiratory center depression resulting in ventilatory failure; the same problem can arise in people with normal lungs following an excessive dose of a narcotic. This situation may particularly arise in the postoperative period, where mucociliary clearance is impaired by the pain of the surgical procedure, but injudicious prescribing of a sedative for a panicky asthmatic patient accounts for all too many cases of iatrogenic hypoventilation. When drug-induced respiratory failure is suspected, the patient can be given one of several narcotic antagonist drugs that can reverse the respiratory depression. However, these agents themselves can cause respiratory depression, and they are of value only as competitors of opiate and other analgesic depressants. The pharmacologic classification of these agents is rather difficult, since their modes of action are complex;[26, 27] unclassified agents are under investigation, for example taloximine.[27]

The narcotic antagonists can reverse narcotic-induced respiratory depression, and their parenteral administration results in prompt increase in respiratory rate and minute volume. However, the effect is shorter lasting (one to four hours) than the depressant effect of the narcotic drug, and repeated doses of the antagonist may be required until the effect of the narcotic finally wears off. The antagonist may also counteract the analgesic effect of the narcotic;

therefore, in postoperative patients who require analgesia, it can be difficult to provide the correct balance of narcotic sedation on one hand, and reversal of respiratory depression by the narcotic antagonist on the other hand.

Narcotic antagonists must not be used to treat respiratory depression that results from causes other than narcotic administration. They are not effective at reversing depression caused by barbiturates and similar sedatives; indeed, some of the narcotic antagonists will potentiate the respiratory depression in such situations. Since it is not always obvious that respiratory depression in a specific patient is due entirely to a narcotic that has been given, the narcotic antagonists must always be given in relatively small dosage, with careful monitoring to evaluate the effect, and with persistent observation to ensure that the depression has been overcome. In such situations, naloxone is the safest agent to utilize, as will be explained.

The only important narcotic antagonists are the three agents discussed as follows.

LEVALLORPHAN (Lorfan). This is the N-allyl analogue of levorphanol (Levo-Dromoran). It is a potent drug, and a dosage of 1 mg given intravenously often suffices in adults. If necessary, one or two additional 0.5 mg doses can be given at 10 minute intervals, but the total dose should not exceed 3 mg. For children, the initial dose is 0.02 mg/kg; for neonates, a dose of 0.05 to 0.1 mg is given by injection into the umbilical vein.

NALORPHINE (Nalline). Nalorphine is the N-allyl analogue of morphine. It has only

TABLE 11–5. NARCOTIC ANTAGONISTS

| | Dosages* | | | | |
| | **Adult (mg)** | | Children | Availability | |
Agent	INITIAL	MAXIMUM	(mg/kg)	(mg/ml)	**Comment**
Levallorphan tartrate† (Lorfan)	1	3	0.02	1	Similar to nalorphine, but more potent
Nalorphine HCl† (Nalline)	5–10	30	0.1	5	Can produce analgesia and respiratory depression
Naloxone HCl (Narcan)	0.2–0.4	1.2	0.01	0.02, 0.4	No analgesic or depressant properties; safest of the narcotic antagonists

*Usually given I.V.; may be given S.C. or I.M.
†Rarely used currently.

one-tenth the potency of levallorphan, and it is given in a dosage of 5 to 10 mg to adults; up to three doses may be given over the course of 30 minutes. Neonates should initially be given from 0.2 mg up to a maximum of 0.5 mg; children require 0.1 mg/kg. This drug is similar to levallorphan in its actions and side effects.

NALOXONE (Narcan). Naloxone is the N-allyl derivative of oxymorphone (Numorphan). Unlike levallorphan and nalorphine, naloxone does not possess agonist opiate properties: it is not an analgesic and it does not itself cause respiratory depression or potentiate barbiturate and other nonnarcotic sedatives. It is the safest and therefore the preferred drug for treating respiratory depression when the cause is uncertain and a narcotic is suspected. If the patient does not improve, then it is unlikely that a narcotic is responsible for the condition—and no harm will have been caused to the patient.

Naloxone is potent and it is rapidly effective; it can be given subcutaneously or intramuscularly as an alternative to intravenous injection, since these routes result in an effect within two minutes. The drug is comparatively very free of adverse effects and, unlike levallorphan and nalorphine, it is not a Scheduled narcotic drug; its greater safety has rendered both levallorphan and nalorphine obsolescent.

The appropriate dose of naloxone for adults is 0.4 mg; repeat dosages can be given if needed at three-minute intervals. Children and neonates require 0.01 mg/kg initially; repeat doses can be given if required. The action of naloxone is somewhat more persistent than that of the other narcotic antagonists, lasting three to five hours. This drug may be of great value other than as a treatment for narcotic-induced respiratory depression. Thus, it may be helpful in the treatment of narcotic addiction, and it may be able to prevent the development of some of the psychic features of narcotic dependency in a patient requiring the prolonged administration of a narcotic analgesic.[28, 29] In a patient with a depressed respiratory center, such as can be anticipated in the presence of chronic obstructive disease, sedative or narcotic therapy may be required; in such a case the simultaneous administration of naloxone may prevent the development of an increase in $PaCO_2$. Since it is not always clinically evident that a respiratory patient is at risk of suffering ventilatory depression when a sedative drug is administered, the patient should be monitored, and naloxone should be given if carbon dioxide retention occurs.

Carbon Dioxide. As described at the beginning of this chapter, carbon dioxide, and the lowered pH that it causes in the blood and the cerebrospinal fluid, serves as a potent respiratory center stimulant. It is also postulated that CO_2 stimulates respiration by acting on specific receptors in the lung.[30] Whatever the full explanation for the actions of CO_2, it is the most effective chemical stimulant of respiration available, and it is occasionally administered for this purpose in respiratory therapy.

As an alternative to the provision of CO_2, it is usually more convenient to arrange for the patient to rebreathe his own expired gas. This can be achieved very simply by having the patient breathe in and out of a small bag; such therapy is adequate for most people who present with symptoms caused by the hyperventilation syndrome. Rebreathing techniques are also advocated by many surgeons as a stimulus to deep breathing and coughing to prevent atelectasis in postoperative patients: simple devices, such as a rubber glove fitted around a mouthpiece, or somewhat more complex equipment, such as the Adler rebreather or the Dale-Schwartz tube, can be used as alternatives to IPPB.[31]

Although the breathing of CO_2 can serve to stimulate respiration in patients with a normal $PaCO_2$, obviously it is inappropriate to use this form of therapy in patients who are already retaining CO_2. Carbon dioxide is therefore in a separate category from the other respiratory stimulants, which are used mainly for the management of patients manifesting hypoventilation. The administration of carbon dioxide in concentrations of 2 to 10 per cent was used to some extent in the past to stimulate deep breathing during the recovery from surgical procedures, but at present IPPB, incentive spirometry or chest physiotherapy are preferred. Carbon dioxide administration could also be used as a test for the degree of narcosis in a patient drugged by morphine, barbiturates or similar agents; if the subject shows a clinical response to 7 to 10 per cent CO_2 administration, by increasing the depth of breathing, then it can be assumed that the depth of narcosis is not too great and that spontaneous recovery will probably ensue.[32] It is of interest that propranolol, a beta-blocking agent, reduces the central response to carbon dioxide.[33] A more practical use of CO_2 is in the treatment of poisoning by noxious gases such as carbon monoxide, since the respiratory stimulation provided by the CO_2 will result in a more rapid blowing off of the noxious gas: 7 to 10 per cent CO_2 can be used for this purpose.[32] In modern respiratory practice, these uses of CO_2 in narcotic or noxious gas poisoning are rarely employed, although anesthesiologists may utilize the approach on some patients.

Some minor uses for CO_2 inhalation include the treatment of hiccups, and for production of vasodilation. The latter action was thought to be of value in cerebrovascular disease, but this is no longer considered to be a valid concept. Much of the therapeutic CO_2 gas used in respiratory work today is employed in pulmonary function studies, particularly in studying the respiratory response of a patient to various concentrations of the gas when evaluating the integrity of respiratory control. When combined with helium gas, the degree of ventilatory response can be used to help differentiate between respiratory center depression and airway obstruction.[34]

Carbon dioxide has a variety of different clinical effects on the brain and circulation as well as on breathing. If a concentration of less than 2 per cent is administered to a normal person, few significant clinical effects may appear. With concentrations of 2 to 5 per cent, the subject may gradually develop a respiratory acidosis; if the peripheral chemoreceptors and the respiratory center are functioning normally, slight hyperventilation will occur, and the $PaCO_2$ will be kept within the normal range. A 5 per cent concentration of CO_2 has a partial pressure of about 35 mm Hg, which is close to that in the normal arterial blood. A concentration of 10 per cent CO_2 has a partial pressure of about 70 mm Hg, and breathing such a gas mixture will result in a progressive increase in $PaCO_2$ toward this level. In practice, such a high concentration usually results in considerable respiratory stimulation, which will be apparent within two minutes; a normal adult breathing 10 per cent CO_2 will respond with a minute volume of about 75 liters.[35] Continued administration of such a high concentration will cause loss of consciousness and convulsions within about 10 minutes. Concentrations higher than 10 per cent have only slightly greater quantitative effects; such CO_2 mixtures can be fatal.[36]

The therapeutic range of CO_2 concentrations is, therefore, in the region of 5 to 8 per cent, with 5 per cent CO_2 in 95 per cent O_2 being the safest and most suitable mixture. Breathing this gas will result in hyperventilation in a normal person; there will be a sensation of deep breathing without the discomfort of true dyspnea. After 10 minutes or so, the patient is liable to undergo general vasodilation, which will cause a fall in blood pressure, and this may be manifested by faintness. Other subjective sensations include dizziness, headache, tingling, a sensation of cold, palpitations, visual dimming, tremors, nausea, restlessness, general discomfort and mental depression.[35-37] Prolonged breathing of CO_2 in a concentration of 5 to 8 per cent will cause central depression, and possibly coma, but convulsions are less likely to appear. Other possible toxic complications include vomiting, disorientation and hypertension, and signs of CNS damage.[36]

Carbon dioxide in air or with oxygen can be obtained for therapeutic or diagnostic use. It is advisable to use no more than a 6 per cent concentration of CO_2 in 94 per cent oxygen; the gas should be administered by a well-fitted nonrebreathing mask, which should be held to the patient's face by an attendant. Adverse effects should be watched for during, and for 10 minutes after, the treatment; the CO_2 administration should not be continued for more than 10 minutes.[37] It must be emphasized that this use of CO_2 as a respiratory stimulant is rarely necessary, and can be used only on a subject capable of normal respiratory responses who is not retaining carbon dioxide. A further benefit from breathing this concentration of carbon dioxide may be achieved since, as discussed in Chapter 4, 6 per cent CO_2 can cause some relaxation of the airways in asthmatics. It is of interest that inhalation of carbon dioxide was advocated in the last century as one of many unproven modalities in the treatment of respiratory disease (see Chapter 1). For further discussion of carbon dioxide, see Chapter 13.

Carbonic Anhydrase Inhibitors. Several diuretic drugs exert their effects by inhibiting the enzyme carbonic anhydrase in the proximal tubules of the kidney. The enzyme catalyzes the first of the two reversible reactions: $CO_2 + H_2O \rightleftarrows H_2CO_3 \rightleftarrows H^+ + HCO_3^-$. As a result of this enzymic activity, the carbon dioxide in the blood is converted rapidly into carbonic acid, which immediately ionizes to provide hydrogen and bicarbonate ions. The hydrogen ion is exchanged for sodium ions, which are then reabsorbed from the ultrafiltrate in the renal tubules. When a carbonic anhydrase inhibitor is administered, the availability of exchangeable hydrogen ions is marked diminished, and there is decreased ability to reabsorb sodium and potassium. As a result, sodium loss occurs, and bicarbonate ions accompany the outflow of the sodium resulting in a loss of this buffer ion. The final consequence of the effective diuresis of sodium bicarbonate from the blood is an alkalinization of the urine and development of metabolic acidosis in the blood. The fall in pH results in a potent stimulation of the respiratory center, and relative hyperventilation occurs until sufficient CO_2 is blown off to match the bicarbonate diuresis, thereby restoring the pH toward normal. However, some patients may not be able to muster an adequate ventilatory response, and respiratory failure may worsen as a result of carbonic anhydrase inhibitor therapy.[38] In spite of this possibility, these drugs were extensively used in the 1950s and 1960s as respiratory stimulants, but they generally produced only transient effects on stimulating an increase in carbon dioxide excretion.

Another value of these drugs in respiratory therapy is to create a rapid bicarbonate diuresis in a patient with a severe metabolic alkalosis. Such a situation can arise when a patient with chronic respiratory failure is placed on a respirator and the excessive stores of CO_2 are blown off too rapidly by overvigorous ventilation. The increased body stores of bicarbonate will remain in this situation to cause a considerable and possible dangerous increase in the pH: when this exceeds 7.6 there is a marked potential for severe epileptiform seizures to occur. If a suitable carbonic anhydrase inhibitor is given intravenously, there is a brisk diuresis of bicarbonate within minutes, and an acid urine may be rapidly converted to an alkaline pH.[39]

ACETAZOLAMIDE (Diamox). Acetazolamide is the best-known carbonic anhydrase inhibitor. It was used formerly as a diuretic; currently, there are many superior diuretics, thus the drug is rarely used now. Acetazolamide is a sulfonamide derivative, and it is usually well tolerated: side effects include drowsiness and paresthesiae, and hypersensitivity reactions similar to those caused by the sulfonamides (Chapter 10) occur occa-

sionally. The drug is still used to decrease intraocular pressure in glaucoma, and it may be a helpful adjunct in the management of some forms of epilepsy. It can be used to alkalinize urine, which can be of value as a means of increasing the excretion of overdoses of salicylate. A further occasional use is in the treatment of periodic paralysis.

Although acetazolamide is rarely used as a respiratory stimulant currently, it may have a respiratory use in the prevention or treatment of high-altitude sickness:[40] the mechanism involved is not entirely worked out, but leads to a decrease of HCO_3^- in the arterial blood and cerebrospinal fluid.[41]

Acetazolamide is available as Diamox, in tablets of 125 and 250 mg and as time-release capsules containing 500 mg. The parenteral solution is best used intravenously, and dosages up to 500 mg can be given. The usual adult dose is 250 to 500 mg a day for diuresis, but alternate-day therapy may be adequate. For other purposes, the dosage may be repeated every four hours if needed when managing an acute problem.

DICHLORPHENAMIDE (Daranide). This drug is not structurally related to acetazolamide, and it differs from the latter in causing an increase in excretion of chloride as well as sodium, potassium, bicarbonate and water. Dichlorphenamide is a more effective diuretic than acetazolamide, and it causes less metabolic acidosis. Although dichlorphenamide is still regarded as a respiratory stimulant by some workers,[42] it is rarely used for this purpose, although it is a preferred carbonic anhydrase inhibitor for the management of glaucoma.

The side effects of dichlorphenamide are similar to those of acetazolamide. The drug is available as 50 mg tablets, and the dose that has been used for respiratory stimulation is 50 to 100 mg twice a day.

Additional carbonic anhydrase inhibitor diuretics are *methazolamide* (Neptazane) and *ethoxzolamide* (Cardrase, Ethamide): these agents are similar to acetazolamide and they may be less likely to cause side effects.

RESPIRATORY DEPRESSANTS

Many different classes of drugs can have an adverse effect on respiration, and drugs of numerous kinds when taken purposefully or accidentally in excessive amount may result in death through respiratory depression. Patients with acute asthma or with any of the chronic obstructive pulmonary diseases are particularly vulnerable to drug-induced respiratory depression, and great care has to be exercised when prescribing a central nervous system depressant drug to such patients. Elderly people, and patients with impaired hepatic or renal function who do not metabolize and excrete drugs in a normal fashion, are also susceptible to this adverse outcome when given the normal dosage of a drug with depressant properties.

Certain classes of drugs are utilized for their depressant effect on the brain and on respiration, the most obvious example being the general anesthetics. Paradoxically, they may be utilized to help patients with respiratory disease in appropriate circumstances: thus, general anesthesia can be used in the management of intractable asthma, as described in Chapter 4, in which the effects of the important general anesthetics on respiration are described (see Table 4–20). Similarly, narcotic drugs and related depressant agents are utilized for their suppressive effect on the cough center, as described in detail in Chapter 9. A number of nonnarcotic antitussives, such as isoaminile and pipazethate, also depress the respiratory center, although several of these agents may actually stimulate respiration, for example benzonatate, chlophedianol, dextromethorphan, noscapine and sodium dibunate (Table 9–11).

Many drugs used in the treatment of psychiatric disorders can have a depressant effect on central nervous activity and may cause respiratory depression in susceptible patients. It is probable that the majority of chronic respiratory disease victims develop neuropsychiatric problems during the course of their illness, and grounds for prescribing psychotherapeutic drug therapy are not unusual. Thus, asthmatic and other respiratory patients frequently complain of anxiety or depression, and many of them have difficulty in sleeping; some develop frank psychoses or severe neuropsychiatric problems. In cases such as these, the physician is faced with a therapeutic dilemma in trying to provide appropriate management without causing harm. In general, psychotherapeutic drugs should be avoided in these patients, particularly those agents with a sedative effect; but when pharmacologic therapy is deemed necessary, an agent with minimal effects on the central nervous system should be selected.

Whenever a drug with respiratory depressant properties is prescribed to a patient with obstructive respiratory disease, the smallest effective dose should be given initially, and any increase in dosage should be made cautiously with appropriate monitoring to ensure that no adverse effects are caused by the drug. Other properties of the drug should be taken into account, such as anticholinergic effects that may have an adverse drying action on the respiratory mucosa. Thus, antihistamines, which have such a drying effect as well as sedative properties (see Chapter 9), should be used with great care in respiratory patients.

In the following sections, psychotherapeutic drugs will be considered with regard to their effects on respiration. It should be recognized that adequate formal evaluations of most of the drugs to be described have not been carried out in patients with respiratory disease; therefore, in all cases, each agent should be prescribed with the appreciation that any individual patient may be susceptible to more profound respiratory depression than would occur in a subject with normal airways. The only recent review that has evaluated the effects of psychotropic drugs on respiration is a comprehensive analysis by Steen. In general, it appears that there is little evidence that any of the antianxiety drugs, antipsychotic drugs, antidepressant drugs or nonnarcotic analgesic drugs have major depressant effects on respiration, while the narcotic, hypnotic and sedative drugs do possess this potentially dangerous property.[43]

Classes of Psychotropic Drugs

Various classifications have been proposed for the drugs that have a predominant effect on the central nervous system, but no scheme is totally satisfactory.[44, 45] In each class of medication, numerous drugs have been marketed, although they differ to only a minor degree from the important well-established drugs in each category.[44, 46] The classification provided here and the representative drugs do not conform to any established order, and an attempt is made to simplify the complex and confusing topic of psychotherapeutic pharmacology. In Table 11–6, some of the main pharmacologic differences between the psychotherapeutic drugs are presented. Individual drugs belonging to the different categories do not

TABLE 11–6. COMPARISON OF PSYCHOTROPIC DRUGS

	Tricyclic Antidepressants e.g. AMITRIPTYLINE	Sedative- Hypnotics e.g. PHENOBARBITAL	Minor Tranquillizers e.g. DIAZEPAM	Antipsychotics e.g. CHLORPROMAZINE
Sleep potentiation	+ or −	+++	++	±
Relief of pain	−	−	+	±
Relief of anxiety	+	++	+++	+ or ++
Relief of mania	−	+	+	+++
Relief of depression	+++	−	−	±
Useful in schizophrenia	−	±	±	+++
Muscle relaxant	−	+	+++	++
Anticonvulsant	−	+++	+++	−
Respiratory depression	±	++	+	− or +
Adrenergic potentiation	+	−	−	−
Adrenergic blockade	−	−	±	++
Antihistaminic	+	−	−	+
Antiserotonin	−	−	±	+++
Anticholinergic	+++	−	−	++
Addiction potential	−	+++	+++	−
Central side effects	++	++	+	+++
Psychomotor side effects	++	+	+	+++
Production of amnesia	±	+	+	+
Useful in alcoholism	−	−	+++	+
Useful in hiccups	−	±	±	++
Preanesthesia adjunct	±	++	+	±

necessarily demonstrate the tabulated properties, but the listed representative agents of each class do possess the characteristics that are contrasted in this table.

Anesthetics and the opioid narcotic analgesics will not be discussed further since their noteworthy properties in respiratory therapy have already been considered in earlier chapters. The less potent analgesics will be described, and then the true psychotropic drugs will be discussed, that is, the sedative-hypnotics, the minor tranquillizers, major tranquillizers and the antidepressants.

Nonopiate Analgesics. A number of analgesic agents, which are of potency comparable to that of morphine, lack the mind-affecting and addictive qualities of the true opioids that were discussed in Chapter 9. The most important of these are presented in Table 11–7, and they are contrasted with the very familiar mild analgesics, acetaminophen, propoxyphene and salicylates, which can be safely given to respiratory patients. The most familiar and potent of these nonopiates is meperidine, which does have addictive properties; pentazocine is also somewhat susceptible to addiction, but this problem has not been described with the remaining agents. Some of the drugs listed have predominant sedative or sleep-inducing properties, and several can cause respiratory center depression; they should

be utilized with appropriate care in patients with respiratory disease.

MEPERIDINE (Demerol). This drug has already been discussed in Chapters 4 and 9. It is less potent as an analgesic than morphine, and it is much less effective when given orally than parenterally. Meperidine possesses sedative and respiratory depressant effects that are comparable to those of morphine, and it can cause depression of neonatal breathing if given to a mother during parturition; this effect can be reversed by use of a narcotic antagonist. Since meperidine is also a drug of addiction and it can cause bronchoconstriction, it offers no real advantages over morphine as an analgesic for respiratory patients.

Side effects of meperidine include dizziness, nausea, vomiting, dry mouth, sweating, visual disturbances, palpitations, weakness, postural hypotension, syncope and euphoria. Potentiation or unfavorable reactions occur when meperidine is combined with major tranquillizers or antidepressants. The drug may cause more side effects in ambulatory patients than in bed patients.

Meperidine can be given to adults orally or intramuscularly in a dosage of 50 to 100 mg every three to four hours. Intravenous administration can cause severe hypotension and tachycardia. When given to a respiratory patient, adverse effects on breathing may be reversed by administering 0.4 mg naloxone

TABLE 11–7. NONOPIATE ANALGESICS

Drug	Adult Dosage (mg)	Analgesic Potency	Antitussive Effect	Respiratory Depression	Addiction Potential	Clinical Notes
Acetaminophen* (Tylenol, etc.)	325–650 P.O.	+	–	–	–	Similar to salicylates, with less gastric irritation; overdose can cause hepatic necrosis
Alphaprodine (Nisentil)	20–60 S.C. 20–30 I.V.	++(+)	+	+	±	Similar to meperidine, but shorter duration of action
Anileridine (Leritine)	25–75 P.O., S.C., I.M.	++(+)	++	++	±	Similar to meperidine, but more effective when given orally
Ethoheptazine (Zactane)	50–150 P.O.	+(+)	–	–	–	Central stimulating effect with parenteral administration may occur
Fentanyl (Sublimaze)	0.025–0.1 I.V., I.M.	++	+++	+++	+	Short-acting and very potent; used as an adjunct to anesthesia, and in neuroleptanaglesia
Meperidine (Demerol)	50–150 S.C., I.M.	++	±	+++	++	Standard alternative to morphine; less effective when given orally
Methotrimeprazine (Levoprome)	5–30 I.M.	++(+)	–	–	–	Phenothiazine derivative, with similar side effects; potent analgesic and sedative; causes hypotension
Pentazocine (Talwin)	20–60 P.O., I.M.	++(+)	–	+++	+	Similar to morphine, but causes less sedation; increases blood pressure; may cause dizziness and psychomimetic effects
Piminodine (Alvodine)	25–40 P.O. 10–20 S.C., I.M.	++	++	++	?	More potent than meperidine, with fewer side effects
Propoxyphene* (Darvon)	65–100 P.O.	+	–	+	±	Moderate analgesic, with abuse potential, although not truly addicting
Salicylates* (Aspirin, etc.)	300–1000 P.O.	+(+)	–	–	–	Can cause respiratory stimulation (see Table 11–1); can cause asthma in hypersensitive patients

*These agents are considered "mild" analgesics, whereas the others in this table are "strong."

parenterally; the dose can be repeated several times if indicated.

ALPHAPRODINE (Nisentil). This is similar to meperidine, but has a more rapid onset and a shorter duration of action. It offers no important advantages to patients with respiratory diseases, but it has the virtue of being relatively nonaddictive.

ANILERIDINE (Leritine). Anileridine is similar to meperidine, but offers the advantage of being relatively more effective when given orally. A suitable oral dose for adults is 25 to 50 mg every four to six hours. It has little, if any, addictive potential.

ETHOHEPTAZINE (Zactane). This drug is related to meperidine, but is much less potent as an analgesic, and it has no addictive potential. Side effects are less frequent with this agent, but include nausea, vomiting, epigastric distress, dizziness and pruritus. Ethoheptazine is suitable for respiratory patients with mild to moderate pain, since it has no respiratory depressant action; indeed, parenteral administration may cause some respiratory stimulation.

FENTANYL (Sublimaze). Fentanyl is a very potent analgesic with a relatively short duration of action. The drug has a morphine-like effect when given in 1/100th of the usual dose of morphine, and it is a powerful respiratory depressant and antitussive. When given intravenously, it can cause muscular rigidity, and apnea may occur: this effect is reversed by giving a short-acting muscle relaxant such as succinylcholine.

Fentanyl has been used as an analgesic for short surgical or endoscopic procedures. It has been given in combination with the major tranquillizer droperidol to produce neuroleptanalgesia (see later, in discussion of droperidol), and it can be used on its own as an adjunct for the induction of various forms of anesthesia. The drug potentiates the action of all other agents that have central depressant effects. Since fentanyl is a hazardous drug for patients with impaired respiratory control, it should be avoided as a routine analgesic in these subjects. A further problem is that fentanyl has been responsible for delayed respiratory depression, which may occur several hours after the patient has recovered from the anesthetic.[46a]

METHOTRIMEPRAZINE (Levoprome). This drug is a substituted phenothiazine that is a potent analgesic and sedative. Methotrimeprazine is suitable for severe intractable pain; 15 to 20 mg is equivalent to 20 mg of morphine or 75 mg of meperidine, but dependency and habituation do not occur, and it is not subject to narcotic controls. Although methotrimeprazine can cause the same side-effects as other nonanalgesic phenothiazines, it is not a respiratory depressant. One of the main untoward effects is orthostatic hypotension and syncope, and in some patients concomitant administration of a vasopressor drug may be necessary. The drug should not be given with other drugs having a psychotropic effect, because potentiation may occur. Care is needed when using this drug in elderly people or patients with heart failure or blood pressure problems, but in standard dosages it does not appear to be a hazard to patients with respiratory insufficiency.

Methotrimeprazine is available for administration only by intramuscular injection; the dosage for adults is 5 to 20 mg every four to six hours. The valuable properties of this sedative-analgesic suggest that it should be utilized more frequently in respiratory patients having intractable pain without cough, such as may occur with metastatic complications of lung cancer.

PENTAZOCINE (Talwin). This is less effective than morphine, but is suitable for the treatment of moderate pain. Although pentazocine appears to have narcotic antagonist properties, it can cause respiratory depression; it should not be used in conjunction with other narcotics, since it may decrease the analgesic effect while not lessening the hazard to breathing. The effects of pentazocine can be reversed by naloxone, but not by levallorphan or nalorphine.

Although the drug is less of a sedative and less habituating than morphine, addiction and abuse can occur. Pentazocine causes many untoward effects, including nausea, vomiting, dizziness, lightheadedness and euphoria; high doses can cause an increase in blood pressure and heart rate, and circulatory depression with shock may follow. In view of all these disadvantages, it is surprising that the drug is so popular, but the fact that it has not been subjected to narcotic control undoubtedly accounts for much of the overenthusiasm that physicians have for prescribing the drug. Because of its marked potential for respiratory depression, pentazocine should be avoided in patients with asthma and other forms of respiratory insufficiency.

PIMINODINE (Alvodine). Piminodine has a structure similar to that of meperidine, and analgesic potency comparable to that of morphine. Although it has less sedative action than does morphine, it causes similar untoward actions, including respiratory depression. There is little reason to recommend the use of this drug in any situation, and it should not be used in respiratory patients.

Sedative-Hypnotics. Although there are no clear pharmacologic distinctions between so-called sedative drugs and hypnotics, it is conventional to employ a number of drugs for their mild, calming effect, although many of them can help induce sleep.[47] Similarly, drugs used in the management of insomnia can also be used for daytime sedation.[48] It is therefore convenient to consider these two types of psychotropic drugs together (see Table 11-6).

All too many respiratory patients complain of restlessness or mild anxiety during the day and impaired sleep at night. The problems may be partly related to the patient's frequent coughing, dyspnea and respiratory discomfort, and to conflicts with respect to cigarette smoking. A substantial component in the restlessness and sleep disturbance may be attributable to bronchodilator therapy: ephedrine, in particular, may cause central stimulation, and for this reason combination preparations based on ephedrine contain sedative doses of phenobarbital or hydroxyzine (see Chapter 5).

Although it is commonly stated that sedatives and hypnotics are contraindicated in asthma and other chronic respiratory diseases,[49, 50] and though some experts blame sedative therapy as a component in many deaths occurring in asthmatics,[51] there is insufficient evidence to condemn all sedative-hypnotic therapy in a blanket fashion. Steen, in his comprehensive review,[43] did not find adequate evidence that appropriate doses of the majority of sedative-hypnotic drugs cause any more respiratory depression than that which accompanies normal sleep. However, there is indisputable evidence in the literature that careless use of sedative drugs in patients with chronic obstructive pulmonary diseases can cause respiratory failure, and the physician should utilize these agents with great circumspection. The best advice is to try to avoid central depressant drugs in asthmatics and other patients with chronic obstructive diseases; but if such therapy is deemed necessary, an agent with a short action and relative freedom from respiratory center depression should be prescribed in minimal dosage, and the response of the patient should be carefully evaluated. As shown in Table 11-6, the sedative-hypnotics do not produce analgesia, and most of them have little, if any, anticholinergic, antihistaminic or adrenergic-blocking properties.

The sedative-hypnotic drugs have inherent disadvantages in all patients, particularly in dependent individuals. Thus, they are habituating, and they are frequently major causes of drug abuse. Patients who claim they feel tired because they do not sleep well may not benefit from most of the hypnotics, since these drugs generally cause a nonrefreshing sleep, and they may leave the patients with a hangover. Deep sleep, which is accompanied by rapid eye movement (REM) is more satisfying than other forms of sleep, but most hypnotics decrease the total amount of REM sleep.[48] It is often thought that a hypnotic that permits adequate REM sleep is the most suitable, but whether this is necessarily so is disputable. A major problem with most agents is that they lose their potency as patients become habituated to them, and the quality of the sleep deteriorates. Thus, as a rule, sleep-inducing drugs should not be used routinely, and should be taken only occasionally to cover a few nights of disturbed rest.

The sedative-hypnotic drugs include some of the barbiturates, and a number of other agents from different pharmacologic classes. The more important of these will be discussed below.

BARBITURATES. These drugs were the first to be used extensively as sleeping agents and for psychotherapeutic purposes. They are all derived from barbituric acid (malonylurea), and they can be used to produce sedation, amnesia, hypnosis and anesthesia. Depending on their chemical structure, their actions may persist only for minutes (ultra short-acting) or as long as a day or more. The long-acting agents enter the brain slowly, and their onset of action is correspondingly delayed; they are used for treating chronic psychoneuroses, and, since they are anticonvulsants, they are employed in the management of epilepsy. The intermediate and short-acting barbiturates are more suited for use as sedatives or hypnotics, but they are regarded as "old-fashioned," and have fallen into relative disfavor. However, since they are inexpensive and their actions are well known, several of these drugs could be used as sedative-hypnotics. Because all the barbiturates are respiratory depressants, they should be used only with great care as sedatives in respiratory patients, and they

TABLE 11–8. IMPORTANT BARBITURATES

Drug	Onset of Sleep (hrs)	Duration of Effect (hrs)	Sedative Dose (mg)	Hypnotic Dose (mg)	Comments
Long-Acting	0.5–1	4–12			
Barbital (barbitone) (Veronal)			65–130	300–600	"Old" sedative and hypnotic
Phenobarbital (Luminal, Eskabarb)			15–30*	100–320	Useful sedative and superior anticonvulsant; present in combination bronchodilator preparations
Intermediate-acting	0.25–0.5	2–8			
Allobarbital (Dial)			30	100–300	Rarely used
Amobarbital (Amytal)			20–40	65–300	Used for occasional sedation and for insomnia
Butabarbital (Butisol)			8–30	50–100*	Used for occasional sedation and for insomnia
Short-acting	0.25–0.5	1–4			
Cyclobarbital (Phanodorm)				100–300	Rarely used
Pentobarbital (Nembutal, Nebralin)			30	100–200*	Used for occasional insomnia or sedation
Secobarbital (Seconal)			15–30	100–300*	Used for occasional insomnia or sedation
Ultra short-acting	0.03	0.2			
Hexobarbital (Evipal, Sombulex)			250–500	250–500	Basal hypnotic, used as anesthesia adjunct
Methohexital (Brevital)			–	–	Similar to thiopental
Thiamylal (Surital)			–	–	Similar to thiopental
Thiopental (Pentothal)			–	–	For intravenous anesthesia

*Preferred drug, with appropriate dosage range.
Note: The anesthetic dose is approximately three times the hypnotic dose; the lethal dose is approximately six times the hypnotic dose.[29]

should probably be avoided as hypnotics in these patients.[52] The important barbiturates are listed in Table 11–8.

The ultra short-acting barbiturates are used intravenously or as retention enemas to produce anesthesia.[29] The most important of these agents, thiopental, was discussed in Chapter 4. One of these ultra short-acting drugs, hexobarbital, is used as a sleeping pill.

Phenobarbital (Luminal) is the prototype barbiturate; it is used as a daytime sedative and in the management of epilepsy. The drug is used in combination with ephedrine and theophylline (Chapter 5), but it is a relatively undesirable drug, since it induces hepatic enzymes that metabolize glucocorticoids, and therefore it can decrease the effectiveness of steroid therapy in asthma.[53] Elderly patients and those in severe pain may react paradoxically to barbiturates with agitation and confusion; it may induce hyperexcitability in children. Although it is a useful sedative, it should not be used as a hypnotic, and in general it should not be used for

sedative purposes in patients with respiratory diseases.

Barbital (Veronal) is one of the oldest barbiturates, and it is rarely used now. It is similar to phenobarbital, but less effective, and differs by virtue of not being metabolized by the liver as are the other barbiturates.

Amobarbital (Amytal) is the best known of the intermediate-acting barbiturates. It can be used as a daytime sedative, but its effect may be variable, lasting two to 8 hours; it is also suitable for use as a hypnotic. Amobarbital offers no advantages for respiratory patients, although it has been combined with ephedrine in bronchodilator preparations.

Butabarbital (Butisol) and *Allobarbital* (Dial) are similar to amobarbital, and offer no added advantages.

Pentobarbital (Nembutal) is a short-acting barbiturate, with an onset of action within half an hour of an oral dose, and an effect that lasts one to four hours. It is used both for sedation and for hypnosis, and it is a relatively popular sleeping drug. It can lose

TABLE 11–9. SEDATIVE-HYPNOTIC DRUGS

Drug	Adult Dosage (mg)	Respiratory Depression	Comments
Short-Acting Barbiturates			
Pentobarbital (Nembutal)	100–200	+	Should be avoided in patients with respiratory disease
Secobarbital (Seconal)	100–200	+	Should be avoided in patients with respiratory disease
Alcohols			
Chloral hydrate (Noctec, Somnos, etc.)	250–1500	±	Inexpensive, but causes gastric irritation; low dosage suitable for many respiratory patients
Chloral betaine (Beta-Chlor)	870–2610	±	Similar to chloral hydrate, but less gastric irritation
Ethanol	Varies	±	Useful as a "nightcap" in some patients
Ethchlorvynol (Placidyl)	500–1000	±	No advantages; several side effects
Triclofos (Triclos)	750–2250	±	Similar to chloral hydrate, but has no aftertaste
Carbamates			
Ethinamate (Valmid)	500–1000	±	Brief duration of effect
Piperidinediones			
Glutethimide (Doriden)	500–1000	±	No advantages; should not be used because it has abuse potential; many side effects
Methyprylon (Noludar)	200–400	±	Similar to barbiturates; several side effects
Quinazolines			
Methaqualone (Parest, Quaalude, Somnafac, Sopor)	150–400	±	Has become a drug of abuse; rarely indicated
Benzodiazepines			
Flurazepam (Dalmane)	15–30	±	One of the best hypnotic agents: effective, safe and results in satisfactory sleep; effectiveness persists
Other benzodiazepines	Varies	±	May be effective and relatively safe

*The lower dosage should be used initially in respiratory patients; larger doses may be needed for sleep. For sedation, the dosage can be repeated up to three or four times a day.

much of its effectiveness if used daily for over two weeks. In common with other barbiturates, it can cause respiratory depression, and it should be avoided in patients with chronic respiratory insufficiency (Table 11–9).

Secobarbital (Seconal) is similar to pentobarbital, and it is a relatively popular sedative and hypnotic; it is also used to decrease apprehension in patients being prepared for surgery. However, it has no advantages over pentobarbital.

Cyclobarbital (Phanodorm) is a short-acting agent, comparable to pentobarbital or secobarbital.

Hexobarbital is an ultra short-acting barbiturate, which can be used intravenously as an anesthetic, or orally (as Sombucaps or Sombulex) as a sleeping drug. Since its hypnotic action is very short lasting, it may be of some use to patients who need help in getting to sleep. However, it is probably no safer than the other barbiturates in patients with chronic respiratory insufficiency.

ALCOHOLS. Although ethyl alcohol itself, in any of its many forms, is often used as a sedative, it cannot be regarded as a reliable or safe drug for calming the anxious patient. A drink of a favored alcoholic beverage at night can undoubtedly help induce sleep in many patients, and this use of a "nightcap" may be better for older people with respiratory disease than any of the other hypnotic drugs. However, the substituted alcohols that are available as sleeping medications may be judged more suitable for most patients (see Table 11–9).

Chloral hydrate is a relatively safe and

long-established hypnotic that can be obtained in a variety of proprietary preparations. It is metabolized rapidly in the body to trichloroethanol; both chloral and its metabolite act on the brain to cause sedation and hypnosis. When taken as a hypnotic, it usually induces sleep within half an hour, and its effect lasts four to eight hours. The drug has an unpleasant taste or odor, which can be minimized by chilling the fluid or by taking it as a capsule. It is less likely than the barbiturates to cause paradoxic agitation in elderly patients, but its effectiveness as a hypnotic tends to decline if chloral is used nightly for over a week. Gastric irritation is its major defect, and several derivatives are available that have less propensity to cause nausea, abdominal distress or vomiting. The most important of these derivatives are *chloral betaine* and *triclofos,* which are much more expensive than chloral hydrate.

Chloral has been reported to be useful and safe as a sedative in asthmatics,[52] and there appears to be no evidence that it is hazardous when given as a sleeping aid to patients with respiratory insufficiency.[43] Thus, the drug can be regarded as an inexpensive, relatively safe hypnotic for occasional use for respiratory patients.

Chloral hydrate is available as elixirs, syrups, capsules and suppositories. The sedative dose for adults is 250 mg, and this dose can be given eight-hourly if required. For use as a hypnotic, 0.5 to 1 gm can be used, and, in general, the smaller dose should be given to respiratory patients.

Ethchlorvynol (Placidyl) is a tertiary acetylenic alcohol. It is comparable to chloral hydrate, but it is less potent and less predictable as a hypnotic. Although this drug was introduced as a sedative, it has no advantages for daytime sedation either. At present, there is no comparative information to suggest that ethchlorvynol offers any advantages for use in patients with respiratory disease, and its overdose potential is a severe disadvantage.

CARBAMATES. When alcohols are esterified with carbamic acid, their hypnotic properties are often increased. Currently, the only carbamate regarded primarily as a sedative-hypnotic is ethinamate, whereas the dicarbamate, meprobamate, is classified as a tranquillizer.

Ethinamate (Valmid) is a rapidly-acting short-duration hypnotic, producing up to four hours sleep. Although not advocated as a sedative, it can be used in the preanesthesia preparation of a patient for minor proce-

dures. Its side effects are similar to those of the barbiturates, but it does not appear to be a respiratory depressant; however, this property of the drug may not have been adequately evaluated. It may, therefore, be suitable as an occasional hypnotic for respiratory patients. The drug is available as 500 mg tablets; one or two tablets before retiring is the adult dose (Table 11–9).

PIPERIDINEDIONES. These agents were investigated because of their chemical relationship to the barbiturates. One of the piperidinediones is actually a central stimulator (bemegride), and was discussed earlier in this chapter. Two piperidinediones are in current use as sedative-hypnotics (see Table 11–9).

Glutethimide (Doriden) is an effective central depressant; in toxic doses it causes less respiratory depression than the barbiturates. It is thus likely to be a relatively safe agent for use in patients with respiratory insufficiency. However, the drug has more side effects: among these are nausea, vomiting, blurred vision, paradoxic excitement, sedation hangover, convulsions following withdrawal, and a number of rare hypersensitivity reactions including purpura, aplastic anemia, agranulocytosis, dermatitis and acute intermittent porphyria. The drug was relatively popular in the 1960s, and it became a drug of abuse; overdosage problems were common, and were difficult to manage, since the drug enters into an enterohepatic circulatory cycle and can cause prolonged coma. At present, glutethimide is not thought to offer sufficient advantages over the better-established sedative-hypnotics to justify its use in respiratory therapy.

Methyprylon (Noludar) is more potent than glutethimide, and is second only to the barbiturates. It causes less respiratory depression than the barbiturates, and it has similar side effects. There is insufficient information available to determine whether the drug is suitable for patients with respiratory insufficiency, but it may be a useful alternative agent. It is available as tablets of 50 and 200 mg, and capsules of 300 mg. The hypnotic dose for adults is 200 to 400 mg.

QUINAZOLINES. These agents are similar in structure to the barbiturates, and are related to the piperidinediones. Only one agent in this class is currently available—methaqualone (Table 11–9).

Methaqualone is a potent drug, with sedative-hypnotic value, and additional anticonvulsant, antispasmodic, local anesthetic (but not analgesic), antihistaminic and anti-tussive properties. Some additional psychic properties are claimed by advocates who have been responsible for converting metha-qualone to a major drug of abuse. Cardiac and respiratory depression are less common with overdosage than are seen after the barbiturates; methaqualone may be rela-tively safe as a hypnotic in respiratory patients, particularly those requiring cough suppression at night. The drug has side effects similar to the barbiturates, but it may be less toxic than glutethimide; however, it is the only hypnotic that may produce convul-sions when taken in acute overdose.

Because of its serious abuse potential, methaqualone cannot be recommended, al-though it may be of value in occasional respiratory patients. Several oral proprietary brands of the drug or of its hydrochloride are marketed; the sedative-hypnotic dose for adults is 75 to 400 mg orally.

BENZODIAZEPINES. These drugs are the most important minor tranquillizers for the management of anxiety, and they can be used equally well as daytime sedatives or as nighttime hypnotics. However, mainly as a result of convention, only one benzodiaze-pine, flurazepam, is regarded as a hypnotic (Table 11–9).

Flurazepam (Dalmane) has gained the reputation of being one of the best hypnotic agents. It is effective within 20 to 45 minutes of oral administration, and it generally re-sults in seven or eight hours of satisfying sleep. It does not decrease the amount of REM sleep, and it does not produce sedation hangover, or rebound problems when with-drawn. Tolerance to its hypnotic effective-ness does not develop as readily with flurazepam as with most other hypnotics. Other advantages of flurazepam are that overdosages are less likely to kill, and respiratory depression is less of a problem than with barbiturates. The drug has a lower abuse potential than the barbiturates, the piperidinediones or methaqualone. Its com-mon side effects are similar to those of the barbiturates, and include ataxia, vertigo and paradoxic reactions.

Flurazepam is marketed as capsules of 15 and 30 mg; the hypnotic dose for adults is 15 to 30 mg. Up to 45 mg can be given safely to most patients, without danger of respiratory depression;[43] however, one group of inves-tigators has reported that this drug in a dosage of 15 mg can cause some central depression of respiration.[54] A related ben-zodiazepine, nitrazepam, may be safer in this respect;[54] this drug is available in Britain as Mogadon. Flurazepam should, nevertheless, be considered as an alternative to chloral hydrate and its derivatives for respiratory patients who need a hypnotic. Because of its valuable properties as a sleeping agent, it should not be used for routine daily sedation. In this respect, most physicians prefer other benzodiazepines for daytime sedation, and indeed many of these other benzodiazepines probably serve as effective hypnotic drugs also.

Tranquillizers. A group of sedative drugs has gained recognition for effectiveness in the management of psychoneuroses that are characterized by symptoms of marked psy-chic distress such as anxiety, tremulousness, apprehension, restlessness, disturbed behav-ior, psychosomatic complaints and social maladaptation. Although many patients presenting with these problems could be managed by psychotherapy or by the use of mild doses of the sedative-hypnotic drugs, it has become conventional to use agents that are promoted by the pharmaceutical industry as "antianxiety drugs" under the aegis of the emotive word "tranquillizer." Respiratory physicians favor the tranquillizer, since they have been conditioned to believe that drugs of this class are less likely than the sedative-hypnotic drugs to cause respiratory center depression in patients with asthma or other chronic obstructive pulmonary disease. In fact, except for barbiturates, there is no evidence to suggest that the sedative-hyp-notics have any greater respiratory depres-sant properties than the tranquillizers. For practical purposes, the two classes of agent can be used interchangeably, and the tran-quillizers could be used as aids to sleep and in the preanesthesia preparation of patients for surgery.

The benzodiazepine group of tranquillizers has gained the advantages of a well-directed promotional campaign that was aimed at the medical and dispensing professions, as well as the public, at an appropriate time in the evolution of psychotherapeutic pharmacol-ogy.[45, 55] The proprietary agents Equanil (Miltown), Librium and Valium have each in succession become glamorized props in the theater of modern psychoneuroses, and at the present time it is virtually futile to try to convince physicians or the public that their confidence in these appurtenances of the brave new world of "pop psychopharma-cology" is simply a mass audience response

TABLE 11-10. TRANQUILLIZERS

Drugs	Adult Dosage* (mg)	Respiratory Depression	Clinical Notes
BENZODIAZEPINES			
Chlordiazepoxide (Librium and generics)	15–100†	±	May cause habituation; cumulative effects can occur; drowsiness is most common side effect
Clorazepate (Tranxene)	15–60	±	Similar to diazepam
Diazepam (Valium)	2.5–10†	±	Popular drug of abuse, but is of legitimate value; probably not significantly superior to chlordiazepoxide, and it has more side effects
Lorazepam (Ativan)	2–4	±	Less likely to cause residual sedation; new agent, similar to oxazepam
Oxazepam (Serax)	10–30	±	Relatively short-acting, with low incidence of adverse effects, and early onset of sedation; useful as a hypnotic
Prazepam (Verstran)	10–30	±	Similar to clorazepate, but has more prolonged effect
DICARBAMATES‡			
Meprobamate (Equanil, Miltown)	200–400	± or +	Less effective than benzodiazepines; drowsiness is most frequent side effect
Tybamate (Solacen, Tybatran)	125–350	± or +	Shorter action than meprobamate
MISCELLANEOUS			
Benactyzine (Phobex, Suavitil)	1–3	–	Mild tranquillizer of uncertain value; has anticholinergic properties
Benzquinamide (Emete-Con)	0.5–1 mg/kg	–	Antiemetic; causes cardiac and respiratory stimulation
Hydroxyzine (Atarax, Vistaril)	25–100	– or ±	Antiemetic, antihistaminic, mild bronchodilator (see Table 4–19)
Phenaglycodol (Ultran)	200–600	–	Mild neurosedative and weak muscle relaxant with low toxicity

*Doses are given 2–4 times a day, depending on drug and on patient.

†Maximum sedative effect may be attained only after 7 days: build-up of effect may occur during this time. Administration 1–2 times/day should suffice thereafter. Higher doses may be tolerated by cigarette smokers.

‡In low or medium dosage used as sedative-hypnotics.

to the phenomenon of insubstantive societal persuasion. Having said this, the most important of these formulated doses of tranquillity will now be considered (Table 11–10).

BENZODIAZEPINES. Hundreds of agents in this class have been synthesized, but only a handful have been marketed. It is claimed they have properties in addition to their antianxiety effects. They are of value as premedication adjuncts prior to surgical anesthesia, and they can be used in the treatment of alcohol withdrawal. They are anticonvulsants, and have muscle-relaxing properties, the nature of which is difficult to define and the quality of which is difficult to substantiate; however, many of these drugs have been used successfully in the management of tetanus.

The main virtues of the benzodiazepines compared with the sedative-hypnotics are that the former drugs are safer and have fewer disturbing side effects, and are relatively ineffective as suicide agents. A tranquillizing dose of a benzodiazepine appears to be less likely to cause drowsiness or loss of mental function than a tranquillizing dose of one of the sedative-hypnotics. However, these quantitative and qualitative virtues are not always recognizable in individual patients who are tried on courses of each type of drug. At present, it seems reasonable to state that the benzodiazepines are the antianxiety drugs of choice,[56] and they are less likely to cause respiratory depression than the sedative-hypnotics. However, standard doses of any of the benzodiazepines are undoubtedly capable of causing various degrees of respiratory depression in patients with chronic obstructive airways diseases.[49, 50] Although these agents can be safely used by many respiratory patients,[57] the patient should be made aware of the extreme hazard associated with increasing the dosage to combat, for instance, the mounting anxiety that so often accompanies worsening bronchospasm. Similarly, the physician should make it an absolute rule never to administer one of these agents to a severely anxious respiratory patient unless the blood gases have been checked. If the patient is hypocarbic, then the causative hyperventilation may be managed appropriately with a tranquillizer, but if there is an increased $PaCO_2$, tranquillizer therapy should be withheld unless the physician is prepared to manage the patient by means of endotracheal intubation.

Chlordiazepoxide (Librium) was the first of the benzodiazepine tranquillizers to be introduced, and it is still fairly popular for the treatment of anxiety, and psychoneuroses such as alcoholism. The oral preparation is slowly absorbed, and variable blood levels are achieved. The half-life of chlordiazepoxide is one to two days, and therefore several days of therapy are required before a plateau level is achieved, and a cumulative effect may then be seen. Adverse effects include drowsiness, ataxia, confusion, rashes, edema, gastrointestinal disturbances, changes in libido, extrapyramidal symptoms, edema, menstrual irregularities, jaundice and agranulocytosis. Large doses may cause hypotension, syncope and central depression; impaired respiration can occur in patients with obstructive airways disease. In some psychiatrically disturbed patients, normal doses can produce paradoxic reactions, including excitement, overstimulation and rage—a disturbing outcome to be attributed to a tranquillizer. Although chlordiazepoxide is effective for the control of acute agitation and delirium tremens, it is not considered a muscle relaxant.

Chlordiazepoxide is available as the base for oral administration, and as the hydrochloride for both oral and parenteral use: the dosage of either preparations is the same. For adults with anxiety, the appropriate dosage is 5 to 25 mg three to four times a day; up to 100 mg can be used in a patient with severe neurosis or alcoholism, or for preoperative preparation. Only the lower dosages should be used in respiratory patients. Since chlordiazepoxide is now available as generic preparations, it is relatively inexpensive, and it can be regarded as the benzodiazepine of choice for use as a tranquillizer or sedative-hypnotic.[58]

Diazepam (Valium) is similar to chlordiazepoxide, but it is more potent and possesses muscle relaxing properties. Unlike chlordiazepoxide, it is suitable for use as an anticonvulsant, and is very effective in the management of status epilepticus. Diazepam is also a more effective hypnotic agent and could be used as a sleeping aid, as is its congener flurazepam. Whether all these advantages suffice to explain the extreme popularity of diazepam as a tranquillizer cannot readily be determined from the literature.

The adverse reactions to diazepam are similar to those of chlordiazepoxide, but even more side effects are listed for the former, including depression, tremor, slurred speech, sleep disturbance, urinary retention, amnesia, diplopia and blurred vision. Diazepam also has a long half-life, and cumulative effects are usual during the first week of therapy. Respiratory depression can occur in elderly subjects and in patients with impaired ventilatory mechanics. The drug does not appear to be substantially superior to chlordiazepoxide as a tranquillizer in the average patient with anxiety, but it may be safer in patients with respiratory insufficiency,[57] particularly when administered orally.

In older patients, both chlordiazepoxide and diazepam are more likely to cause central depression, since their metabolic elimination is decreased in the elderly. Smokers appear to have an increased tolerance for these drugs as a consequence of increased metabolism; similarly, alcoholics and abusers of tranquillizers have increased tolerance.

The adult dosage is 2 to 10 mg up to four times a day by mouth. Intramuscular doses can be given; usually 2 to 10 mg is suitable, with repeated doses, if necessary, of up to 30 mg in an eight hour period. Diazepam can be given intravenously, taking five minutes for each 1 ml: more rapid injections can cause severe hypotension.

Clorazepate (Tranxene) is similar to diazepam, with little important difference in properties or side effects other than the fact that it is not considered as effective a muscle relaxant or anticonvulsive. Moreover, the drug is relatively expensive. The oral dosage for adults is 15 to 60 mg per day in two to four divided doses.

Oxazepam (Serax) may offer some advantages over diazepam: it has comparable properties, but fewer side effects. It has a shorter half-life, and cumulative properties are less likely to occur; it is also less likely to cause ataxia. Oxazepam is somewhat less expensive than its congeners, and it should be considered a prime choice for a traquillizer. However, it has not been shown to offer any advantages to respiratory patients.

Recently, *lorazepam* (Ativan) and *prazepam* (Verstran) have been introduced; there is insufficient experience with these agents to permit recommendations for their preferential use.

DICARBAMATES. Early in this century, it was discovered that phenoxypropanediol (Antodyne), which is a simple ether of glycerol, could cause skeletal muscle relaxation without loss of consciousness. A number of other so-called relaxants, with a related chemical structure, have been developed since then. One of the first to be carefully studied was *mephenesin:* it has been shown to depress nervous transmission through spinal and supraspinal polysynaptic pathways, and to prolong synaptic recovery time. This drug also has a mild sedative effect, and it protects the brain against the stimulatory action of analeptics.

The effectiveness of mephenesin was enhanced by converting it to a carbamate ester: this is more slowly absorbed and is metabolized less rapidly than mephenesin. Other carbamates were synthesized, and several have been introduced as muscle relaxants, although their value falls short of being impressive. In spite of the fact that derivitives of glycerol are muscle relaxants, there is no evidence that glycerol itself or the expectorant glyceryl guaiacolate (guaifenesin, Chapter 3) have similar actions. The important glycerol derivatives currently marketed as muscle relaxants are methocarbamol (Robaxin) and chlorphenesin (Maolate). These agents do not have significant central depressant effects, and none of them are credited with expectorant properties.

Meprobamate (Equanil, Miltown) is variously classified chemically as a substituted dicarbamate or as a propanediol, and it is a simple aliphatic compound related to mephenesin. When introduced, meprobamate originally enjoyed the popularity that diazepam subsequently usurped. It is a less effective sedative, relaxant and anticonvulsant than the benzodiazepines. Currently, it is used as a sedative-tranquillizer, and it has little hypnotic activity. It is perhaps most useful for anxious patients who also complain of muscle tension or spasm, and it is effective when there is also mild depression. Adverse effects are not common, but include drowsiness, ataxia, slurred speech, blurred vision, vertigo, paresthesiae, euphoria, paradoxic excitment, nausea, vomiting, diarrhea, tachycardia, arrhythmias, hypotension, syncope, rashes, leucopenia, purpura, edema, fever, hyperpyrexia, bronchospasm, oliguria, anaphylaxis, porphyria and other hypersensitivity responses. Although there seem to be a large number of adverse effects, meprobamate is probably no more toxic than other tranquillizers. The drug has not been reported to be particularly dangerous to respiratory patients, but it probably has a potential for ventilatory depression similar to the benzodiazepines; however, it may be more dangerous when an overdose is taken.

The adult oral dose of meprobamate is 200 to 400 mg, and up to 2400 mg can be taken a day; it is available only as tablets and capsules. The drug is now available as generic preparations, and it is therefore relatively inexpensive.

Tybamate (Tybatran) is similar to meprobamate, but is more effective as a tranquillizer and has a shorter action. It may, therefore, be safer in respiratory patients, but at present there is no evidence to suggest that this is the case. Up to 3 gm a day of the oral preparation can be given to adults in divided doses. However, there seem to be insufficient practical advantages to justify the preferential use of this relatively expensive dicarbamate.

MISCELLANEOUS. Various other agents have been classified as tranquillizers, but they are usually considered with regard to their other properties, for example the antihistamines (see Chapter 9).

Hydroxyzine has been considered earlier (Chapters 4, 5 and 9), and it merits further consideration in this chapter. Because of its antihistaminic and bronchodilator properties, it is a useful sedative-hypnotic or tranquillizer for anxious patients with bronchospastic diseases. It is also used as an antispasmodic and an antiemetic, and is effective in the management of urticaria. The various central properties of the drug are of value in the preanesthesia preparation of patients for surgery, and it should be regarded as a drug of choice for this purpose in patients with ventilatory inadequacy. Slight respiratory depression has been seen with hydroxyzine,[59] but this may be less a problem than with other tranquillizers, since mild respiratory stimulation has also been attributed to the drug.[43] The various prepara-

TABLE 11–11. CLASSES OF ANTIPSYCHOTIC AGENTS*

Drug	Examples	Adult Dosage* (mg)	Sedative Effects	Antiemetic Effects	Anti-cholenergic Effects	Extra-pyramidal Side Effects
PHENOTHIAZINES						
Dimethylamino-alkyls	Chlorpromazine	10–100	+++	+	+	++
Piperazinyl-alkyls	Fluphenazine	0.3–2	+	++	±	+++
Piperidyl-alkyls	Thioridazine	10–200	+++	−	++	+
THIOXANTHENES						
Dimethylamino derivative	Chlorprothixene	10–125	++	+	+	++
Piperazinyl derivative	Thiothixene	2–15	+	++	±	++
BUTYROPHENONES						
Piperidyl derivative	Haloperidol	0.25–15	±	+	±	+++
DIBENZODIAZEPINES						
	Clozapine		++	+	++	−
RAUWOLFIA ALKALOIDS						
	Reserpine	0.1–5	++	−	−	+

*Dosage schedules vary, but these agents are usually given 3–4 times a day.

tions of hydroxyzine that are available are presented in Table 4–19. The appropriate adult dosage is 25 to 100 mg three or four times a day.

Other drugs that have been classified as tranquillizers include *benactyzine* (Suavitil, Phobex), *benzquinamide* (Emete-Con), and *phenaglycodol* (Ultran): none of these is as potent as the agents discussed earlier in this section. Benzquinamide is of interest in that it is an antiemetic, and it may cause respiratory stimulation.[43] Benactyzine is claimed to have a mild antidepressant effect; it is made available in combination with meprobamate in Deprol.

Antipsychotic Drugs. Numerous drugs are of value in the treatment of schizophrenia, manic-depressive states and other psychoses. Although these drugs are also known as *major tranquillizers,* and sometimes as *ataractics* or *neuroleptics,*[60] their antipsychotic properties are of greater relevance.[45, 55] Many elderly people, especially during the course of a severe acute or debilitating illness, develop psychotic reactions and require treatment with one of these drugs. Respiratory patients who experience severe stress may undergo a psychotic break, and their psychologic vulnerability leads to the not infrequent need for antipsychotic drug therapy on respiratory care units.

The antipsychotic agents differ from the minor tranquillizers in several important respects: the former are not addictive, they have numerous disturbing side effects, they are of less value as sedatives or hypnotics and they have little tendency to produce respiratory depression (Table 11–6). By and large, overdosages with these drugs are less likely to be fatal than are suicidal attempts with the sedative-hypnotic drugs.[61] Thus, the antipsychotic agents are of less concern to the respiratory clinician, since they are unlikely to present major therapeutic dilemmas when they are needed by patients with chronic obstructive airways diseases.

A number of different pharmacologic classes of antipsychotic drugs are recognized (Table 11–11), and these are discussed in the following section.

PHENOTHIAZINES. The most important agents used in the mangement of the psychoses are the phenothiazines; these agents are of particular value in schizophrenia and other chronic psychotic illnesses. The phenothiazines have various other important therapeutic properties, including sedative, antiemetic and anticholinergic activities. Several of these agents also have antihistaminic properties; these were discussed in Chapter 9 (see Table 9–23). The most widely used of the two dozen or so available phenothiazines is the well-known agent chlorpromazine.

Chlorpromazine (Thorazine; Largactil in the United Kingdom) is a dimethylamino phenothiazine. It is used as an antipsychotic and an antiemetic, and has been used as an adjunct to anesthesia. It has more sedative properties than most of the other phenothiazines, but it has little tendency to cause respiratory depression. In common with many of the major tranquillizers, it often causes extrapyramidal reactions, including bizarre movements (dyskinesias, dystonias), parkinsonism and akathisia (motor restlessness).[47] Some of these reactions may persist for an indefinite period after drug therapy is discontinued, for example tardive dyskinesia. The anticholinergic effects of chlorpromazine may cause drying of respiratory secretions, and since the drug has a minor blocking effect on alpha-adrenergic receptors, it may be of adjunctive value in some forms of asthma. Toxic problems include cholestatic jaundice, dermatologic reactions and blood dyscrasias. A major virtue of chlorpromazine and similar antipsychotic agents is that overdosage rarely results in death.

Fluphenazine (Permitil, Prolixin) is an example of the piperazine class of phenothiazines. It is less sedating than chlorpromazine, but is more likely to cause extrapyramidal effects. Fluphenazine is the most potent of the phenothiazines.

Thioridazine (Mellaril) is the prototype of the piperidine compounds, and may currently be the most widely used antipsychotic agent. It has potency similar to that of chlorpromazine, but it has virtually no antiemetic effects, and it causes less extrapyramidal reactions. However, as is common with these agents, the incidence of anticholinergic effects is inversely proportional to the incidence of extrapyramidal effects.

THIOXANTHENES. These drugs are very similar in structure to the phenothiazines, and each major phenothiazine has a thioxanthene analogue. Incidentally, these drugs are not related to the methylxanthines (Chapter 6). The main thioxanthenes are subclassified as dimethylamino derivatives and piperazine derivatives.

Chlorprothixene (Taractan) is similar to chlorpromazine, but is slightly less potent. It has less sedative effect, but its other properties and side effects are comparable.

Thiothixene (Navane) is similar to fluphenazine, but is less potent. It is more effective as an anti-emetic and produces fewer extrapyramidal side effects than does fluphenazine.

BUTYROPHENONES. The only agent in this class that is used as antipsychotic is *haloperidol* (Haldol). This drug resembles the piperazine phenothiazines, such as fluphenazine, in action. It is a very potent agent, and is of considerable value in schizophrenia, manic psychoses and delirium; it is of particular value in the treatment of the stress psychoses that so often occur in patients undergoing intensive care unit treatment. Haloperidol has less sedative action than most other antipsychotic drugs, and although it is an antiemetic, it lacks anticholinergic effects, but it does cause extrapyramidal reactions. A particularly important property of haloperidol, and other butyrophenones, is its ability to potentiate sedatives and analgesics.

Haloperidol is available as tablets and as ampules for intramuscular injection. The appropriate dosage range for adults with delirium is 0.25 to 15 mg; usually smaller doses are given, and are repeated or increased if necessary.

Droperidol (Inapsine) is a butyrophenone that is not used as an antipsychotic, but it resembles haloperidol in many ways, including its ability to potentiate sedatives and analgesics. It produces marked sedation, little or no amnesia, and is an antiemetic; it does cause extrapyramidal reactions, and it can cause hypotension secondary to vasodilation resulting from blockade of alpha-adrenergic receptors. The importance of this drug is that it has been used in combination with the narcotic analgesic fentanyl (Sublimaze, described earlier in this chapter) as an adjunct to anesthesia. The droperidol in this situation causes dissociative anesthesia, and the combination of the two drugs produces *neuroleptanalgesia*.[62] This state is characterized by the patient being calm and conscious, yet detached from and indifferent to the environment, with no desire to move. In this condition, the patient may be able to tolerate and cooperate with endoscopy and minor surgical procedures, although for some patients the subsequent recall of the event may be unpleasant. The combination of droperidol and fentanyl with local anesthesia has been successfully employed to produce neurolept analgesia for bronchoscopies.[63] The two drugs could also be used to produce neuroleptic anesthesia, as a prelude to the administration of a general anesthetic, particularly for neurosurgical procedures in which the general anesthesia can be discontinued to allow the patient to cooperate with the surgeon during the operation.[62]

A fixed combination of the two drugs is marketed, as Innovar, which contains fentanyl 0.05 mg/ml and droperidol 2.5 mg/ml.

The premedication dosage of Innovar ranges from 0.5 to 2 ml I.M.; as an adjunct to general anesthesia with nitrous oxide it is usually given in increments of 1 to 2 ml every five minutes until anesthesia is achieved.[62] Since droperidol is long-acting, postprocedure problems may occur; these include extrapyramidal effects and hypotension. More disturbing is that some patients under Innovar neuroleptanalgesia develop respiratory depression either because fentanyl depresses the respiratory center or because droperidol causes the patient to "forget" to breathe. The effect of fentanyl can be reversed by naloxone; if the fentanyl produces rigidity, a muscle relaxant such as succinylcholine can be given.[62] Extrapyramidal reactions (such as uncontrolled movements of the tongue, neck or body) that are caused by droperidol can be treated with antiparkinsonism agents—which help reverse the extrapyramidal reactions caused by any antipsychotic drug: diphenhydramine (Benadryl) 10 to 50 mg I.M. may suffice (see Chapter 9).

DIBENZODIAZEPINES. This class of antipsychotic drugs has not been introduced in the U.S. However, *clozapine* (Leponex) is an investigational agent with the unique quality of causing no extrapyramidal side effects.

RAUWOLFIA ALKALOIDS. For hundreds of years, the alkaloids of the plant *Rauwolfia serpentina* have been used in herbal medicine. One of the main alkaloids is *reserpine,* which is relatively nonpotent as an antipsychotic agent and as an antihypertensive drug. The drug is not an antiemetic and it lacks anticholinergic effects, but it resembles the phenothiazenes in other properties. A major problem with reserpine is that it can cause depression; sedation, bradycardia and nasal stuffiness are additional major side effects. Reserpine probably has little effect on respiration.

MISCELLANEOUS. Several less important agents are used in the treatment of psychoses. These include the investigational diphenylbutylpiperidines (for example pimozide, Orap), dibenzoxazepines (for example loxapine, Loxitane), and the indolics (for example molindone, Moban).

Antidepressant Drugs. Although depression is often part of an anxiety state or a psychosis, many depressed patients respond more favorably to specific antidepressant drugs.[64, 64a] Two classes of drugs (the monoamine inhibitors and the tricyclics) have been found to be particularly effective (Table 11–12).

MONOAMINE OXIDASE INHIBITORS (MAOI). These drugs were introduced before the tricyclics, but because of their many side effects they are rarely used currently. The MAO inhibitors block the oxidative deamination of natural monoamines by monoamine oxidase in the brain and other organs (see Chapter 4), and as a result, mood-elevating amines accumulate in the brain. The MAO inhibitors also abolish REM sleep, lower blood pressure and help relieve angina. Their toxic potential is greater than that of any other group of psychotherapeutic drugs and includes hepatotoxicity, orthostatic hypotension, central stimulation (tremors, insomnia, convulsions) and peripheral neuropathy. They potentiate other sympathomimetic amines, including those present in precursor form in foods such as cheese and beer, and can cause severe hypertensive crises. The MAO inhibitors are thus quite unsuited for patients who receive sympathomimetic bronchodilator therapy.

The first MAOI antidepressant to be introduced was iproniazid; although this agent is the isopropyl derivative of isoniazid (INH), it is not effective against tuberculosis, but it is much more effective as a mood elevator in depressed patients. The agents that are most commonly used at present are as follows:

Phenelzine (Nardil) is sometimes helpful in cases of mild endogenous depession. The usual adult dosage is 20 mg three times a day. It is a mild sedative, but apparently has no adverse effect on respiration.

Isocarboxazid (Marplan) is probably comparable in effect to phenelzine, and has no added advantages.

Tranylcypromine (Parnate) is similar to, but more rapidly acting than, phenelzine.

TRICYCLIC COMPOUNDS. These agents are similar in structure to the phenothiazines, but they are of no value in agitated patients. The tricyclic agents are more effective than the MAO inhibitors, and are the drugs of choice for all forms of depression, but are probably more effective in endogenous rather than reactive depression. They act by blocking the re-uptake of norepinephrine by adrenergic nerve terminals; and, as was pointed out in Chapter 4, some of the tricyclic compounds may be of value in asthma.[65]

The tricyclic antidepressants all have potent anticholinergic effects, and can cause

TABLE 11–12.   ANTIDEPRESSANTS

Drug	Adult Dosage* (mg/day)	Sedative Effects
MONOAMINE OXIDASE INHIBITORS		
Isocarboxazid (Marplan)	10–30	+
Phenelzine (Nardil)	15–90	+
Tranylcypromine (Parnate)	10–30	±
TRICYCLICS		
Amitriptyline (Elavil, Endep)	75–300	+++
Desipramine (Norpramin, Pertofrane)	75–300	+
Doxepin (Adapin, Sinequan)	75–300	+++
Imipramine (Tofranil, Imavate, Janimine, Presamine)	75–300	++
Nortriptyline (Aventyl, Pamelor)	40–150	+
Protriptyline (Vivactil)	15–60	±

*Can be given in single or divided doses.

hypotension, tachycardia and electrocardiographic abnormalities; overdosage may result in prolonged and serious arrhythmias, which can be fatal. The anticholinergic drug, physostigmine, may reverse some of these adverse effects. Although the usual doses do not depress respiration, and may help relieve bronchospasm, overdosages can cause respiratory depression. Other side effects include dizziness, constipation, urinary retention, sweating, headache, weakness, fatigue, mania, tremors, delusions, confusion, hallucinations, insomnia, cholestatic jaundice, rashes, blood dyscrasias and endocrine effects. A number of these agents are currently in use (Table 11–12). They are all rather similar, and they may not produce a noticeable effect for 7 to 21 days.[65] Usually, once-a-day dosage suffices, since they are long-acting.

Amitriptyline (Elavil) is probably the most favored of the tricyclic antidepressants. It has a tendency to cause more sedation, and possibly more confusion in elderly people, than other tricyclics; also, it stimulates appetite. The usual adult dosage is 50 to 100 mg before bedtime initially, with a subsequent dosage up to 200 to 300 mg per day; split doses can be given, but more often a single evening dose is best.

Imipramine (Tofranil, Presamine) is the prototype tricyclic agent. Although effective in the treatment of depression, it is not necessarily of value in accompanying anxiety. Abrupt stopping of treatment with the drug may produce withdrawal symptoms (headache, malaise, anorexia) and akathisia. The drug is available as the hydrochloride and as the pamoate; they are similar in properties. The usual adult dosage is 50 to 100 mg given as a single dose in the evening, but 200 to 300 mg a day may be required.

Desipramine (Norpramin, Pertofrane) may be more suitable for elderly people, since it causes less daytime sedation than the other tricyclics.

Doxepin (Adapin, Sinequan) has the advantage of little anticholinergic activity, and may be safer than other tricyclics in patients with cardiac arrhythmias.

Nortriptyline (Aventyl) is similar to amitriptyline and imipramine.

Protriptyline (Vivactil) tends to cause central stimulation, and may decrease the appetite in some people.

PARALYZING AGENTS

Although tranquillizers and related compounds may relieve muscle spasm, they do not reduce the patient's ability to move voluntarily. General anesthetics can abolish consciousness, volition and pain perception, but produce full abolition of muscular tone only when the level of anesthesia becomes profound. In surgical anesthetic practice, more satisfactory patient management is attained by using lighter general anesthesia in combination with muscle paralysis; a number of agents are used to produce this degree of immobilization.

Paralyzing drugs are also of value in the occasional patient requiring intensive respiratory care. Severe diseases causing neuromuscular hyperactivity may require the judicious administration of adequate doses of these drugs; tetanus or severe intractable seizure activity are examples of life threatening conditions that may necessitate this form of pharmacologic control. The paralyzing drugs may also be used to facilitate a difficult endotracheal intubation, or to manage laryngeal spasm. An occasional role for these agents is to prevent struggling, fighting or gross tachypnea in a patient who is being managed with ventilatory support following endotracheal intubation. Additional special uses of pharmacologic paralysis are to relax large muscles when reducing a fracture, or to prevent spasms from occurring during electroshock treatment.

In the practice of respiratory care, the need for adjunctive drug-induced muscle relaxation or paralysis is infrequent, and few intensivists obtain much experience in their use. Since these agents can be difficult to use optimally, it is preferable to seek the assistance of an anesthesiologist who is thoroughly conversant with their use. The respiratory clinician can often avoid the need to employ these drugs by giving the patient who requires relaxant therapy large amounts of sedative-hypnotic or tranquillizing agents, perhaps with an opiate drug. In any case, when a paralyzing agent is utilized, the patient should be sedated or narcotized, since the subjective experience of pharmacologic paralysis is extremely unpleasant. If the patient who is paralyzed recovers consciousness, great care should be taken by all attendants to reassure the patient and to avoid injudicious talk or behavior: it is all too easy to overlook the fact that a totally paralyzed subject can be rational, comprehending, and "scared stiff."

The earliest paralyzing agent to be used was the well-known South American Indian arrow poison, generally called *curare*. Since the time of the introduction of this drug into modern medicine, a number of additional synthetic agents have become available, and considerable understanding of their mechanisms of action has developed. Nevertheless, there is still debate and controversy regarding the basic actions and uses of these potent drugs.[66] The subject is complex; the following discussion will be simplified and maintained at a practical level: much more extensive discussions can be found in standard pharmacology and anesthesiology textbooks.[29, 42, 62, 67]

Mechanisms of Action of Paralyzing Agents

Contraction of the voluntary muscles is initiated by efferent impulses arriving along their supplying motor nerves. The complex mechanism involved in neuromuscular transmission is comparable to that which occurs in the propagation of nerve impulses along the axons, and the pharmacologic block of transmission at the muscles is comparable to the mechanism by which local anesthetics prevent neuronal conduction.

The resting potential of the nerve supplying a muscle is determined by the relative permeability of the cell membrane to sodium and potassium ions. The terminal junctional membrane of the motor neuron endplate, which is closely juxtaposed to the sarcoplasm of the muscle fiber, contains synaptic vesicles filled with acetylcholine, which is the basic neurotransmitter. When an impulse is propagated along the motor nerve, the action potential serves to release acetylcholine, which diffuses instantly into the subneural space between the terminal junctional membrane and the muscle; the neurotransmitter attaches to receptors in the sarcoplasm, and increases the membrane permeability. As a consequence, Na^+ ions diffuse into the muscle and K^+ ions migrate out; the resulting wave of depolarization initiates muscular contraction.[68] It is probable that alterations in calcium ion flux also play an important role in the process. Repolarization, and relaxation, of the muscle occurs when acetylcholine is released from the muscle receptor as a result of hydrolysis by the enzyme acetycholinesterase.

Paralyzing agents work by blocking the neurotransmission caused by acetylcholine, and they are therefore called "neuromuscular blocking drugs," which is a more precise term than "muscle relaxants."[70] The paralyzing agents in current use are believed to work either by serving to produce prolonged depolarization at the neuromuscular junction or by competing with acetylcholine for receptor sites: in either case, further release of acetylcholine by the neuron will not be able to effect further muscular contraction. Less effective paralysis can be produced by other pharmacologic mechanisms.[66] Thus, drugs such as hemicholinium can be used to prevent the synthesis of new acetylcholine in the neurons, or the depolarizing action at the sarcoplasmic receptors can be prolonged by the use of synthetic anticholinesterases that prevent the breakdown of acetylcholine and thereby do not permit opportunity for the muscle to return to the repolarized state required for subsequent reactivation and contraction. Finally, the release of acetylcholine from the nerve terminals can be prevented by miscellaneous means, for example, by low calcium, high magnesium or phosphate, botulinum toxin and various antibiotics such as the aminoglycosides (see Chapter 10). Some natural toxins may have a curare-like blocking action: thus, the snake venom α-bungarotoxin produces a slow but virtually irreversible postjunctional neuromuscular block.[69]

When a parenteral dose of a curare-like neuromuscular blocking agent is administered, the effect is dose dependent. Small doses in an alert patient result in unpleasant sensations of lightheadedness, weakness and blurred vision, accompanied by specific motor dysfunction such as ptosis, diplopia, dysarthria and dysphagia. Larger doses cause the experience of heaviness and weakness in the extremities, followed by total limb paralysis. The respiratory muscles are the last to be affected; breathlessness and a choking sensation are usually experienced before total apnea supervenes. During recovery, the diaphragm recovers first, followed usually by the face, arms and legs, trunk, hands and feet, and pharynx. When pharmacologic paralysis of a respiratory patient is required, large doses must be used to inhibit diaphragmatic movement, and adverse systemic effects can be expected. Usually, the central nervous system is not directly affected, but the cardiovascular system is susceptible to the pharmacologic actions of these drugs. Repeated doses or large doses of any neuromuscular blocking agent may produce quite different effects from the single doses given to facilitate a procedure such as intubation.[66-68]

Nondepolarizing Agents (Table 11–13). The original paralyzing drug, curare, acts by competing with acetylcholine for the muscle receptor, and thus causes paralysis by nondepolarizing (or antidepolarizing) competitive block: such agents are sometimes called stabilizing blockers. When given in large doses to paralyze respiration, hypotension may occur, but spontaneous recovery usually ensues; however, hypertension may be seen as an alternative, and either bradycardia or tachycardia can occur. Curare is believed to release histamine in the lungs; thus, the drug could produce bronchospasm, and although this is unlikely to be a major problem, it is generally advised that curare should be avoided in asthmatics.[68] It should be recognized that there is still some controversy about whether tubocurarine, the active principle of curare, does, in fact, cause bronchoconstriction.[70]

At present, four competive blocking agents are available, and each will be discussed briefly.

TUBOCURARINE (curare). This is the active alkaloid of the root of the South American plant *Chondodendron tomentosum*. "Curare" is derived from the original Indian word for the poison extract; extracts of curare subsequently introduced include d-tubocurarine (tube curare), calabash (gourd curare) and pot curare; these names are related to the ways in which the extracts were formerly packaged.[29]

Tubocurarine is still used as an anesthetic adjunct, the appropriate intravenous dose being 6 to 9 mg, followed in five minutes by 3 to 6 mg more, if necessary. After intravenous administration, an effect is seen within a few seconds and is maximal within three minutes; after intramuscular injection, it takes 10 to 15 minutes for muscle paralysis to develop. General anesthetics such as ether, cyclopropane, halothane and methoxyflurane potentiate the relaxing effect of the drug, allowing reduction in the dosage of tubocurarine; a similar effect may be seen in patients treated with aminoglycoside antibiotics. Ether is particularly effective as a potentiator, and only 2 to 3 mg of tubocurarine may be needed when ether anesthesia is employed. In the absence of potentiating anesthesia, it takes about 20 to 30 mg of tubocurarine to produce sufficient relaxation to allow endotracheal intubation.

For maintenance paralysis in anesthesia or for a ventilated respiratory patient, one-fourth to one-third of the initial dose can be given every 45 to 60 minutes. In children, a

TABLE 11–13. THE NEUROMUSCULAR BLOCKING DRUGS

Drug	Onset of Action (Minutes)	Usual Duration of Effect (Minutes)	Breakdown or Excretion	Single Dose (I.V.)	Adult Dosage Infusion Dosage (I.V.)	Usual Dose (mg)	Reversal of Action by Neostigmine	Side Effects
NON-DEPOLARIZING AGENTS								
d-Tubocurarine (curare, Tubadil, Tubarine)	1–3	Usually 45–90 (full recovery takes longer)	Excreted mainly by the kidney	6–9 mg, then 3–6 mg if necessary in 5 min.	2–3 mg every 45–60 mins.	12–30	Yes	Hypotension or hypertension. Bradycardia or tachycardia. Histamine release may occur. Myasthenia gravis is exacerbated by curariform agents.
Gallamine (Flaxedil)	1.5–2	15–30	Excreted entirely by the kidney	2–2.5 mg/kg + 0.3–1.2 mg/kg if necessary	—	80–150	Yes	Vagal block: tachycardia, hypertension. Effect is prolonged in renal insufficiency. No histamine release or ganglionic blockade produced.
Pancuronium (Pavulon)	1–3	Up to 50 (full recovery takes longer)	Excreted by kidney	0.08–0.1 mg/kg	0.01–0.02 mg/kg every 20–40 min	4–6	Yes	Slight tachycardia; slight hypertension possible.
Metocurine (Metubine)	1–3	Less than 50	Excreted mainly by kidney	Variable e.g. 0.13–4 mg/kg	—	10–30	Yes	Similar to tubocurarine; less cardiovascular effects than tubocurarine or pancuronium
DEPOLARIZING AGENTS								
Succinylcholine (suxamethonium, Anectine)	1	5 (in most people)	Hydrolyzed by pseudocholinesterase: absent in 1:3000 people	Variable: e.g. 0.6–2 mg/kg	0.5–10 mg/min	60–100	No	Variable cardiovascular effects due to vagal and sympathetic stimulation. Prolonged paralysis occurs in sensitive people. Causes fasciculations; may result in muscle pain. Increases serum potassium.
Decamethonium (Syncurine)	1	20	Excreted by kidney	0.03–0.06 mg/kg	—	3–6	No	Similar to succinylcholine, but prolonged paralysis does not occur.

dose of 0.2 to 0.25 mg/kg produces apnea. When the drug infusion is stopped, full muscular power usually returns in 15 to 50 minutes. The drug has a complex excretory mechanism, which involves mainly the kidney and partly the liver.

Tubocurarine is marketed as its chloride, both in generic forms and as proprietary preparations (such as Tubadil and Tubarine). It is available as solutions of 3 mg/ml and 15 mg/ml.

GALLAMINE. Gallamine is a synthetic curarizing agent that produces nondepolarizing block; it has about one-sixth the potency of tubocurarine, and it tends to have a shorter-lasting effect. It differs in some other respects from tubocurarine; of particular note is that it causes a block of the vagus nerve to the heart and may cause tachycardia and some hypertension: it can be used with halothane to counteract the tendency of the latter to cause bradycardia. Unlike tubocurarine, it is excreted entirely by the kidney, and its effect is prolonged in renal failure. It is alleged not to release histamine, and it may be safer than tubocurarine for patients who are likely to develop bronchospasm.

A problem with the use of gallamine is that its dose varies considerably in different patients. It is potentiated by general anesthetics that are more potent than nitrous oxide, and dosage has to be carefully evaluated in individual circumstances. The usual initial intravenous dosage for both adults and children is 2 to 2.5 mg/kg, followed by doses of 0.3 to 1.2 mg/kg; no more than 150 mg should be given. Its effect usually appears within 1.5 to 2 minutes and lasts 15 to 30 minutes.

The drug is available as gallamine triethiodide (Flaxedil), and it is marketed in solutions of 20 mg/ml and 100 mg/ml.

PANCURONIUM. This is a synthetic agent that is similar to tubocurarine, although it is five times more potent and longer acting. It offers several advantages: it does not release histamine, does not cause ganglionic blockade, and it has a vagolytic effect. Thus, the drug is unlikely to cause hypotension; it tends to increase the heart rate, but this effect is slight. At present, it appears to be the drug of choice for use in patients in respiratory care units.[66a]

Pancuronium is particularly recommended for inducing muscle relaxation to permit endotracheal intubation. Following intravenous injection, peak relaxation occurs within two to three minutes, and lasts for up to 50 minutes. The adult dosage is 0.08 to 0.1 mg/kg followed, if necessary, by 0.01 to 0.02 mg/kg every 20 to 40 minutes. In children, the dosage is 0.06 to 0.1 mg/kg, followed by 0.01 to 0.06 mg/kg as needed.

The drug is available as pancuronium bromide (Pavulon) in solutions of 1 mg/ml and 2 mg/ml.

METOCURINE. Metocurine is more potent than tubocurarine, and has a shorter duration of action. It is available as dimethyl tubocurarine iodide (Metubine), but it is rarely employed; one major disadvantage of the drug is that the appropriate dosage is very variable, and considerable familiarity with metocurine is required if it is to be used effectively and safely. However, when used correctly it can be of value, particularly in patients with cardiovascular instability for whom metocurine may be safer than tubocurarine or pancuronium.[71]

Depolarizing Agents (Table 11–13). An alternative group of muscle relaxants produces blockade to neuromuscular transmission by acting in a fashion similar to acetylcholine. These drugs depolarize the postjunctional sarcolemmal membrane and cause an initial contraction that is manifested by fasciculations (twitching) of the skeletal muscles. Although repolarization occurs in the normal fashion, the drug continues to occupy the receptor site and renders it unavailable for further stimulation; relaxation persists until the drug is removed by hydrolysis and the receptor is again susceptible to cholinergic activation. The usual type of short-lasting depolarization is known as Phase 1 block; if large doses of the drug are used, the receptor behaves as though it is blocked by a nondepolarizing competitor; and this state is described as Phase 2 block.[67, 68] The mechanism of action of the depolarizing agents is not well understood, and the fact that they appear to produce a prolonged action similar to that resulting from the nondepolarizing blocking agents has led to the inadequate term of "dual block" being applied to the action of the depolarizing agents.[68]

SUCCINYLCHOLINE (suxamethonium). This is the only important depolarizing agent. The drug causes a rapid development of paralysis (preceded by fasciculations) within one minute of a dose being given intravenously; in most people the effect largely wears off after five minutes, and is completely over within 10 minutes. Hydrolysis of the drug is produced by serum pseudocholinesterase, an enzyme produced by the liver. Inadequate amounts of the enzyme are produced by individuals with severe diseases, such as hepatic insufficiency, anemia, electrolyte imbalance or advanced malnutrition, and in such patients the effect of succinylcholine is prolonged. About 95 per cent of the population is homozygous for normal pseudocholinesterase, the remaining 5 per cent being either homozygous for an abnormal form of the enzyme or heterozygous for two abnormal forms: the abnormal enzymes produce hydrolysis of succinylcholine only very slowly.[68] About one in 3000 of the population have sufficient intrinsic abnormality of pseudocholinesterase to be liable to prolonged paralysis following succinylcholine administration.[67] Simple biochemical tests are available for detecting succinylcholine sensitivity.

The paralysis resulting from succinylcholine differs from that caused by the curariform agents, in that the facial and pharyngeal muscles are only slightly affected. The drug can cause both vagal and sympathetic stimulation, and complex changes in heart rate and hypertension may result; hyperkalemia (such as occurs after severe injury) predisposes patients to life-threatening arrhythmias when succinylcholine is used. There is a possibility of succinylcholine causing bronchospasm in susceptible patients, but this is uncommon. The vagus-mediated muscarinic effects (salivation, increased bronchial secretions and bradycardia) can be prevented or counteracted by giving atropine. A frequent postoperative complaint, particularly in patients who ambulate early, is pain and stiffness in the trunk msucles, probably resulting from muscle trauma caused by the initial muscle spasms that precede the onset of paralysis. A hazardous complication may result from the increased intragastric pressure that occurs during the paralytic stage due to the fasciculations: this may predispose patients to vomiting and aspiration.

The dose of succinylcholine can be very variable; initially, an adult should be given 0.6 to 1.1 mg/kg. For a continuous infusion, a 0.1 to 0.2 per cent solution can be used, and the rate of administration may be between 0.5 to 10 mg/minute. In children 1.1 mg/kg is given initially, and 0.3 to 0.6 mg/kg can be given subsequently. The drug is available as succinylcholine chloride as a generic preparation and under various trade names, such as Anectine, Quelicin, Sucostrin and Sux-Cert. It is marketed as solutions of 20, 50 and 100 mg per ml.

TABLE 11–14. POTENTIATION AND ANTAGONISM OF EFFECTS OF PARALYZING DRUGS

	Nondepolarizing Agents e.g. Tubocurarine	Depolarizing Agents e.g. Succinylcholine
PATHOPHYSIOLOGIC FACTORS		
Increased temperature	↑	↓
Decreased temperature	↓	↑
Acidosis	↑	↓ or ↑
Alkalosis	↓	↑ or ↓
Liver disease	↓	↑
Renal insufficiency	↑	↑
Malnutrition, severe illness, anemia		↑
Myasthenia syndromes	↑	
DRUGS		
Inhalational anesthetics	↑	↓
Intravenous anesthetics	↑	
Various antibiotics (e.g. aminoglycosides)	↑	↑
Anticholinesterases	↓	↑
Acetylcholine	↓	↑
Magnesium sulfate	↑	
Hypokalemia, hyponatremia	↑	↓
Calcium chloride	↓	↓
Catecholamines	↓	↑
Phenothiazines		↑
Nondepolarizing agents	↑	↓
Depolarizing agents	↓	↑
Antiarrhythmia drugs	↑	

DECAMETHONIUM (Syncurine). This is a depolarizing agent that is excreted by the kidney and is not hydrolyzed by cholinesterases. It is longer-acting than succinylcholine, with an effect persisting for about 20 minutes. In other respects, it is similar to succinylcholine, but it is less frequently used.

In general, the depolarizing agents are less desirable than the curariform drugs, and the only advantage of succinylcholine is its short action. Decamethonium does not offer this brevity of effect, and therefore the curariform drugs are preferred.

Agents that modify the Neuromuscular Blocking Drugs

The effects of the neuromuscular blocking drugs can be influenced by other drugs and by certain physiologic conditions (Table 11–14). The paralyzing actions of the depolarizing agents, such as succinylcholine, can be potentiated by anticholinesterase drugs, such as neostigmine (Prostigmin), pyridostigmine (Mestinon, Regonol), edrophonium (Tensilon) and hexafluorenium (Mylaxen). Acetylcholine will similarly potentiate the action of the depolarizers. Various antibiotics, phenothiazines and magnesium sulfate have been reported to cause a more prolonged action of these drugs; hypothermia has a similar potentiating effect. In contrast, the nondepolarizing agents, such as tubocurarine, have their effects diminished by anticholinesterase drugs, acetylcholine and lowered temperature; in addition, the curariform action is decreased by catecholamines and by concomitant administration of depolarizing agents. The effects of the depolarizing drugs are similarly diminished by concomitant administration of nondepolarizing agents, and also by anesthetics such as ether and halothane. The nondepolarizing agents, in contrast, are potentiated by ether or halothane, and more so by enflurane and isoflurane; they may also be potentiated by intravenous anesthetics such as thiopentone.[70] The nondepolarizing agents are also potentiated by various antibiotics, local anesthetics, quinidine, beta-adrenergic blocking agents and magnesium sulfate. Acidosis and hypokalemia enhance the action of tubocurarine.

While the action of the curariform drugs can be reversed by administering anticholinesterase drugs, that of succinylcholine cannot be antagonized by these agents. In general, the curariform drugs are easier and safer to use, and may be less hazardous. However, the short action of succinylcholine (at least, in the majority of patients) makes it more suitable for short-term paralysis, such as may be required to enable endotracheal intubation to be carried out. For control of a fighting patient on a respirator, the longer and more predictable action of a curariform drug such as pancuronium renders it more suitable for use.

Whenever the use of a paralyzing drug is considered for a respiratory patient, a physician experienced in the use of these agents should participate in the management. If a curariform drug is utilized, its action can be reversed by the intravenous administration of neostigmine methylsulfate 1 to 3 mg (0.08 mg/kg in children); if an excessive amount of the nondepolarizing drug had been given, neostigmine may not be successful. A problem with the use of neostigmine or other anticholinesterases is that they have muscarinic actions, and can cause bradycardia, bronchospasm and increased oropharyngeal secretion; concomitant atropine should be administered to forestall these effects.

REFERENCES

1. Solliday, N. H., Chandrasekhar, A. J., Nam, K. I., Cugell, D. W. and Bazley, E. S.: The lazy respiratory center—or how to recognize a tired horse. Chest 66:71–76, 1974.
2. Whipp, B. J.: Physiological consequences of carotid body resection in man: a frame of reference. Respiratory Therapy 5:29–30, Nov./Dec., 1975.
3. Comroe, J. H.: The peripheral chemoreceptors. In Handbook of Physiology, Section 3 Respiration. Vol. 1. W. O. Fenn and H. Rahn (Eds.). Washington, D.C., American Physiological Society, 1964.
4. Winter, B.: Surgical treatment of asthma, chronic bronchitis and emphysema by bilateral carotid body resection. Respiratory Therapy 5:18–28, Nov./Dec., 1975.
5. Rudolf, M., Banks, R. A. and Semple, S. J. G.: Hypercapnia during oxygen therapy in acute exacerbations of chronic respiratory failure. Lancet 2:483–486, 1977.
6. Pierson, D. J.: Respiratory stimulants: review of the literature and assessment of current status. Heart and Lung. 2:726–731, Sept./Oct., 1973.
7. Woolf, C. R.: The use of "respiratory stimulant" drugs. Chest 58:49–53, 1970.
8. Bickerman, H. A. and Chusid, E. L.: The case against the use of respiratory stimulants. Chest 58:53–56, 1970.
9. Moser, K. M., Luchsinger, P. C., Adamson, J. S., McMahon, S. M., Schlueter, D. P., Spivack, M. and Weg, J. G.: Respiratory stimulation with intravenous doxapram in respiratory failure. N. Engl. J. Med. 288:427–432, 1973.

10. Anon: Respiratory stimulants. Br. Med. J. 2:522–523, May, 1972.
11. Wang, S. C. and Ward, J. W.: Analeptics. Pharmac. Ther. B. 3:123–165, 1977.
12. Vandam, L. D.: Medullary stimulants. In Drugs of Choice 1976–1977. W. Modell (Ed.). St. Louis, The C. V. Mosby Company, 1976. Ch. 13.
13. Winnie, A. P.: Chemical respirogenesis: a comparative study. Acta Anaesth. Scand. Suppl. 51:1–32, 1973.
14. Gawley, T. H., Dundee, J. W., Gupta, P. K. and Jones, C. J.: Role of doxapram in reducing pulmonary complications after major surgery. Br. Med. J. 1:122–124, Jan., 1976.
15. Editorial: A new stimulant for ventilatory failure? Lancet 1:753–754, 1973.
16. Fritts, H. W. and Rochester, D. F.: Respiratory stimulants and obstructed airways. N. Engl. J. Med. 288:464–465, 1973.
17. Miller, W. F., Archer, R. K., Taylor, H. F. and Ossenfort, W. F.: Severe respiratory depression: role of a respiratory stimulant, ethamivan, in the treatment. J.A.M.A. 180:905–911, 1962.
18. Brewis, R. A. L. and Hodges, N. G.: Long-term and short-term effects of oral prethcamide in chronic ventilatory failure. Br. Med. J. 2:764–766, June, 1970.
19. Lambertsen, C. J.: Effects of drugs and hormones on the respiratory response to carbon dioxide. In Handbook of Physiology. Sect. 3. Respiration. Vol. 1. W. O. Fenn and H. Rahn (Eds.) Washington, D. C., American Physiological Society, 1964.
20. Zwillich, C. W., Pierson, D. J., Hofeldt, F. D., Lufkin, E. G. and Weil, J. V.: Ventilatory control in myxedema and hypothyroidism. N. Engl. J. Med. 292:662–665, 1975.
21. Lyons, H. A.: Centrally acting hormones and respiration. Pharmac. Ther. B. 2:743–751, 1976.
22. Sutton, F. D., Zwillich, C. W., Creagh, C. E., Pierson, D. J. and Weil, J. V.: Progesterone for outpatient treatment of Pickwickian syndrome. Ann. Intern. Med. 83:476–479, 1975.
23. Orenstein, D. M., Boat, T. F., Stern, R. C., Doershuk, C. F. and Light, M. S.: Progesterone treatment of the obesity hypoventilation syndrome in a child. J. Pediatr. 90:477–479, 1977.
24. Aranda, J. V., Gorman, W., Bergsteinsson, H. and Gunn, T.: Efficacy of caffeine in treatment of apnea in the low-birth-weight infant. J. Pediatr. 90:467–472, 1977.
25. Putnam, J. S., Kaufman, L. V., Michaels, R. M., Canter, H. G. and Katz, S.: Methylphenidate therapy in primary alveolar hypoventilation. Chest 64: 137–140, 1973.
26. Lewis, J. W., Bentley, K. W. and Cowan, A.: Narcotic analgesics and antagonists. Ann. Rev. Pharmacol. 11:241–270, 1971.
27. Brown, E. B.: Drugs and respiratory control. Ann. Rev. Pharmacol. 11:271–284, 1971.
28. Martin, W. R.: Naloxone. Ann. Intern. Med. 85:765–768, 1976.
29. Collins, V. J.: Principles of Anesthesiology. Philadelphia, Lea and Febiger, 2nd ed., 1976.
30. Guz, A.: Does carbon dioxide excite ventilation by stimulating receptors within the lungs of mammals? Am. Rev. Respir. Dis. 115: #6 Pt. 2:239–243, 1977.
31. Ziment, I.: Intermittent positive pressure breathing. In: Respiratory Care: A Guide To Clinical Practice. G. G. Burton, G. N. Gee and J. E. Hodgkin (Eds.). Philadelphia, J. B. Lippincott Company, 1977. Ch. 23.
32. Comroe, J. H.: Physiology of Respiration. Chicago, Year Book Medical Publishers Incorporated, 2nd ed. 1974.
33. Mustehin, C. P. Gribbin, H. R., Tattersfield, A. E. and George, C. F.: Reduced respiratory response to carbon dioxide after propranolol: a central action? Brit. Med. J. 2:1229–1231, Nov., 1976.
34. Grant, J. L., Lucier, E. and Mahnke, M. L.: Estimation of ventilatory drive with carbon dioxide and helium. Ann. Intern. Med. 74:62–66, 1971.
35. Wollman, H. and Dripps, R. D.: The therapeutic gases: oxygen, carbon dioxide, and helium. In The Pharmacological Basis of Therapeutics. L. S. Goodman and A. Gilman (Eds.). 3rd ed. New York, The Macmillan Company, 1965.
36. Lambertsen, C. J.: Therapeutic gases: oxygen, carbon dioxide and helium. In Drill's Pharmacology in Medicine. J. R. dePalma (Ed.), 4th ed, New York, McGraw Hill Book Company, 1971.
37. Egan, D. F.: Fundamentals of Respiratory Therapy. 3rd ed. St. Louis, The C. V. Mosby Company, 1977.
38. Coudon, W. L. and Block, A. J.: Acute respiratory failure precipitated by a carbonic anhydrase inhibitor. Chest 69:112–113, 1976.
39. Drug Spotlight: Choosing diuretics for optimal results. Patient Care, June 15, 1976, pp. 22–50.
40. Hackett, P. H., Rennie, D. and Levine, H. D.: The incidence, importance and prophylaxis of acute mountain sickness. Lancet 2:1149–1155, 1976.
41. Kroneberg, R. S. and Cain, S. M.: Effects of acetazolamide and hypoxia on cerebrospinal fluid bicarbonate. J. Appl. Physiol. 24:17–20, 1968.
42. Martindale: The Extra Pharmacopoeia. London, The Pharmaceutical Press, 27th ed., 1977.
43. Steen, S. N.: The effects of psychotropic drugs on respiration. Pharmac. Ther. B. 2:717–741, 1976.
44. Honingfeld, G. and Howard, A.: Psychiatric Drugs: A Desk Reference. New York, Academic Press, 1973.
45. Hollister, L. E.: Drugs for emotional disorders: current problems. J.A.M.A. 234:942–947, 1975.
46. Cain, N. N. and Cain, R. M.: A compendium of psychiatric drugs, Part II. Drug Therapy, February, 1975, pp. 77–83.
46a. Adams, A. P. and Pybus, D. A.: Delayed respiratory depression after use of fentanyl during anesthesia. Br. Med. J. 1:278–279, Feb., 1978.
47. Drugs for psychiatric disorders. Med. Lett. Drugs Ther. 18:89–96, 1976.
48. Help for the patient who can't sleep. Patient Care, February 1, 1976, pp. 98–133.
49. Brewis, R. L. A.: Respiratory disorders. In Textbook of Adverse Drug Reactions. D. M. Davies (Ed.). Oxford, Oxford University Press, 1977. Ch. 8.
50. Mindham, R. H. S.: Hypnotics and sedatives. In Meyler's Side Effects of Drugs. A Survey of

Unwanted Effects of Drugs Reported in 1972-1975. M. N. G. Dukes (Ed.). Amsterdam, Excerpta Medica. Vol. VIII, 1975. Ch. 4.

51. Clark, T. J. H.: Acute severe asthma. *In:* Asthma. T. J. H. Clark and S. Godfrey (Eds.). Philadelphia, W. B. Saunders Company, 1977.

52. Bickerman, H. A.: Pharmacologic therapy in the management of pulmonary emphysema. *In* Pulmonary Emphysema. A. L. Barach, and H. A. Bickerman (Eds.) Baltimore, The Williams and Wilkins Company, 1956. Ch. 6.

53. Editorial: Barbiturates in asthma. Brit. Med. J. 3:490, Aug., 1972.

54. Geddes, D. M., Rudolf, M. and Saunders, K. B.: Effect of nitrazepam and flurazepam on the ventilatory response to carbon dioxide. Thorax 31:548–551, 1976.

55. Katz, R. L.: Sedatives and tranquillizers. New Engl. J. Med. 286:757–760, 1972.

56. Kiely, W. F.: Psychiatric syndromes in critically ill patients. J.A.M.A. 235:2759–2761, 1976.

57. Zsigmond, E. K., Flynn, K. and Martinez, O. A.: Diazepam and meperidine on arterial blood gases in healthy volunteers. J. Clin. Pharmacol. 14:377–381, 1974.

58. Choice of a benzodiazepine for treatment of anxiety or insomnia. Med. Lett. Drugs Ther. 19:49–50, 1977.

59. Gasser, J. C. and Bellville, J. W.: Interaction of the effects of hydroxyzine and pentazocine on human respiration. Anesthesiology 43:599–601, 1975.

60. Hollister, L. E.: Mental disorders—antipsychotic and antimanic drugs. New Engl. J. Med. 286:984–987, 1972.

61. Jacobsen, E.: The properties of psychotropic drugs. *In* Modern Psychiatric Treatment. T. P. Detre and H. G. Jarecki. Philadelphia, J. B. Lippincott Company, 1971. Ch. 14.

62. Cullen, S. C. and Larson, C. P.: Essentials of Anesthetic Practice. Chicago, Year Book Medical Publishers, Inc. 1974. Ch. 17.

63. Keller, R., Waldvogel, H. and Herzog, H.: Neurolept analgesia for bronchoscopic examinations. Chest 67:315–319, 1975.

64. Treating depression. Patient Care, March 1, 1977, pp. 20–77.

64a. Biggs, J. T.: Clinical pharmacology and toxicology of antidepressants. Hosp. Practice 13:79–84, 1978.

65. Greenblatt, D. J. and Shader, R. I.: Rational use of psychotropic drugs. IV. Antidepressants. *In* Drug Therapy Reviews Vol. 1. R. R. Miller and D. J. Greenblatt (Eds.). New York, Masson Publishing USA, Inc., 1977, pp. 73–84.

66. Lamid, S. and Wang, R. I. H.: Neuromuscular blocking agents. Drug Therapy, Feb. 1974 pp. 123–129.

66a. Roizen, M. F. and Feeley, T. W.: Pancuronium bromide. Ann. Intern. Med. 88:64–68, 1978.

67. Lee, J. A. and Atkinson, R. S.: A Synopsis of Anaesthesia. Bristol, John Wright and Sons Ltd., 7th ed., 1973.

68. Flynn, R. E.: Controlled ventilation: neuromuscular blocking agents. *In* Current Respiratory Care. K. F. MacDonnell and M. S. Segal (Eds.). Boston, Little, Brown and Company, 1977. Ch. 14.

69. Rogers, H., Spector, R. and Trounce, J. R.: An Introduction to Mechanisms in Pharmacology and Therapeutics. London, William Heinemann Medical Books Ltd., 1976.

70. Gautier, H. and Vincent, J.: Muscle relaxants and breathing. Pharmac. Ther. B. 2:463–469, 1976.

71. Fogdall, R. P.: Metocurine—a "new" muscle relaxant. West. J. Med. 128:148–149, Feb., 1978.

CHAPTER
12

AGENTS USED IN PULMONARY DIAGNOSTIC STUDIES

The development of fiberoptic bronchoscopy and the accessibility of the tracheobronchial tree to endoscopy have resulted in a decline in the need for agents used in radio-contrast studies, and an increased need for drugs used in inducing topical anesthesia of the airways to facilitate endoscopy. In recent years, techniques using radionuclide studies of the lungs have assumed an increasingly important role in the diagnosis of both ventilation and perfusion abnormalities; a variety of agents have been introduced. Another new diagnostic area, of increasing relevance, is that based on the physiologic reaction to inhalational provocative agents, utilizing suitable drugs and industrial chemicals or antigens. The classes of drugs employed in these various studies constitute the basis for this chapter.

RADIOGRAPHIC DIAGNOSTIC AGENTS

Two classes of agents are utilized in radiodiagnostic studies of the lungs: (A) contrast media, and (B) radionuclides.

Contrast Media

Radiopaque contrast media produce radiologic visualization of the gas-filled airways or the blood vessels. The contrast technique used in displaying the anatomy of the airways is known as bronchography, whereas blood vessels are displayed by angiography.

Bronchography has been rendered less important by the development of bronchoscopy, and relatively few radiographic contrast studies are carried out currently compared with the era preceding the introduction of fiberoptic bronchoscopy. A further common use for bronchography in the past was to display the presence of bronchiectasis, and other chronic bronchopulmonary abnormalities caused by infection, in the evaluation of a patient for resectional surgery. In the modern era of respiratory therapy, chronic persistent "surgical" infections are relatively rare, and resection is a comparatively uncommon form of therapy.

Because bronchography is undergoing a decline, little attempt has been made to develop new contrast agents; the number of products in use has declined[1] and fewer choices of such agents are currently available. Most bronchographic studies are carried out using propyliodone, which presently has to be imported from the United Kingdom. No major U.S. pharmaceutical manufacturer produces any bronchographic contrast agent currently.

Hazards of Bronchography. Minor complications are common with bronchography, but serious reactions are rare, and deaths are extremely rare, amounting to only about 0.02 per cent. The serious complications that are seen occur mainly as a result of the accompanying general or local anesthesia necessary for the bronchographic procedure.[1, 2] The agent can be introduced into the tracheobronchial tree through an endoscope, by instillation down the pharynx through the open larynx, or, more satisfactorily, by injection through a cannula introduced into the trachea via puncture of the cricothyroid membrane.[3]

The instillation of significant volumes of contrast media into the lungs results in a loss of functioning alveoli. The vital capacity is reduced as a direct consequence, and ventilation-perfusion imbalance is caused, which results in a fall in PaO_2 and an increase in tidal volume and minute ventilation.[2] Patients with reactive airways develop increased airway resistance, and breathlessness or chest discomfort is usually experienced; susceptible patients may develop wheezing or frank asthma. The incidence of severe complications is higher in children.[2, 4]

Following the bronchographic procedure, postural drainage, percussive therapy and supervised coughing or aspiration of the tracheobronchial tree should be provided. Atelectasis can occur, and secondary complications may follow, although pneumonia is a rare consequence. Many patients develop nonpulmonary reactions, including fever, headache, nausea, vomiting and urticaria. The complications of iodism (Chapter 3) may appear in susceptible patients: rashes, salivary gland swelling and a flu-like illness with burning sensation of the nose, throat or eyes have been reported.

Originally, radiopaque metallic powders were used in bronchography, with barium and bismuth being the most favored; barium sulfate may still have a following today. Later, iodinated poppyseed oil was introduced, and subsequently organic iodides in aqueous solution or oily suspensions became popular. At present, it is generally agreed that no ideal medium is available, but oily contrast media are recognized as more inert and in general more suitable than water-soluble media or aqueous suspensions. The water based agents can produce more severe inflammatory reactions, whereas oily media can persist in the lungs and induce local fibrosis or granuloma formation. There is no evidence to implicate bronchographic contrast media in the subsequent development of lung cancers.[4] Although iodinated oils are no longer used, their replacement with suspensions of organic iodides in oils has not entirely eliminated the risk of lipoid granuloma formation.

Most radiologists and pulmonologists agree that bronchography should be used in only very exceptional circumstances, and

TABLE 12–1.   PRECAUTIONS TO OBSERVE IN BRONCHOGRAPHIC STUDIES

Precaution	Reason
Do not study patients with severe respiratory insufficiency, active pulmonary infection, active bronchospasm, or unstable asthma.	Condition may be severely exacerbated acutely, and subsequent pulmonary problems may develop.
Avoid iodine-containing media in patients who have iodine allergy.	Iodism may be produced, e.g. coryza, lacrimation, swollen salivary glands, rash, flu-like syndrome.
Do not study both lungs at same time.	Avoid possibility of causing bilateral pulmonary complications.
Be prepared to treat acute reactions.	Bronchospasm, severe coughing, vomiting, fever, hypoxemia, laryngeal edema, anaphylaxis can occur.
Use local or general anesthesia with great care.	Anesthetic complications are more frequent and dangerous than those resulting from the contrast agents.
Avoid in younger children, particularly those under the age of 2.	Good studies are difficult to obtain, and complications are frequent.
Follow procedure with respiratory and/or chest physical therapy.	Contrast medium that is not expelled from the lungs may cause acute or chronic reactions.
Avoid in patients with labile medical conditions, such as cardiac arrhythmia or frequent seizures.	Underlying medical problems may be exacerbated during the procedure.

that precautions should be observed (Table 12–1). Small children are less suitable for such studies, and bronchography should not be done in infants under the age of two. The procedure is also contraindicated in unstable asthma, and iodinated contrast media must not be given to patients with known allergy to iodides. Contrast studies of the lung should not be carried out while acute bronchopulmonary infection or bronchospasm is present. It may be advisable to administer a small test dose of the contrast medium before a full amount of the agent is delivered into the lung. No more than 20 ml of contrast agent should be used, and the radiographer should be alert to the early development of reactions, while efforts should be made after bronchography to clear the lungs of residual contrast material.

Properties of Contrast Agents. The agents used in bronchography are selected for their ability to fulfill the following requirements: high degree of radiopacity, stability and lack of toxicity, ease of elimination, suitably high viscosity to ensure uniform distribution, appropriate properties of adherence to respiratory mucosa and to mucus, and ease and safety of use.[5]

Most of the contrast media used in bronchography are iodine-containing organic compounds; the greater the percentage of iodine, the greater the contrast that is obtained. More recently, barium compounds and tantalum have been used, whereas an older contrast agent, thorium dioxide, which has some radioactivity, has fallen into disfavor. Probably, the majority of bronchographic studies in the U.S. are carried out with the British proprietary contrast agent Dionosil. No studies have been carried out on this agent or on other organic drugs containing iodine to determine whether they possess similar mucokinetic properties to those attributed to the organic iodide expectorant drug Organidin (see Chapter 3); likewise, there is no information as to whether Organidin could be used as a bronchographic contrast agent!

Individual Contrast Agents. The most important agents that have been used over the years in the U.S. and in Europe will be discussed in the following section. The practical methods of using each agent are similar, and certain basic principles should be observed; the main agents of relevance are presented in Table 12–2.

IODINATED OIL. Iodine can be combined with vegetable oils in various ways.[5] An early product, iodized oil (ethiodized oil, Ethiodol) was made by adding iodine to the ethyl esters of the fatty acids of poppyseed oil. A very viscous derivative, Lipiodol

TABLE 12–2. BRONCHOGRAPHIC AGENTS

Agent	Disadvantages
CRYSTALLINE ORGANIC IODIDES	
In aqueous solution	
Iopydol } (Hytrast)*† Iopydone }	Clears slowly from lungs, and causes reactions
Propyliodone (Dionosil Aqueous)	Not so suitable for peripheral airways
In oily suspension	
Iodopyridine*	Too toxic for general use
Propyliodone (Dionosil Oily)†	May cause pneumonitis
IODINATED OILS	
Ethiodized oil (Ethiodol)	Too toxic for general use
Iodinated arachis oil	Too toxic for general use
+ chlorinated arachis oil	
(Iodochlorol)*	
Iodinated poppyseed oil (Lipiodol)	Frequent side effects, including granulomas
Iodinated sesame oil (Iodipin)*	Frequent side effects, including granulomas
Iodinated oil with sulfanilamide	May cause methemoglobinemia and other side effects
(Visciodol)*	
PARTICULATE SUSPENSIONS	
Barium sulfate (Micropaque,	May impact in airways; can persist in lung indefinitely
Steripaque)†	
Bismuth carbonate*	Too toxic for general use
Thorium oxide*	Radioactive
Tantalum*	Explosive; may persist in lung indefinitely

*Agents that are not generally available.
†Agents that are favored by many experts.

Ultra-Fluid, was an inferior contrast agent containing 35 to 39 per cent iodine, and had too high an incidence of side effects; it is no longer used in bronchographic studies.

For bronchography, organic iodides, in a concentration of 37 to 50 per cent, are suspended in oil, providing a more viscous medium. The available products are those made from poppyseed oil (Lipiodol Viscous), sesame oil (Iodipin) and arachis oil (which is also combined with chlorine in Iodochlorol).[5] These agents produce good central bronchograms, but the more peripheral airways are poorly demonstrated, and elimination of the bronchographic medium is relatively difficult because it tends to inspissate distally.

Lipiodol Viscous, which contains about 50 per cent iodine, is the iodized oil most readily available currently. The preparation is injected through a cannulated syringe into the airways, and about 12 ml is instilled into each lung. Any Lipiodol that is accidentally swallowed should be removed by inducing vomiting or by gastric lavage. Use of this agent can be hazardous in patients with chronic airways disease, since the product can result in exacerbation of the obstruction. Moreover, retention of the oily product can lead to lipoid pneumonia, fibrosis and granuloma formation. Most experts feel that the iodinated oils should be avoided because of the relatively high incidence of local and general reactions and in fact these products are not approved for use in bronchography in the U.S.

IODINATED OIL WITH INERT POWDERS. Over the years, various preparations have been tried that contain inert powders added to the iodinated oil to increase its viscosity and thereby to prevent the contrast medium from entering the alveoli too readily. The powders that have obtained the most attention have been talc, magnesia and sulfonamide powder. Sulfanilamide was added to various iodinated oils and marketed as Lipiodol-sulfanilamide, Sulphodiol, Visciodol and so on. Although these products did offer advantages, they also led to various complications, such as methemoglobinemia.[2, 5] The selection of sulfanilamide as a thickening agent was based on its antibacterial properties that were considered to be of value in preventing postbronchographic infection. None of these viscous products are available at present.

PROPYLIODONE (Dionosil). Propyliodone is the propyl ester of iodopyracet (Diodrast). It is the only iodine-containing drug currently favored for use as a contrast agent in bronchography; indeed, it is the only one currently approved by the FDA.[3] It appears to be safer than any other iodine-containing agent, because it does not liberate its iodine content and therefore it is less likely to cause allergic reactions. The drug is available both as a 60 per cent suspension in peanut, arachis or other vegetable oil and as a 50 per cent aqueous suspension: each is of consistency appropriate to provide a uniform, widely dispersed coating of the tracheobronchial mucosa. The aqueous preparation results in better coating of the proximal bronchi, whereas the oily preparation results in an overall greater intensity of contrast with better peripheral filling. The oily product is more likely to cause pneumonitis,[2] although it causes less immediate airway irritation. The drug can be absorbed, and it undergoes breakdown by hydrolysis to diodone (iodopyracet); about 50 per cent of the administered amount appears in the urine as this product, while the rest of the agent is usually expelled in the expectorated sputum. Total clearance of the agent usually occurs within two days, and residues do not persist in the lungs.

Both forms of Dionosil are generally safe; the drug does not cause serious inflammatory or granulomatous reactions, in contrast to the iodized oils. Nevertheless, it should be used with caution in patients with chronic airways disease; these patients are particularly likely to develop dyspnea, coughing, and possibly some atelectasis and fever. Other possible side effects include arthralgias, eosinophilia, headache, dyspnea, sore throat and rash. The usual dose of the drug is 0.75 to 1 ml per year of age or 0.2 ml/kg up to a maximum of 20 ml. Accidental injection of this contrast agent into the soft tissues causes a severe prolonged inflammatory reaction that can be aborted by antibiotic and glucocorticoid therapy.[2] The oily preparations should be favored for most bronchographic studies, since they are better tolerated and cause less coughing and therefore result in better bronchograms. The oily preparation contains about 34 per cent iodine, and therefore provides better contrast than the aqueous suspension, which contains about 28 per cent iodine. Leading experts in North America regard propyliodone as the only satisfactory bronchographic contrast agent; Fraser and Paré recommend the aqueous preparation.[5a]

IOPYDOL AND IOPYDONE. These are iodine-containing agents that are used in combination in aqueous suspension in the British preparation Hytrast. They are cleared more slowly than propyliodone and are more dangerous. The combination (iopydol 46 per cent, iopydone 30.5 per cent, with various amounts of methylcellulose) was used in the United Kingdom for bronchography, but it has not been used in the U.S. in recent years. These agents contain a higher concentration of iodine (50 per cent) than does Dionosil; therefore, Hytrast produces superior contrast images. Peripheral filling is not easily obtained, since the product is viscous; however, since Hytrast does not undergo hydrolytic breakdown, any peripheral pooling of the agent may be followed by crystallization in the terminal bronchioles, resulting in an inflammatory reaction.

Hytrast has been marketed in the plain aqueous form and with methylcellulose, which makes it more viscous. Both these products result in incidences of inflammatory consequences similar to those accompanying the use of oily propyliodone. Hytrast is more likely to cause segmental collapse of the small airways of children, particularly in asthmatics, and more often when general anesthesia with oxygen supplementation is used.[2] Although Hytrast is considered to be a superior agent in Europe[5], it is not in favor in the United States.

BARIUM SULFATE. This is used extensively for radiographic examination of the stomach and intestines. For gastric studies, 300 gm of the compound are suspended in 400 ml water. A similar solution can be used as a bronchographic agent, since it is relatively inert and does not cause hypersensitivity reactions, while it produces relatively good contrast radiographs of the tracheobronchial tree. Large amounts of the compound can result in bronchial blockage, particularly in patients with obstructive airways disease, and inflammation could result. Barium particles may persist in the lungs, resulting in chronic abnormalities in subsequent chest x-rays; chronic damage, with fibrosis and granulomatous reactions, can occur, although rarely. In spite of its virtues, barium sulfate has never been widely used as a bronchographic agent, mainly because it cannot be marketed in a stable form, and the mixture has to be constituted freshly for each examination.[2]

Bismuth subcarbonate could also result in good contrast studies, but it is toxic to the lung tissue, and is therefore not suitable for bronchography.

TANTALUM POWDER. Tantalum powder has been used in laboratory investigations and has resulted in some excellent contrast studies.[6] The agent is delivered by inhalation rather than instillation, and it does not reach and coat abnormal areas reliably.[3] Unfortunately, the material is combustible and therefore cannot be employed in clinical practice. Although some studies have shown it to be inert and safe in patients with various pulmonary diseases,[6] other investigators have found that prolonged retention of the powder in the lungs can occur, with consequent pulmonary opacification.[7]

MISCELLANEOUS AGENTS. Agents of various types have been used by various investigators in bronchographic studies. Such drugs include the iodine-containing contrast agents, *Gastrografin* and *Pulmidol* (propyldocetrizoate);[5] none have proved to be of adequate safety or value. Pulmidol has a high iodine content and a high viscosity; it did not produce good peripheral airway filling, and it was very toxic. None of these agents offer sufficient advantages for them to be considered competitors of the established contrast media.

Radionuclides

Nuclear medicine has provided a dramatically successful means for investigating abnormalities of pulmonary vascular perfusion and bronchoalveolar ventilation as part of the routine evaluation of respiratory problems in the clinical setting.[8, 9] Perfusion studies are widely used throughout the U.S. and ventilation studies are becoming available; combined scanning studies are essential to enable a complete interpretation to be made of a suspected pulmonary vascular abnormality. The technique finds its greatest utility in the diagnostic evaluation of pulmonary embolus.[10] The equipment, specialized knowledge and technical competence required for such studies are being acquired to an increasing extent, and the respiratory physician is expected to have some familiarity with the radiopharmaceuticals utilized in nuclear medicine.

The equipment that is needed to carry out pulmonary scanning studies varies from comparatively inexpensive rectilinear scanners to complex computerized scintillation cameras, which may be utilized with multiple detector systems of great sophistication. The facility in which any nuclear studies are carried out must conform with rigid safety precautions; in appropriately run units, patients undergoing scanning procedures are exposed to minimal radiation risks. Furthermore, the overall risk of adverse reactions to radionuclide pulmonary studies in both children and adults is extremely small. Nuclear studies of the lung are simpler to perform, less dangerous and offer greater versatility than do the angiographic techniques that are available for studying the pulmonary vasculature. At present, the cost of carrying out scanning or photoscintiphotography studies of the lung compares favorably with that of angiographic techniques. For all these reasons, lung scanning has, to a considerable extent, replaced pulmonary angiography.

Individual Radiopharmaceuticals. The earliest studies in pulmonary radionuclide imaging used albumin labeled with a radioactive isotope of iodine. Since that time other agents and carriers have been introduced: among the isotopic radionuclides are technetium (which is produced artificially from molybdenum or uranium and is used as sodium pertechnetate), and, less frequently, indium and gallium. Carriers are often derived from albumin, using specially produced macroaggregates or microspheres; other agents include sulfur-colloid, and ferrous and ferric hydroxide. More sophisticated radionuclides include isotopes of the inert gases nitrogen, xenon and krypton, as well as oxygen, which are given by inhalation. An additional technique is to administer labeled particles by aerosolization for studies of airway patency and structure.

The more important of these agents will be discussed in the following section (see also Table 12-3).

IODINE-131 LABELED ALBUMIN. One of the first radioactive labels used in clinical diagnostic medicine was the radioisotope iodine 131 (^{131}I). This was combined with human serum albumin to provide a suitable tracer for studies of blood volume and distribution. Since 1964, Taplin has extended his initial concept of using macroaggregates of albumin (MAA) for studies of the pulmonary circulation.[11] These particles

TABLE 12-3. RADIOPHARMACEUTICALS USED FOR PERFUSION LUNG SCANNING

Agent	Dosage	Physical Half-Life†	Biologic Half-Life*	Particle Size	Total Body Radiation Dose	Comments
Iodine-131 Macroaggregated Albumin (MAA^{131}I)	150–300 μCi	8.1 days	2–9 hrs	10–90 μ	+++	Inferior lung scans produced; thyroid affected unless blocked by SSKI
Technetium-99m Macroaggregated Albumin (MAA^{99m}Tc)	2–4 mCi	6 hrs	2–9 hrs	5–100 μ	+	Agent of choice Not retained in lung in COPD
Technetium-99m Albumin Microspheres	2–4 mCi	6 hrs	7–15 hrs	20–40 μ	+	An agent of choice More uniform particles Remain longer in lung in COPD; safer than MAA in presence of right-to-left shunt
Technetium-99m Ferric Hydroxide	2–4 mCi	6 hrs	27 hrs	3–50 μ	++	Iron hydroxide particles remain in the lung for a relatively long time and may cause severe reactions; deaths have occurred
Indium-113m Ferric Hydroxide	0.5–3 mCi	1.7 hrs	27 hrs	5–60 μ	++	Indium is an alternative to technetium; causes similar reactions
Xenon-133 in Saline	5–20 mCi	5.3 days	30 secs	Gas in solution	+(++)‡	Requires scintillation camera system or multiple probe system; safe in pulmonary hypertension
Gallium-67 Citrate	1–4 mCi	3.2 days	2–3 wks	Molecular	++	For demonstrating lung cancer, lymphoma, abscess, sarcoid, and some pneumonias

†Time for radioactivity to decrease by 50%.
*Time for amount of agent in lung to decrease by 50%.
‡Radiation dose to body depends on dose administered.

range in sizes from 5 to 100 μ; following their introduction into a peripheral vein, the particles are dispersed throughout the blood circulating in the lung, and they become trapped in the small pulmonary vessels. The labeled particles persist in their positions until they become broken up and dispersed, usually within two to nine hours; during that time adequate rectilinear scanning can be carried out. The dispersed particles are phagocytosed by the reticuloendothelial system, mainly in the liver.

The disadvantages of the technique are related both to the macroaggregates and to the radioiodine. Calculations show that in the average patient, less than 0.5 per cent of the small vessels in the lungs are plugged by the MAA particles, and no harm would be expected to occur. In practice, the large majority of patients tolerate the procedure well, but deaths have been reported following administration of radionuclide-tagged MAA to patients with severe pulmonary hypertension or diffuse obliterative pulmonary vascular disease, presumably because the additional vascular blockade by the MAA causes an acute severe exacerbation of the pulmonary vascular pressure.[12]

The half-life of ^{131}I is about eight days; therefore, the body is exposed to an appreciable amount of radiation. For this reason, relatively small doses of the labeled MAA are given, and the resulting lung scan lacks high definition. A further disadvantage of radioiodine is that it is sequestered by the thyroid gland, which could be damaged as a result; prior administration of Lugol's solution (SSKI, 10 drops three times a day for 10 days) is used to block the gland's uptake of [131]I.

IODINE-131 LABELED MICROSPHERES. Denatured human albumin can be prepared as microspheres of a homogeneous size, with a diameter of 20 to 40 μ. The microspheres are more resilient and remain in the lung for a longer time than do the soft macroaggregates.[10] These labeled spheres provide an alternative carrier to MAA, but technetium (^{99m}Tc) is preferred as a label.

TECHNETIUM-99M LABELED ALBUMIN. Technetium is derived from molybdenum; its 99m nuclide is used in pertechnetate ^{99m}Tc, which is reduced with agents such as ascorbic acid or stannous chloride. It offers a number of technical characteristics that make it particularly suitable for lung-scanning.

The main advantage ^{99m}Tc has over ^{131}I is

that the former has a much shorter physical half-life, of about six hours; it results in much less overall body irradiation than does ^{131}I, and ^{99m}Tc labeled albumin does not accumulate in the thyroid gland. Larger dosages of ^{99m}Tc can be used with complete safety, and the resulting lung scans are technically superior to those obtained with [131]I.[13]

Both macroaggregated albumin and albumin microspheres have been labeled with ^{99m}Tc; the MAA product may remain in the lungs as long as the microspheres do, but the retention time of the microspheres may be markedly increased in obstructive lung disease.

TECHNETIUM-99M LABELED IRON HYDROXIDE. Both ferrous and ferric hydroxide have been labeled with ^{99m}Tc; these products appear to remain in the lungs for a much longer time than do the albumin carriers.[10] The iron hydroxide carriers appear to be more prone to cause adverse reactions, and their use is declining.[14]

INDIUM LABELED NUCLIDES. Indium-113m ([113m]In) can be used in comparable fashion to technetium. Some workers have employed other nuclides, such as mercury isotopes, but there is no evidence that these agents are superior to ^{99m}Tc or [113m]In for displaying the pulmonary vasculature. Indium has a number of technical virtues, the main one being that it results in excellent lung scans with comparatively slight radiation.

GALLIUM-67. It has been found that this isotope (^{67}Ga) is preferentially concentrated by hypermetabolic tissues in the lung. It therefore can be used both to display and differentiate pulmonary lesions, such as carcinomas, lymphomas, abscesses and sarcoidosis; ^{67}Ga scans help differentiate such lesions from pulmonary embolism or pneumonitis.[15] The labeled agent, gallium-67 citrate, is injected intravenously, and a scan is carried out 48 to 72 hours later. Carcinomas as small as 1.5 cm in diameter can be revealed by this technique.

Other radionuclides that have been used in similar fashion to ^{67}Ga include preparations of mercury-197 ([197]Hg), selenium-75 (^{75}Se) and labeled bleomycin.[10] Interesting developments can be expected with these "tumor-seeking" radionuclides in the future.

XENON-133 IN SALINE. Xenon is an inert gas that is three times more soluble in water than is oxygen. The half-life of ^{133}Xe is very short, and therefore this diagnostic agent is very safe to use. Xenon-133 dissolved in

TABLE 12–4. RADIOACTIVE GASES USED FOR VENTILATION STUDIES

Agent	Dosage	Physical Half-Life	Radiation Dose	Comments
Xenon-133	0.5–30 mCi	5.3 days	+++	Clinically useful
Xenon-135	0.2 mCi/l	9.1 hr	+++	Under investigation
Xenon-127	0.5–10 mCi	36.4 days	++	Under investigation
Nitrogen-13	5 mCi	10 min	+	Under investigation
Oxygen-15	5 mCi	2 min	+	Under investigation
Krypton-81m	5 mCi	13 sec	+	For experimental use only

saline can be given as an intravenous injection, and 90 per cent of this is removed by the pulmonary vasculature during its first circulation through the lungs. Imaging during breath-holding gives a picture of the circulation, and for this purpose a multiple-detector system or a gamma camera is used while the patient holds his breath at total lung capacity for about 15 seconds. When breathing resumes, the xenon is liberated from the blood vessels and is then distributed throughout the lungs, and imaging will reveal the ventilatory distribution. Xenon-133 in saline is safe to use in patients with pulmonary hypertension.

RADIOACTIVE GASES. Inhalation of a labeled gas is used to obtain a scintiphotographic display of the ventilatory distribution within the airways. The patient breathes in a mixture of air with a labeled gas, such as ^{133}Xe, and a number of photoscans are taken to demonstrate the initial distribution of the gas and the rate of washout from the different lung regions.[9, 10, 15]

The gases that have been used in ventilation studies include isotopes of xenon, oxygen and nitrogen (Table 12–4). Other radioactive gases, such as isotopes of krypton, have been used as research tools.

ISOTOPE-LABELED AEROSOLS. The radionuclide agents used to display the pulmonary circulation can also be given by aerosol to display the airways.[8–10, 17] In obstructive disease, much of the aerosol is deposited in the more central airways, with relatively little reaching the peripheral parts of the lung. Radioaerosols may provide a more sensitive indication of early chronic obstructive disease than do other common diagnostic procedures.[18] The rate of clearance of the deposited aerosol can be followed by obtaining sequential scans; this technique has proved to be of value in the study of the activity of the mucociliary escalator.[19]

Technetium-99m labeled albumin or sulfur colloid, and neutralized indium-113m chloride have been used in aerosol studies.[10] The

agent can be delivered by an air-compressor–driven nebulizer, IPPB, or ultrasonic nebulizer. The techniques are relatively cumbersome, and the results are of variable quality. Such studies, however, have been of secondary interest, and have revealed that less than 10 per cent of a measured dose of an agent that is put in an IPPB nebulizer is actually deposited in the lungs.[10, 20]

The value of radioaerosol diagnosis has not been determined as yet, but the technique offers some important advantages. Thus, the radionuclide can be given as a simple aerosol, and does not require introduction by a transtracheal catheter or by endoscopy. The radioaerosols do not cause allergic reactions or pharmacologic side effects, and no persistent or late consequence need to be expected. Whereas bronchographic media can be given only to the anesthetized respiratory tract, radioactive aerosols are tolerated by the unprepared mucosa—although a bronchodilator should be given if the patient has reactive airways. Thus, while one can expect a further decline in the use of bronchography and radiopaque contrast media, an increase in techniques using both the established and innovative labeled aerosols will undoubtedly occur.

ADDITIONAL AGENTS. A large number of carriers and radionuclides have been evaluated in nuclear medicine, and many of these have undergone investigation in studies of the pulmonary circulation, airway function and parenchymal structure.[20a] Among the carriers that have been reported are sulfur-colloid in an albumin coagulum, sulfur-colloid in a gelatin coagulum, phosphate-albumin coagulum, stannous oxide, aluminum oxide and strontium carbonate. Various agents have also been prepared as microspheres, including gelatin and dextran. Inert agents have also been used as microspheres, and apparently they have been quite safe: included in this group are polystyrene, plastic and ceramic products. An alternative preparation that is similar but more biologic is lipid droplets as microspheres. Among the radionuclides that have been used are bromine (^{82}Br), carbonate (^{11}CO$_3$), chromium (^{51}Cr), gold (^{198}Au), rubidium (^{97}Ru), silver (^{111}Ag) and strontium (^{87}Sr). Undoubtedly, other agents could, and will, be used in the very productive field of radiopharmaceutics.

LOCAL ANESTHETICS

Local anesthetic agents are of particular interest in respiratory therapeutics as a means of providing topical anesthesia of the respiratory tract to permit procedures such as endoscopy, minor surgery, or special investigations such as bronchography. Other topical uses of local anesthesia include the treatment of sore throats and the management of coughs (see Chapter 9); for coughs, topical (aerosol) administration, or intravenous or oral delivery can be used for suitable agents. A further important use is to relieve pleural or costal pain by giving a local infiltration of an anesthetic or by inducing a nerve block. Local anesthetics might be expected to be of benefit in the treatment of asthma and other forms of bronchospasm, but are actually of little value in such therapy (see Chapter 4).

Mechanism of Action. Nervous conduction by pain fibers depends upon a noxious stimulus affecting the permeability of the axonal membrane to ionic passage; the exact mechanism involved in this phenomenon has not been fully elucidated.[21, 22] Sodium ions, which exist in relative excess in the perineural fluid, diffuse along the concentration gradient into the activated nerve fiber. The resting electric gradient is negative on the inside of the membrane and positive on the outside; the difference in potential across the neuronal membrane is 50 to 90 millivolts. The entry of sodium ions into the neurons decreases this potential to zero, following which there is a reversal of polarity. At this stage of depolarization, potassium ions move along their concentration gradient across the neuronal membrane into the perineural space. The local axonal changes in ionic flux are transmitted in relay fashion along the nerve fiber as an action potential, and when this reaches the appropriate part of the brain, the organism experiences pain and usually responds with an appropriate reflex action. During the recovery of the nerve fiber, sodium is pumped out by an energy-demanding biochemical process, and potassium

reenters to restore the neuron to its resting state.

Local anesthetics are known to act by stabilizing the neuronal membrane, thereby making it relatively impermeable to ionic flux.[23] It is probable that this stabilizing action is dependent on the anesthetic reacting with a lipoprotein receptor site on the internal surface of the neuronal membrane.[24] During the reaction, calcium ions are displaced from the receptor site, and thus calcium plays an important role in local anesthetic action. The effects of local anesthetics are entirely reversible, and normal neuronal function returns within one to three hours.

Pharmacology of Local Anesthetics. Most of the local anesthetics in use today are either nonnitrogenous hydroxy esters (such as benzocaine, butacaine, cocaine, hexylcaine, procaine and tetracaine) or amino compounds (such as dibucaine and lidocaine); an important exception is dyclonine, which is a ketone. The differences in chemical constitution are not reflected in characteristic anesthetic properties, and the various agents have similar effects and side effects. Other classes of local anesthetic agents are recognized, some of which are very simple (for example, phenol); others are mainly reserved for alternative therapeutic uses (for example, benzonatate as a cough suppressant). Many of the local anesthetics also demonstrate additional properties to some degree – particularly antihistaminic, anticholinergic and curare-like effects.

The side effects of most local anesthetic agents can be serious, but the marketed drugs all offer good therapeutic:toxic ratios, and therefore dangerous side effects can usually be avoided. In general, the agents available are given primarily by injection for infiltration around nerve fibers. When given topically, it is advisable to use only about one-third of the established maximum safe dosage used for infiltration.

The topical agents can cause local tissue irritation, and in susceptible patients attempted anesthesia of the respiratory tract may cause bronchospasm. All local anesthetics with the exception of cocaine are vasodilators, and this action enhances their rate of absorption. An acid environment, such as is caused by pus, inactivates these agents. If too large a dose of a topical anesthetic is given, absorption into the systemic circulation may occur to a degree sufficient to produce toxic reactions. The initial effect is usually one of central excitation, which may be manifested by agitation, yawning, nausea, vomiting and twitching; higher serum levels cause seizures. Large doses of longer-acting agents are more likely to result in severe adverse effects. Other possible adverse effects include cardiovascular depression, hypotension, syncope and arrhythmias. Rarely, allergic or idiosyncratic reactions occur: these include rashes, eczema, edema, bronchospasm, methemoglobinemia and agranulocytosis.

In Table 12–5, the most important properties of the major agents used for topical anesthesia are compared. The concentrations and amounts used in practice vary markedly, but the total dosage should be kept close to that recommended. The onset of action of most agents occurs in less than five minutes, but some drugs (such as dibucaine) may take as long as 15 minutes; however, various factors influence this, including the dosage used, the method of adminstration, the amount of mucus in the airways, and the condition of the respiratory mucosa. The durations of action and the relative potencies and toxicities of these drugs also depend on such factors as the dosage and amount used, the use of adjuvants (such as epinephrine), and the biochemical and pathophysiologic status of the airways. In general, the least amount of the most dilute solution that is effective should be employed. The local anesthetics are metabolized in different ways, according to their chemical structure: most esters are hydrolyzed by plasma cholinesterase and the metabolites are excreted in the urine, whereas other esters and the amides are metabolized in the liver.

It is of interest that the local anesthetics may have an antimicrobial action, the mechanism of which is not certain. Of the agents that have been evaluated, dyclonine, hexylcaine and tetracaine have the most pronounced effect, whereas that of lidocaine and procaine is less, and cocaine is without any significant antimicrobial properties.[25, 26] These considerations are relevant, since antimicrobial anesthetics should be avoided in bronchoscopies when specimens will be cultured for bacteria and fungi.[25]

The effects of local anesthetics on ciliary activity and mucociliary clearance have been examined in some detail.[19, 27, 28] Lidocaine and procaine, in low concentrations, cause ciliary incoordination, whereas most of the other agents used in bronchoscopy stimulate ciliary mobility in low concentrations, but inhibit activity in high concentrations. Hex-

ylcaine causes impaired ciliary activity for over 24 hours and also causes epithelial cellular destruction.

Individual Local Anesthetics. A relatively small number of the available local anesthetics are suitable for inducing topical anesthesia in the upper or lower respiratory tract.[23] (Table 12–5).

BENZOCAINE. Benzocaine is a relatively weak anesthetic that is insoluble in water and is not suited for anesthetizing the tracheobronchial tree. It can be used in tablet form or as a solution for the treatment of painful oropharyngeal conditions (see Chapter 9). Benzocaine 14 per cent is the main constituent of the popular topical anesthetic Cetacaine; the additional components are 2 per cent butyl aminobenzoate, 2 per cent tetracaine, 0.5 per cent benzalkonium chloride and 0.005 per cent cetyl dimethyl ethyl ammonium bromide. This product is available as an aerosol spray, a liquid, an ointment and a gel, and one form or another is of value for anesthetizing the nose or throat prior to nasotracheal intubation.

BUTACAINE. This is of use for upper respiratory tract anesthesia but is not used for the tracheobronchial tree.

COCAINE. Cocaine is the only important naturally occurring local anesthetic. It is an alkaloid derived from the leaves of the Andean plant *Erythroxylon coca;* chemically, it is a benzoic acid ester of methyl ecgonine. Cocaine is of little value for infiltration anesthesia or for nerve blocks, and its use is restricted to surface application to mucosae.

Cocaine is absorbed rapidly through the tracheobronchial mucosa, but some delay results from its property of causing vasoconstriction by releasing norepinephrine from storage granules in the neuronal synapses. In spite of its systemic absorption and its central stimulant and addictive propensities, the drug is safe and effective when used as a respiratory tract anesthetic for bronchoscopy; occasional side effects include transient moderate hypotension, tachycardia, nausea and euphoria. Since it is very effective, well tolerated and has no antibacterial action, many physicians consider it the anesthetic of choice for bronchoscopic procedures. Adequate anesthesia usually lasts for about 20 minutes, and additional protection against cocaine toxicity is provided by premedication with a barbiturate or diazepam.[29]

The drug can be used as a 10 per cent solution to anesthetize the pharynx, larynx

TABLE 12–5. TOPICAL AGENTS FOR AIRWAY ANESTHESIA

Drug	Concentrations Used PER CENT	Maximal Dosage for Adults* (mg)	Onset of Action (min)	Length of Action (hr)	Relative Potency	Relative Toxicity	Antimicrobial Potency	Comments
Benzocaine (Americaine, Cetacaine)	1–20	300	1	0.5–1	1	1		Used for throat anesthesia; poorly soluble in water; used in combination preparations
Butacaine (Butyn)	1–2	100	1	1	4	3		Used in nose, throat and mouth procedures
Cocaine	2–20	230	1	1–2	4	4	−	Central stimulant, addictive, vasoconstrictor; valuable for bronchoscopy
Dibucaine (Nupercaine)	0.5–2	50	15	4–6	15	12		Most toxic agent; rarely used
Dyclonine (Dyclone)	0.5–1	70	10	1	4	1	+	No cross-sensitivity with other local anesthetics, since it is a ketone
Hexylcaine (Cyclaine)	1.5	250	5	0.5	3	1	+	May cause mucosal irritation; impairs mucociliary clearance
Lidocaine (Xylocaine)	2–10	250	3	1	3	1.5	±	Most frequently used agent for bronchography and bronchoscopy; systemic absorption can result in toxicity (e.g. seizures)
Piperocaine (Metycaine)	2–10	250	1	1.5	3	2		Used for nasal anesthesia
Procaine (Novocain)	2–10	300	4	1	1	1	±	Standard local anesthetic; *not* effective topically
Tetracaine (Amethocaine, Pontocaine)	0.5–1	60	9	0.75	10	8	+	Very potent; must be used with care

*Larger doses may be safe if given over the course of a procedure.

and trachea, and then a 4 per cent solution can be used to facilitate endoscopy of the segmental bronchi. If no more than a total of 2 ml of the 10 per cent solution is aerosolized, some of which can be diluted to a 4 per cent solution, the safe dose of 200 mg will not be exceeded. In fact, a dose as large as 300 mg is probably safe in adults with normal hepatic function, but a dosage of 3.3 mg/kg should be regarded as maximal.[30]

DIBUCAINE. Dibucaine is the most potent and most toxic of the local anesthetics, and has an effect that can last for several hours. The drug should not be considered suitable for routine procedures; in fact, it is rarely indicated in view of its toxic actions on the respiratory mucosa.[31]

DYCLONINE. Dyclonine differs from most other local anesthetics, since it is a ketone. If a patient has known allergy to one of the other agents, dyclonine can be employed without any risk of a hypersensitivity reaction. The drug is potent, but relatively nontoxic, and it can be effectively administered by ultrasonic nebulization in preparation for intubation and bronchography.[32] Dyclonine can also be given as a 0.5 per cent gargle for anesthetizing the throat, following which lidocaine may be used for the preparation of the lower respiratory tract.[29]

HEXYLCAINE. Hexylcaine is relatively toxic to the respiratory mucosa, and can result in a prolonged impairment (24 hours) of mucociliary clearance. It cannot be recommended for tracheobronchial anesthesia.

LIDOCAINE (lignocaine in the United Kingdom). Lidocaine is the most popular and most valuable local anesthetic, and is probably employed by the majority of physicians for topical anesthesia of the respiratory tract. Lidocaine is also of considerable value, when given intravenously, in the treatment of ventricular arrhythmias. Although systemic therapy may result in adverse effects, topical administration is usually well accepted.

Because lidocaine is a widely used anesthetic, it has been subjected to many studies. It has been given intravenously and by instillation in order to relieve bronchospasm (Chapter 4) and to suppress coughing (Chapter 9); other agents, such as procaine, may be of similar value when given intravenously.[33] Lidocaine instillation into the tracheobronchial tree generally has little effect on airway mechanics, but nebulization of the drug may cause an increase in airway resistance in susceptible patients.[34] Although a fall in PaO_2 has also been described,[35] other investigators have found no significant alteration of airway caliber or of blood gases with topical lidocaine usage.[36]

The appropriate dose of lidocaine for tracheobronchial anesthesia is no more than 250 mg, although some experts use more;[37] however, the dosage should be kept below 6 mg/kg.[38] When lower dosages are employed, toxic blood levels are not achieved[39-41]. A recommended method of inducing tracheobronchial anesthesia is by the ultrasonic nebulization of 4 to 7 ml of 4 per cent lidocaine.[42] Alternative methods of nebulization may be as effective, and IPPB may be even more effective.[43] In Canada, lidocaine is available as a 10 per cent solution in a Freon-powered aerosol.[41]

The use of lidocaine in respiratory therapy merits further consideration in appropriate circumstances. As an example, the drug has been reported to be of value when given topically to improve patient tolerance of an artificial airway during mechanical ventilation.[36] Since the drug is also very effective when given by infiltration, intramuscular injection of up to 50 ml of the 0.5 per cent solution is useful for the management of chest wall pain due to radiculitis, fractured rib or thoracotomy. Lidocaine is also marketed as a jelly, ointments and viscous solutions for intranasal, oropharyngeal and esophageal anesthesia. The 2 per cent jelly is useful for anesthetizing the nasal passages prior to nasal intubation. Preparations containing epinephrine in concentrations of 1:250,000 to 1:50,000 can be used: the sympathomimetic prevents bronchospasm, and by causing vasoconstriction it decreases the rate of absorption of the lidocaine, and also serves to prevent mucosal bleeding.

PIPEROCAINE. This is useful for producing nasal anesthesia, but is not used as a tracheobronchial anesthetic.

PROCAINE. Although procaine was used in Dautrebande's original formulation of Aerolone (Chapter 5), this agent is not effective when given topically. The drug is similar to lidocaine when given by infiltration, and it is a standard injectable local anesthetic. However, it currently has no specific use in inhalation therapy.

TETRACAINE. Tetracaine is one of the most potent of the local anesthetics; deaths have resulted from its topical tracheobronchial administration. It is too toxic to the respiratory mucosa for use with bronchography or bronchoscopy,[31] but it may be of occasional value for anesthesia in minor respiratory tract surgical procedures. However, many workers have had unfavorable experiences, even with careful use of this agent.[30, 44]

BENZONATATE (Tessalon, Chapter 9). Benzonatate is chemically related to tetracaine, with the addition of a long-chain glycol. Its conventional use is as an antitussive,[33] but oral, intramuscular and direct endotracheal administration have been used as adjuncts to bronchoscopy or intubation. The use of benzonatate as a topical airway anesthetic merits further evaluation.

Use of Local Anesthetics in Bronchoscopy. The major use of topical anesthesia of the respiratory tract is in laryngoscopy and bronchoscopy. For laryngoscopy, the anesthetic of choice is 4 per cent lidocaine, or, as an alternative, 4 per cent cocaine.[29] Usually, the solution is first sprayed into the oropharynx, and then transmucosal block of the superior laryngeal nerves is attained by applying swabs soaked in the anesthetic to the pyriform sinuses. The anesthetic can then be diluted to 2 per cent for spraying of the epiglottis and for injecting through the laryngeal aperture. As an alternative, Cetacaine can be used: three or four seconds of spraying the solution should produce adequate anesthesia of the mouth, pharynx and larynx. Some surgeons favor the simultaneous use of percutaneous infiltration with procaine or lidocaine to block the superior laryngeal nerves: overdosage can be avoided by the control in dosage allowed by the injections, and superior anesthesia is obtained.

For bronchoscopy, similar techniques are employed. Lidocaine 4 per cent or 4 to 10 per cent cocaine are most often favored, but some physicians still use 0.5-1 per cent tetracaine. Additional anesthetic will need to be instilled into the more distal airways once the bronchoscope has been introduced into the trachea. Although aerosolization of local anesthetics has been recommended, using various nebulizers, ultrasonic nebulization, or IPPB, there is no definitive evidence to prove that these techniques result in anesthesia superior to that obtained by the methods described here.

DRUGS USED IN PROVOCATIVE INHALATION TESTS

Although the diagnosis of asthma is usually made from the history or pulmonary function studies, including response to bronchodilators, there are patients who present a confusing history and inconclusive routine studies. In such cases, it is sometimes useful to evaluate the patient's response to an inhalational drug (such as one of those listed in Table 12–6) that will stimulate a bronchospastic response in susceptible airways.[45] Numerous irritant drugs can be employed for this purpose (see Table 1–34 and Table 9–17), but for basic evaluation, it is customary to use physiologic agents, including parasympathomimetic drugs and histamine.[46] For more sophisticated studies, specific industrial irritants or organic allergens may

TABLE 12–6. INHALATIONAL PROVOCATION AGENTS

Drugs	Allergens From Animal and Plant Sources	Industrial Agents Organic	Inorganic
Cholinergic agents	Pollens and spores	Piperazine	Platinum salts
carbachol	Fungal extracts	Sulfonamides	Chrome salts
methacholine	Housedust	Toluene diiso-	Nickel salts
Histamine	House mite extract	cyanate	Vanadium pentoxide
Citric acid	Animal danders	Epoxy resins	
Other agents:	Avian extracts	Phthalic anhydride	
Table 1–34	Antibiotics and	Ethylene diamine	
Table 9–17	precursors	Polyvinyl fumes	
	Proteolytic enzymes		
	Flour and grain dust		
	Castor bean dust		
	Wood dusts		
	Cotton derivatives		

be used if the patient's history and routine allergy tests (such as skin tests) suggest that such studies may be of value.[47-49] Provocative tests are also used by investigators to help elucidate the genetics and mechanisms of bronchospasm and to evaluate methods of airway protection using therapeutic drugs or maneuvers.[50]

Only those pulmonary function laboratories in which the medical director or personnel have adequate experience should embark on provocation studies.[49] Inhalational challenges require careful, patient and adequately controlled methodology, which is beyond the resources of the majority of pulmonary function laboratories. A specially air conditioned area is needed to prevent the aerosolized drug, chemical or antigen from contaminating the general area, and a high level of quality control is required to generate meaningful results. Some patients who are exposed to such inhalational challenges may develop severe reactions, and therapeutic measures to cope with such events must be instantly available.

Appropriately carried out inhalational challenges will reliably produce significant bronchospasm in virtually all unprotected asthmatic patients. Sometimes, however, a patient reacts dramatically to one challenge agent but not to another, whereas on a subsequent occasion the relative response thresholds may change. For this reason, testing with at least two challenge drugs may be required, and when indicated, more specific environmental agents should be nebulized. When a patient's relatives are tested, a proportion will tend to show a smaller reaction to the challenge drug that affected the asthmatic patient, but this reaction will be greater than that of a completely normal person. The finding of such a lesser reaction implies that the relative has a susceptibility to asthma; such information may be of value in the evaluation of a subject who is contemplating entering an occupation where there is a relatively high risk of chemical- or antigen-induced asthma being contracted.

Each bronchospasm-inducing drug is usually given as an aerosol of the agent or its salt dissolved in saline. Organic dust products and chemicals can be prepared as solutions for aerosolization, or they can be given as powders for inhalation. Lactose powder can be used as an excipient when using powdered agents in challenge studies.[49] Finally, challenge studies can be carried out with chemical fumes, utilizing a suitable environmentally isolated study chamber.

Individual Challenge Drugs
(Table 12–7)

Parasympathomimetic Drugs. The effect of the neurotransmitter acetylcholine on cholinergic receptors in the causation of bronchospasm was explained earlier (see Chapter 4 and Figure 4–1).

ACETYLCHOLINE (Miochol). Acetylcholine produces two types of neurogenic response when it is released from membrane-bound vesicles in cholinergic presynaptic nerve terminals. Its *nicotinic* actions, resembling those of nicotine, are seen at motor endplates in voluntary muscles and in the synapses of the autonomic ganglia: these actions are not blocked by atropine. The *muscarinic* actions of acetylcholine occur at the postganglionic neuroeffector junctions of the parasympathetic system; this effect on the bronchial muscles causes bronchospasm. The action is similar to that of muscarine, derived from the poisonous mushroom, and

TABLE 12–7.   STANDARD BRONCHIAL PROVOCATION DRUGS

Agents	Properties	Dosage (mg/ml)	Comment
CHOLINERGIC AGENTS			
Carbamylcholine (carbamoylcholine, carbachol, Carcholin)	One of the most potent choline esters; muscarinic effects greater than nicotinic	0.25–40	Stable agent with long shelf-life
Methacholine (Mecholyl)	Similar to acetylcholine; muscarinic action only	0.075–25	Generally preferred over carbamylcholine
HISTAMINE			
Histamine phosphate	May cause more stimulation of bronchial mucosa than cholinergic agents	0.02–20	Alternative to cholinergic agents

it is blocked by atropine. Acetylcholine is a quarternary ammonium compound, and it is broken down by the blood and tissue enzyme, acetylcholinesterase. It is considered unsuitable as a therapeutic or diagnostic agent, and therefore synthetic analogues are used in provocation tests.

CARBAMYLCHOLINE (carbachol). Carbamylcholine is one of the most potent of the synthetic choline esters. Rather than being derived from acetic acid as is acetylcholine, carbamylcholine is derived from carbamic acid, and the ester link is less susceptible to enzymic hydrolysis by cholinesterases; it therefore has a relatively prolonged effect. The drug has both muscarinic and nicotinic action, with relatively greater nicotinic properties; systemic administration results in predominant stimulation of the gastrointestinal and urinary tracts. Therapeutically, the drug is used mainly in the treatment of glaucoma, and it is readily available as ophthalmic solutions.

For inhalation challenges, it has been recommended for use in concentrations of 0.025 per cent to 4 per cent in propylene glycol.[51] The solution can be inhaled for five seconds with a vital capacity maneuver, followed by a five seconds breath-hold. The initial challenge should be made with the most dilute solution, and if no response is obtained, progressively more concentrated solutions can be tried. Although carbamylcholine is favored by some workers, it is used to a lesser extent than the other major parasympathomimetic drug, methacholine.

METHACHOLINE (Mecholyl). Methacholine is prepared by acetylating methylcholine; it is relatively resistant to hydrolysis by cholinesterases, and therefore it has a longer action than does acetylcholine. It has insignificant nicotinic action, and its muscarinic potency is 10 to 20 times that of acetylcholine. Its action is blocked by atropine, and its effects are prolonged by cholinesterase inhibitors such as neostigmine and physostigmine. Oral administration of the drug has little effect on the respiratory tract, whereas parenteral or inhalational administration causes bronchoconstriction and secretion by the bronchial glands. Inhalation of the drug does not have adverse cardiac effects in patients with cardiopulmonary problems.[52]

Methacholine bromide is supplied as tablets, whereas the chloride is used in solution. Aerosolized solutions are administered in concentrations varying from 0.075 to 25 per cent; most investigators use the range of 0.25 to 5 per cent (2.5 to 50 mg/ml diluent). Some experts recommend 10 breaths of the lowest selected concentration, followed by a two hour wait before trying a higher concentration, if need be: concentrations used may be 0.075, 0.15, 0.31, 0.62, 1.26, 2.5, 5, 10 and 25 mg/ml.[53] For practical purposes, it is advised that the powder be made up into three standard solutions of 0.25, 2.5 and 25 mg/ml, since adequate studies can be accomplished with these concentrations.

The greater familiarity with methacholine suggests that this should be the cholinergic drug of choice for inhalation challenge.

Histamine. As explained in Chapters 4 and 9, histamine is a major mediator involved in inflammatory reactions, including those of asthma. It can be used as an alternative to the cholinergic agents in aerosol provocation tests. The drug is used in other diagnostic studies, including investigations of gastric responses, circulatory behavior and skin reactivity. There are no important analogues utilized in bronchial provocation, but betazole and betahistine are available for gastric stimulation and for the treatment of Meniere's disease respectively.

Histamine phosphate is marketed as a solution, and it is aerosolized in concentrations of 0.02 to 10 mg/ml in similar manner to that described for methacholine: concentrations recommended are 0.03, 0.06, 0.12, 0.25, 0.5, 1, 2.5, 5 and 10 mg/ml.[53] A useful standard concentration for experimental work is provided by a 1.6 per cent solution of histamine phosphate.[54] Some patients who do not respond to metacholine will respond to histamine, but the significance of this is not known.[53]

Other Inhalational Challenges. Many agents have been used[46–48, 55], and the more important ones are listed in Table 12–6. A recent review provides additional details about bronchoconstrictive agents such as serotonin, angiotensin, kallidin, eledoisin, bradykinin, fibrinopeptides, various ions, and prostaglandins.[56]

REFERENCES

1. Weigen, J. F. and Thomas, S. F.: Complications of Diagnostic Radiology. Springfield, Ill., Charles C Thomas, 1973.
2. Ansell, G. (Ed.): Complications of Diagnostic Radiology. Oxford, Blackwell Scientific Publications, 1976. Ch. 12.
3. Forrest, J. V. and Sagel, S. S.: Bronchography. In: Special Procedures in Chest Radiology. S. S. Sagel (Ed.). Philadelphia, W. B. Saunders Company, 1976. Ch. 3.

4. Ansell, G.: Contrast media toxicity. *In:* Recent Advances in Radiology. T. Lodge and R. E. Steiner (Eds.). Edinburgh, Churchill Livingstone, 1975. Ch. 19.

5. DiGugliemo, L.: Radiocontrast agents for bronchography. *In:* International Encyclopedia of Pharmacology and Therapeutics: Radiocontrast Agents. Sect. 76. Vol. 2. P. K. Knoefel (Ed.). Oxford, Pergamon Press, 1971. Ch. 10.

5a. Fraser, R. G. and Paré, J. A. P.: Diagnosis of Diseases of the Chest. Philadelphia, W. B. Saunders Company, 2nd Ed., 1977, p. 217.

6. Nadel, J. A., Wolfe, W. G., Graf, P. D., Youker, J. E., Zamel, N., Austin, J. H. M., Hinchcliffe, W. A., Greenspan, R. H. and Wright, R. R.: Powdered tantalum: a new contrast medium for roentgenographic examination of human airways. N. Engl. J. Med. 283:281–286, 1970.

7. Friedman, P. J. and Tisi, G. M.: "Alveolarization" of tantalum powder in experimental bronchography and the clearance of inhaled particles from the lung. Radiology 104:523–535, 1972.

8. Moser, K. M.: Clinical applications of ventilation/perfusion scintiphotography. *In:* Textbook of Pulmonary Diseases. G. L. Baum (Ed.). Boston, Little, Brown and Company, 2nd ed. 1974. Ch. 4.

9. Wagner, H. N.: The use of radioisotope techniques for the evaluation of patients with pulmonary disease. Am. Rev. Respir. Dis. 113:203–218, 1976.

10. Secker-Walker, R. H.: Nuclear medicine in lung disease. *In:* Special Procedures in Chest Radiology. S. S. Sagel (Ed.). Philadelphia, W. B. Saunders Company, 1976. Ch. 6.

11. Taplin, G. V., Dore, E. K., Poe, N. D., Swanson, L. A. and Greenberg, A.: Pulmonary arterial perfusion and aerated space assessment by scintiscanning. *In:* Frontiers of Pulmonary Radiology. M. Simon, E. J. Potchen and M. J. LeMay (Eds.). New York, Grune and Stratton, 1969, pp. 33–75.

12. Child, J. S., Wolfe, J. D., Tashkin, D. and Nakano, F.: Fatal lung scan in a case of pulmonary hypertension due to obliterative pulmonary vascular disease. Chest 67:308–310, 1975.

13. Adelstein, S. J. and Holman, B. L.: Pulmonary scintigraphy. Postgrad. Med. 54:69–74, 1973.

14. Ackery, D. M. and Sterling, G. M.: Radioisotopes in the study of pulmonary function and disease. *In:* Recent Advances in Respiratory Medicine, I. T. B. Stretton (Ed.). Edinburgh, Churchill Livingstone, 1976. Ch. 1.

15. Niden, A. H., Mishkin, F. S., Khurana, M. M. L. and Pick, R.: ⁶⁷Ga lung scan: an aid in the differential diagnosis of pulmonary embolism and pneumonitis. J.A.M.A. 237:1206–1211, 1977.

16. Wagner, H. N. and Strauss, H. W.: Radioactive tracers in the differential diagnosis of pulmonary embolism. Prog. Cardiovasc. Dis. 4:271–282, 1975.

17. Shibel, E. M., Landis, G. A. and Moser, K. M.: Inhalation lung scanning evaluation—radioaerosol versus radioxenon techniques. Dis. Chest 56:284–289, 1969.

18. Ramanna, L., Tashkin, D. P., Taplin, G. V., Elam, D., Detels, R., Coulson, A. and Rokaw, S. N.: Radioaerosol lung imaging in chronic obstructive pulmonary disease: comparison with pulmonary function tests and roentgenography. Chest 68:634–640, 1975.

19. Wanner, A.: Clinical aspects of mucociliary transport. Am. Rev. Respir. Dis. 116:73–125, 1977.

20. Ziment, I.: Why are they saying bad things about IPPB? Respir. Care 18:677–689, 1973.

20a. Taplin, G. V. and McDonald, N. S.: Radiochemistry of macroaggregated albumin and newer lung scanning agents. Sem. Nucl. Med. 1:132–152, 1971.

21. de Jong, R. H.: Neural blockage by local anesthetics. J.A.M.A. 238:1383–1385, 1977.

22. de Jong, R. H.: Local anesthetic mechanisms. Anesthesiology Review. March, 1974, pp. 18–23.

23. Lamid, S. and Wang, R. I. H.: The range of local anesthetics. Drug Therapy. Aug., 1975, pp. 103–118.

24. Covino, B. G. and Vassalo, H. G.: *In:* Local Anesthetics. Mechanisms of Action and Clinical Use. New York, Grune and Stratton, Inc., 1976.

25. Bartlett, J. G., Alexander, J., Mayhew, J., Sullivan-Sigler, N. and Gorbach, S. L.: Should fiberoptic bronchoscopy aspirates be cultured? Am. Rev. Respir. Dis. 114:73–78, 1976.

26. Weinstein, M. P., Maderazo, E., Tilton, R., Maggini, G. and Quintiliani, R.: Further observations on the antimicrobial effects of local anesthetic agents. Curr. Ther. Res. 17:369–374, 1975.

27. Okeson, G. C. and Divertie, M. B.: Cilia and bronchial clearance: the effects of pharmacologic agents and disease. Mayo Clin. Proc. 45:361–373, 1970.

28. Corssen, G. and Allen, C. R.: A comparison of the toxic effects of various local anesthetic drugs on human ciliated epithelium in vitro. Tex. Rep. Biol. Med. 16:194–202, 1958.

29. Snow, J. C.: Anesthesia: In Otolaryngology and Ophthalmology. Springfield, Ill., Charles C Thomas, 1972.

30. Yrigoyen, E. and Fujikawa, Y. F.: Flexible fiberoptic bronchoscopy: anesthesia, technique and results. West J. Med. 122:117–122, Feb., 1975.

31. Corssen, G. and Allen, C. R.: Cultured human respiratory epithelium: its use in the comparison of the cytotoxic properties of local anesthetics. Anesthesiology. 21:237–243, 1960.

32. Martin, B. H., Israel, J. and Stovin, J. J.: Anesthesia and intubation for bronchography. Radiology. 104:536, 1972.

33. Aviado, D. M., Koelle, G. B., Lish, P. M., Sheffner, A. L. and Salem, H. (Eds.): *In:* International Encyclopedia of Pharmacy and Therapeutics. Antitussive Agents Vol. III. Pergamon Press, Oxford, 1970, Ch. 12.

34. Miller, W. C. and Awe, R.: Effect of nebulized lidocaine on reactive airways. Am. Rev. Respir. Dis. 111:739–741, 1975.

35. Salisbury, B. G., Metzger, L. F., Altose, M. D., Stanley, N. N. and Cherniack, N. S.: Effect of fiberoptic bronchoscopy on respiratory performance in patients with chronic airways obstruction. Thorax 30:441–446, 1975.

36. Wilbur, H. O. and Ouellette, T. R.: Topical anesthesia to improve patient tolerance of artificial airways during mechanical ventilation. Resp. Care. 21:617–619, 1976.

37. Padfied, A.: Risks of lignocaine in bronchography. Br. Med. J. 3:690, Sept., 1973.

38. Anon: Risks of lignocaine in bronchography. Br. Med. J. 3:344, Aug., 1973.

39. Chu, S. S., Rah, K. H., Brannan, M. D. and Cohen, J. L.: Plasma concentration of lidocaine after endotracheal spray. Anesth. Analg. 54:438–441, 1975.

40. Karvonen, S., Jokinen, K., Karvonen, P. and Hollmen, A.: Arterial and venous blood lidocaine concentrations after local anaesthesia of the respiratory tract using an ultrasonic nebulizer. Acta. Anaesthesiol. Scand. 20:156–159, 1976.

41. Pelton, D. A., Daly, M., Cooper, P. D. and Conn, A. W.: Plasma lidocaine concentrations following topical aerosol application to the trachea and bronchi. Can. Anaesth. Soc. J. 17:250–255, 1970.

42. Christoforidis, A. J., Tomashefski, J. F. and Mitchell, R. I.: Use of an ultrasonic nebulizer for the application of oropharyngeal, laryngeal and tracheobronchial anesthesia. Chest 59:629–633, 1971.

43. Chinn, W. M., Zavala, D. C. and Ambre, J.: Plasma levels of lidocaine following nebulized aerosol administration. Chest 71:346–348, 1977.

44. Credle, W. F., Smiddy, J. F. and Elliott, R. C.: Complications of fiberoptic bronchoscopy. Am. Rev. Respir. Dis. 109:67–72, 1974.

45. Aas, K.: The Bronchial Provocation Test. Springfield, Ill., Charles C Thomas, 1975.

46. Spector, S. L. and Farr, R. S.: Bronchial inhalation procedures in asthmatics. Med. Clin. N. Amer. 58:71–84, 1974.

47. Pepys, J. and Hutchcroft, B. J.: Bronchial provocation tests in etiologic diagnosis and analysis of asthma. Am. Rev. Respir. Dis. 112:829–859, 1975.

48. Pepys, J.: Nonimmediate asthmatic reactions. *In:* Bronchial Asthma: Mechanisms and Therapeutics. E. B. Weiss and M. S. Segal (Eds.). Boston, Little, Brown and Company, 1976. Ch. 17.

49. Davies, R. J. and Pepys, J.: Occupational asthma. *In:* Asthma. T. J. H. Clark and S. Godfrey (Eds.). Philadelphia, W. B. Saunders Company, 1977. Ch. 10.

50. Austen, K. F., and Lichtenstein, L. M. (Eds.): Asthma: Physiology, Immunopharmacology and Treatment. New York, Academic Press, 1973. (See pages 51–53, 169–184, 294–314.)

51. Swinburne, A. J., Utell, M. J., Shigeoka, J. W., Speers, D. M., Gibb, F. R., Morrow, P. E. and Hyde, R. W.: Simplified quantitative assessment of airway reactivity using an inhaled parasympathomimetic agent. Am. Rev. Respir. Dis. 115 #4, Pt. 2:169, 1977.

52. Grieco, M. H. and Pierson, R. N.: Cardiopulmonary effects of methacholine in asthmatic and normal subjects. J. Allergy 45:195–207, 1970.

53. Spector, S. L. and Farr, R. S.: Bronchial provocation tests. *In:* Bronchial Asthma: Mechanisms and Therapeutics. E. B. Weiss and M. S. Segal (Eds.). Boston, Little, Brown and Company, 1976. Ch. 43.

54. Empey, D. W., Laitinen, L. A., Jacobs, L., Gold, W. M. and Nadel, J. A.: Mechanisms of bronchial hyperreactivity in normal subjects after upper respiratory tract infection. Am. Rev. Respir. Dis. 113:131–139, 1976.

55. Murphy, R. L.: Industrial diseases with asthma. *In:* Bronchial Asthma: Mechanisms and Therapeutics. E. B. Weiss and M. S. Segal (Eds.). Boston, Little, Brown and Company, 1976. Ch. 17.

56. Simonsson, B. G. and Svedmyr, N.: Bronchoconstrictor drugs. Pharmac. Ther. B 3:239–303, 1977.

RESPIRATORY GASES

AIR AND NITROGEN

The lungs provide the route of access and elimination for the gases involved in metabolism (oxygen and carbon dioxide), just as the bowel serves as the route of access and elimination for the solids and liquids involved in nutrition. By and large, the respiratory gases cannot be used to treat abnormal disease states of the lung itself (any more than ordinary food or drink is used to treat disease of the bowel), although the appropriate distribution of gases within the respiratory tract serves to provide the distention that prevents the lungs from collapsing. Air, at all altitudes at which man can live, contains the same fixed proportions of gases (Table 13–1), and the lungs have evolved in harmony with the proportions and properties of the main gases in the ambient atmosphere. Thus, the fact that air contains about 78 per cent nitrogen and 21 per cent oxygen is appropriate to normal pulmonary

function, and any gross alteration in these proportions can lead to malfunction of the lungs.

Nitrogen (N_2) is essentially an inert gas that is not utilized metabolically by any body tissue: the amount of nitrogen that leaves the lungs during normal breathing is therefore equal to the amount that enters. The blood and tissues also contain a fixed amount of nitrogen, which appears to have no significant role in the functioning of the tissues. If a subject is given a nitrogen-free atmosphere to breathe (either pure oxygen, or oxygen and helium, or oxygen and an anesthetic gas), all the nitrogen will be washed out of the body:[1] during this process of denitrogenation, over 6.5 liters of nitrogen can be removed from the normal adult, 5.5 liters of which comes from the air in the lungs, and 1 liter from the tissues. Such a nitrogen washout will decrease the partial pressure of the gas in the lungs, and in sequential fashion there will be a progressive reduction of

TABLE 13–1. APPROXIMATE COMPOSITION AND PARTIAL PRESSURES OF COMPONENTS OF AIR AT SEA LEVEL

Component	Dry Air		Alveolar Air		Arterial Blood Partial Pressure (torr)	Venous Blood Partial Pressure (torr)
	Partial Pressure (torr)	Per Cent	Partial Pressure (torr)	Per Cent		
Nitrogen	590.0	78.09	569	74.8	573	573
Oxygen	158.0	20.95	104	13.7	100	40
Carbon Dioxide	0.2	0.03	40	5.3	40	46
Argon, Neon, etc.	6.8	0.93	(<1)	(<0.1)	(<1)	(<1)
Water Vapor	–	–	47	6.2	47	47
	760	100	760	100	760	706

·partial pressure of nitrogen in the blood, in the tissues, and from any compartment in which gas is trapped. Therefore, breathing nitrogen-free gas can lead to the progressive extraction of nitrogen from a distended bowel, from a pneumothorax or from subcutaneous emphysema. The resolution of these abnormal states can be therapeutically speeded by having the patient breathe 100 per cent oxygen for a few hours; such therapy can be recommended if the trapped gas is causing clinical or physiologic distress (see discussion later in this chapter).

Pure oxygen, when breathed for several hours, gradually replaces the inert nitrogen in every part of the lung. If, subsequently, any regional airway obstruction occurs in the lung, the oxygen will be rapidly absorbed into the pulmonary blood supply, and progressive atelectasis will occur: this is one of the major complications that may occur with oxygen therapy. One can regard the normal presence of nitrogen in the lung as providing internal scaffolding, serving to prevent areas of atelectasis from developing. The rate at which nitrogen is "washed out" from the lungs when breathing oxygen is measured in the pulmonary function laboratory to provide an index of the homogeneity of air distribution in the lungs and to indicate the presence of areas of maldistribution.

Air given under hyperbaric conditions can lead to manifestations of nitrogen toxicity. Nitrogen produces effects similar to those of oxygen on various tissues when breathed under hyperbaric conditions, but the toxicity of hyperbaric nitrogen results in manifestations similar to those of alcohol intoxication or to subanesthetic concentrations of nitrous oxide.[1] Usually, these findings do not appear until the ambient pressure reaches 4 or 5 atmospheres, and a lethal outcome will result if nitrogen is administered as a component of air breathed in at a pressure of about 10 atmospheres. Another type of nitrogen toxicity can occur when a hyperbaric atmosphere is reduced too rapidly to normobaric. Thus, when a diver surfaces too rapidly, the decrease in pressure of the nitrogen can result in the serious condition known as caisson worker's disease or the bends. This results from bubbles of nitrogen forming when the pressure is reduced in tissues that have been supersaturated with the gas. The minute bubbles form mainly in muscles, joints, bones and nervous tissue, and can cause severe musculoskeletal pains, visual disturbances, cerebral damage, neurologic impairment and infarcts in bone (Table 13–2). This syndrome can appear acutely in divers, and it must be treated by rapid recompression followed by very slow decompression back to atmospheric pressure.

Thus, although nitrogen is not regarded as an important therapeutic gas, its absence or its presence in excess can each cause health hazards. Its presence in ambient air leads to this "fixed combination drug" being ideally constituted, and although the air that the majority of us breathe would not meet FDA standards of purity, this combination gas is nevertheless used as a major drug in respiratory therapy. Unfortunately, when purified and piped into hospital rooms or compressed into cylinders, it can become relatively expensive: indeed, compressed air of requisite purity may be more expensive than compressed oxygen, since ordinary ambient air is not always safe for human consumption, and therefore has to be subjected to expensive cleansing processes, or it is generated artificially as oxygen and nitrogen that are then combined in the appropriate proportions (Table 13–3). Consideration of the expense involved in the use of medical air provides an important reason for avoiding overprescribing this drug; for example, if a patient requires domiciliary IPPB therapy, an electrically driven device should be ordered in preference to one that has to be powered by tanks of compressed air.

OXYGEN

Oxygen has become one of the most commonly used and misused drugs in hospital practice. The increasing use of oxygen 30 years ago was a major factor leading to the development of the American paramedical specialty of Inhalation Therapy, which evolved into the wider-based and less pharmacologically oriented specialty of Respiratory Therapy. At present, few practitioners think of oxygen as a drug, and as a result it is used with far less precision than most other potent drugs in clinical therapeutics. The relative expense of oxygen may well necessitate that this agent be dispensed using clearer indications and more control in the future.

Availability of Oxygen

As shown in Table 13–1, oxygen constitutes about 21 per cent of ambient air at sea level, and its concentration remains virtually the same at all altitudes where free life exists.

TABLE 13–2. EFFECTS OF DIFFERENT CONCENTRATIONS OF NITROGEN

Concentration	Pressure	Adverse Effects
78% (normal air)	1 atmos	Inert; no toxicity
20% (with 80% O_2)	1 atmos	Progressive atelectasis in lungs Progressive absorption of gas from inner ear and sinuses
78% (normal air)	Over 2 atmos	High pressure effects: similar to alcohol intoxication Decompression sickness: muscle and joint pains, visual disturbances, neurologic damage, bone infarcts

TABLE 13–3. AVAILABILITY OF COMPRESSED GASES IN CYLINDERS

Gas	Symbol	Color Code	H	G	M	E	D	B	A	DD	BB	AA
Oxygen	O_2	Green	+	+	+	+	+	+	+			
Carbon dioxide	CO_2	Gray		+	+	+	+	+	+			
Nitrogen	N_2	Black		+		+	+					
Air		Yellow		+		+	+					
Nitrogen/oxygen	N_2/O_2	Black and green		+	+	+	+					
Carbon dioxide/ oxygen	CO_2/O_2	Gray and green		+	+	+	+	+	+			
Helium	He	Brown		+	+	+	+	+	+			
Helium/oxygen	He/O_2	Brown and green		+	+	+	+	+	+			
Nitrous oxide	N_2O	Light blue	+	+	+	+	+	+	+			
Cyclopropane	$(CH_2)_3$	Orange or chrome								+	+	+
Ethylene	C_2H_4	Red		+	+	+	+	+	+			

TABLE 13–4. AVAILABILITY OF OXYGEN IN CYLINDERS

Cylinders					Available Amount of Oxygen* (APPROXIMATE HOURS)		
Size	Empty Weight (Pounds)	Pounds	Oxygen Content Liters	Cubic Feet	1 Liter Flow Rate	2 Liter Flow Rate	4 Liter Flow Rate
A	2.5	0.25	75.7	2.5	1.2	0.6	0.3
B	5.75	0.5	151	5	2.3	1.2	0.6
D	10.25	1.31	360	13	6	3	1.5
E	15	2.25	624	22	10	5	2.5
M	66	11.00	3028	107	48	24	12
G	100	18.44	5299	187	86	43	21
H	135	20.00	6907	244	112	56	28

Note: an H cylinder should provide at least 50 IPPB treatments, each lasting 15–20 minutes.
*Allowance is made for the fact that tanks are not completely emptied in practice.

Most of the oxygen that is utilized in therapeutics is provided in hospitals from central sources where it is stored as either gaseous or liquid oxygen. The gas is piped into hospital rooms for delivery to individual patients at a standard pressure of 50 pounds per square inch at the gauge (psig, that is, pressure in excess of one atmosphere).[2] For emergency use, for patient transportation, and for therapeutic use outside the hospital, oxygen is available as compressed gas in cylinders of various sizes (Table 13–3). It is important to know how much gas is present in a cylinder, and how long a cylinder will supply a given flow of oxygen (see Table 13–4): many patients receiving domiciliary oxygen utilize more than two large cylinders a week, which constitutes a not inconsiderable expense. In addition to cylinder gas, domiciliary oxygen is available in portable supplies that the patient can carry when walking; this necessitates using a liquid oxygen reservoir from which the "walker" unit can be refilled. More recently, an important new concept has entered the market: this is the oxygen-enricher, which utilizes a molecular sieve to preferentially concentrate the oxygen of the room air for delivery to the patient.[3] This device can be run on household electricity, and it can readily supply a flow rate equivalent to over 4 liters of 100 per cent oxygen per minute, which will satisfy the requirements of almost all hypoxemic patients who require chronic oxygen supplementation (Table 13–5).

For special purposes, oxygen can be provided under higher pressure, as hyperbaric oxygen. The therapeutic and practical pressures that are utilized lie between 2 and 4 atmospheres (1 atmos = 760 torr = 760 mm Hg); special hyperbaric chambers are required for the patient, in some cases with

TABLE 13–5. DEVICES FOR PROVIDING DOMICILIARY OXYGEN*

	Average Monthly Cost for Continuous O$_2$ Delivery (DOLLARS)				
	1L/MIN	2L/MIN	3L/MIN	4L/MIN	Comments
GAS CYLINDERS					
H tanks	126	216	306	411	Small additional costs involved.
PORTABLE O$_2$ DEVICES†					
Linde Walker	138	228	318	408	Device is obtained on lease.
Ecol Stroller	172	269	367	457	Device is obtained on lease.
Erie Traveller	109	199	284	379	Initial purchase cost is $194.
Mada 1313	109	199	284	379	Initial purchase cost is $196.
O$_2$ ENRICHERS					
Bendix Broix Bunn DeVilbiss Marx	Monthly operating costs average $20–30 Purchase price averages $2200–2500 Rental price averages $270/month				

*Adapted from information provided by William A. Dasher, M.D.
†Reservoir supply also required.
The variety of devices and the relative costs are in a state of flux; the information listed is of comparative value but is susceptible to considerable change.

their attendants, to enter for therapy. The use of hyperbaric oxygen is assuming greater importance, both in scientific and industrial work below the surface of the sea, and in hospital therapeutics for which this form of treatment may become more commonplace in the future.

At altitudes above sea level, oxygen is breathed in as a hypobaric gas; although its concentration remains about 21 per cent, its partial pressure decreases progressively with elevation, to levels less than 1 atmos. Oxygen is therefore required by many respiratory patients in mountainous cities, such as Denver, whereas they may not require oxygen supplementation if they descend to sea level. Similarly, respiratory patients who fly in commercial aircraft may require oxygen administration, since the pressurization results in an atmosphere comparable to that of a mile-high habitation.

Trained or acclimatized healthy people can adapt to a surprisingly low concentration of oxygen, but persistent habitation cannot be tolerated at an altitude greater than about 17,000 ft. The highest elevation that can be tolerated without oxygen supplementation, for at least more than a few minutes, is somewhere in the region of 30,000 ft. above sea level, which is coincidentally the highest elevation on earth. At such a level, the expected partial pressure oxygen in the ambient air is less than 50 torr.[1, 4] It is significant that trained mountaineers can function effectively in the most exacting

circumstances, such as prevail near the summit of Mt. Everest, with a PaO_2 of less than 30 torr. Quite obviously, the average lowlander could not tolerate such a poor level of oxygenation, and patients with chronic diseases would be fatally incapacitated. Nevertheless, the extraordinary range of oxygen tensions in the arterial blood that are compatible with function makes it difficult to select a value for PaO_2 that should be regarded as the lower level of normal; indications for oxygen therapy should not be based solely on criteria related to PaO_2, as will be explained later.

Physiology of Oxygen Transport

Although the oxygen content in inspired gas determines the amount of oxygen that is potentially available, it is the partial pressure (PO_2) that provides the driving force of oxygen transport into the lungs and tissues. At sea level, normal dry air contains 21 per cent oxygen at a pressure of $0.21 \times 760 = 159.6$ torr (i.e. 159.6 mm Hg). The air in the trachea during inspiration is completely humidified with water vapor, which exerts a partial pressure of 47 torr at body temperature. Therefore, the partial pressure of oxygen in the inspired air (P_IO_2) cannot be greater than $160 - 47 = 113$ torr. In the lungs, the presence of carbon dioxide further decreases the partial pressure of oxygen in the alveoli (P_AO_2), and in practice the average alveolar pressures of the gases in the normal lung at sea level are approxi-

TABLE 13–6. VARIABLES AFFECTING PaO₂

Variable	Comment
Oxygen concentration (F_IO_2)	Directly affects PaO_2
Oxygen tension (PO_2)	Directly affects PaO_2
Hypoventilation	Causes rise in $PaCO_2$ and reciprocal fall in PaO_2
Hyperventilation	Causes fall in $PaCO_2$ and reciprocal rise in PaO_2
Physiologic shunt (i.e., venous admixture)	May exceed normal 3–5% and decrease PaO_2
Pathologic shunt (e.g., cardiac defect, pulmonary arteriovenous fistula)	Causes variable decrease in PaO_2 that is not overcome by F_IO_2 of 100%
Lung disease (V/Q inequality, variable shunts, diffusion defects)	Cause variable decrease in PaO_2 that may be largely overcome by F_IO_2 of 100%
Age	PaO_2 falls with age. In sitting position: $PaO_2 = 104.2 - (0.27 \times$ age in years)
Position	PaO_2 is less in supine position: $PaO_2 = 109 - (0.43 \times$ age in years)

TABLE 13–7. NORMAL VALUES FOR PaO$_2$ IN DIFFERENT SITUATIONS

Variable	PaO$_2$ Range (torr)	Approximate Hemoglobin Saturation (%)
AGE:		
Neonate	98–106	97–98
Young adult	85–100	96–98
Middle aged	75–90	95–97
Elderly	60–80	91–96
ALTITUDE (young adult):		
Sea level (e.g., Los Angeles)	85–100	97–98
One mile high (e.g., Denver)	65–75	92–95
POSITION (young adult):		
Sitting	90–100	97–98
Supine	85–95	96–97
Asleep	70–85	95–96

mately $P_AO_2 = 100$ torr, $P_ACO_2 = 40$ torr, $P_AH_2O = 47$ torr, $P_AN_2 = 570$ torr (Table 13–1).

Oxygen rapidly crosses the alveolar-capillary membrane into the pulmonary circulation, while carbon dioxide diffuses out with similar facility. The arterial blood that leaves the lung normally contains oxygen exerting a partial pressure of 95 to 100 torr, and values of arterial oxygen tension (PaO$_2$) in excess of 95 torr are considered to be normal in healthy young adults breathing air at sea level. However, the value of the PaO$_2$ is affected by several variables in addition to the concentration of oxygen in the ambient air and the barometric pressure. These variables are tabulated in Table 13–6, and the expected ranges of PaO$_2$ under various situations are presented in Table 13–7 with the corresponding Hb saturations. It should be noted that there is a progressive decline of PaO$_2$ with age, and, as an approximation, the following formula[5] can be used:

$$\text{Predicted mean arterial PO}_2 = 102 - \frac{\text{age}}{3}.$$

The arterial PaO$_2$ is always less than the alveolar P_AO_2, because of the diffusion gradient (related to regional factors that prevent complete equilibration by diffusion across the alveolar-capillary membrane) and the normal venous admixture (since 3 to 5 per cent of the cardiac output constitutes a normal physiologic shunt by bypassing the pulmonary circulation to mix with oxygenated blood entering the left side of the heart), as illustrated in Figure 13–1. The difference between P_AO_2 and PaO$_2$ is known as the alveolar-arterial oxygen (A−aO$_2$) gradient or difference, and may be expressed as $P_{A-a}O_2$

or (A−a)PO$_2$, as will be discussed later in this chapter.

Most of the oxygen that enters the blood is carried in combination with hemoglobin in the red blood cells, but an important fraction enters into simple solution in the plasma. It has been calculated that, in theory, each gram of normal hemoglobin (Hb) can carry a maximum of 1.39 ml of oxygen in the form of oxyhemoglobin (HbO$_2$).[5] In practice, it has been shown that the Hb usually carries only about 1.31 ml/gm.[5] In most texts the commonly accepted value for oxygen saturation lies between these two figures, and therefore 1.34 ml of oxygen per gram of hemoglobin is the customary value that is generally accepted. Normal blood, which contains 15 gm Hb/100 ml, will therefore carry a maximum of $15 \times 1.34 = 20.1$ ml of oxygen in the form of HbO$_2$. The amount of oxygen actually carried by Hb depends upon the partial pressure of oxygen that the blood is exposed to, and the relationship between the Hb saturation and the PO$_2$ is demonstrated by the familiar sigmoid curve illustrated in Figure 13–2.

Hemoglobin has evolved in harmony with man's environmental relationship, and its properties are ideally adapted to efficiently take up a maximal amount of oxygen at the relatively high P_AO_2 that exists in the lungs, and to yield a high proportion of this when perfusing poorly oxygenated tissues with a low PO$_2$. In the resting healthy body, the tissues are well oxygenated, and thus only a small proportion of the oxygen bound as HbO$_2$ is released. However, under metabolic, physiologic, pathologic or environmental stress, the tissue oxygenation demands are much greater, and the tissue PO$_2$ is low,

Oxygen Cascade

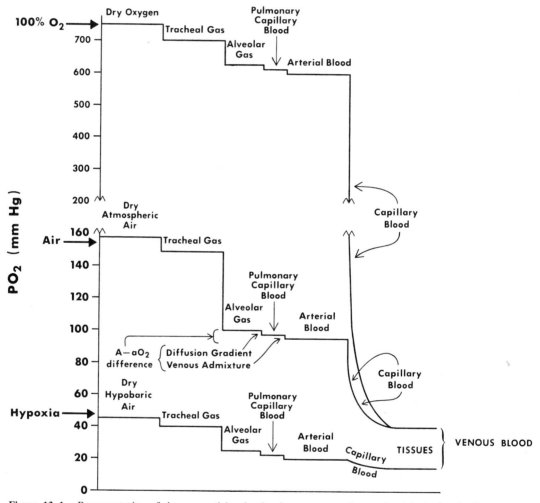

Figure 13–1. Representation of the sequential reduction in oxygen tension at physiologically significant stages of gas transport from the environment to the tissues under conditions of normoxia, hyperoxia or hypoxia. From: A Guide To The Interpretation of Pulmonary Function Tests. L. N. Ayers, B. J. Whipp and I. Ziment. Published by Projects in Health, Inc. New York, N.Y. 1974.

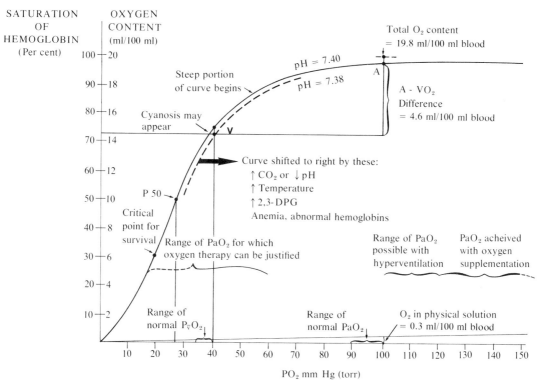

Figure 13–2. Oxygen-Hemoglobin Dissociation Curve
Note: A = typical point on the curve for normal arterial blood (young healthy adult, sea level)
V = typical point on the curve for normal venous blood
P50 = PO_2 at which hemoglobin is 50% saturated

which places it on the steep part of the dissociation curve; as a consequence, a relatively large proportion of the oxygen is given up by the Hb.

The dissociation curve possesses other remarkable features.[1, 5, 6] It is moved to the right when exposed to increased temperature or to acidity (the Bohr effect) as may occur from tissue activity. As shown in Figure 13–2, the conditions usually found in the venous blood environment result in a rightward shift of the dissociation curve; this physiologic property of Hb ensures that slightly more oxygen is released from the Hb and delivered to the tissues. Among various factors that affect the affinity of Hb for O_2, one of the more important is the molecule 2,3-diphosphoglycerate (2,3-DPG), which is produced in the red blood cells by anaerobic glycolysis and is present in the red blood cells in a concentration equal to that of hemoglobin. The molecule 2,3-DPG, in common with other ligands such as carbon dioxide, binds preferentially to the deoxygenated form of Hb and stabilizes it, decreasing its capacity to combine with oxygen. In this way, 2,3-DPG, carbon dioxide and certain other molecules cause a shift in the Hb dissociation curve to the right.

As shown in Table 13–8, a number of clinical conditions can result in a shift of the

TABLE 13–8. FACTORS THAT INFLUENCE O_2-Hb DISSOCIATION CURVE

Increased Affinity for O_2 (CURVE SHIFTED TO LEFT)	Decreased Affinity for O_2 (CURVE SHIFTED TO RIGHT)
Alkalemia (pH ↑, $PaCO_2$ ↓)	Acidemia (pH ↓, $PaCO_2$ ↑)
Hypothermia	Fever
Abnormal Hb (e.g., fetal, Hb Rainier)	Abnormal HB (e.g., Hb Kansas)
Carboxyhemoglobin	Anemia
Methemoglobin	Aldosterone
Decreased ADP or ATP	Exercise
Cirrhosis	Inorganic ions
Decreased 2,3-DPG: transfused bank blood decreased inorganic phosphate hexokinase deficiency male sex hypothyroidism polycythemia	Increased 2,3-DPG: hypoxia, angina increased inorganic phosphate pyruvate kinase deficiency female sex thyrotoxicosis mongolism cortisone congenital heart disease cardiac failure anemia

TABLE 13–9. EFFECT OF DEPTH OR HEIGHT ON OXYGEN CARRIAGE*

	3 Atmos (66 ft. Below Sea Surface)		2 Atmos (33 ft. Below Sea Surface)		1 Atmos (Sea Level)		Approx. 2/3 Atmos (10,000 ft. Altitude)		Approx. 1/2 Atmos (20,000 ft. Altitude)		Approx. 1/3 Atmos (30,000 ft. Altitude)	
	100% O$_2$	21% O$_2$	100% O$_2$	21% O$_2$	100% O$_2$	21% O$_2$	100% O$_2$	21% O$_2$	100% O$_2$	21% O$_2$	100% O$_2$	21% O$_2$
Ambient dry air P$_I$O$_2$ (torr)	2280	480	1520	319	760	160	523	110	349	73	226	47
Arterial blood PaO$_2$ (torr)	2026	350	1313	230	640	100	420	53	260	37	125	20
Hemoglobin saturation (%)	100	100	100	100	100	97	100	85	100	70	99	30
HbO$_2$ (ml O$_2$/100 ml blood)†	20.1	20.1	20.1	20.1	20.1	19.5	20.1	17.1	20.1	14.1	19.9	6.0
Dissolved O$_2$(ml/100 ml blood)‡	6.2	1.1	4.6	0.6	2.1	0.3	1.4	0.2	1.0	0.1	0.7	<0.1
Total O$_2$ content, CaO$_2$ (ml/100 ml arterial blood)	26.3	21.2	24.7	20.7	22.2	19.8	21.5	17.3	21.1	14.2	20.6	6.0

*Values are approximate. It should be noted that the figures given by different authorities vary considerably: the actual values depend on factors such as acclimatization.

†Assuming 15 gm Hb/100 ml blood, and a maximum uptake of 1.34 ml O$_2$/gm Hb.

‡Assuming about 0.3 ml dissolved O$_2$/100 ml blood for every increase in PaO$_2$ of 100 torr.

dissociation curve, and it is possible to envisage the future use of pharmacologic agents that could cause a rightward shift in the tissues, thereby increasing the amount of O_2 delivered.

Oxygen in the Blood

The tissues require a surprisingly small tension of oxygen to supply them with adequate oxygen; a tissue PO_2 in the region of 1 torr may be sufficient. However, as shown in Figure 13–1, there is a steep cascade of oxygen partial pressures from the atmosphere to the tissues, and environmental or pathologic conditions can markedly interfere with the normal values at each stage.

When room air is breathed at sea level, 19.8 ml of oxygen are present in each 100 ml of arterial blood; when breathing 100 per cent oxygen, the amount carried is increased only to 22.2 ml/100 ml of blood (Table 13–9). The reason for the small increase is that room air with a P_1O_2 of 160 torr results in a PaO_2 of about 100 torr with about 97 per cent saturation of the Hb, while close to 100 per cent saturation is achieved with a PaO_2 of about 200 torr. This latter level is usually reached when 40 per cent oxygen (at a PaO_2 of about 300 torr) is breathed (Table 13–10), and additional oxygen in the ambient atmosphere will not result in any further binding of O_2 to Hb. However, oxygen does enter the blood in simple solution in the plasma, the amount that is dissolved being in direct proportion to the partial pressure of the oxygen to which the blood is exposed. For each increase in PO_2 of 100 torr, about 0.3 ml of oxygen is dissolved in each 100 ml of blood. Arterial blood, following exposure to room air in the lungs, normally contains about 0.3 ml of dissolved O_2 per 100 ml of

blood (when the PaO_2 is about 100 torr); when breathing 100 per cent O_2, the resulting PaO_2 may be close to 650 torr, and the amount of dissolved oxygen reaches about 2.1 ml per 100 ml of blood (Table 13–9).

When air or oxygen is breathed under increased pressure, additional oxygen can enter the blood in solution. As shown in Table 13–9, the administration of air at 3 atmospheres of pressure results in 1.1 ml of oxygen being dissolved in every 100 ml of arterial blood.[1, 5] If pure oxygen is breathed at this hyperbaric pressure, about 6.2 ml of oxygen will enter each 100 ml of blood. In the normal resting adult, the tissues require a total of about 250 ml of oxygen per minute, and the normal arterial-venous difference for oxygen (the volume of O_2 extracted by the tissues) amounts to about 6 ml O_2/100 ml arterial blood. Thus, it would be possible for the oxygen needs of the body to be supplied by the amount of oxygen dissolved in the blood when breathing 100 per cent O_2 at 3 atmospheres of pressure. Since oxygen is transferred even more readily from simple solution along the concentration gradient than it is from combination with Hb, it is possible to oxygenate a patient using hyperbaric O_2 even if there is no Hb in the blood. In clinical practice, there is no pathologic condition in which the blood contains no Hb, but severe deficiency can be present in profound anemia, and severe impairment of oxygen-carrying ability can occur when Hb is converted to carboxyhemoglobin by carbon monoxide poisoning. There are, therefore, clinical conditions in which the administration of 100 per cent O_2 at 3 or 3.5 atmospheres of pressure can provide for oxygenation in the pathologic absence of the normal amount of or function of Hb.

Hypoxemia and Hypoxia

There are several categories of abnormal conditions for which oxygen therapy may be justified. The most common and important indication is hypoxemia, and an analysis of this concept must first be discussed.

Hypoxemia. When the PaO_2 of the arterial blood is less than normal, then hypoxemia can be diagnosed. In practice, there is some difficulty in deciding what lower level of PaO_2 provides the dividing line between normal and abnormal, but for practical purposes it is convenient to take the hypoxemic threshold as being 60 torr for a normal middle aged adult at sea level. However, it

TABLE 13–10. EFFECT OF F_1O_2 ON PaO_2 IN NORMAL LUNGS AT SEA LEVEL

F_1O_2 (per cent)	P_1O_2 (torr)	PaO_2* (torr)
21	160	100 ± 5
30	228	150 ± 10
40	304	200 ± 15
50	380	250 ± 20
60	456	315 ± 25
70	532	380 ± 30
80	608	460 ± 30
90	684	540 ± 30
100	760	620 ± 30

*These values are approximate.

TABLE 13-11. USE OF OXYGEN TO DIFFERENTIATE CAUSES OF HYPOXEMIA

Cause of Hypoxemia	Mechanism Involved	Clinical Examples	P_AO_2	PaO_2	$PaCO_2$	$PaO_2 +$ $PaCO_2$ on Room Air	$P_{A-a}O_2$ on Room Air	$P_{A-a}O_2$ on 100% O_2	Rate of Rise of PaO_2 on 100% O_2	PaO_2 After Inhalation Therapy*
	NORMAL		100–110	85–100	38–42	110–135	5–30	10–125		
Decreased oxygen intake	Decreased P_IO_2	Altitude, nitrous oxide inhalation	↓	↓–↓↓↓	↓	<120	N	N	Rapid, toward normal	Remains low
	Hypoventilation	Narcosis, weakness, COPD, respiratory insufficiency, obesity	↓	↓–↓↓↓	↑	110–130	N or ↑	N or ↑	Variable response, up to >400 torr	May increase or may fall
Ventilation: perfusion imbalance ($\dot{V}/\dot{Q}\downarrow$)	$\dot{V}\downarrow$	Airway obstruction, atelectasis	N or ↓	↓–↓↓↓	variable	<120	↑	N or ↑	Slow, usually to >400 torr	May increase
	V = 0 (i.e., R to L shunt)	Anatomic, e.g., pulmonary A-V fistula, atrial septal defect	↓	↓–↓↓↓	N or ↓	<110	↑	↑	Rapid, to <400 torr (<200 torr if original PaO_2 <50 torr)	No change
		Physiologic, e.g., pneumonia	↓	↓–↓↓↓	N or ↓	<110	↑	↑	Fairly rapid, may reach 400 torr	May increase, but does not reach normal
	$\dot{Q}\downarrow$	Pulmonary embolism	N or ↓	↓–↓↓	→	<110	↑	↑	Rapid, but may not reach 400 torr	No change or slight increase
Diffusion defect	Alveolar-capillary block (usually with some $\dot{V}/\dot{Q}$ imbalance)	Sarcoidosis, interstitial pneumonia	N or ↓	→	N or ↓	<120	↑	N or ↑	Delayed increase, to 400 torr	No change or slight increase

Note: ↓ = below expected normal for age, etc.
↑ = above expected normal for age, etc.
N = within normal expected range

→↓ , →↑↑ = moderately decreased or increased
→↓↓↓ , →↑↑↑ = markedly decreased or increased

P_IO_2 = partial pressure of oxygen in the inspired air
P_AO_2 = alveolar partial pressure of oxygen
PaO_2 = arterial partial pressure of oxygen
$PaCO_2$ = arterial partial pressure of carbon dioxide

*Includes IPPB, aerosol therapy, bronchodilators, coughing, physical therapy (breathing room air)

should be recognized that in different patients evidence of oxygen insufficiency may be detectable at levels as high as 75 torr, or may not appear until the PaO_2 falls to about 45 torr.

The causes of hypoxemia may be analyzed in many different ways,[7-9] but the most familiar classification is that shown in Table 13–11. Most, but not all, types of hypoxemia can be improved by the administration of oxygen, and, as illustrated in Table 13–11, the effects of the administration of 100 per cent O_2 for about 20 minutes can produce different responses depending on the cause of the hypoxemia. The categories of hypoxemia represent basic situations, and in clinical practice a patient with respiratory disease usually manifests a mixed picture. The rate of relief of the hypoxemia with O_2 supplementation can give a further clue to the etiology of the defect, and although it is usually impractical and unnecessary to take multiple specimens of arterial blood to monitor the rate of increase in PaO_2, following the changes with an oximeter can be of practical value.

It is convenient to use the alveolar-arterial gradient of oxygen as a basis for evaluating the etiology of hypoxemia.[10, 11] The gradient can be determined to a satisfactory approximation from this alveolar gas equation:

$$P_AO_2 = P_IO_2 - P_ACO_2 \frac{(1 - (1 - R)F_IO_2)}{R}$$

Where P_AO_2 = partial pressure of oxygen in alveolar air

P_IO_2 = partial pressure of oxygen in inspired air

P_ACO_2 = partial pressure of carbon dioxide in alveolar air

F_IO_2 = fraction (%) of oxygen in inspired air

R = respiratory quotient.

For practical purposes, it can be assumed that

$P_ACO_2 = PaCO_2$ (i.e., partial pressure of carbon dioxide in arterial blood)

and $1 - (1 - R)F_IO_2 = 1 - (1 - 0.8)0.21$
$= 1 - 0.042 = 0.958 = 1$ approximately

$\therefore PaO_2 = P_IO_2 - \frac{PaCO_2}{R}$ approximately.

Since $R = 0.8$, unless the clinical state is very abnormal,

$P_AO_2 = P_IO_2 - \frac{PaCO_2}{0.8}$ approximately,

or $P_AO_2 = P_IO_2 - (PaCO_2 \times 1.25)$.
(Equation 1)

From this formula, the P_AO_2 can be derived if the partial pressure of O_2 in the administered gas is known. The $PaCO_2$ is determined from a sample of the arterial blood. Since the PaO_2 can be determined from the same sample, the $P_{A-a}O_2$ can be readily calculated; this is the alveolar-arterial gradient, or difference, of oxygen.

A further mathematical relationship is of value in the analysis of hypoxemia. The alveolar-arterial gradient can be considered to be approximately equivalent to the difference between the theoretically possible sum of the PaO_2 and $PaCO_2$ and the actual sum of these values, using the theoretic ideal situation in which $PaO_2 = 100$ torr and $PaCO_2 = 40$ torr. The less accurate calculation of the gradient derived from these figures differs somewhat from the $P_{A-a}O_2$ gradient derived from the alveolar gas equation, and it is therefore convenient to use slightly different terminology to emphasize this difference. Thus,

$$(A-a)PO_2 = 140 - (PaO_2 + PaCO_2).$$
(Equation 2)

(Note: this equation applies only if the subject breathes room air.) Utilizing this theoretic relationship, or the alveolar-arterial gradient $(P_{A-a}O_2)$ as derived from the alveolar gas equation, the gradient normally lies between 5 and 15 torr in younger people, and can rise to up to 30 torr in normal older people.[12]

Two examples will illustrate the application of these two formulas in the practical analysis of hypoxemia.

Example 1: A patient breathing 21 per cent O_2 (with a P_IO_2 of 149 torr) on blood gas analysis has a PaO_2 of 90 torr and a $PaCO_2$ of 40 torr. What is the gradient?

(1) Using Equation 1:
$P_AO_2 = 149 - (40 \times 1.25)$
$= 149 - 50 = 99$
$\therefore P_{A-a}O_2 = 99 - 90$
$= 9$ torr.

(2) Using Equation 2:
$(A - a)PO_2 = 140 - (90 + 40)$
$= 140 - 130$
$= 10$ torr.

Example 2: A patient breathing 21 per cent O_2 ($P_1O_2 = 149$ torr) on blood gas analysis has a PaO_2 of 90 torr and a $PaCO_2$ of 12 torr. What is the gradient?

(1) Using Equation 1:
$$P_AO_2 = 149 - (12 \times 1.25)$$
$$= 149 - 15 = 134$$
$$\therefore P_{A-a}O_2 = 134 - 90$$
$$= 44 \text{ torr.}$$

(2) Using Equation 2:
$$(A - a)PO_2 = 140 - (90 + 12)$$
$$= 140 - 102$$
$$= 38 \text{ torr.}$$

Thus, similar enough results are obtained using either equation, particularly when the blood gases are not very abnormal. In Example 2, there is an increase in the gradient demonstrated by either calculation, indicating the presence of venous admixture. If, when using Equation 2, the calculated $(A-a)PO_2$ is less than 10 torr—particularly if the $PaCO_2$ exceeds 40 torr—then it is probable that the patient is breathing oxygen; an alternative explanation would be that the blood gas analysis is technically incorrect.[12]

Both the total response and the rate of response of the PaO_2 to breathing 100 per cent O_2 can be of value in elucidating the cause of the hypoxemia, as demonstrated in Table 13–11. A further value of performing this test is that the PaO_2 on 100 per cent O_2 can be used to calculate the amount of a right-to-left shunt.[13] Normally, when breathing 100 per cent O_2 at 760 torr, the resulting PaO_2 should be in the range of 590 to 650 torr (Table 13–10). Any lesser value implies the presence of a shunt, and the degree of shunting is calculated from the following equation:

$$\% \text{ shunt} = (670 - PaO_2) \times 5\%$$
approximately.

This estimate is reasonably accurate for subjects at sea level if the PaO_2 exceeds 200 torr.

Example: A patient at sea level is given 100 per cent O_2 to breathe by a closed system, with venting of expired gas. After 20 minutes, the PaO_2 is 420 torr. How large is the right-to-left shunt?

$$\% \text{ shunt} = (670 - 420) \times 5\%$$
$$= 250 \times 5\%$$
$$= 12.5\% \text{ approximately.}$$

Since the normal shunt does not exceed 5 per cent, the result of this calculation implies that certain areas of this particular patient's lungs are perfused but not ventilated.

Hypoxia. As explained above, hypoxemia is defined by measuring the PaO_2. In contrast, hypoxia is not measurable, but is inferred from clinical determinations of signs and symptoms, which can be supplemented by laboratory data.[14] Hypoxia implies that insufficient oxygen is delivered to the tissues, and this results in abnormalities or insufficiency in function. The causes of tissue hypoxia can be analyzed in several ways,[8, 14, 15] but the conventional classification is that provided in Table 13–12.

Many authors still refer to "hypoxia" as "anoxia," although the former term is generally more appropriate. Usually, hypoxia is associated with hypoxemia, and in most cases at least one of the causes of hypoxemia listed in Table 13–11 can be found in patients with hypoxia. Thus, although hypoxemia and hypoxia have different meanings, they are frequently found together, with hypoxemia being a frequent cause of hypoxia. The other major causes can be categorized as follows.

ANEMIC HYPOXIA. This is seen in conditions in which the hemoglobin content of the blood is decreased (anemia, hemorrhage, hemolysis, sickling), or where its oxygen-carrying power is impaired, as in carbon monoxide poisoning when the hemoglobin is converted to carboxyhemoglobin. Various other abnormal hemoglobinopathies may decrease the ability of the Hb to bind O_2. Usually, in all these cases, the cardiac output increases, and the O_2-Hb dissociation curve shifts to the right, as an adaptive response.[6, 9] The primary treatment should be directed at the hematologic problem, but oxygen therapy has a palliative effect. In a few circumstances, hyperbaric oxygen may be indicated, such as when a patient presents with severe anemia and for technical or personal reasons cannot receive transfusions.

CIRCULATORY HYPOXIA. This is seen when the oxygenated blood is delivered to the tissues in inadequate amounts. Circulatory hypoxia can be a result of decreased cardiac output, of hypotension, or of insufficiency of the arterial supply to the tissues resulting from vascular disease, thrombosis, trauma, or edema of the perivascular tissue. The administration of oxygen is unlikely to be of more than minor benefit, although in some cases (particularly tissue ischemia),

TABLE 13–12. CAUSES OF HYPOXIA

Category	PaO$_2$	PvO$_2$	Cardiac Output	O$_2$-Hb Dissociation Curve Shifted	Effective Hemoglobin	Primary Tissue Problems	Examples	Treatment		
								Increase F$_1$O$_2$	Hyperbaric O$_2$	Other
Hypoxemic	↓	N or ↓	N, ↑ or ↓	To right	N	No	See Table 13–11	Always	No	Respiratory therapy
Anemic (isotonic)	N	N or ↓	N, ↑ or ↓	To right or to left	↓	No	Anemia, hemorrhage, abnormal hemoglobin, sickling, carboxyhemoglobin, methemoglobin	Always	In some cases	Transfuse, treat primary problem
Circulatory (stagnant, hypokinetic)	N or ↓	↓	↓	To right	N	No	Heart failure, hypovolemia, shock, tissue ischemia	Always	No	Treat cardiac and circulatory problems
Cellular (histotoxic)	N or ↓	N or ↑	N or ↓	To left	N	**Yes**	Cyanide and other forms of poisoning	Always	Theoretical value	Use antidote and general support
Demand (over-utilization)	N or ↓	↓	↑	To right	N	**Yes**	Exercise, fever, hypermetabolic stress	May help	No	Manage primary problem
Increased oxygen affinity	N	N	N	**To left**	↓	No	Massive transfusion, hypothermia (see Table 13–8)	Yes	No	Treat primary problem

Note: ↑ = increase, ↓ = decrease, N = normal. Primary causes are in bold face type.

hyperbaric oxygen therapy can be of critical value. Circulatory hypoxia may be diagnosed in ill patients by finding that the partial pressure of oxygen in the mixed central venous pool ($P\bar{V}O_2$) is decreased below the normal 35 to 40 torr.[16, 17] This problem can arise in hypoxemic patients, who require ventilatory support, when positive end-expiratory pressure (PEEP) is utilized: the PaO_2 may be increased, but the resulting mechanical decrease in venous return and in cardiac output may lead to a fall in $P\bar{V}O_2$. Thus, the alleviation of hypoxemia may produce hypoxia, and sampling of blood from a balloon-tipped flow-directed Swan-Ganz catheter may be required to demonstrate the creation of this complication.

CELLULAR HYPOXIA. Cellular hypoxia is caused by the poisoning of the intracellular enzymes involved in tissue metabolism. Usually, this occurs as a result of accidental or deliberate exposure to a poison such as cyanide; effective treatment may not be available before the patient succumbs. Although oxygen administration may not be very effective, an F_IO_2 of 100 per cent should be utilized. If the opportunity is presented, it may be possible to sustain life by using hyperbaric oxygen therapy while treating the poisoning with antidotal or supportive measures.

DEMAND HYPOXIA. Demand hypoxia is an invariable complication of excessive stress, such as results from maximum exercise. It may also occur in hypermetabolic states such as marked fever or thyrotoxic storm, and in these conditions the O_2-Hb dissociation curve undergoes an adaptive shift to the right.[6, 9] The administration of supplemental oxygen can benefit patients who are suffering from pathologic demand hypoxia.

INCREASED OXYGEN AFFINITY HYPOXIA. This can occur when the O_2-Hb dissociation curve is markedly shifted to the left, so that the oxygen that is picked up in the lungs is poorly released in the tissues.[15] The most important practical cause of this problem is the massive transfusion of banked blood, which has a decreased 2,3-DPG content (see Table 13–8). The condition may be suspected when a patient with a normal PaO_2 manifests evidence of hypoxia following a massive transfusion.[6, 9] Other causal factors of this form of hypoxia are very unlikely to present any clinically detectable abnormalities of oxygen transport.

Manifestations of Hypoxia. Tissue hypoxia, rather than arterial hypoxemia, causes abnormal symptoms. The manifestations of hypoxia differ according to whether the exposure is acute, or gradual and chronic; individuals show varying degrees of susceptibility, depending on whether they are fit and active, or debilitated and physiologically disadvantaged.

It is a common experience that many healthy people who go to a mountainous resort experience symptoms caused by the hypoxic environment, but it is also well known that individuals differ markedly in their reactions to the decreased P_IO_2. However, all individuals will experience some symptoms and will demonstrate some signs of hypoxia once the PaO_2 reaches a critically low range (Table 13–13).[18] These manifestations are likely to occur to some degree when the PaO_2 falls below 45 to 50 torr: at this point, the O_2-Hb dissociation curve is steep, and considerable desaturation of the hemo-

TABLE 13–13. CORRELATION OF OXYGENATION WITH SYMPTOMS

Range of PaO₂ (torr)	Approximate SaO₂* (per cent)	Clinical Correlation
>250	100	Oxygen toxicity may develop
150–200	100	Obtained with F_IO_2 of about 30–35%
100–150	98–100	Rarely indicated therapeutically
95–100	97–98	Normal young adult at sea level
80–90	94–96	Normal elderly, or young person during sleep
70–80	92–94	Elderly person during sleep
55–65	88–91	Mild respiratory failure; start of steep portion of the O_2-Hb dissociation curve
50–55	84–88	May warrant chronic O_2 therapy
40–50	75–84	Usually necessitates vigorous treatment
30–40	60–75	Acute: may cause loss of consciousness / Chronic: potentially hazardous
20–30	36–60	Tolerable only in acclimatized mountaineer for short time
<20	<35	Hypoxic brain damage or death likely to occur

*SaO₂ = percentage saturation of hemoglobin with oxygen

TABLE 13–14. POSSIBLE SYMPTOMS AND SIGNS OF SIGNIFICANT HYPOXEMIA

	Acute*	Chronic†
Respiration	Breathlessness, tachypnea, hyperventilation, Cheyne-Stokes breathing, respiratory depression	Shortness of breath, dyspnea on effort, intolerance of increases in hypoxia (e.g., from altitude)
Pulmonary	Liability to pulmonary edema	Pulmonary hypertension
Cardiovascular	Increased cardiac output, vasodilation, palpitations, tachycardia, arrhythmias, hypotension, faintness, angina, acute cardiac failure	Cor pulmonale, decreased cardiac output, myocardial insufficiency, arrhythmias, unstable blood pressure
Central nervous	Euphoria, sleep disturbance, slurred speech, headache, impaired judgment, lassitude, inappropriate behavior, poor concentration, confusion, diplopia, papilledema, retinal hemorrhages, restlessness, lethargy, seizures, obtundation, coma, cerebral edema	Intellectual impairment, psychoneuroses, depression, paranoia, memory loss, insomnia, restlessness, irritability, tiredness, headache, papilledema
Neuromuscular	Fatigue, weakness, tremor, asterixis, hyperactive reflexes, incoordination	Myoclonic jerking, fatigue
Renal	Sodium retention, fluid retention	Edema, renal insufficiency
Other	Lactic acidosis, acidemia, cyanosis, diaphoresis, nausea, vomiting, cool extremities, shock	Polycythemia, vasodilation, plethora, clubbing, liver failure, tendency to venous thrombosis, poor tissue repair

*Acute hypoxia may cause a variety of serious syndromes, including mountain sickness (soroche).
†Chronic hypoxia may be tolerated for years by healthy high altitude dwellers, but may be a serious problem for patients with lung disease. Symptoms and signs are less marked than in acute hypoxemia.

globin can readily occur. The common manifestations of hypoxemia are listed in Table 13–14, and include neuropsychiatric, cardiovascular and respiratory problems in particular.

Acute hypoxia can produce the syndrome of high-altitude or mountain sickness (also known as acute soroche), the most important adverse outcome of which may be pulmonary edema.[1, 4, 19] This complication may be preventable, to some extent, by giving acetazolamide (Diamox), as discussed in Chapter 11, but once the condition develops, the best treatment is to evacuate the victim to a lower altitude. Cautious visitors who gradually ascend to high altitude can become acclimatized to the hypobaric atmosphere; indeed, high mountain climbers cannot perform their spectacular ascents unless slow acclimatization has first been attained. Permanent high altitude dwellers show a complex of adaptive responses, including marked polycythemia, which eventually may result in detrimental complications, such as severe pulmonary hypertension with cardiac failure: the complex is known as chronic mountain sickness, chronic soroche, or Monge's disease.[1] It is of interest that natives of high altitude villages who visit lower levels may be at particular risk of developing high altitude pulmonary edema on return to their native habitation.[4]

In patients with respiratory diseases who live below 6000 feet, the syndrome of chronic hypoxia that evolves is similar to, but usually less dramatic than, chronic soroche (see Table 13–14). Dyspnea, neuropsychiatric problems and exercise limitation are generally the main complaints of these patients.[14] However, polycythemia, pulmonary hypertension and cor pulmonale are the complications that warn of a decreased life expectancy, and these findings provide major indications for oxygen therapy.[20] Cyanosis is not a reliable sign of severe hypoxia, since it is often difficult to detect, particularly in pigmented people, and it may be absent if the patient has concurrent anemia: at least 5 gm of deoxygenated hemoglobin must be present in each 100 ml of arterial blood for cyanosis to be visible. The presence of polycythemia makes it easier to detect cyanosis, but many of these patients have sluggish blood flow (in part because of the increased viscosity of the blood), and this may lead to increased extraction of oxygen in the tissues, thereby causing "stagnant hypoxia"; this can occur even if the PaO_2 is normal.

In the final analysis, the most reliable index of hypoxia in the vast majority of respiratory patients is provided by blood gas analysis, since there is usually accompanying hypoxemia. Certainly, the basis for providing rational oxygen therapy must be the finding of either a reduced PaO_2 or a reduced PvO_2 that improves with the administration of oxygen, although there are a number of situations in which oxygen therapy may be justifiably initiated in the presence of a normal oxygen tension in the blood.[21]

Indications for Oxygen Therapy

Oxygen is given to numerous patients, in emergencies and as part of hospital therapy, on empirical grounds, and it is often difficult to prove that any benefit results. However, since oxygen is relatively inexpensive and harmless in such circumstances, its use need not be condemned. Nevertheless, it is reasonable to base therapy on rational physiologic principles,[8] and some of these will be considered in this section. It will be useful to consider oxygen therapy under several subcategories.

Acute Therapy (Table 13–15). Oxygen is of value in the acute management of both respiratory and nonrespiratory disorders. In the majority of cases there will be subjective or objective evidence of respiratory distress, including dyspnea, shortness of breath, hypoventilation or hyperventilation, or cyanosis. In respiratory diseases, the finding of a decreased PaO_2 and an increase in

TABLE 13–15. INDICATIONS FOR ACUTE OXYGEN THERAPY

HYPOXEMIC CONDITIONS (see Table 13–11)
  Obstructive airways diseases
  Restrictive pulmonary diseases
  Pulmonary emboli
  Alveolar filling diseases
  Pulmonary interstitial diseases
  Respiratory depression/failure
  Insufficient ambient oxygen
  Right-to-left shunt

HYPOXIC CONDITIONS (see Table 13–12)
  Cardiac failure
  Severe cardiac arrhythmias
  Circulatory insufficiency
  Complicated myocardial infarction
  Tissue ischemia
  Severe anemia or hemoglobinopathy
  Increased work of breathing
  Increased tissue requirements for oxygen

CONDITIONS REQUIRING NITROGEN WASHOUT
  Pneumothorax
  Pneumomediastinum
  Subcutaneous emphysema
  Post-pneumoencephalography
  Acute gaseous intestinal distention
  Pneumatosis coli
  General anesthesia

$(A-a)PO_2$ will be present, and there will be evidence of hypoxemia or hypoxia (see Tables 13–11 and 13–12). When respiration is severely depressed, ventilatory support will usually be required; this may necessitate endotracheal intubation and the use of a respirator.

Oxygen therapy may be of value for the nonrespiratory problems presented in Tables 13–11 and 13–12; in particular, acute cardiac decompensation usually merits oxygen administration as part of the overall management. Thus, O_2 is generally considered to be indicated for acute heart failure, early myocardial infarction, angina with arrhythmias, and hypotension secondary to cardiac disease. Although oxygen therapy can be of benefit in patients with complicated myocardial infarction, there is probably nothing to be gained by giving supplemental O_2 to patients with uncomplicated infarction or with routine angina.[22, 23] On the other hand, hypoxemia should be considered as a possible cause of impaired myocardial function or arrhythmias of uncertain etiology.[24]

A special value of high concentration oxygen administration is to treat patients with air collections trapped in the tissues; for example, pneumothorax, pneumomediastinum, subcutaneous emphysema, postpneumoencephalography or distended bowel.[25] The oxygen in such loculated gas pockets is absorbed fairly rapidly, leaving mainly nitrogen in the trapped gas. When 100 per cent oxygen is breathed, the nitrogen is washed out of the lungs, and the decreased P_AN_2 results in nitrogen being progressively washed out of the blood. The fall in PaN_2 allows the more rapid movement of N_2 along the concentration gradient from the tissues into the blood. Consequently, there is an increased rate of removal of nitrogen from the trapped gas, and more rapid resolution of the problem can be produced. One interesting example of this use of oxygen is for the disease pneumatosis coli, in which multiple gas-filled cysts appear in the submucosa of the colon: high concentrations of inspired O_2 have been reported to provide effective therapy.[26]

Chronic Therapy (Table 13–16). In recent years, there has been a tremendous increase in prescriptions for oxygen therapy for home use by patients with chronic respiratory insufficiency. Reports have shown that O_2 supplementation can result in subjective improvement in such patients, and can lead to an increase in exercise tolerance.[27-29] Furthermore, long-term therapy

TABLE 13–16. CONSIDERATIONS IN CHRONIC OXYGEN THERAPY*

DISEASE CRITERIA
Chronic respiratory insufficiency
Chronic pulmonary hypertension
Chronic heart failure with hypoxia
Other causes of hypoxia

PHYSIOLOGIC CRITERIA
PaO_2 below 50–55 torr, breathing room air, at rest
Significant fall in PaO_2 (to below 50–55 torr) during exercise or for prolonged periods during sleep
($P\overline{v}O_2$ below 35 torr

CLINICAL CRITERIA
Breathlessness or dyspnea at rest or on effort
Pulmonary hypertension
Cor pulmonale
Secondary polycythemia
Hyperirritable myocardium (with arrhythmias attributable to hypoxia)

PRACTICAL CRITERIA
Maximum respiratory therapy must be used to optimize pulmonary status
Smoking should be discontinued
Oxygen administration should be demonstrated to produce subjective or objective alleviation of physiologic or clinical abnormalities.
The patient must be capable of improving life style as a result of the benefits of chronic oxygen therapy.

OBJECTIVES
To improve PaO_2 or $P\overline{v}O_2$ to appropriate level
Reversal of symptoms and signs of hypoxia
Improvement of exercise tolerance and self-reliance

Appropriate use of oxygen:
a. Lowest rate of delivery that is effective
b. As necessary for acute symptomatic relief
c. For at least 8–18 hours/day for relief of chronic complications
d. Avoidance of adverse effects of oxygen

*One or more criteria in each category should be met if the use of chronic oxygen therapy is to be justified for any individual patient. The use of oxygen therapy in other conditions, such as psychogeriatric abnormalities, requires further evaluation.

can decrease polycythemia and pulmonary hypertension, and thereby alleviate complicating cor pulmonale. The judicious use of oxygen as part of a domiciliary respiratory therapy regimen may decrease the need for frequent hospital admissions, and there is a possibility that it can prolong useful and worthwhile life.

Unfortunately, this expensive form of therapy can be greatly overused, and therefore attempts to establish criteria and guidelines have been made.[20, 30] At present, the value of chronic oxygen administration for hypoxemic patients on a nationwide basis has not been fully evaluated, and the cur-rently available suggestions may require future modification.

Most authorities feel that chronic oxygen therapy is justifiable in patients in stable condition who demonstrate a PaO_2 of less than 50 to 55 torr at rest while breathing air.[30] Several blood gas samples may need to be analyzed to establish a representative PaO_2, and all patients who may be candidates for chronic O_2 should be given appropriate respiratory therapy and should be required to stop smoking so as to allow the PaO_2 to reach an optimal level. In patients for whom nocturnal hypoxemia is suspected to be a major problem, sleep studies may be required; electrocardiographic monitoring may reveal nocturnal cardiac arrhythmias, but the critical requirement is the finding of a reduced PaO_2 during various phases of sleep. Careful evaluation is necessary in such patients to determine whether the sleep hypoxemia is truly significant. In other patients, some additional special studies may be required to document hypoxemia, including monitoring the PaO_2 during exercise, and more rarely it may be advisable to monitor the PvO_2 for evidence of hypoxia.[31]

In some patients, less severe degrees of hypoxemia may produce clinical evidence of tissue hypoxia, including polycythemia, pulmonary hypertension, cor pulmonale, or impaired exercise tolerance that can be improved with oxygen. In other patients, a case may be made for oxygen supplementation, in the absence of hypoxemia or other complications, when the basic respiratory effort that the patient is forced to make to effect gaseous exchange is far above normal; this type of pattern may be seen in emphysematous "pink puffers," and although by present criteria they often do not qualify for chronic oxygen therapy, it may be worth determining whether supplemental oxygen decreases the respiratory effort and improves the overall status of such a patient.

The use of supplemental oxygen has its greatest application in patients with various types of chronic obstructive pulmonary disease, but other entities, such as severe restrictive disease, may merit chronic O_2 administration. In general, these latter diseases result in the patient having a greatly increased minute ventilation, and relatively high rates of flow of oxygen may be required compared with the low flows (1 to 4 liters per minute) that suffice for most patients with obstructive diseases.[29]

Certain patients with nonrespiratory diseases may benefit from chronic oxygen therapy. Thus, cardiac diseases causing a low PaO_2 should be treated with the appropriate cardiotonic regimen, and oxygen supplementation should be prescribed if evidence of hypoxia or hypoxemia persists. In a few other diseases, the availability of home oxygen for occasional emergency use may be justified, for example, in patients subject to frequent seizures accompanied by apnea, patients with a hereditary predisposition to sudden hematologic crises (such as sickle cell anemia), individuals susceptible to upper airway obstruction (such as those with angioneurotic edema), and possibly others. However, the vast majority of patients who require home oxygen therapy are those with pulmonary disease, and this is as true for dwellers at moderately high altitudes as it is for sea level populations.

Whenever chronic oxygen therapy is thought to be indicated, the physiologic basis should be evaluated and documented. Of equal importance are considerations based on practicality. Thus, the expense and inconvenience of chronic O_2 cannot be justified if the patient or attendants detect no demonstrable benefit from the oxygen. As an example, many geriatric patients, in the terminal years or months of their lives, may present some indications for oxygen therapy, but if no health benefits or improvements in their life style result, the extraordinary expense that could accrue throughout the nation from this form of management would render oxygen supplementation unacceptable. The greatest justifications for oxygen therapy can be demonstrated in those individuals for whom measurable parameters (such as PaO_2 or hematocrit) can be utilized to demonstrate improvement, or where obvious and meaningful improvements in life style (for example, restoration of relative independence, or return to work or social interactions) can clearly be brought about. Thus, the social and practical considerations in chronic oxygen therapy are as important as the physiologic and clinical factors.

When chronic oxygen therapy is prescribed, it should be stressed to the patient that administration for at least eight hours a day (or night) will probably be required to bring about any sustained improvement in the hypoxic complications of the disease. Thus, polycythemia may be brought under control by eight hours a day of oxygen therapy, but it may require 15 to 18 hours of administration each day to reduce pulmonary hypertension.[33, 34] Although it is often taught that intermittent oxygen therapy is harmful,[35] it is clear that most patients use their oxygen in this fashion according to their individual needs, and it is rare to see any adverse outcome of this practice. It is reasonable for incapacitated patients to use oxygen for the sole purpose of obtaining relief when breathless or when exercising; many patients probably use their oxygen in this fashion for not more than a total of one hour a day. There is thus great variation in the way oxygen is prescribed for long-term use, and even greater variation in the ways in which individual patients choose to use their domiciliary supply.

Hyperbaric Oxygen. Although the administration of oxygen under high pressure has been used in therapeutics for many years, its value in general medicine has not been fully established.[36] Surprisingly, few clear and practical indications for its use have emerged in spite of considerable experience, particularly in naval and diving medicine. Although this form of therapy is unlikely to become generally available, all regions of the country should have accessible hyperbaric treatment facilities. The need is greatest wherever recreational or industrial underwater diving is prevalent, since decompression sickness provides a major indication for hyperbaric therapy.[37, 38]

As explained earlier in this chapter and as shown in Table 13–9, hyperbaric oxygen exposure results in two important improvements in oxygen carriage: significant amounts of oxygen are carried in simple solution in the plasma, and the high partial pressure of oxygen in the blood creates a powerful driving force that helps push O_2 into the tissues. Hyperbaric oxygen therapy therefore has several major values (see Tables 13–12 and 13–17): (a) it compensates for inadequate O_2 carriage by hemoglobin; (b) it improves the oxygenation of ischemic tissue; (c) it exposes tissues to the pharmacologic effect of hyperbaric oxygen, which is attributable to the presence of very active, oxidizing, free radicals that may also be responsible for toxic effects on the host; (d) it helps produce reabsorption of air trapped in the tissues.

Hyperbaric oxygenation of the blood results in several physiologic effects.[36, 39] There is a generalized constriction of the hyperoxygenated arterioles, and although this decreases tissue perfusion, the considerable increase in PaO_2 ensures that the organs do receive increased amounts of O_2. There is usually some evidence of vagal stimulation during hyperbaric therapy, and this is likely to be manifested by slowing of the heart rate, with a slight reduction in cardiac output. The blood pressure generally increases, and after a short time the arteriolar constriction in some organs, such as the brain, tends to diminish. This may result, in part, from secondary vasodilation caused by both the increased production of tissue CO_2 and the diminished carriage of CO_2 by Hb, which results since oxyhemoglobin has less affinity for CO_2.[5] Although the tissue CO_2 may rise as a consequence of these effects, the pH of the blood does not usually change.

A further important physiologic effect of hyperbaric therapy is the compression of fluid or gas trapped in tissues or in loculated collections. This effect can be beneficial if tissues are edematous or if their blood supply is compromised by the gaseous pressure, and the mechanical effect of exposure to the hyperbaric atmosphere can improve tissue perfusion, with better oxygenation as a direct physical consequence.

The main indications for hyperbaric treatment are tabulated in Table 13–17; some additional dubious indications are also listed. In general, treatments are provided for about one to two hours one to three times a day in chronic conditions, or for as long as is safe (usually a session of two to four hours) in acute conditions. Most therapy is carried out at about 3 to 3.5 atmos, but pressures used range from 2 to 4 atmos.

The use of hyperbaric oxygen to treat decompression sickness is perhaps its most important role.[38] Although the painful complications of too rapid decompression, known as "the bends," are believed to result from bubbles of nitrogen forming in the fat of tissues (as discussed earlier in this chapter), the etiology is, in fact, probably more complex.[40] The other well-established indications for hyperbaric therapy are carbon monoxide poisoning,[28, 36, 41] gas gangrene caused by *Clostridia*,[42, 43] and the treatment of burns.[43, 44] Certain conditions are treated with hyperbaric oxygen in other countries far more commonly than is the case in the U. S., for example, myocardial infarction complicated by arrhythmias, pulmonary edema, or shock.[36, 45] The use of hyperbaric therapy in the management of chronic osteomyelitis,[43]

TABLE 13–17.   POSSIBLE INDICATIONS FOR HYPERBARIC OXYGEN

Indications	Examples of Clinical Values	
	ESTABLISHED	CONTROVERSIAL
Inadequate or ineffective hemoglobin	Carbon monoxide poisoning Severe acute anemia or hemorrhage (when blood transfusion cannot be given immediately)	Sickle cell crisis Methemoglobinemia Neonatal hypoxemia
Organ or tissue ischemia	Burns (of skin, or inhalational) Chronic osteomyelitis Pressure sores, skin ulcers Myocardial infarction, complicated Ischemic tissue transplants	Regional arterial insufficiency (with threatened gangrene, stroke, blindness or loss of skin graft) Frostbite, severe tissue trauma Snakebite (regional therapy of limb) Amniotic fluid embolism, fat embolism
For gas exchange in tissues	Decompression sickness (bends) Air embolism	Adynamic ileus (i.e., bowel distention)
Inadequate pulmonary gas exchange	Neonatal asphyxia	Severe adult respiratory distress syndrome Massive pulmonary embolus Shock syndromes Emphysema Drowning
For hyperoxic effect	Gas gangrene (anaerobic myonecrosis) Cyanide poisoning Adjuvant to radiotherapy Actinomycosis	To reverse some features of senility Severe tissue poisoning (e.g., alcohol or barbiturate overdose)
Special circumstances	To facilitate surgical correction of arterial insufficiency To facilitate cardiac surgery in cyanotic heart disease, etc. To evaluate a worker for environmental toleration	

pressure sores,[46] skin ulcers,[46] tissue transplants (for example, skin grafts),[36, 43] air embolism,[38] neonatal asphyxia[36] and actinomycosis[47] is probably accepted more readily outside the U.S. In rare circumstances, hyperbaric O_2 may be life-saving in patients with severe anemia or after hemorrhage or hemolysis,[48] or in sickle cell anemia,[49] particularly if blood transfusion is not feasible for individual or technical reasons. Another fairly well-established use for hyperbaric oxygen is as an adjuvant to radiotherapy for carcinomas: the hyperbarism results in the production of free radicals of oxygen that act synergistically with the radiation to kill the hypermitotic cells of the malignant growth.[50]

A number of years ago, hyperbaric oxygen was considered to be of possible value in various forms of respiratory distress syndromes, both adult and neonatal;[36, 51] however, the current practice of intensive respiratory care is more successful, and at present there is no indication for hyperbaric management. Some surgeons favor carrying out, in hyperbaric operating chambers, certain forms of surgery that expose vital tissues to the risk of intraoperative hypoxia: vascular surgery and the correction of cyanotic heart defects are the main indications that have been advocated for this type of intervention.[36, 39, 43] A final use of hyperbaric oxygen is to reverse some of the mental and possibly some of the vascular deterioration associated with senility;[52] this is undoubtedly a potential area for popular abuse, and far more controlled evaluative work will be required to determine its true value.

Administration of Oxygen

Numerous devices of various degrees of complexity can be used to provide oxygen (Table 13–18). For lower concentrations, nasal cannulas should be employed: these devices are simple, inexpensive, easy to use, well tolerated and suitable for most patients.[53, 54] The amount of oxygen delivered can be quite variable, and is dependent on factors such as the flow rate, the positioning of the prongs, and the patient's rate and depth of respiration, that is, factors that affect the inhalation flow rate and the duration of the inhalation. The smaller the tidal volume, the greater the resulting F_IO_2 will be;[55] children and small adults will therefore automatically obtain relatively high concentrations of oxygen. The cannula can be effective even in mouth-breathers, be-

cause the gas is drawn into the mouth by the current of inspired ambient air;[15] however, the F_IO_2 will be somewhat less in such cases than it would be if the patient inhaled through the nose. Similarly, malpositioning of the prongs of the cannula—which is not uncommon in practice—can cause a reduction in the F_IO_2.[56] In dyspneic patients, high flow rate and large tidal volume are common, and the resulting dilution with ambient air produces a significant decrease in the expected F_IO_2.[51] Despite the various practical problems, the majority of patients who require oxygen can achieve a satisfactory PaO_2 with flows of 1 to 4 liters per minute; occasional patients may need up to 8 liters per minute. Flow rates greater than 7 or 8 liters per minute tend to produce nasal mucosal drying and discomfort, and the higher flows can result in an unpredictable increase in F_IO_2.

More reliable control of the F_IO_2 is achieved by using a nasopharyngeal catheter or a venturi mask. There is relatively little indication for catheters, however, since they are irritating and are more of a nursing burden, requiring replacement in the alternate nasal passage every day to prevent pharyngeal damage.[54] The venturi masks were introduced in an effort to provide a more reliable F_IO_2, using a device that is more acceptable to patients and attendants than the catheter. The engineering features of the venturi masks ensure that a relatively narrow range of F_IO_2 is achievable with an individual device; the delivery flow rate of the oxygen can be altered without causing a significant alteration in the resulting F_IO_2.[14, 55] However, it is important to realize that although the manufacturers claim that the 24, 28, 35 and 40 per cent venturi masks are reliable, the actual F_IO_2 delivered may vary by 1 to 2 per cent or even more from the stated concentration.[57, 58] Venturi masks in current use are engineered to provide either 24, 28, 35 or 40 per cent oxygen, with the F_IO_2 being relatively independent of the oxygen flow rate used as long as this exceeds the stated minimum. It has been recommended that 6 l/min flows (rather than 4 l/min) be used for the 24 and 28 per cent masks, and 10 l/min flows (rather than 8 l/min) for the 35 and 40 per cent masks.[58] Campbell has recently described the use of a 60 per cent venturi mask that could be of value in severely hypoxic patients who can be managed without endotracheal intubation.[59] Venturi masks may cause

TABLE 13–18. OXYGEN CONCENTRATIONS DELIVERED BY VARIOUS DEVICES*

Device	Oxygen Source (liters/min)	Air/O₂ Entrainment Ratio	F_IO_2 Range (per cent)	Expected† F_IO_2 (per cent)	Comments
NASAL CANNULA‡	1	Varies	21–24	24	Sufficient for most pa-
	2	"	23–28	28	tients
	3	"	27–34	32	Suitable for many hy-
	4	"	31–37	36	poxic patients
	5–6	"	32–44	40–44	Uncomfortable and
	7–8	"	35–50	45–48	unreliable for flows
	>8	"	40–60	Variable	greater than 6 liters/ min
SIMPLE MASK§	3–4	Varies	25–32	28–30	Less convenient alter-
	5–6	"	30–45	35–42	native to cannula;
	7–8	"	40–60	44–54	provides greater hu-
	>8	"	55–65	55–60	midification
MASK WITH RESERVOIR§ (e.g. partial rebreathing)	5	Varies	35–50	50	For higher F_IO_2; un-
	7	"	35–75	70	comfortable; only
	10	"	65–100	99	for short-term use
NON-REBREATHING MASK§	4–10	"	40–100	Variable	
VENTURI MASK‖	4–6	20:1	(total flow 84 l/min)	24	Not always as reliable
	4–6	10:1	(total flow 44 l/min)	28	as claimed; relative-
	8–10	5:1	(total flow 48 l/min)	35	ly expensive and in-
	8–10	3:1	(total flow 32 l/min)	40	convenient
FACE TENT	4–8	Varies	30–50	Variable	Useful for high humid-
	8–10	"	45–65	Variable	ity
OXYGEN TENT	10–20	Varies	30–60	50	Rarely used currently
CROUP TENT	7–10	Varies	60–80	Variable	For temperature and humidity control
NEBULIZER UNITS	"100%"	Varies	70–90	100	Fairly reliable; for use
	"60–70%"	"	45–60	60–70	with mask and wide
	"40%"	"	25–35	40	delivery tube
IPPB	"Airmix"	Varies	40–90+	40	Overoxygenation can
	"100%"	0	100	100	readily occur
VENTILATORS	21–100	Varies	21–100	21–100	Allow for precise F_IO_2

*All values are approximate, and are based on numerous reports in the literature.
†This F_IO_2 may be achieved by average adult with normal breathing pattern.
‡Nasal catheters provide similar F_IO_2 to cannula with great reliability, and greater discomfort.
§F_IO_2 achieved is greatly affected by closeness of the fit of the mask.
‖Actual F_IO_2 delivered by venturi mask may differ from expected F_IO_2 by about 2%.

discomfort, and some patients experience a sense of claustrophobia. In common with all face masks, they interfere with talking, drinking, eating, and expectorating, and with IPPB treatments, and are therefore frequently removed: in contrast, the simple nasal cannula can remain in place during these common activities. A further disadvantage of venturi masks is that they are relatively wasteful of oxygen, and are therefore not suited for home use. Thus, although venturi masks can, in theory, produce precise oxygenation, in practice they may fail to fulfill their purpose, and all too often one sees the mask on the patient's forehead or neck rather than covering the nose and mouth. Whenever precise and careful use of a nasal cannula can be guaranteed (such as in an intensive care unit or for a compliant patient at home), the need for a venturi mask is correspondingly diminished.

Simple masks of different types are useful for providing humidity with oxygen; in fact, the oxygen is often a secondary consideration, while the humidity or aerosol therapy becomes the main objective.[2, 60, 61] The closer the fit to the patient's face that the mask provides, the less dilution there will be with ambient room air, and the higher the F_IO_2 that will be achieved. All types of face masks possess the practical disadvantages of the venturi mask, but if a precise F_IO_2 is not essential, simple face masks are more convenient and less expensive than venturi masks. Although a venturi mask is not currently used to provide an F_IO_2 greater than 40 per cent (one probably will be in the future[59]), face masks are available that can result in concentrations of O_2 up to 100 per cent. In resuscitative work, very tight-fitting molded masks can be used to deliver the highest concentrations, but such masks are not suitable for use for more than a few hours at most.

When an aerosol or humidity device is used as part of the oxygenation setup, considerable variations in the F_IO_2 may result.[62-64] It is important for therapists to be familiar with the equipment and to employ it correctly; appropriate checks should be made periodically, and when the F_IO_2 is supposed to be carefully controlled, it should be measured at intervals with an oxygen analyzer.

If less precise oxygenation will suffice, and relatively dense humidity is required, a face tent, or even a hood or an oxygen tent, can be used.[60] The value of oxygen-tent therapy has been challenged in recent years, and the alleged benefits have not stood up to careful examination. As a consequence, tent therapy has become rare in adult patient management, and is used less commonly for children.[2] The main value of a tent is to provide a therapeutic oxygen-enriched mist for a child who will not accept a nasal or facial device. Croupettes or croup tents are in a different category, and are of definite value in the management of neonatal respiratory disease.[59]

When higher concentrations of oxygen are needed for more than a short time, the patient will generally need to be intubated with an endotracheal tube, and then any desired F_IO_2 can be reliably delivered by a modern ventilator. Since the delivery of an F_IO_2 of more than 60 per cent may cause adverse effects after 48 to 72 hours, there is relatively little need for reliable masks to provide higher concentrations of oxygen. If 60 per cent or more oxygen is required, then it is often best to intubate and ventilate the patient; effective oxygenation may be carried out with less than 60 per cent O_2 when the appropriate rate and depth of ventilatory control are employed, but if higher concentrations of oxygen are needed to correct hypoxemia, techniques such as positive end-expiratory pressure (PEEP) may need to be added. If a patient cannot be adequately oxygenated with a ventilator and adjuvant techniques such as PEEP, consideration should be given to the possible use of a membrane oxygenator. However, use of this device presents tremendous logistic problems, and the outlook for a patient who requires this type of management is currently very poor.

When conventional methods of oxygenation prove inadequate, then hyperbaric oxygenation or a membrane oxygenator ("artificial lung"),[65, 66] or even the use of fluorocarbon liquids or emulsions[67] in the lungs or to replace circulating blood, can be considered. However, these approaches are rarely available or are impractical, and criteria for their use in the management of severe hypoxemia are still evolving. At present, they have no role in general respiratory therapy.

Adverse Effects of Oxygen

Serious complications of oxygen can be divided into various categories, each of which may be thought of as a stage in the development of "oxygen toxicity" or "oxygen poisoning" (Table 13–19).

Physiologic Effects. When oxygen is given to a patient with chronic respiratory failure or a depressed respiratory center, the resulting improvement in the PaO_2 may cause abolition of the hypoxia that is responsible for driving respiration. As a result, relative hypoventilation occurs, causing a rise in the $PaCO_2$. In some patients, this will act as a stimulus to breathing, and a period of relative hyperventilation may ensue. This type of breathing pattern is sometimes clinically apparent as Cheyne-Stokes breathing. In patients with chronic obstructive pulmonary disease (COPD), the $PaCO_2$ may continue to rise, and eventually the patient becomes somnolent; in extreme cases of "CO_2 narcosis" obtundation may develop, and apnea may occur. This unfortunate outcome is all too frequent when an unsophisticated patient or attendants increase the rate of flow of the oxygen supply without taking the patient's blood gases or clinical status into consideration.

This physiologic effect of oxygen is an unpredictable outcome of O_2 therapy, but all hypoxic or hypercarbic patients should be regarded as potential candidates for CO_2 narcosis. It is probable that there is in these patients a depression of the normal respiratory center responsiveness to CO_2, whereas the carotid body peripheral chemoreceptors remain sensitive to oxygen; therefore, relieving the hypoxia removes the prime respiratory stimulus. Regrettably, there is no simple test available for determining whether a patient's breathing is dependent on the hypoxic drive. If this state is suspected, then low-flow (1 to 2 liters/minute) O_2 should be initiated, and the clinical response and blood gases should be monitored; if deterioration appears, use of a respiratory stimulant such as doxapram should be considered (see Chapter 11).

Oxygen Intolerance. If normal volunteers

TABLE 13–19. OXYGEN TOXICITY SYNDROMES

Syndrome	Rapidity of Development	Oxygen Concentration	Cause	Manifestations	Comment
PHYSIOLOGIC EFFECT	Minutes or hours	20–60%	↑ PaO_2	Respiratory depression ("CO_2 narcosis")	Only in patients with respiratory failure
OXYGEN INTOLERANCE					
Physiologic	Minutes	60–100%	↑ PaO_2	Tachycardia, decreased cardiac output, hypotension, arteriolar constriction	These reactions are very variable, and have a complex etiology
Pathologic	Hours	90–100%	↑ F_1O_2	Symptoms of ear, sinus and tracheobronchial discomfort	Earliest finding is decreased tracheobronchial mucociliary clearance. For other features, see Table 13–20
OXYGEN IRRITATION					
Physiologic	Hours or days	70–100%	↑ F_1O_2	Absorption atelectasis	May result in abnormal chest x-ray, blood gases and pulmonary function tests
Pathologic	Days	90–100%	↑ F_1O_2 + ↑ PaO_2 (uncertain)	Tracheobronchitis or bronchopneumonia	Causes bronchoscopic or chest x-ray changes; see Table 13–21
OXYGEN DAMAGE					
Normobaric	Days	90–100%	↑ F_1O_2 + ↑ PaO_2 (uncertain)	Pulmonary damage	Early and late pulmonary changes have been defined (see Table 13–21)
Hyperbaric	Hours	100%	↑ PaO_2	Central nervous system damage, e.g., convulsions	Effect due to high PaO_2 (> 1200 torr)
RETROLENTAL FIBROPLASIA	Hours or days	>40%(?)	↑ PaO_2	Insidious development of blindness in premature neonates	Full etiologic explanation is uncertain

are kept in an atmosphere of 100 per cent O_2, each will eventually develop severe discomfort.[68] Symptoms usually appear within 2 to 16 hours, but some people tolerate the experience for over 36 to 48 hours before complaining. The initial abnormality in normal people has been shown to be an impairment of ciliary activity, with a decreased rate of mucociliary clearance.[69] The initial symptom is usually substernal discomfort, which is exacerbated by deep breathing. Subsequently, a dry cough becomes progressively more pronounced, and the tracheal irritation increases. Eventually, there is marked pain on inspiration, which may have a pleural quality, and the subject becomes dyspneic. Similar changes in the upper airways may result in a sensation of nasal stuffiness and a sore throat; eye irritation and ear discomfort are other early complaints[70] (see Table 13–20). The chest x-ray and pulmonary function tests may remain normal until the symptoms become pronounced. Complete reversal of these symptoms of oxygen intolerance will rapidly

occur if the subject returns to an atmosphere of air.[68]

Oxygen intolerance does not occur when normal people are exposed to an F_1O_2 of less than 60 per cent at normobaric pressure, such as pertains at sea level. Individual susceptibility varies, but the development of symptoms tends to be a function of both F_1O_2 and length of exposure.[71] Clearly, many hypoxemic patients who require high concentrations of oxygen to correct their low PaO_2 have tolerated more than 60 per cent O_2 for many days, and it is possible that the damaged lung may be less susceptible to the pathologic consequences of oxygen intolerance.[70] However, all individuals are at some risk when exposed to the higher concentrations of oxygen.

Manifestations of oxygen intolerance may be detectable in organs other than the lung. The normal physiologic effect of an F_1O_2 in excess of 60 per cent is caused by the correspondingly elevated PaO_2, which would be over 450 torr in the normal person at sea level. The main effects are vascular, and are

TABLE 13–20. ACUTE EFFECTS OF HIGH CONCENTRATIONS OF NORMOBARIC OXYGEN*

Effect On	Site of Action	Result	Outcome
RESPIRATION	1. Peripheral chemoreceptors (e.g., carotid body)	Depression of respiratory drive	Increase in tissue CO_2 and in $PaCO_2$, which may then stimulate ventilatory drive
	2. Decreased amount of deoxygenated hemoglobin	Decreased carriage of CO_2	
	3. Abolition of hypoxic drive (in COPD)	CO_2 narcosis	Hypoventilation, apnea
HEART	1. Vagal receptors	Slight bradycardia	Decrease in cardiac output†
	2. Cardiac muscle	Slight depression	
REGIONAL CIRCULATION	1. Cerebral vessels	Arteriolar constriction	Uncertain†
	2. Coronary vessels	Arteriolar constriction	Uncertain†
	3. Peripheral circulation	Arteriolar constriction	Slight hypertension†
	4. Retinal circulation‡	Arteriolar constriction	Impaired visual fields
	5. Conjunctival vessels	Vasodilation	Conjunctivitis
	6. Pulmonary circulation	Vasodilation	Improved $\dot{V}/\dot{Q}$ match, reduction of pulmonary hypertension
EAR, SINUSES	Air in body cavities	Replaced by oxygen, which is then absorbed	Ear pain and sinus pain
AIRWAYS	Respiratory mucosa of nose, throat, trachea and bronchi	Irritation	Impaired mucociliary clearance, mucosal swelling and inflammation
LUNG PARENCHYMA	Poorly ventilated zones	Nitrogen washout, followed by O_2 absorption	Microatelectasis, atelectasis
PULMONARY FUNCTION	Airways and parenchyma	Decreased compliance	Decrease in vital capacity
BLOOD	1. Erythrocyte membrane	Damage	Hemolysis
	2. Kidneys (?)	Fluid retention††	Decrease in hematocrit and serum albumin

*The time taken for the eventual effects to develop is very variable.
†These effects are rarely of clinical significance.
‡In premature neonates, retinal vascular proliferation may occur (retrolenta fibroplasia).
††Initial fluid retention is usually followed by a diuresis.

manifested in the regional circulation (Table 13–20). Hyperoxia causes some vasoconstriction of most systemic arterioles, but the resulting changes of perfusion in the cerebral and coronary vessels (which have been subjected to the most study) do not appear to be of clinical significance.[15] It is noteworthy that the high F_IO_2 results in an increase in oxygenated hemoglobin in the blood, and this has less capacity to carry CO_2 than does deoxygenated Hb (the Haldane effect); consequently CO_2 increases in the tissues and in the blood. As a result, secondary vasodilation may be produced, which can overwhelm the vasoconstriction caused by the hypoxemia. Furthermore, the Haldane effect may result in an increased CO_2 drive to respiration in normal subjects, which accounts for the initial hyperventilation that people with normal respiratory control experience when breathing 60 to 100 per cent O_2.[15]

Although most blood vessels constrict as a result of hyperoxia, the pulmonary blood vessels dilate. This effect can be beneficial in respiratory patients, who often have pulmonary hypertension, and accounts for much of the improvement that oxygen therapy brings about in cor pulmonale. In this respect, the eye is comparable to the lungs, since both the conjunctival vessels and the retinal vessels dilate; normal subjects may develop conjunctivitis as part of the oxygen intolerance syndrome.

A further outcome of oxygen excess is that nitrogen is "washed out" of air collections in the body, as described earlier. The oxygen content of the inner ear and sinuses initially increases, but after a while some absorption of the oxygen occurs, creating negative pressure in these closed spaces. The patient may then experience a "vacuum headache," due to ear and sinus pain.[25] A similar effect can occur in the lungs, and absorption microatelectasis may develop as part of the oxygen intolerance syndrome.

Other organs may demonstrate a response

to the high PaO_2. Hyperoxia causes vagal stimulation, which results in slight bradycardia, reversible by atropine. There may also be a direct depressant effect on the heart, or an aortic body reflex, resulting in a slight decrease in cardiac output.[15, 25] An initial retention of fluid has been reported following 100 per cent oxygen administration, and this is subsequently followed by a diuresis; the explanation is unknown.[72] Secondary changes in hematocrit and in serum albumin may occur as a result of the fluid shifts.

One of the important consequences of 100 per cent O_2 administration that has been reported in some subjects is hemolysis.[72] This occurs in susceptible people because O_2 can damage the cell membrane of erythrocytes.

Oxygen Irritation. This is a more advanced consequence of exposure to a high F_IO_2; the syndrome is mainly recognizable as a pulmonary entity (Table 13–19 and 13–21). This stage of oxygen toxicity emerges as a continuum from the syndrome of oxygen intolerance, and differs only in that there is objective evidence of pulmonary damage.[68, 73] The chest x-ray will show areas where microatelectases merge into atelectatic streaks; there will also be patches of bronchopneumonia. Subjects show signs, symptoms or bronchoscopic evidence of tracheobronchitis, but usually there is no evidence of infection. Pulmonary function tests will be abnormal at this stage;[9, 68] the most reliable indication of pulmonary involvement is the decrease in vital capacity. Other findings that may be present include decreased compliance, reduced functional residual capacity, and evidence of shunting. Some of these abnormalities may persist for

several days after the subject has been returned to a normal respiratory environment.

Oxygen Damage. This is the final stage of oxygen toxicity. It is a syndrome that was originally described by Lorrain Smith in 1899, and it has become a subject of intense interest and controversy in the past decade. There are many practical difficulties that have prevented the development of a clear understanding of this interesting consequence of hyperoxygenation. Animal studies cannot be transposed to the human condition, since the human lung is relatively resistant to oxygen damage when compared with the usual laboratory animals.[73] Studies on humans have been difficult to interpret, and ethical considerations have prevented definitive experimental investigations in this area.[74, 75]

The lung has a limited ability to react to severe noxious events, and the results tend to present with similar pathologic findings. Experimental oxygen damage is very similar in appearance to that produced by viral infections, and other insults that the sick human lung is exposed to may produce similar results. Most patients who require prolonged courses of oxygen therapy at a high F_IO_2 will also require intubation, respirator support, airway suctioning, tracheobronchial topical drug therapy and so on; furthermore, their lungs are liable to be exposed to fluid overload or hypovolemia, infection, embolization and so on. All of these adverse factors may contribute to the eventual pathology of the lung, from which an attempt has to be made to define the contribution of the oxygen.[68, 70]

A clear understanding has emerged about

TABLE 13–21. PULMONARY TOXICITY CAUSED BY HIGH CONCENTRATIONS OF OXYGEN

Site	Early Effects	Late Effects
AIRWAYS	Nasal stuffiness, sore throat, substernal discomfort, pain on inspiration, cough, dyspnea*	Tracheobronchitis, bronchopneumonia, atelectasis†
PARENCHYMA	Exudative phase: atelectasis, alveolar and interstitial edema, intra-alveolar hemorrhage, fibrinous exudation, hyaline membrane, destruction of endothelial cells and Type I alveolar cells‡	Proliferative phase: hyperplasia and proliferation of Type II alveolar cells, fibroblast proliferation, lymphocytic infiltration, septal cell swelling, capillary hyperplasia, fibrosis‡
PULMONARY FUNCTION	Decreased compliance, shunting, reduced vital capacity, reduced functional residual capacity	Decreased diffusing capacity, increased $P_{A-a}O_2$, decreased expiratory flow rate

*Oxygen intolerance syndrome
†Oxygen irritation syndrome
‡Oxygen damage syndrome (early and late)

some of the features of end-stage pulmonary oxygen toxicity. Etiologically, it is known that the condition is brought about only if the lung is exposed continuously to more than 60 per cent O_2 for more than two days. Although a high F_IO_2 is a major factor, this alone is not toxic, since astronauts and other volunteers have tolerated many days of 100 per cent O_2 at a pressure of one-third of an atmosphere[71] (about 250 torr), which should result in a PaO_2 of about 125 torr (Table 13–9). It is known that a high PaO_2 (perhaps in excess of 450 torr) is required to produce the full development of oxygen toxicity. At the present state of knowledge, it would appear that the syndrome depends on the combination of a high F_IO_2 causing a high PaO_2 continuously for several days; individual susceptibility varies considerably, and it is thought that many patients with damaged lungs are more resistant to the toxic effects.[70] In addition, it is known that if the F_IO_2 is increased gradually over several days, or if a high F_IO_2 is interrupted with intermittent breathing of gas with a much lower F_IO_2, then "acclimatization" of the lungs to the toxic effects of oxygen may develop.[72]

The pathologic features of oxygen toxicity can be divided into an early exudative phase and a late proliferative phase, the details of which are tabulated in Table 13–21. The final outcome may be fibrotic scarring, but in clinical practice many other secondary abnormalities, such as infection, will usually be prominent.[73]

Although severe damage to organs other than the lungs is unusual, there is one special situation where extrapulmonary oxygen toxicity is a major and dramatic problem. If excessive oxygen is administered to a pre-mature newborn infant, the developing retinal vessels undergo initial constriction, with suppression of normal retinal vascularization and destruction of endothelial cells. Subsequently the remaining endothelial cells undergo a disorganized vascular proliferation, that destroys the immature retina.[76, 77] The resulting condition, *retrolental fibroplasia*, results in blindness. Unfortunately, it has not become clear what the exact limits of oxygen tolerance are for the neonatal retina, but it is probable that exposure to sufficient oxygen to cause a PaO_2 in excess of 150 torr for more than a few hours causes the disease. Many books claim that if no more than 40 per cent oxygen is given to the premature neonate, oxygen toxicity can be avoided. However, it is wise to monitor the PaO_2, and to avoid causing an unnecessary elevation. Since the premature lung may also be very susceptible to oxygen damage (for example, pulmonary dysplasia), cautious use of oxygen is particularly important in neonates, who have experienced many months of conditioning to a relatively hypoxic environment.

Hyperbaric Oxygen Toxicity. This has features that distinguish it from normobaric oxygen toxicity (Table 13–22). The various syndromes associated with hyperbaric gas exposure are related to the high F_IO_2 and high PaO_2, to the high arterial pressure of the inert gases (particularly nitrogen), and to the mechanical risks associated with compression and decompression.

Hyperbaric 100 per cent O_2 results in an acceleration in development of the various syndromes of normobaric oxygen toxicity. When exposure to over 2 atmos is experienced, most patients develop severe symp-

TABLE 13–22. HAZARDS OF HYPERBARIC EXPOSURE

Air*	100% O_2†	Either‡
Decompression sickness ("caisson disease," "bends"):	Pulmonary oxygen toxicity syndromes (see Table 13–19)	Growth of emphysematous bullae
Painful bones and joints	Central nervous system toxicity:	Rupture of lung blebs, cysts or bullae (causing pneumo-thorax, etc.)
Skin irritation	Anxiety, nervousness	
Eye irritation, decreased visual fields	Nausea, vertigo, tinnitus	Sinus, ear or dental pain
Air-embolism ("chokes")	Paresthesias	Rupture of ear drum
Headache, weakness, paresis	Twitching (mainly facial)	Intestinal pain (i.e., bowel distention)
Debility, fatigue, shock	Diaphragmatic spasms	Pneumoperitoneum in female
	Myoclonus	Bone infarcts
Nitrogen narcosis or nitrogen intoxication	Convulsions	
	Flash fires	

*Oxygen toxicity will also occur if pressure is sufficient to cause a $PaO_2 > 1200$ torr.
†Decompression sickness is less likely to occur with hyperbaric O_2.
‡These are the general effects of "barotrauma," caused by exposure to any hyperbaric environment.

TABLE 13–23. CAUSES OF TISSUE DAMAGE IN OXYGEN TOXICITY

Basic Effect	Outcome
Oxidation of sulfhydryl bonds	Inactivation of enzymes and coenzymes, e.g., dehydrogenases, cytochrome oxidase, flavoproteins, glutathione, nicotinamide adenine nucleotide, coenzyme A
Peroxidation of double bonds in lipids	Damage to cell membranes of erythrocytes, resulting in hemolysis
Degradation of neurotransmitters of brain	Depletion of gamma-aminobutyric acid (GABA), resulting in a decrease in the seizure threshold
Radiomimetic effect	Potentiation of radiosensitivity of malignant neoplasms

*Damage to these agents may account for cellular death of lung tissues and of anaerobic bacteria.

toms of oxygen intolerance or oxygen irritation within a few hours, and soon afterwards the features of oxygen damage will appear unless the exposure is discontinued. However, it appears that these aspects of oxygen toxicity are comparable to the results of more prolonged exposure to normobaric oxygen in high concentration.

As was described by Paul Bert in a monumental study in 1878, oxygen at a partial pressure greater than about 1200 torr can cause a unique central nervous system syndrome.[73] The first manifestations are likely to be anxiety and nonspecific distress; paresthesias of the face and limbs may then appear. Next, the muscles of the eyelids and face may be susceptible to twitching, and myoclonus may affect other muscle groups, including the diaphragm. Finally, the subject develops convulsions, followed by coma and death.[9, 73]

CAUSES OF OXYGEN TOXICITY. As already explained, some of the hazards of oxygen are related to physiologic effects of an increased PaO_2, and others are caused by the action of a high concentration of O_2 in the gases in the lungs. The direct tissue damage, particularly that seen in the nervous system with hyperbaric oxygen, is more difficult to explain, and involves complex biochemical mechanisms.[78, 79] Probably the basic toxic element in high concentration oxygen administration is the presence of highly active free oxygen radicals. These are normally destroyed by the enzyme superoxide dismutase, which is produced principally by the Type II pneumocytes. It is relevant that damaged lungs, resulting from a variety of insults including excessive oxygen, lose Type I alveolar cells, following which there is a proliferation of Type II cells. If high concentrations of oxygen therapy are given to a patient with damaged lungs, the excess of Type II cells may account for the relative lack of susceptibility of the lungs to further damage by the oxygen.[9, 73]

The adverse effects of oxygen are directed mainly at enzymes and coenzymes that contain oxidizable sulfhydryl bonds, at double bonds in lipids and at certain neurotransmitters (see Table 13–23). A wide range of enzymes may be inactivated, while damage to the lipid membrane of erythrocytes can result in hemolysis. The neurotransmitter gamma-aminobutyric acid (GABA) is found principally in the central nervous system, and its depletion in severe oxygen toxicity may account for the development of seizures.

Certain factors have been found to exacerbate the development of oxygen toxicity, while others have a prophylactic effect.[80] From Table 13–24, the most relevant deduction to be made is that continuous therapy with 60 to 100 per cent oxygen should not be initiated in a patient if avoidable; if unavoidable, the high concentrations should not be maintained for longer than two days. It has been shown that stepwise increases in F_IO_2 over the course of several days enable the tissues to become acclimatized to oxygen, and the toxic manifestations can be averted.[72, 73] Alternatively, it may be possible to interpose periods (perhaps of 10 to 20 minutes) on a low F_IO_2 every few hours during a course of high F_IO_2 administration; this is not often possible in practice, and it may not serve a useful purpose, but nevertheless it is worthy of consideration particularly when using hyperoxia to help resolve a pneumothorax.

Various anabolic hormones and hypermetabolic states increase the risk of developing oxygen toxicity, whereas hypoendocrine or hypometabolic states may have some prophylactic value.[73, 80] Certain ions, in particu-

TABLE 13-24. FACTORS MODIFYING RATE OF DEVELOPMENT OF OXYGEN TOXICITY

Factor	Exacerbating	Prophylactic*
Exposure to F_IO_2 of 100%	Continuous therapy for over 2 days	Intermittent exposure or acclimatization
Hormones	Glucocorticoids, ACTH, epinephrine, insulin, thyroid	Hypothyroidism, adrenergic blocking drugs, hypophysectomy, adrenalectomy
Clinical status	Hyperthermia, convulsions	Immaturity, starvation, hypothermia
Metallic ions	Copper, iron	Cobalt, manganese, nickel
Drugs and miscellaneous factors	CO_2 inhalation, paraquat, vitamin E deficiency, dextroamphetamine, X-irradiation, aspirin, atropine, viral infection	Antioxidants, chlorpromazine, gamma-aminobutyric acid, ganglionic blocking drugs, reserpine, glutathione, trishydroxymethylaminomethane (THAM), sodium bicarbonate, vitamins C, E and K, general anesthetics, cysteine, anticonvulsants

*The majority of these prophylactic measures have not been subjected to clinical evaluation, and apart from intermittent exposure or acclimatization to oxygen, none can be regarded as of practical value at present.

lar copper and iron, appear to exacerbate the condition, whereas cobalt, manganese and nickel may be protective.[79] Among exacerbating factors are hypercarbia (which may be a major problem in patients with respiratory failure) and viral infections.[81] Findings that glucocorticoids and viral pneumonia can exacerbate oxygen toxicity make it difficult to recommend rational therapy for severe viral pneumonia: many physicians treat this condition with glucocorticoids as well as high concentrations of oxygen; some of the adverse outcomes may be attributable to the iatrogenic component.

Experimentally, prophylaxis can be provided by antioxidants, including vitamin E, which appears to prevent red cell hemolysis by hyperoxygenation.[73, 79] Another method of prophylaxis is to provide additional substrate when it is known that depletion occurs as a result of oxygen toxicity: succinate, glutathione, GABA and other agents have been effective in experimental animals.[9, 80] Many other agents have been suggested,[5, 82] but their practical value remains to be proved.

Safe Administration of Oxygen

Oxygen must be given for a clear purpose; in most cases it is administered as treatment for either hypoxemia or hypoxia. When treating hypoxemia, the blood gases must be utilized as the basis for initiating treatment and for evaluating the outcome. In general, a PaO_2 of at least 60 torr is required, and it is unusual for greater than 100 torr to be necessary. At present, there is a huge grey zone of ranges of PaO_2: values below 100 torr are considered to suffice in most clinical situations, and values in excess of 1500 torr are required in hyperbaric treatment. The need for a level of PaO_2 in the zone of 100 to 1500 torr is relatively uncertain, and represents an area for further evaluation.

General rules in the administration of oxygen are presented in Table 13-25, but the most important rule is to avoid giving more O_2 than is required, particularly if this necessitates administering more than 60 per cent O_2. Physicians, respiratory therapists, nurses and patients must treat oxygen as a drug, employing precise amounts when indicated, and utilizing clinical and laboratory evaluation to help adjust the dosage.

When treating hypoxemia, there is much less precision available in the guidelines (Table 13-26). Certainly, there is a suspicion that oxygen is of benefit in many conditions, even though the explanation offered may be weak; a good example is the use of oxygen to treat elderly patients with neuropsychologic deterioration. In patients such as these, even though hypoxemia does not exist, 2 liters per minute of oxygen for a month has been reported to improve memory, despite the change in PaO_2 being unremarkable.[83] Certainly, a great deal more knowledge is required before one can provide clear criteria

TABLE 13–25. SAFE USE OF NORMOBARIC OXYGEN THERAPY IN HYPOXEMIC PATIENTS

Precautions	Comment
1. Give only enough oxygen to bring PaO_2 up to 60–70 torr.	The value of a PaO_2 in excess of 70 torr has not been shown.
2. Avoid giving in excess of 60% O_2 for longer than 2 days.	Concentrations of 60–95% O_2 are probably safe for at least 2 days.
3. Do not give more than 95% O_2, if possible, so as to prevent the development of atelectasis.	The presence of 5% N_2 in gas in the lungs tends to prevent atelectasis.
4. If high concentrations of O_2 are used to help produce resolution of a pneumothorax, etc., give the O_2 intermittently, or progressively increase the F_1O_2 every few hours.	Two hours of O_2 followed by 10–20 minutes on room air will prevent the adverse effects of high F_1O_2. Acclimatization to hyperoxia may be produced by progressively increasing the F_1O_2.
5. Avoid irritating airways with the oxygen stream.	Avoid high flow rates through the nose, and provide adequate humidification.
6. If high concentrations of O_2 are required to correct hypoxemia, consider alternate forms of respiratory care, and decrease high F_1O_2 as soon as possible.	Intubation with respiratory support using large tidal volumes or sighing or PEEP may result in adequate oxygenation with a lower F_1O_2.
7. Monitor clinical state frequently when giving oxygen to patients with abnormal control of respiration.	Too much O_2 in a patient with respiratory failure or a depressed respiratory center may cause CO_2 narcosis or even apnea.
8. Monitor blood gases frequently when tight control is needed.	Blood gas monitoring provides precise information as to how PaO_2 and $PaCO_2$ are affected by F_1O_2.
9. When hypoxic features persist in spite of correcting PaO_2 seek explanation (e.g., monitor $P_{\bar{v}}O_2$).	Anemia, abnormal hemoglobin, low cardiac output, tissue ischemia, etc. may be cause of hypoxia.
10. Ensure patient and attendants use equipment correctly; devices must be comfortably placed and functioning appropriately.	Intermittent oxygen therapy, or variations in F_1O_2, can have deleterious effect on control of breathing, unless carefully supervised.
11. When giving IPPB or aerosol therapy, or when suctioning, be wary of changes in F_1O_2, and PaO_2, and take corrective action if necessary; monitor F_1O_2 if in doubt.	IPPB may deliver an unexpectedly high F_1O_2. Bronchodilators may cause fall in PaO_2. Suctioning may cause severe fall in PaO_2; prior increase in F_1O_2 for a few minutes is of prophylactic value.

TABLE 13–26. SAFE USE OF OXYGEN THERAPY IN HYPOXIC PATIENTS

Precautions	Comment
NORMOBARIC THERAPY	
1. Evaluate cause of hypoxia and correct primary abnormality.	In cardiac failure, cardiac therapy may be more important than O_2 therapy.
2. Correct other contributory abnormalities.	See Precaution 9, Table 13–25.
3. Beware of O_2 suppressing hypoxic drive in patient with unsuspected respiratory insufficiency.	When there is doubt, monitor blood gases. Use particular caution if $PaCO_2$ is elevated.
4. Consider possible value of elevating PaO_2 to above 100 torr, when using normobaric oxygen.	In some patients, there may be benefits from a high PaO_2 (above 200–400 torr), but this has not been clearly defined (e.g., in ischemia).
HYPERBARIC THERAPY	
1. Observe safety precautions to prevent overdosage.	In general, not more than 3.5 atmos should be given for not more than 1–2 hours at a time.
2. Avoid preventable barotrauma to lungs, ears and sinuses.	Treat bronchospasm, mucus retention, otitis, and nasal mucosal swelling before initiating each treatment.
3. Use extra precautions in patients who are at particular risk of complications.	Patients who have anxiety, claustrophobia, nausea or seizure history are at particular risk.
4. Utilize regional hyperbaric treatment where possible, rather than exposing whole body to hyperbaric environment.	Regional therapy may be adequate for ischemic injury or infection, or snakebite on a limb.
5. Avoid risk of fire or explosion.	This has been a major hazard in hyperbaric O_2 work.

and advice for the treatment of hypoxic problems.

When hyperbaric treatment is used, expert technicians and physicians must supervise the procedure. A number of elementary precautions should be taken, as suggested in Table 13–26. Patients with upper respiratory tract infection or congestion are at particular risk of barotrauma to the ears or sinuses, and if hyperbaric management cannot be delayed, an oral or topical mucosal constrictor should be given (see Chapter 9). Several other precautions should be routinely observed, such as when patients are likely to vomit, panic or convulse in the hyperbaric chamber: many of these patients may be unsuitable for hyperbaric treatment.

One of the most important precautions to take whenever oxygen is used is to avoid the risk of fire: too many patients refuse to recognize the need to avoid open flame near an oxygen source. The risk is particularly great when hyperbaric oxygen is used; severe flash fires have occurred. In this regard, oxygen is one of the few drugs that can be as mortally dangerous to the physician and allied health worker as it is to the recipient of the therapy.

CARBON DIOXIDE

The relationship between carbon dioxide (CO_2) and oxygen was discussed earlier in this chapter, and some of the therapeutic properties of CO_2 were reviewed in Chapters 4 and 11. Additional basic aspects of CO_2 pharmacology will be presented in the following section.

Carbon dioxide is the normal end-product of the metabolic processes, in both animals and plants, which take place with the release of energy. The resulting CO_2 has to be eliminated; the respiratory route of excretion is well adjusted to perform this function in concert with the simultaneous ventilatory function of taking in oxygen.[1, 7] In the normal human, ventilation adequate to produce an arterial oxygen tension of 95 to 100 torr will be sufficient to eliminate CO_2 from the blood at a rate that keeps the arterial carbon dioxide tension ($PaCO_2$) close to 40 torr. It is important to recognize that while this figure of 40 torr is appropriate for the normal individual, it is not essential to the body's well being, and a reasonably healthy life can be lived with a much higher $PaCO_2$. Furthermore, if a patient is given supple-

mental O_2, an even higher $PaCO_2$ may prove to be tolerable, and it is possible for respiratory patients on chronic oxygen therapy to adjust to a $PaCO_2$ in excess of 100 torr. The key factor in the body's acceptance of an abnormal $PaCO_2$ is the corresponding change in blood buffers that is required for the preservation of the arterial pH.

The normal resting body produces a smaller volume of CO_2 (200 ml/min) than the 250 ml/min of oxygen that it requires. The ratio of CO_2:O_2 is 200:250 = 0.8; this is the respiratory quotient (R.Q.), and it is largely determined by the total food substrates made available in the diet. During stress, such as occurs with heavy exercise, the CO_2 production may increase 1000 per cent, and unless the overall excretory mechanism is functioning adequately, a marked rise in $PaCO_2$ can occur. However, any increase in CO_2 in the blood stimulates the peripheral chemoreceptors, while the respiratory center is also stimulated directly by the CO_2 in the blood and in the cerebrospinal fluid, as explained in Chapter 11. As a result, the respiratory rate and depth are increased to match the requirements for CO_2 elimination.

The CO_2 produced in the tissues diffuses readily into the capillary blood, where it goes into solution in the plasma. A small proportion of the CO_2 is bound to plasma proteins as carbamino groups, but the greatest proportion diffuses into the erythrocytes. In the red cells, the CO_2 is rapidly converted into carbonic acid (H_2CO_3) by the enzyme carbonic anhydrase; this reaction occurs 13,000 times more rapidly than it would in the absence of the enzyme. The resulting H_2CO_3 then dissociates into hydrogen ions (H^+) and bicarbonate ions (HCO_3^-). The HCO_3^- diffuses along the concentration gradient out of the erythrocytes into the plasma and is replaced by chloride ions (Cl^-), which diffuse into the red blood cells. Part of the CO_2 in the red cells binds with the deoxygenated hemoglobin to form carbamino groups; this process is facilitated by the action of CO_2 on the O_2-Hb dissociation curve, which is thereby shifted to the right and gives up more O_2 as a consequence. Furthermore, reduced Hb serves CO_2 transport by binding more carbon dioxide than does oxygenated Hb at any partial pressure.

In the lungs, the CO_2 that is dissolved in the plasma rapidly diffuses along the concentration gradient into the alveolar space, and the whole process that took place in the tissues is rapidly reversed. The CO_2 that is carried as HCO_3^- and as carbamino groups is thereby made almost instantaneously available for excretion into the alveoli. The partial pressures of carbon dioxide therefore fall progressively from the tissues to the venous blood; the $PaCO_2$ is lower in the alveolar air, and is much lower in the ambient atmosphere. The relationship between the PCO_2 and PO_2 at various sites in the pathway is shown in Table 13–1.

Relationship of $PaCO_2$ to pH

Each day, the body produces about 20,000 mEq of acid made up of CO_2 and other metabolic acids. The amount of acid tolerated in the arterial blood is controlled within very narrow limits, and the hydrogen ion activity in the blood usually lies between 10^{-7} to 10^{-8} mole/l. The H^+ content is conveniently expressed as a negative logarithm, with the notation pH; the arterial blood pH lies close to 7.40. The pH is determined by both the amount of acid and the amount of buffering base, and the following relationships can be recognized:

$$H^+ \text{ concentration} = K \frac{\text{total acid}}{\text{total base}} \left(\begin{array}{l}\text{where K is}\\\text{a constant}\end{array}\right)$$

$$\therefore \qquad pH = pK + \log \frac{\text{base}}{\text{acid}}.$$

In the arterial blood, the most important base is bicarbonate, and the most important acid is carbonic acid. Therefore

$$pH = pK + \log \frac{HCO_3^-}{H_2CO_3}.$$

There is a fixed relationship between the amount of CO_2 dissolved in the plasma and the concentration of H_2CO_3, and it can be shown that[2]:

$$PaCO_2 \times 0.03 = \text{mM } CO_2/\text{liter plasma}$$

Furthermore:

$$[H_2CO_3] = \text{mM } CO_2/\text{liter plasma}$$
$$\therefore [H_2CO_3] = PaCO_2 \times 0.03$$
$$\therefore \qquad pH = pK + \log \frac{[HCO_3^-]}{PaCO_2 \times 0.03}.$$

In arterial blood:

$$pH = 6.1 + \log \frac{24}{40 \times 0.03}$$
$$= 6.1 + \log \frac{24}{1.2}$$
$$= 6.1 + \log 20$$
$$= 6.1 + 1.3$$
$$= 7.4.$$

Thus, the ratio of bicarbonate to CO_2, which is normally 20:1, controls the pH, which is normally in the range of about 7.37 to 7.43 in the arterial blood. The control of bicarbonate is carried out by the kidney, which can slowly adapt to changes in HCO_3^- concentration; when HCO_3^- is present in excess, the normal slow rate of renal excretion can be hastened by using a carbonic anhydrase inhibitor as explained in Chapter 11. In contrast, the control of CO_2 is susceptible to much more rapid and finer control by the lungs. The overall effect of ventilation on the $PaCO_2$ is so firmly related that hypoventilation can be defined as an increase in $PaCO_2$ beyond normal limits (greater than 45 torr), and hyperventilation as a decrease in $PaCO_2$ beyond normal limits (less than 35 torr). The relative controlling effect of the kidneys and lungs on pH can be conceptually represented by this formula:

$$pH = pK + \log \frac{\text{kidney function}}{\text{lung function}}.$$

Thus, the production and elimination of CO_2 is linked by mathematic relationships to both the PaO_2 and the pH. The relationship of $PaCO_2$ and pH is mathematically related to the HCO_3^- content of the arterial blood, and a change in any one of these will produce corresponding changes in the other two, and will bring about secondary changes in the $PaCO_2$. Both the direct manipulation of $PaCO_2$ and the indirect manipulation of HCO_3^- have been utilized to effect changes in ventilation, as described in detail in Chapter 11. In similar fashion, the ventilatory response of a subject to different concentrations of inhaled CO_2 can be used diagnostically in the evaluation of respiratory control.

Pharmacologic Effects of CO_2

Some of the pharmacologic properties of carbon dioxide have already been detailed in

TABLE 13–27. PHYSICAL PROPERTIES OF RESPIRATORY GASES

	Air	Nitrogen	Oxygen	Carbon Dioxide	Helium
Molecular weight	28.96	28	32	44	4
Physical state in cylinder at 70° F	Gas	Gas	Gas	Liquid*	Gas
Density (gm/l at 0° C and 1 atmos)	1.293	1.250	1.429	1.977	0.178
Specific gravity (air = 1)	1.00	0.97	1.14	1.53	0.14
Viscosity (in poises)	183	178	201	148	194
Solubility coefficient in blood at 38° C	–	0.0130	0.0230	0.47	0.0087

*Carbon dioxide undergoes sublimation.

Chapter 11. Carbon dioxide is about 1.5 times heavier than air, and 1 part is soluble in 1.2 parts of water at body temperature (see Table 13–27). It is alleged that CO_2 (or HCO_3^- or H_2CO_3), probably by virtue of its rapid diffusibility across membranes, promotes the absorption of water by mucous membranes, and this could account for the popularity of aerated beverages: these carbon dioxide–containing solutions appear to relieve thirst more rapidly than does plain water.[84] However, the solution of bicarbonate may stimulate the stomach to secrete more acid, which liberates the CO_2 and promotes eructation. Other important physical properties of CO_2 are its noncombustibility and its low thermal conductivity, which allows the solidified gas to remain relatively stable as dry ice, as compared with ice produced from water. Other pharmacologic effects of CO_2 on various tissues and organs of the body are summarized in Table 13–28.

It is somewhat discouraging to find that CO_2 is regarded less highly today than it was formerly, and that it has a diminishing role in

respiratory therapy. When concentrations in excess of 5 to 7 per cent are breathed in for any length of time, various toxic manifestations may develop, and these become more severe if the administration of the gas is continued (Table 13–29). Concentrations of CO_2 in excess of 10 per cent are more hazardous, and mixtures of 30 per cent CO_2 in air or oxygen can rapidly lead to convulsions, coma and death. Thus, whenever CO_2 is given by inhalation, the patient must be carefully monitored for the development of toxic complications, and courses should be administered for a limited time. In general, concentrations of CO_2 in excess of 7 per cent should be avoided: such concentrations are difficult to justify with our current knowledge, and they are undoubtedly hazardous.[2, 15, 25]

HELIUM

Helium (He) is obtained from some of the natural gas fields, such as those near Amarillo, Texas. This unique gas is a

TABLE 13–28. THERAPEUTIC USES OF CARBON DIOXIDE

System Affected	Effect	Possible Clinical Values*
Respiratory System	Stimulation of depth of respiration	Prevention of atelectasis
	Increase in minute ventilation	To hasten recovery from inhalational anesthesia
	Stimulation of coughing	To improve mucokinesis
	Bronchodilation	Adjuvant in asthma
	To correct hypocarbia	Management of hyperventilation
	To inhibit diaphragmatic spasm	Treatment of hiccups (singulus)
Circulation	Cerebral vasodilation	Prophylaxis of developing stroke
	Ophthalmic artery dilation	Treatment of threatened ophthalmic artery occlusion
Central Nervous System	Depression of mental state	Treatment for anxiety neurosis
Blood	Shift of O_2-Hb dissociation curve to right	Decreases affinity of Hb for carbon monoxide: useful in CO poisoning

*Most of the claimed benefits are of dubious value in clinical practice.

TABLE 13–29. TOXIC EFFECTS OF CARBON DIOXIDE*

RESPIRATION	Initial stimulation, then depression.
CIRCULATION	Vasodilation by direct action on blood vessels. Vasoconstriction due to sympathetic activity resulting from hypothalamic stimulation.
CORONARY VESSELS	Vasoconstriction or vasodilation.
CEREBRAL VESSELS	Vasodilation, causing headache.
HEART	Arrhythmias, including ventricular fibrillation.
CENTRAL NERVOUS SYSTEM	Anxiety, dizziness, confusion, mental depression; analgesia, paresthesias, tremors, fasciculations, twitching, convulsions, coma.
OTHER	Perspiration, flushing, dilated pupils, dimming of vision, diplopia, nausea, vomiting, hypertension, exhaustion.

*Toxic effects can be produced by breathing concentrations of carbon dioxide in excess of 5%. More rapid onset of symptoms and more severe toxicity occur when higher concentrations are used.

relatively limited natural resource, and its use in clinical medicine is necessarily restricted by its potential scarcity and its increasing cost. It is similar to argon and neon in that it is an inert gas with no natural physiologic function or pharmacologic toxicity. However, its special properties have made it of value in respiratory diagnosis and therapeutics; it has no other important applications in clinical medicine.

The most important physical property of helium is its low density, which is about one-seventh that of nitrogen and one-eighth that of oxygen: in other words, it has a low specific gravity, which is only 0.14 that of air (Table 13–27). Although it is sometimes stated that it has a low viscosity, this is not so; in fact, its viscosity is slightly greater than that of air. Other properties of importance are its high acoustic velocity (which results in a curious distortion of the voice of a person breathing a high concentration of the gas), and its high rate of diffusion and low solubility. An important property of helium is its ability to diffuse heat. Divers immersed in a high concentration of the gas tend to lose so much body heat that they develop severe shivering. The relevant properties of helium are summarized in Tables 13–27 and 13–30.

The gas is often used in place of nitrogen in combination with 20 per cent oxygen in commercial diving, since the mixture of He-O_2 has only one-third the specific gravity of air, and it therefore offers several advantages.[15] The danger of inert gas narcosis and of decompression sickness is greatly reduced

TABLE 13–30. IMPORTANT PROPERTIES OF HELIUM*

Property	Effect	Therapeutic Implications
Low density	Low driving pressure required	Less energy expenditure needed to work or breathe in He-O_2 than in 100% O_2 or air
	Readily moves through obstructed airways	Useful in various types of airway obstruction
	Poor vehicle for suspended droplets	Unsuited for use in aerosol therapy
High acoustic velocity	Alters conduction of sound	Causes change in voice in person breathing He-O_2
Inertness	No adverse tissue effects	He-O_2 is safer than air for breathing under hyperbaric conditions
		Suitable for diagnostic studies, e.g., in determination of functional residual capacity (FRC)
Low solubility	Does not enter tissues readily	Hyperbaric He-O_2 unlikely to result in "bends" on decompression
High diffusibility	Readily conducts heat	Divers in He-O_2 atmosphere lose heat and may shiver violently
Low flammability	He-O_2 unlikely to support combustion	He-O_2 safer than O_2-N_2 in explosive situations

*Helium is used in combination with 20–30% oxygen (He-O_2).

with He compared with that associated with nitrogen. The low density of the gas gives the mixture of He and O_2 a low resistance, which allows breathing at hyperbaric pressures under the sea to occur with relatively little effort; exertion is considerably easier under these circumstances than it would be in an atmosphere of hyperbaric air. Helium is less soluble in tissues than is nitrogen; bubbles of helium are unlikely to appear in joints and other organs during decompression. The relative safety from developing the bends makes possible a shorter decompression time for divers.

In terrestrial therapeutics, the advantage of the He-O_2 mixture is that the critical velocity for the development of turbulent flow is three times that for air.[2] When He-O_2 is breathed through a restricted orifice, less effort is needed because the specific gravity of the mixture is low, and laminar flow is preserved, thereby decreasing the problem of resistive drag. Patients with increased airway resistance will have to make less respiratory effort when breathing He-O_2 than they are required to make when breathing air. This is certainly true when there is upper airway obstruction, such as occurs in epiglottitis or carcinoma of the larynx. However, as pointed out in Chapter 4, it is arguable whether this difference is of relevance in the distal airways. Although experts such as Barach,[85] Segal,[85] Motley[86] and Egan[2] claim that breathing a mixture of 80 per cent He and 20 per cent O_2 is of considerable benefit in severe asthma, there appears to be little general support for this form of therapy. Even if one does accept that He-O_2 can be of value, it is doubtful whether the difficulty and expense involved in using this form of therapy can be justified now that so many alternative ways of managing asthma are available. Pragmatic difficulties abound when helium therapy is employed: a special flowmeter must be used, a closed system is required to avoid wasting the precious gas, and a continuous positive pressure setup should be employed for maximal benefits.[85]

The persuasive writings of Barach and others lead one to conclude that helium can be a valuable adjunct in the management of severe asthma. However, it is questionable whether this form of therapy has a role in medicine today; practical considerations ensure that it can be readily available only in centers specializing in this form of treatment. Nevertheless, it would not be unreasonable for the Respiratory Therapy Department of the average hospital to have a tank of 80 per cent helium—20 per cent oxygen available for the emergency management of upper airway obstruction or severe unremitting asthma.

In general, the use of helium in hospitals is confined to its employment in respiratory diagnosis. The gas is used by pulmonary function laboratories in determining the functional residual capacity (FRC) and, secondarily, the total lung capacity (TLC). Otherwise, most of the helium utilized for respiratory purposes is employed in the diving world, where its value cannot be denied.

OTHER GASES

Carbon monoxide, neon and *xenon* are used for certain diagnostic tests of pulmonary function. However, they are used in small concentrations, and under such circumstances they have no pharmacologic benefits or side effects. They will therefore not be considered further.

REFERENCES

1. Guenter, C. A.: The respiratory environment. *In* Pulmonary Medicine. C. A. Guenter and M. H. Welch (Eds.). Philadelphia, J. B. Lippincott Company, 1966. Ch. 1.
2. Egan, D. F.: Fundamentals of Respiratory Therapy. St. Louis, The C. V. Mosby Company, 2nd ed. 1973. Ch. 8.
3. Brown, H. V. and Ziment, I.: Evaluation of an oxygen concentrator in patients with chronic obstructive pulmonary disease. Respiratory Therapy (In press).
4. Hecht, H. H.: A sea level view of altitude problems. Am. J. Med. 50:703-708, 1971.
5. Nunn, J. F.: Applied Respiratory Physiology. London, Butterworths, 2nd ed., 1977. Ch. 12.
6. Klocke, R. A.: Oxygen transport and 2,3-diphosphoglycerate (DPG): Chest 62 (5, Suppl. Pt. 2):79S-85S, 1972.
7. Guenter, C. A.: Respiratory function of the lungs and blood. *In* Pulmonary Medicine. C. A. Guenter and M. H. Welch (Eds.). Philadelphia, J. B. Lippincott Company, 1977. Ch. 4.
8. Andrews, J. L.: Physiology and treatment of hypoxia. Clin. Notes Resp. Dis. (published by the American Thoracic Society.) Vol. 13. # 2, Fall, 1974.
9. Baldwin, G. R.: Oxygen: therapeutics, toxicity and advances. *In* Current Respiratory Care. K. F. McDonnel and M. S. Segal (Eds.). Boston, Little, Brown and Company, 1977. Ch. 10.
10. Snider, G. L.: Interpretation of the arterial oxygen and carbon dioxide partial pressures: a simplified approach for bedside use. Chest 63:801-806, 1973.
11. Shapiro, A. R., Virgilio, R. W. and Peters, R. M.: Interpretation of alveolar-arterial oxygen tension difference. Surg. Gynec. Obstet. 144:547-552, 1977.

12. Hodgkin, J. E.: Blood gas analysis and acid-base physiology. *In* Respiratory Care: a Guide to Clinical Practice. G. G. Burton, G. N. Gee and J. E. Hodgkin (Eds.). Philadelphia, J. B. Lippincott Company, 1977. Ch. 12.

13. Hyde, R. W.: Clinical interpretation of arterial oxygen measurements. Med. Clin. N. Amer. 54:617–629, 1970.

14. Daniele, R. P. and Rogers, R. M.: Oxygen and nonventilatory therapy of respiratory failure in COPD. Postgrad. Med. 54:145-154, Sept., 1973.

15. Lambertsen, C. J.: Therapeutic gases: oxygen, carbon dioxide, and helium. *In* Drill's Pharmacology in Medicine. J. R. DiPalma (Ed.). New York, McGraw Hill Book Company, 4th ed., 1971. Ch. 55.

16. Gray, B. A.: Clinical applications of mixed venous oxygen measurements. *In* Respiratory Intensive Care. R. M. Rogers (Ed). Springfield, Ill., Charles C Thomas, 1977. Ch. 14.

17. Mithoefer, J. C., Holford, F. D. and Keighley, J. F. H.: The effect of oxygen administration on mixed venous oxygenation in chronic obstructive pulmonary disease. Chest 66:122-132, 1974.

18. King, T. K. C. and Briscoe, W. A.: Abnormalities of blood gas exchange in COPD. Postgrad. Med. 54:101-108, Sept., 1973.

19. Rennie, D.: Give me air!—But not much. N. Engl. J. Med. 297:1285-1287, 1977.

20. Flick, M. R. and Block, A. J.: Chronic oxygen therapy. Med. Clin. N. Amer. 61:1397-1408, 1977.

21. Hedley-Whyte, J. and Winter, P. M.: Oxygen therapy. Clin. Pharmacol. Ther. 8:696-737, 1967.

22. Lal, S., Savidge, R. S. and Chhabra, G. P.: Oxygen administration after myocardial infarction. Lancet 1:381-383, 1969.

23. Rawles, J. M. and Kenmure, A. C. F.: Controlled trial of oxygen in uncomplicated myocardial infarction. Br. Med. J. 1:1121-1123, May, 1976.

24. Ayres, S. M. and Grace, W. J.: Inappropriate ventilation and hypoxemia as causes of cardiac arrhythmias: the control of arrhythmias without antiarrhythmic drugs. Am. J. Med. 46:495-505, 1969.

25. Wollman, H. and Smith, T. C.: The therapeutic gases: oxygen, carbon dioxide, and helium. *In* The Pharmacologic Basis of Therapeutics. L. S. Goodman and A. Gilman (Eds.). New York, Macmillan Publishing Co., Inc., 5th ed., 1975. Ch. 43.

26. Down, R. H. L. and Castleden, W. M.: Oxygen therapy for pneumatosis coli. Br. Med. J. 1:493-494, March, 1975.

27. Petty, T. L., Stanford, R. E. and Neff, T. A.: Continuous oxygen therapy in chronic airway obstruction: observations on possible oxygen toxicity and survival. Ann. Intern. Med. 75:361-367, 1971.

28. Altschuler, S. L.: Oxygen therapy in pulmonary disease: oxygen use and toxicity. Med. Clin. N. Amer. 57:851-860, 1973.

29. Lilker, E. S., Karnick, A. and Lerner, L.: Portable oxygen in chronic obstructive lung disease with hypoxemia and cor pulmonale: a controlled double-blind cross-over study. Chest 68:236-241, 1975.

30. Block, A. J. et al.: Oxygen administration in the home. (Official statement of American Thoracic Society.) Am. Rev. Respir. Dis. 115:897-899, 1977.

31. Jöbsis, F. F.: Intracellular metabolism of oxygen. Am. Rev. Respir. Dis. 110, #6, Pt. 2:58-63, 1974.

32. Mithoefer, J. C.: Indications for chronic oxygen therapy in chronic obstructive pulmonary disease. Am. Rev. Respir. Dis. 110, #6, Pt. 2:35-39, 1974.

33. Burrows, B.: Arterial oxygenation and pulmonary hemodynamics in patients with chronic airways obstruction. Am. Rev. Respir. Dis. 110, #6, Pt. 2:64-70, 1974.

34. Block, A. J.: Low flow oxygen therapy: treatment of the ambulant outpatient. Am. Rev. Respir. Dis. 110, #6, Pt. 2:71-84, 1974.

35. Campbell, E. J. M.: Respiratory failure: the relation between oxygen concentrations of inspired air and arterial blood. Lancet 2:10-11, 1960.

36. Ledingham, I. M.: Hyperbaric oxygen. *In* Recent Advances in Surgery. S. Taylor (Ed.). London, J. and A. Churchill Ltd., 7th ed., 1969. Ch. 10.

37. Strauss, R. H. and Prockop, L. D.: Decompression sickness among scuba divers. J.A.M.A. 223:637-640, 1973.

38. Davis, J. C., Dunn, J. M., Hagood, C. O. and Bassett, B. E.: Hyperbaric medicine in the U.S. Air Force. J.A.M.A. 224:205-209, 1974.

39. Ashfield, R.: Hyperbaric oxygen. *In* Scientific Foundations of Anaesthesia. C. Scurr and S. Feldman (Eds.). Philadelphia, F. A. Davis Company, 1970. Sect. IIB, Ch. 6.

40. Elliott, D. H., Hallenbeck, J. M. and Bove, A. A.: Acute decompression sickness. Lancet 2:1193-1199, 1974.

41. Winter, P. M. and Miller, J. N.: Carbon monoxide poisoning. J.A.M.A. 236:1502-1504, 1976.

42. Editorial: Gas gangrene and hyperbaric oxygen. Br. Med. J. 3:715, Sept., 1972.

43. Pascale, L. R. and Wallyn, R. J.: Surgical applications of the hyperbaric chamber. Surg. Clin. N. Amer. 48:63-70, 1968.

44. Hart, G. B., O'Reilly, R. R., Broussard, N. D., Goodman, D. B. and Yanda, R. L.: Treatment of burns with hyperbaric oxygen. Surg. Gynec. Obstet. 139:693-696, 1974.

45. Glauser, S. C. and Glauser, L. M.: Hyperbaric oxygen therapy: size of infarct determines therapeutic efficacy. Ann. Intern. Med. 78:77-80, 1973.

46. Fischer, B. H.: Topical hyperbaric oxygen treatment of pressure sores and skin ulcers. Lancet 2:405-409, 1969.

47. Manheim, S. D., Voleti, C., Ludwig, A. and Jacobson, J. H.: Hyperbaric oxygen in the treatment of actinomycosis. J.A.M.A. 210:552-553, 1969.

48. Myking, O. and Schreiner, A.: Hyperbaric oxygen in hemolytic crisis. J.A.M.A. 227:1161-1162, 1974.

49. Kylstra, J. A.: Hyperbaric oxygen. *In* Advances in Respiratory Care and Physiology. T. B. Caldwell and F. Moya (Eds.). Springfield, Ill., Charles C Thomas, 1973. Ch. 15.

50. Editorial: Oxygen and radiotherapy. Br. Med. J. 4:125-126, Oct., 1974.

51. Patrick, T. R., Manning, G. T., Oforsagd, P. A. and Trapp, W. G.: The correction of severe

hypoxemia in adult respiratory distress syndrome with hyperbaric oxygenation (OHP). Chest 58:483–490, 1970.

52. Editorial: Hyperbaric oxygen seems to aid aged patients. J.A.M.A. 231:238-240, 1975.
53. Cherniack, R. M. and Hakimpour, K.: The rational use of oxygen in respiratory insufficiency. J.A.M.A. 199:146-150, 1967.
54. Kory, R. C., Bergmann, J. C., Sweet, R. D. et al.: Comparative evaluation of oxygen therapy techniques. J.A.M.A. 179:767-772, 1962.
55. Shapiro, B. A., Harrison, R. A. and Trout, C. A.: Clinical Applications of Respiratory Care. Chicago, Year Book Medical Publishers, Inc., 1975.
56. Nicogossian, A., Chusid, E. L. and Miller, A.: Effect of positioning of nasal cannulae on efficacy of oxygen therapy. Respir. Care 16:171-172, 1971.
57. Gibson, R. L., Comer, P. B., Beckham, R. W. and McGraw, C. P.: Actual tracheal oxygen concentrations with commonly used oxygen equipment. Anesthesiology 44:75-77, 1976.
58. Friedman, S. A., Weber, B., Briscoe, W. A., Smith, J. P. and King, T. K. C.: Oxygen therapy: evaluation of various air-entraining masks. J.A.M.A. 228:474-478, 1974.
59. Campbell, E. J. M. and Minty, K. B.: Controlled oxygen therapy at 60% concentration: why and how. Lancet 1:1199-1203, 1976.
60. Bushnell, S. S.: Respiratory Intensive Care Nursing. Boston, Little, Brown and Company, 1973. Ch. 6.
61. Pierce, A. K.: Acute respiratory failure. In Pulmonary Medicine. C. A. Guenter and M. H. Welch (Eds.). Philadelphia, J. B. Lippincott Company, 1977. Ch. 5.
62. Cohen, J. L., Demers, R. R. and Saklad, M.: Air-entrainment oxygen masks: a performance evaluation. Resp. Care 22:277-282, 1977.
63. Hayes, S.: Variations in oxygen output from adjustable nebulizers. Respir. Care 22:1188, 1977.
64. Powers, W. E.: Oxygen therapy: appropriate use of nebulizers. Am. Rev. Respir. Dis. 116:547, 1977.
65. Zapol, W. M. and Kitz, R. J.: Buying time with artificial lungs. N. Engl. J. Med. 286:657-658, 1972.
66. Editorial: Extracorporeal oxygenation for acute respiratory failure. Br. Med. J. 3:340, Aug., 1975.
67. Clark, L. C., Becattini, F. and Kaplan, S.: Can fluorocarbon emulsions be used as artificial blood? Triangle 11:115-122, 1972.
68. Clark, J. M. and Lambertsen, C. J.: Pulmonary oxygen toxicity: a review. Pharmacol. Rev. 23:37-133, 1971.
69. Sackner, M. A., Landa, J., Hirsch, J. and Zapata, A.: Pulmonary effects of oxygen breathing: a 6-hour study in normal men. Ann. Intern. Med. 82:40-43, 1975.
70. Sackner, M. A.: Oxygen therapy: a history of oxygen usage in chronic obstructive pulmonary disease. Am. Rev. Respir. Dis. 110, #6, Pt. 2:25-34, 1974.
71. Menn, S. J. and Tisi, G. M.: Oxygen as a drug: chemical properties, benefits, and hazards of administration. In Respiratory Care: a Guide to Clinical Practice. G. G. Burton, G. N. Gee and J. E. Hodgkin (Eds.). Philadelphia, J. B. Lippincott Company, 1977. Ch. 18.
72. Barach, A. L. and Segal, M. S.: Oxygen therapy in cardiopulmonary disease with a review of oxygen toxicity. Ann. Allergy 30:113-121, 1972.
73. Winter, P. M. and Smith, G.: The toxicity of oxygen. Anesthesiology 37:210-241, 1972.
74. Editorial: Lung damage by oxygen. Lancet 2:1292-1293, 1970.
75. Hedley-Whyte, J.: Causes of pulmonary oxygen toxicity. N. Engl. J. Med. 283:1518-1519, 1970.
76. Nichols, C. W. and Lambertsen, C. J.: Effects of high oxygen pressure on the eye. N. Engl. J. Med. 281:25-30, 1969.
77. Patz, A.: Retrolental fibroplasia. Surv. Ophthalmol. 14:1-29, 1969.
78. Mathewson, H. S.: Pharmacology for Respiratory Therapists. St. Louis, The C. V. Mosby Company, 1977. Ch. 7.
79. Tysinger, D. S.: Oxygen: Part III. Resp. Therapy 7:24-25, Sept./Oct., 1977.
80. Smith, B. E.: Oxygen toxicity. In Advances in Respiratory Care and Physiology. T. B. Caldwell and F. Moya (Eds.). Springfield, Ill., Charles C Thomas, 1973. Ch. 16.
81. Ayers, L. N., Tierney, D. F. and Imagawa, D.: Shortened survival of mice with influenza when given oxygen at one atmosphere. Am. Rev. Respir. Dis. 107:955-961, 1973.
82. Clark, J. M.: The toxicity of oxygen. Am. Rev. Respir. Dis. 110, #6, Pt. 2:40–50, 1974.
83. Krop, H. D., Block, A. J., Cohen, E., Croucher, R. and Shuster, J.: Neuropsychologic effects of continuous oxygen therapy in the aged. Chest. 72:737-743, 1977.
84. Martindale: The Extra Pharmacopoeia. London, The Pharmaceutical Press, 27th ed., 1977. p. 1041.
85. Barach, A. L. and Segal, M. S.: Helium-oxygen therapy in bronchial asthma. In Bronchial Asthma: Mechanisms and Therapeutics. E. B. Weiss and M. S. Segal (Eds.). Boston, Little, Brown and Company, 1976. Ch. 65.
86. Motley, H. L.: Helium-oxygen therapy. Respir. Care 18:668-670, 1973.

APPENDIX

Costs of Respiratory Drugs

The following tables provide some insights into the costs of various formulations of major respiratory drugs and of a number of other drugs that may be of importance in the management of respiratory diseases.

The formation provided on the costs of drugs has been obtained from Facts and Comparisons, published by Facts and Comparisons, Inc., St. Louis. The costs of individual drugs and specific preparations are susceptible to periodic changes, and the information tabulated can be regarded only as a current guideline. Actual dollar prices for drugs are not given; the relative costs listed are based on the "cost index," which is the ratio of the average wholesale costs for equivalent quantities of different products. In other words, if the figures for a particular drug vary from 12 to 240, the wholesale cost of the most expensive product is twenty times that of the least expensive. The products with lowest cost figures are the least expensive, and therefore to be preferred if suitable for the individual patient's needs.

A number of variables can affect the expense of an individual drug. The following considerations should be kept in mind:

1. Brand name drugs are usually more expensive than drugs that are produced under their generic names.
2. The manufacturer that introduces a drug usually continues to charge more for the well-known brand-name product even though competitive manufacturers market the drug at lower cost under less identifiable brand names.
3. Over-the-counter (OTC) preparations are usually much less expensive than equivalent drugs that require a prescription.
4. Simple tablets and capsules are usually far less expensive than other preparations. Special formulations, such as drops suitable for infants, are usually very expensive. Parenteral preparations are comparatively expensive, and there are added costs incurred through the use of syringes and needles, and the use of nursing personnel. The expense of an aerosol drug is increased enormously when a respiratory therapist delivers the medication with relatively complex apparatus.
5. Dispensed drugs are more expensive than wholesale drugs, and the dispensing of a relatively short course of a drug results in an increase in the cost of each dose.
6. A drug that is formulated in small dosage is relatively costly when compared with the same drug formulated in units of much larger dosage.

The information provided in each table offers comparative guidance, and it should help the physician determine which preparation of a specific drug can be obtained by a patient at the most reasonable cost for that class of therapeutic agent.

APPENDIX TABLE 1. RELATIVE COSTS OF MUCOKINETICS

| | Basic Dose | | Relative Costs Per Basic Dose | | | |
| | | | LIQUIDS | | TABLETS | |
Drug	mg	Availability	Generic	Brand	Generic	Brand
Guaifenesin	100	OTC	4+	6–15		7–10
Hydriodic acid	70	OTC		7–8		
Iodides		R	28+			3–48
Iodinated glycerol	60	R		19–26		26
SSKI	300	R	1+	2–20	6+	7

Mucokinetics are discussed in Chapter 3.

APPENDIX TABLE 2. RELATIVE COSTS OF SYMPATHOMIMETIC BRONCHODILATORS

Preparation	Basic Dose mg	Availability*	Relative Cost Per Basic Dose
INJECTION			
Epinephrine 1:1000	0.5	R	6.5+
Epinephrine long-acting	0.5	R	37–59
Ethylnorepinephrine	0.5	R	40
Terbutaline	0.5	R	24–32
ORAL			
Ephedrine tablets, capsules	25	R, OTC	1–32
Ephedrine syrups	25	OTC	16+
Isoproterenol tablets, glossets	10	R	20
Metaproterenol tablets	20	R	24
Metaproterenol syrup	20	R	42
Protokylol tablets	2	R	16
Terbutaline tablets	5	R	31–47
AEROSOLS – Solutions			
Epinephrine	0.2	R, OTC	0.4–2.1
Isoproterenol	0.125	R	1–2
Bronkosol	0.34	R	3
Aerolone	0.125	R	2
AEROSOLS – Metered			
Epinephrine	0.2	OTC	2–4.5
Isoetharine (+Phenylephrine)	0.34	R	4
Isoproterenol	0.125	R	1–5
Isoproterenol (+Phenylephrine)	0.125	R	3–5
Metaproterenol	0.65	R	4

*R = require a prescription; OTC = available without prescription.
Sympathomimetic bronchodilators are discussed in Chapter 5.

APPENDIX TABLE 3. RELATIVE COSTS OF EPHEDRINE-BARBITURATE COMBINATIONS

| Preparation | Unit | Content Per Unit | | | Avail-ability† | Relative Cost |
		EPHEDRINE *mg*	BARBITURATE *mg*	ANTI-HISTAMINE *mg*		
Aladrine	Tablet/Liquid	8.1	S 16.2		R*	12/15
Benadryl with Ephedrine	Tablet	25		D 50		19
D-Asma	Tablet/Syrup	8.1	S 16.2		R*	17/17
Ectasule III/Jr/Sr	Capsules	15/30/60	A 8/15/30		R	19/20/24
Efed	Tablet	8.1	S 16.2		R*	18
Ephedrine and Amytal	Pulvule	25	A 50		R*	13
Ephedrine and Nembutal	Pulvule	25	P 25		R	17
Ephedrine and Seconal	Pulvule	25	S 50		R*	13
Pyribenzamine with Ephedrine	Tablet	12		T 25	R	14
Slo-Tedrin A	Capsule	30	A 15		R	21

*Available as Schedule III drugs.
†R = require a prescription.
A = amobarbital, P = pentobarbital, S = secobarbital, D = diphenhydramine, T = tripelennamine.
Ephedrine-barbiturate combinations are discussed in Chapter 5.

APPENDIX TABLE 4. SUMMARY OF RELATIVE COSTS OF THEOPHYLLINE AND DERIVATIVES*

Drug	Preparations	Range of Relative Costs†
THEOPHYLLINE	tablets	6–18
	capsules	12–18
	elixirs, syrups	12–75
	time-release (oral)	10–31
	suppositories	18–83
	rectal units	356–711
AMINOPHYLLINE	tablets	2–7
	liquids (oral)	20–43
	time-release (oral)	14
	injection (I.V.)	22–126
	rectal units	32–79
	suppositories	5–23
DYPHYLLINE	tablets	11–16
	elixirs	42–65
	time-release (oral)	12
	injections	11–93
OXTRIPHYLLINE	tablets	16–24
	elixir	28

*All preparations require a presciption.
†Based on cost of 100 mg theophylline equivalent.
Theophylline and its derivatives are discussed in Chapter 6.

APPENDIX TABLE 5.   RELATIVE COSTS OF THEOPHYLLINE PREPARATIONS*

Preparation	Liquids	Capsules or Tablets	SR Oral Forms	Suppositories	Enema
Aerolate	32		10–31		
Aqualin				21–83	
Bronkodyl	51	12–18			
Elixicon	34				
Elixophyllin	48	14			
Fleet					356–711
Glynazan		11			
Lanophyllin	16				
Panophylline	75				
Slo-Phyllin	47	7–11	11–31		
Somophyllin		12–18			
Synophylate	28	9	10		
Tega-Bron	39				
Theobid			13–21		
Theo-dur			10–15		
Theofort	24				
Theolair		12–15			
Theo-Lix	31				
Theolixir	49				
Theolline	18				
Theon	35				
Theophyl	39	9			
Theospan	51	6	10		
Various	12+				

*All preparations require a prescription. Costs are based on 100 mg dose.
Theophylline preparations are discussed in Chapter 6.

APPENDIX TABLE 6.   RELATIVE COSTS OF THEOPHYLLINE COMBINED WITH EXPECTORANT†

Preparation	Formulation	Theophylline mg	Expectorant mg	Relative Cost Per Basic Dose
Asbron G Inlay	Tablet/Elixir	300*	G 100	22/65
Asma	Syrup	150	G 90	50
Elixophyllin K1	Elixir	80	KI 130	43
Glynazan	Liquid	180*	G 150, NaC 300	73
Hylate	Tablet/Syrup	400*	G 100	20/84
Quibron	Capsule/Elixir	150	G 90	26/75
Slophyllin GG	Capsule/Syrup	150	G 90	21/21
Synophylate-GG	Tablet/Syrup	300*	G 90/100	20/65
Theo-Col	Capsule/Elixir	150	G 90	9/20
Theo-Guaia	Capsule/Elixir	100	G 100	21/32
Theokin	Tablet/Elixir	448.5**	KI 450	27/23
Theo-Organidin	Elixir	120	IG 30	56
TSG-KI	Elixir	300*	KI 100	23

†All these preparations require a prescription. Basic dose is equivalent to 100 mg theophylline.
*As theophylline sodium glycinate.
**As theophylline calcium salicylate.
 G = guaifenesin. IG = iodinated glycerol. KI = potassium iodide, NaC = sodium citrate.
Theophylline combinations are discussed in Chapter 6.

APPENDIX TABLE 7.   RELATIVE COSTS OF THEOPHYLLINE-EPHEDRINE COMBINATIONS†

Preparation	Unit	Content Per Unit THEOPHYLLINE mg	EPHEDRINE** mg	Availability††	Relative Cost Per Basic Unit
Asmadil	Capsule	260	P-E 50	R	37
Asma-lief	Tablet	130	E 24	OTC	4
Asminyl	Tablet	130	E 32	R	14
Bronchobid	Capsule	260	P-E 50	R	33
Emerox-O.D.	Capsule	260	P-E 50	R	27
Luasmin	Capsule	200*	E 30	R	28
Marax	Tablet/Syrup	130	E 25	R	24/88
Tedfern	Tablet	130	E 24	R	13
Tedral	Tablet/Suspension	130/195	E 24/36	OTC	19/60
Tedral-25	Tablet	130	E 24	R	21
Tedral S.A.	Tablet	180	E 48	R	40
Teephen	Tablet/Suspension	130/195	E 24/36	OTC	4/30
Thalfed	Tablet	120	E 25	OTC	9
Thedirzem	Tablet	100	E 25	OTC	9
Theotabs	Tablet	130	E 24	OTC	5
Thephen	Tablet	130	E 24	OTC	3

†These preparations also contain various amounts of sedative.
*Theophylline sodium acetate.
**E = ephedrine, P-E = pseudoephedrine.
††R = require a prescription, OTC = available without prescription.
Theophylline combinations are discussed in Chapter 6.

APPENDIX TABLE 8.   RELATIVE COSTS OF THEOPHYLLINE-EPHEDRINE WITH OTHER CONSTITUENTS

Preparation	Unit	Content Per Unit THEOPHYLLINE mg	SYMPATHOMIMETIC mg	EXPECTORANT mg	ANTIHISTAMINE mg	Availability	Relative Cost Per Unit
Asma Kets	Tablets	130	E 2–4		C 2	OTC	15
Broncholate	Capsule/Elixir	125	E 25*	G 100		R	19/63
Broncomar	Tablet/Elixir	100/150	P-E 30/30*	G 100/150		OTC/R	25/67
Bronkaid	Tablet	100	E 24	G 100		OTC	14
Bronkolixir	Elixir	45	E 36*	G 150		OTC	54
Bronkotabs	Tablet	100	E 24*	G 100		OTC	18
Duovent	Tablet	130	E 24*	G 100		R	21
Isuprel Compound	Elixir	45	E 12* I 2.5	KI 150		R	134
Luftodil	Tablet	100	E 24*	G 200		R	28
Mudrane G G	Elixir	60	E 12*	G 78		R	62
Quadrinal	Tablet/Suspension	130†	E 24*	KI 320		R	24/44
Quibron Plus	Capsule/Elixir	150	P-E/E 30*/25*	G 100		R	27/77*
Sudolin	Tablet	50	P-E 15*		Ph 15	R	12
Tedral Expectorant	Tablet	130	E 24*	G 100			21
Tedral Anti-H	Tablet	130	E 24*		C 2	OTC	23
Verequad	Tablet/Suspension	130††	E 24*	G 100		OTC	24/44
Wesmatic (Forte)	Tablet	120	E 16*	(G 100)	C 2	R	12(14)

*Sedative also present.
†As theophylline calcium salicylate.
††As theophylline sodium glycinate.
Note: R = require a prescription.   OTC = available without prescription.
        E   = ephedrine.   G   = guaifenesin.   C = chlorpheniramine
        P-E = pseudoephedrine.   KI = potassium iodide   Ph = phenyltoloxamine
Ephedrine combinations are also discussed in Chapter 5.
Theophylline combinations are discussed in Chapter 6.

APPENDIX TABLE 9. RELATIVE COSTS OF AMINOPHYLLINE PREPARATIONS†

Preparation	Liquids	Tablets	Injections	Rectal Suppositories	Rectal Liquids
Aminodur		14*			
Lixaminol	20				
Mini-Lix	43				
Rectalad					53–79
Somophyllin	31				32
Various		2–7	22–126	5–23	

†All preparations require a prescription. Costs are based on doses equivalent to 100 mg theophylline.
*Time-release preparation.
Aminophylline is discussed in Chapter 6.

APPENDIX TABLE 10. RELATIVE COSTS
OF DYPHYLLINE PREPARATIONS*

Preparation	LIQUIDS	TABLETS	Time Release (ORAL)	INJEC-TIONS
Airet	65	16	12	
Circair		11		
Dilin				71
Dilor	42	11–13		50
Dyflex		11–12		
Emfabid			12	
Lufyllin	56	12–16		93
Neothylline	42	11–15		49
Various				11+

*All preparations require a prescription. Costs are based on doses equivalent to 100 mg theophylline.
Dyphylline is discussed in Chapter 6.

APPENDIX TABLE 11. RELATIVE COSTS OF PREPARATIONS OF
DYPHYLLINE AND EXPECTORANT†

Preparation	Unit	DYPHYLLINE BASIC DOSE mg	GUAIFENESIN mg	EPHEDRINE (+BARBITURATE) mg	Relative Cost Per Unit
Air Tab-GG	Tablet	200	200		23
Dilor-G	Tablet/Liquid	200	200		27/40
Dyflex-G	Tablet	200	200		23
Dyline-GG	Tablet/Liquid	200	200		16/32
Emfaseen	Capsule/Liquid	200	100		23/68
G-Bron	Elixir	100	100		45
Lufyllin-GG	Tablet/Elixir	200	100/200		7/116
Lufyllin-EPG	Tablet/Elixir	100	200	16	36/52
Neospect	Tablet	100	200	25	29
Neothylline	Capsule/Elixir	100	50		12/19
Phyldrox	Tablet	100		25	6

†All preparations require a prescription.
Dyphylline is discussed in Chapter 6.

APPENDIX TABLE 12.   RELATIVE COSTS OF GLUCOCORTICOIDS*

Drug	Basic Dose mg	Relative Costs Per Basic Dose ORAL (TABLET)	PARENTERAL (I.V.)
Hydrocortisone	20	28–143	100–626
Prednisone	5	9–89	
Prednisolone	5	31–77	35–529
Triamcinolone	4	38–246	82–204
Methylprednisolone	4	129–227	385–454
Dexamethasone	0.75	21–194	27–283
Betamethasone	0.6	188–197	210

*All preparations require a prescription.
Glucocorticoids are discussed in Chapter 7.

APPENDIX TABLE 13.   RELATIVE COSTS OF ANTIHISTAMINES

Drug	Basic Dose mg	Availability*	Relative Costs Per Basic Dose TABLETS OR CAPSULES Generic	Brand
Bromodiphenhydramine	25	R		18
Brompheniramine	4	R	2–3+	3–9
Carbinoxamine	4	R		8–13
Chlorpheniramine	4	OTC, R	2+	2–10
Cyproheptadine	4	R		25
Dexchlorpheniramine	2	R		9–11
Dimethindene	1	R		9–12
Diphenhydramine	50	R	3–6+	6–18
Diphenylpyraline	2	R		10–11
Doxylamine	12.5	R		9–14
Methapyrilene	25	OTC, R	4+	7–9
Methdilazine	8	R		38–64
Promethazine	25	R	2–4+	10–23
Pyrilamine	25	OTC	1–4+	5–9
Trimeprazine	2.5	R		20–22
Tripelennamine	25	R	4+	3–11
Triprolidine	2.5	R		8

*R = require a prescription, OTC = available without prescription.
Antihistamines are discussed in Chapter 9.

APPENDIX TABLE 14.   RELATIVE COSTS OF ANTITUSSIVES

	Basic Dose mg	Availability*	Relative Cost Per Basic Dose LIQUIDS Brand	TABLETS OR CAPSULES Generic	Brand
Benzonatate	100	R			24
Chlophedianol	25	R	22		
Codeine	5	C II		3–5+	4–6
Dextromethorphan	15	OTC	33–62		15–48†
Hydrocodone	5	C II			29
Levopropoxyphene	50	R	25		15
Noscapine	15	OTC	25		20

*C II = Controlled substance, Schedule II. R = require a prescription. OTC = available without prescription.
†Combination preparations
Antitussives are discussed in Chapter 9.

APPENDIX TABLE 15. RELATIVE COSTS OF DECONGESTANTS

Drug	Basic Dose mg	Availability*	Relative Cost Per Basic Dose Sprays Generic	Brand
Epinephrine	1	OTC	6+	13
Ephedrine	10	OTC		1–17
Naphazoline	0.5	OTC	1–2+	9–17
Oxymetazoline	0.5	OTC		23–40
Phenylephrine	5	OTC	1–2+	2–79
Tetrahydrozoline	1	R		11–75
Xylometazoline	1	OTC		16–44

*R = require a prescription, OTC = available without prescription.
Decongestants are discussed in Chapter 9.

APPENDIX TABLE 16. RELATIVE COSTS OF PSEUDOEPHEDRINE DECONGESTANT PREPARATIONS

Prescription	Unit	Content Per Unit Pseudo- ephedrine mg	Antihistamine mg	Availability*	Relative Cost Per Unit†
Actagen	Tablet	60	T 2.5	R	7
Actamine	Tablet	60	T 2.5	R	5
Actifed	Tablet/Syrup	60	T 2.5	R	16/30
Allerid-D.C.	Capsule	120	Ch 6	R	30
Anamine	Capsule/Syrup	120	Ch 8	R	31/112
Chlorafed	Capsule/Liquid	120	Ch 8	R	32/64
Chlor-Trimeton Decongestant	Tablet	60	Ch 4	OTC	15
Codimal-L.A.	Capsule	120	Ch 8	R	35
Corphed	Tablet	60	T 2.5	R	8
Cotrol-D	Tablet	60	Ch 4	R	17
Deconamine	Tablet/Elixir	60	Ch 4	R	18/34
Disophrol	Tablet	60	D 2	R	20
Drixoral	Tablet	120	D 6	R	39
Eldefed	Tablet	60	T 2.5	R	8
Fedahist	Tablet/Syrup	60	Ch 4	OTC	18/38
Fedrazil	Tablet	30	CC 25	OTC	12
Isochlor	Tablet/Liquid	25	Ch 4	R	18/28
Novafed A	Capsule/Liquid	120	Ch 8		38/80
Phenergan-D	Tablet	60	P 6.25	R	25
Poly-Histine-Dx	Capsule/Elixir	120/60	B 12/8	R	35/34
Pseudo-Hist	Capsule/Liquid	65/60	Ch 10/8	R	30/80
Rhinosyn	Syrup	120	Ch 4	OTC	58
Rinade	Capsule	120	Ch 8	R	35
Rondec	Tablet/Syrup	60	Ch 4	R	26/23
Sherafed	Tablet/Syrup	60	T 2.5	R	12/24
Sudachlor	Capsule	65	Ch 10	R	30
Sudahist	Tablet	60	T 2.5	R	11
Suda-Prol	Tablet/Syrup	60	T 2.5	R	6/18
Symptafed	Capsule	65	Ch 10	R	29
Triphed	Tablet	60	T 2.5	R	8
Tri-Sudo	Tablet	60	T 2.5	R	7

B = brompheniramine, Car = carbinoxamine, CC = chlorcyclizine, Ch = chlorpheniramine, D = dexbromphen-
iramine, P = promethazine, T = triprolidine.
*R = require a prescription, OTC = available without prescription.
Pseudoephedrine decongestants are discussed in Chapter 9.

APPENDIX TABLE 17. RELATIVE COSTS OF CODEINE CONTAINING PREPARATIONS

Constituents Per Basic 5 ml Dose

Preparation	Formu-lation	CODEINE mg	DECONGESTANT mg	ANTI-HISTAMINE mg	EXPECTO-RANTS mg	Narcotic Schedule	Relative Cost Per Basic Dose
Ambenyl	Liquid	10		B 4, D 9	Several	5	28
Calcidrine	Syrup	8.4	E 4.2		CaI 152	5	29
Cetro Cirose	Liquid	10			Several	5	20
Cheracol	Syrup	11			G 15	5	32
Codalex	Syrup	10	Ph 10		Several	5	21
Co-Histine DH	Elixir	10	PP 19			5	17
Copavin	Pulvule	15	Pa 15			3	38
Cosanyl	Syrup	11	P-E 30			5	18
Emprazil-C*	Tablet	15	P-E 20			3	30
J-Histine DH	Elixir	10	Ph 10	Ch 2		5	14
Hycoff-X	Liquid	10	P-E 30		G 100	5	21
Neozyl	Liquid		P-E 10	Ch 2		5	21
Novahistine	Elixir	10	PP 19		G 100	5	32
Nucofed	Syrup	20	P-E 60			3	44
Phenhist	Liquid	10	P-E 10	Ch 2		5	18
Robitussin A-C	Liquid	10			G 100	5	26
Ryna-C	Syrup	10	P-E 30	Ch 2		5	26
Spen-Histine	Liquid	10	PP 19		G 100	5	11
Terpin hydrate w Codeine	Elixir	10			TH 8	5	10+
Tolu-Sed	Syrup	10			G 100	5	26
Tusscidin A-C	Syrup	10			G 100	5	26
Tussi-Organidin	Liquid	10		Ch 2	IG 30	5	23
Winstamine-MW	Syrup	7.5	Ph 10	Pr 5		5	23

DECONGESTANT: E = ephedrine, Pa = papaverine, Ph = phenylephrine, P-E = pseudoephedrine, PP = phenyl-propanolamine.

ANTIHISTAMINE: B = bromodiphenhydramine, Ch = chlorpheniramine, D = diphenhydramine, Pr = prometh-azine.

EXPECTORANT: CaI = calcium iodide, G = guaifenesin, IG = iodinated glycerol, TH = terpin hydrate.

*Emprazil-C contains aspirin 200 mg, phenacetin 150 mg and caffeine 30 mg.

Codeine is discussed in Chapter 9.

APPENDIX TABLE 18. RELATIVE COSTS OF PENICILLINS

Drug	Basic Dose	Relative Cost of Basic Dose ORAL Tablets or Capsules	Liquids*	PARENTERAL
Penicillin G	800,000 u.	4–28		17–69
Procaine penicillin	800,000 u.			15–23
Bicillin	800,000 u.	83–85		122–151
Penicillin V	500 mg	4–25	8–38	
Phenethicillin	500 mg	28–30		
Methicillin	500 mg			90–111
Nafcillin	500 mg	36–39	53	191–211
Oxacillin	500 mg	31–42	43	170–248
Cloxacillin	500 mg	38–44	63	
Dicloxacillin	500 mg	42–70	87–113	
Ampicillin	500 mg	10–38	20–50	64–568
Hetacillin	500 mg	44–45	45–61	
Amoxicillin	500 mg	57–64	61–73	
Carbenicillin	500 mg	50		90–158
Ticarcillin	500 mg			117–132

*Does not include pediatric drop or chewable preparations.

Note: All antibiotics for systemic administration require a prescription.

Penicillins are discussed in Chapter 10.

APPENDIX TABLE 19.   RELATIVE COSTS OF CEPHALOSPORINS*

Drug	Oral Tablets, Capsules etc.	Liquids	Parenteral
Cephaloridine			5
Cephalexin	1	1	
Cefazoline			5–7
Cephradine	1	1–2	3–4
Cephapirin			3

*Basic dose = 100 mg.
Cephalosporins are discussed in Chapter 10.

APPENDIX TABLE 20.   RELATIVE COSTS OF TETRACYCLINES*

Drug	Oral Tablets or Capsules	Liquids	Parenteral
Tetracycline†	3–18	11–49	320–495 (I.M.)
			248–358 (I.V.)
Chlortetracycline	40		401 (I.V.)
Oxytetracycline	4–50		323–366 (I.V.)
Minocycline	53–64	53–54	357–363 (I.V.)
Doxycycline	20–43	33–39	380–386 (I.V.)
Demeclocycline	56–70	78	
Methacycline	41–46	55	

*Basic dose = 500 mg.
†Does not include special formulations.
Tetracyclines are discussed in Chapter 10.

APPENDIX TABLE 21.   RELATIVE COSTS OF AMINOGLYCOSIDE AND POLYMYXIN ANTIBIOTICS

Drug	Basic Dose	Parenteral	Oral
Streptomycin	500 mg	2–3+	
Neomycin	500 mg	10–33	1–4
Kanamycin	500 mg	45–60	7
Gentamicin	80 mg	52–102	
Tobramycin	80 mg	44	
Amikacin	300 mg	41–124	
Colistin	100 mg		17
Colistimethate	100 mg	61–95	
Polymyxin B	1,000,000 u.	32–66	

Aminoglycoside and polymyxin antibiotics are discussed in Chapter 10.

APPENDIX TABLE 22.   RELATIVE COSTS OF OTHER ANTIBIOTICS

Drug	Basic Dose mg	Oral Tablets or Capsules	Liquids†	Parenteral	
Chloramphenicol	100	22–182	281	180–495	
Erythromycin	500	13–53	44–73	6–20	(I.V.)
				458	(I.M.)
Troleandomycin	500	60	75		
Lincomycin	100	68–73	77	333–359	
Clindamycin	100	204–221	279	1109–1347	
Vancomycin	100		951	1164	

†Does not include drops.
These antibiotics are discussed in Chapter 10.

APPENDIX TABLE 23.   RELATIVE COSTS OF SULFONAMIDE PREPARATIONS

Preparation	Oral Tablets	Suspensions	Parenteral
Various Sulfonamides	2–10	4–17	18–39
Trimethoprim-Sulfonamide	47–60	69–78	

Sulfonamides are discussed in Chapter 10.

APPENDIX TABLE 24.   RELATIVE COSTS OF ANTITUBERCULOSIS DRUGS

Drug	Standard Dose gm	Tablet	Syrup	Parenteral
Isoniazid	0.3	3–9	28	109
Ethambutol	1	77–94		
PAS	10	34–72		
Streptomycin	1			2–52
Rifampin	0.6	214		
Viomycin	2			500
Pyrazinamide	1.5	80		
Ethionamide	0.5	57		
Capreomycin	1			697
Kanamycin	0.5			45–60

Antituberculosis drugs are discussed in Chapter 10.

APPENDIX TABLE 25. RELATIVE COSTS OF SELECTED PSYCHOTHERAPEUTIC DRUGS

Drug	Basic Dose	Oral Form	Availability*	Cost Per Basic Dose GENERIC	Cost Per Basic Dose BRAND
ANTIANXIETY AGENTS					
Chlorazepate	7.5 mg	capsules	IV		400–800
Chlordiazepoxide	5 mg	capsules	IV	23–78+	23–290
Diazepam	2 mg	tablets	IV		141–373
Doxepin	25 mg	capsules	R		483–1478
Hydroxyzine	25 mg	tablets	R		212–956
Meprobamate	200 mg	tablets	IV	19–38+	31–282
Oxazepam	10 mg	tablets	IV		324
Prazepam	10 mg	tablets	IV		485
ANTIDEPRESSANTS					
Amitriptyline	75 mg	tablets	R		11–20
Desipramine	75 mg	tablets	R		12–14
Imipramine	10 mg	tablets	R	3–8+	7–23
Nortriptyline	75 mg	capsules	R		16–20
Protriptyline	15 mg	tablets	R		9–12

*R = require a prescription, IV = Schedule IV drugs.
Psychotherapeutic drugs are discussed in Chapter 11.

APPENDIX TABLE 26. RELATIVE COSTS OF SELECTED SEDATIVE-HYPNOTIC DRUGS

Drug	Basic Dose	Oral Form	Schedule	Cost Per Basic Dose GENERIC	Cost Per Basic Dose BRAND
VARIOUS					
Chloral hydrate	500 mg	capsules	IV	8–14+	9–30
Chloral betaine	500 mg	tablets	IV		64
Ethchlorvynol	500 mg	capsules	IV		42–84
Ethinamate	500 mg	capsules	IV		28
Flurazepam	30 mg	capsules	IV		34–56
Mephobarbital	150 mg	capsules	II		21–28
BARBITURATES					
Phenobarbital	16 mg	tablets	IV	1–8+	1–12
Mephobarbital	32 mg	tablets	IV	1+	1–10
Barbital	65 mg	tablets	IV	3+	3+
Amobarbital	30 mg	tablets	II	1–5+	5–13
Butabarbital	15 mg	tablets	III	1–5+	1–10
Secobarbital	100 mg	capsules	II	6–15+	18–32
Pentobarbital	100 mg	capsules	II	6–15+	22–39

Sedative-hypnotic drugs are discussed in Chapter 11.

INDEX

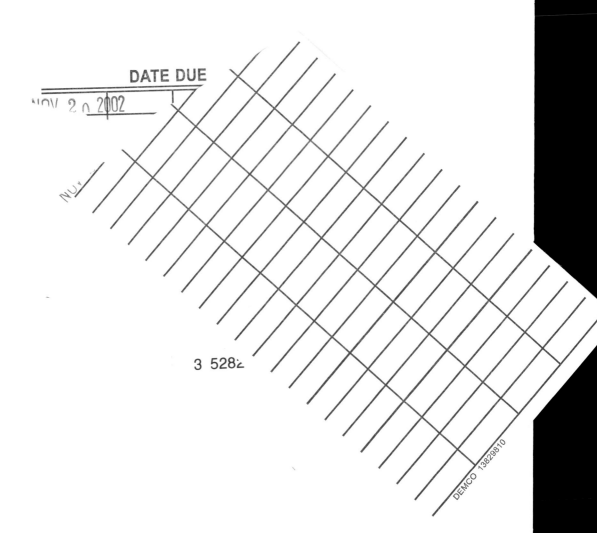